DECISION MAKING IN

Adult Neurology

Clinical Decision Making Series

Berman:
 Pediatric Decision Making
Bready, Smith:
 Decision Making in Anesthesiology
Bucholz, Lippert, Wenger, Ezaki:
 Orthopaedic Decision Making
Callaham, Barton, Schumaker:
 Decision Making in Emergency Medicine
Cibis, Tongue, Stass-Isern:
 Decision Making in Pediatric Ophthalmology
Cohn, Doty, McElvein:
 Decision Making in Cardiothoracic Surgery
DeCherney, Polan, Lee, Boyers:
 Decision Making in Infertility
Greene, Johnson, Maricic:
 Decision Making in Medicine
Karlinsky, Lau, Goldstein:
 Decision Making in Pulmonary Medicine
Korones, Bada-Ellzey:
 Neonatal Decision Making
Levine:
 Decision Making in Gastroenterology
Marsh:
 Decision Making in Plastic Surgery
Nichols, Hyslop, Bartlett:
 Decision Making in Surgical Sepsis
Ramamurthy, Rogers:
 Decision Making in Pain Management
Resnick, Caldamone, Spirnak:
 Decision Making in Urology
Schein:
 Decision Making in Oncology
van Heuven, Zwaan:
 Decision Making in Ophthalmology
Weisberg, Strub, Garcia:
 Decision Making in Adult Neurology

Adult Neurology

Second Edition

Leon A. Weisberg, M.D.

Professor and Director of Neurology
Vice-Chairman Department of Psychiatry and Neurology
Tulane University School of Medicine
New Orleans, Louisiana

Richard L. Strub, M.D.

Chairman, Department of Neurology
Ochsner Clinic
New Orleans, Louisiana

Carlos A. Garcia, M.D.

Professor of Neurology and Pathology
Medical Director, Muscular Dystrophy Clinic
Louisiana State University School of Medicine
New Orleans, Louisiana

B.C. Decker
An Imprint of Mosby–Year Book, Inc.

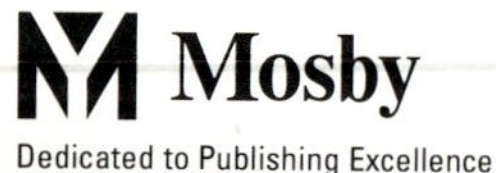 **Mosby**
Dedicated to Publishing Excellence

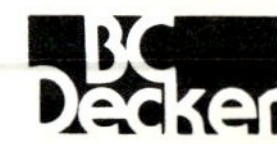

Executive Editor: Susan M. Gay
Senior Managing Editor: Lynne Gery
Manufacturing Supervisor: Theresa Fuchs
Project Supervisor: Arofan Gregory

SECOND EDITION

Printed in the United States of America

Mosby–Year Book, Inc.
11830 Westline Industrial Drive
St. Louis, Missouri 63146

NOTICE: The authors and publisher have made every effort to ensure that the patient care recommended
herein, including choice of drugs and drug dosages, is in accord with the accepted standard and practice at
the time of publication. However, since research and regulation constantly change clinical standards, the
reader is urged to check the product information sheet included in the package of each drug, which includes
recommended doses, warnings, and contraindications. This is particularly important with new or infrequently
used drugs.

ISBN 1-55664-371-3

93 94 95 96 97 CL/MY 9 8 7 6 5 4 3 2 1

PREFACE

Traditionally, the best means of teaching clinical medicine has been a tutorial system. The system is one by which the experienced clinician imparts the skills and the art of his or her trade to the young physician by evaluating patients at the bedside and in the clinic. Reading textbooks and journal articles, listening to lectures, and attending conferences may help supplement these practical clinical skills with more didactic material, but rarely does such material give insight into the decision-making process used by the seasoned practitioner. In our traditional teaching we usually think in terms of categories of disease. The physician then feels obligated to exclude all categories even if the probability of their presence is extremely low. By using clinical decision analysis, the physician may reduce diagnostic uncertainty and avoid unnecessary and excessive diagnostic procedures and therapeutic interventions.

This book is one effort to bridge the gap between didactic learning and practical experience. Decision trees (*algorithms*) are used to help teach the student to think in the same fashion as the experienced clinician. The basic factor that separates the student's approach to a patient's problem from that of the practicing physician is the clinician's knowledge of and experience with the diseases. The student knows the names and basic pathophysiology of the disease, but is as yet unskilled in arriving at the diagnosis given the patient's symptoms and signs.

It is the goal of this book to guide the reader (whether student, new practitioner preparing for board certification, or experienced clinician seeking a review of current trends) through the decision-making process that leads from symptoms and signs to diagnosis.

Leon A. Weisberg, M.D.
Richard L. Strub, M.D.
Carlos A. Garcia, M.D.

CONTENTS

DECISION MAKING IN

Adult Neurology

INTRODUCTION

The information contained in standard neurology textbooks is organized according to established clinical and pathologic disease categories. This is a useful classification *if* the student or neurologist already knows what is wrong with the patient and wishes to compare this individual with the entire spectrum of patients who have this particular disease. In other cases, this disease specific textbook organization is not helpful, because it is not known what is precisely wrong with the patient and the diagnostic clues available to the clinician are isolated neurologic symptoms, abnormal neurologic signs, or abnormal neurodiagnostic findings. From this database, the neurologist must perform detective work to determine the most probable diagnosis. Under these circumstances of diagnostic uncertainty, the neurologist does not know exactly which textbook chapter should be consulted.

As the initial step, neurologists must consider the kaleidoscope of neurologic conditions that may cause specific neurologic abnormalities. The extensive list of possibilities is the differential diagnosis. The neurologist must determine the probability of any of these diseases being the cause of the patient's condition, and which neurodiagnostic studies should be performed to confirm this suspicion. The intuitive thought process by which neurologists determine the most likely diagnostic possibility is referred to as "problem solving."

To demonstrate this process, let us analyze this hypothetical situation. The neurologist is confronted with the patient, Mr. Jones, who has a bewildering and perplexing constellation of neurologic symptoms and signs. The neurologist's goal is to determine what exactly is wrong with Mr. Jones and to establish the preferred course of action (admit to hospital, perform more extensive neurodiagnostic studies, intervene therapeutically with medical or surgical treatment, observe the patient's subsequent course without intervention). To achieve this goal, the neurologist must analyze systematically and effectively the clinical data. This requires clinical judgment so that cost, patient discomfort, and patient risk are minimized but all reasonable diagnostic possibilities are considered. It is necessary to analyze Mr. Jones' neurologic symptoms and signs to determine the most likely diagnostic possibilities, and then decide which neurodiagnostic studies and therapeutic strategies are warranted. *Decision analysis* is the process by which neurologists analyze the clinical problem systematically and sequentially (serially) in an effort to reduce diagnostic uncertainty and arrive at the most likely diagnosis.

Clinical decision analysis is an intricate, complex, and systematic process; however, it is frequently performed almost automatically by experienced clinicians. Before clinical judgment is reduced to an automatic intuitive process, this process must be performed systematically and analytically many times. To achieve this goal, it is possible to structure decision analysis into logical and sequential rules. These are defined as *decision trees* or *clinical algorithms*. The basic principle of algorithms is that inherent in the diagnostic process is logical sequential thought analysis. By the use of algorithms, the "art of neurology" may be transformed into an analytic, sequential, rational process.

Decision trees, or algorithms, are basic analytical frameworks for displaying logical sequences for problem solving. The clinical problem may be simple (straightforward) or complex (multifaceted, vague, ambiguous); however, by creating these decision trees, systematic analysis is possible. Decision trees emphasize *sequential* and serial clinical strategies. This approach considers multiple alternative choices that exist under conditions of diagnostic uncertainty. The cardinal feature of decision trees is a determination of how diagnostic tests are ordered in *series* rather than in parallel (simultaneously). The *next* neurodiagnostic test should be determined by the result of the previous test. This avoids redundant diagnostic tests. Decision trees may be *qualitative,* so that they identify, structure, and set boundaries for the clinical problem and indicate the most appropriate subsequent course of action. Some decision trees are complex or densely foliated; others are simple, well-pruned trees. These latter use linear thought processing and may be effective only for certain simple clinical problems, whereas intuitive thinking (using complex neural networks) may be required for more complex clinical decision analysis, in which cases decision trees may be more difficult to structure and design. The purpose of decision trees is to structure clinical problem solving into a logical and sequential rational process. It is hoped that readers will find the decision trees in this book helpful in their neurologic clinical decision making and that familiarity with the process will inspire them to develop their own algorithms.

The ideal decision tree employs *quantitative* methods, including probability analysis. This requires calculating sensitivity (true positive rate) and specificity (true negative rate) of a particular neurologic sign or neurodiagnostic result. With this quantitative information, mathematical probability determinations for a specific neurologic disease may be calculated. For example, it may be possible to use this quantitative analysis to determine the probability of the diagnosis of multiple sclerosis, herpes simplex encephalitis, bacterial meningitis, or aneurysmal subarachnoid hemorrhage when certain clinical and laboratory results are known. Quantitative decision analyses are most useful in straightforward clinical problems; however, probability analysis may be more difficult in complex clinical situations, and this leads to higher levels of diagnostic uncertainty. It would be ideal if simple decision trees could be used as building blocks for solving more complex clinical problems. This would establish certain logical and rational bases for dealing effectively with specific clinical problems. These could be analyzed easily, rationally, and clearly by the least or most experienced clinicians, using a decision tree or algorithm as the common frame of reference.

References

McNeil BJ, Keeler E, Adelstein SJ. Primer on certain elements of medical decision making. N Engl J Med 1975; 293:211.

Pauker SG, Kassirer JP. Therapeutic decision making: A cost-benefit analysis. N Engl J Med 1975; 293:229.

Riegelman RK. Minimizing medical mistakes: The art of medical decision making. Boston: Little, Brown, 1991.

Sox HC, Blatt MA, Marton KI. Medical decision making. Boston: Butterworths, 1988.

Weinstein MC, Fineberg HV. Clinical decision analysis. Philadelphia: WB Saunders, 1980.

SYMPTOMS AND SIGNS

NEUROLOGIC LOCALIZATION: LESIONS ABOVE FORAMEN MAGNUM

Leon A. Weisberg, M.D.

On the basis of an assessment of a patient's neurologic symptoms and signs, clinicians should be able to answer two questions: (1) is there a lesion localizable within the nervous system? and (2) if such a lesion exists, what is its location in the neuroaxis? As the initial step in neurologic localization, determine the relation of the lesion to the foramen magnum: above, below, contiguous (at the craniocervical junction). Lesions *below* the foramen magnum usually cause motor and sensory symptoms with variable involvement of arms, trunk, and legs. This pattern depends on the level of spinal cord compression. Cervical lesions cause involvement of arms and legs; thoracic lesions cause leg involvement only. Patients with *craniocervical junction lesions* may present with a bewildering array of symptoms due to upper spinal cord and lower cranial nerve conditions. Craniocervical junction lesions include syringomyelia, foramen magnum tumors, and base of the skull lesions (e.g., Arnold-Chiari malformation). Lesions *above* the foramen magnum may be divided into those above (supratentorial) and those below (infratentorial) the tentorium.

A. Lesions that are contiguous with the foramen magnum may extend into the posterior fossa (involvement of cranial nerves IX to XII) or the cervical spinal cord (upper motor neuron signs including spasticity, Babinski signs, hyperactive deep tendon reflexes [including clonus] initially detected in the legs and later in the arms, pain and temperature sensation impairment below the level of the lesion, and sometimes weakness and wasting in the arms). Lesions involving the spinal cord frequently cause autonomic disturbances with bowel, bladder, and sexual dysfunction.

B. Lesions involving infratentorial structures (brain stem, cerebellum, and fourth ventricle) may be intra-axial (within the cerebellum or brain stem) or extra-axial (in the tentorium or cerebellopontine [CP] angle). Cerebellar lesions originate in the vermis (midline) or hemispheres (lateral). Because of the motor representation of body regions within the cerebellum, vermal lesions cause gait and lower limb ataxia, whereas hemispheric lesions cause unilateral cerebellar dysfunction resulting in ataxia and dysmetria ipsilateral to the lesion. Brain stem lesions may cause unilateral or bilateral, symmetric or asymmetric cranial nerve, corticospinal, and cerebellar disturbances. CP angle lesions initially cause unilateral auditory, vestibular, trigeminal, or facial nerve dysfunction; later they may expand to compress the brain stem and cerebellum. Tentorial lesions may expand inferiorly to compress the cerebellum and cause gait ataxia, or expand superiorly into the occipital lobe to cause visual symptoms. Tentorial lesions may cause unusual gait impairment that may initially be incorrectly diagnosed as of psychogenic origin; they may also cause ventricular compression to result in hydrocephalus. Intraventricular fourth ventricular lesions (ependymomas, cysts) and aqueduct of Sylvius lesions usually cause symptoms and signs of intracranial hypertension due to obstructive hydrocephalus. With aqueductal compression, clinical signs of the dorsal midbrain syndrome (upward gaze paresis, dilated pupils with poor light response but relatively preserved near response) may occur.

C. Supratentorial lesions may be focal or diffuse. Lateralized lesions may be cortical (frontal, temporal, parietal, occipital) or subcortical (internal capsule, thalamus, basal ganglia). Cortical lesions may involve the dominant temporal lobe to cause language (aphasic) disorders, or the parietal lobe to cause spatial disorientation (right-left confusion) or constructional apraxia. Occipital lesions may result in visual disturbances (homonymous hemianopia). Frontal lesions may cause changes in personality and behavior without accompanying cognitive impairment. Seizures are common with cortical lesions and uncommon with subcortical or infratentorial lesions.

Neurologic signs depend on the specific supratentorial region involved. Medial frontal lobe involvement results in leg paresis; lateral convexity lesions cause paresis of the face and arm with relative sparing of the legs. Subcortical internal capsular lesions may cause dysarthria but usually not aphasia; capsular lesions may produce motor (pure motor hemiparesis) or sensory (pure sensory syndrome) disturbance with equal involvement of the face, arm, and leg. Thalamic lesions may also cause hemisensory disturbances. Unilateral basal ganglia lesions may result in hemiballismus, hemichorea, hemidystonia, or hemiparkinsonism, depending on the subcortical structures predominantly affected. If consciousness is impaired and there are no focal neurologic signs or intracranial hypertension, consider diffuse encephalopathy usually due to toxic or metabolic disturbances. If consciousness is normal and there are signs of intracranial hypertension, consider an obstructive intraventricular lesion. Midline supratentorial lesions may be intraventricular and obstruct the lateral or third ventricle; these lesions cause intracranial hypertension without localizing signs. Extraventricular midline juxtasellar lesions may produce endocrine (hypothalamic-pituitary) or visual (optic chiasmal or optic nerve) symptoms.

In some cases, the disorder may be diffuse and involve either gray or white matter regions. Clinical disturbances that indicate gray matter dysfunction include dementia, seizures, aphasia, agnosia,

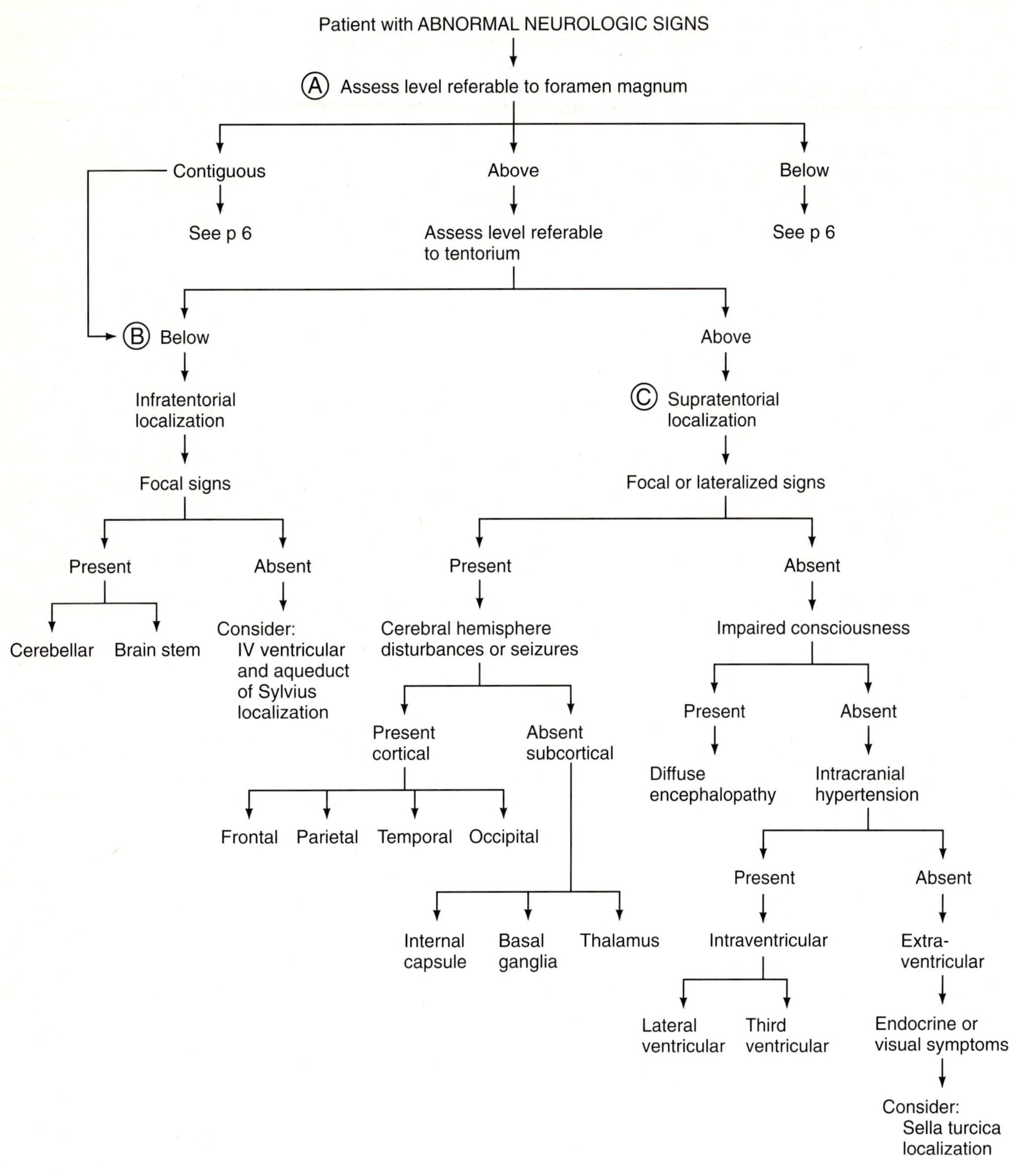

apraxia, and visual field deficit. Clinical clues to white matter dysfunction include spasticity, weakness of upper motor neuron type, ataxia, sustained clonus, Babinski signs, or optic atrophy.

References

Brazis PW, Masdeu JC, Biller J. Localization in clinical neurology. Little, Brown, 1985.
DeJong RN. The neurologic examination. New York: Hoeber, 1970.

NEUROLOGIC LOCALIZATION: LESIONS BELOW FORAMEN MAGNUM

Leon A. Weisberg, M.D.

Lesions below the foramen magnum may involve the spinal cord (myelopathy) or spinal root (radiculopathy). They may cause both sensory and motor and autonomic disturbances. Spinal cord lesions may cause upper motor neuron (UMN) signs (weakness, spasticity, hyperactive deep tendon reflexes [DTRs], reduced superficial abdominal reflexes, clonus, Babinski signs) due to lateral corticospinal tract involvement and lower motor neuron signs (weakness, hypotonia, reduced DTRs, absence of pathologic reflexes, fasciculations) due to anterior horn cell dysfunction. Spinal cord lesions may cause loss of all sensory modalities as seen with complete cord transection, ipsilateral loss of vibration and position sensation with contralateral pain, and temperature impairment due to cord hemisection (Brown-Séquard syndrome); a shawl-like sensory pattern due to compression of centrally crossing sensory fibers as in syringomyelia; saddle-area anesthesia due to conus medullaris or cauda equina lesions; or loss of pain and temperature sensation with sparing of proprioception and vibration sensation due to anterior spinal artery infarction.

A. The presence of both sensory and motor disturbances suggests a spinal cord lesion; if there are only motor findings, a spinal cord compressive lesion is unlikely. Motor dysfunction alone may be seen in motor system disease, e.g., primary lateral sclerosis or HIV-1 myelopathy. In rare instances of spondylitic myelopathy, there may be motor signs without sensory signs; however, with spinal cord compression caused by a herniated disc, there are usually motor and sensory findings. If there are motor findings alone (with fasciculations and distal weakness), consider anterior horn cell disease or motor neuropathy. If weakness is proximal with normal sensation and normal reflexes, consider neuromuscular junction or muscle disease (myopathy).

B. Spinal root lesions involve both the dorsal root, causing sensory disturbances (which often are the initial symptom), and ventral roots, causing motor symptoms. They are usually the result of a herniated disc and are accompanied by neck or back pain. These lesions are most common in the cervical and lumbar regions and uncommon in the thoracic region. The distribution of motor, reflex, and sensory abnormalities depends on the specific root being compressed. For example, in the cervical region, C5, C6, and C7 nerve roots are compressed by herniated intervertebral discs, whereas L4, L5, and S1 roots are most likely compressed in the lumbosacral region. When the cervical roots are compressed, there may

initially be radiculopathy and later myelopathy. Less commonly, the thoracic nerve roots or thoracic spinal cord may be compressed. This may result in an anesthetic band encompassing the thoracic or abdominal region. In patients with these sensory disturbances, look for the vesicular skin eruptions of herpes zoster, which may cause similar sensory symptoms and may simulate a thoracic compressive cord or root lesion. In thoracic myelopathy, sensory symptoms are accompanied by spasticity and hyperactive DTRs (including clonus) in the legs, Babinski signs, and absent superficial abdominal reflexes. With an upper thoracic lesion, both upper and lower abdominal reflexes are absent; with a lower thoracic lesion, upper superficial abdominal reflexes are intact and lower abdominal reflexes absent. With a lower thoracic lesion, when the patient attempts to sit up, the umbilicus moves upward owing to intact upper abdominal muscles and paretic lower abdominal muscles (Beevor sign). If the spinal cord is compressed, there is usually sphincter dysfunction with motor and sensory abnormalities below the lesion. Cervical lesions may cause both arm and leg dysfunction; thoracic lesions involve the legs only.

C. Lesions involving the conus medullaris (the lowest portion of the spinal cord) cause sphincter dysfunction with sensory disturbances involving the sacral region (bottom of the feet and buttocks [saddle area]). Cauda equina lesions involve multiple lumbar and sacral spinal roots to cause leg weakness and wasting; there is a sensory impairment corresponding to the radicular pattern. If a patient has bilateral leg weakness but no sphincter disturbances, check DTRs carefully. The finding of sustained clonus and positive Babinski signs suggests spinal cord rather than radicular localization.

D. If weakness is confined to one leg with accompanying UMN signs, consider a parasagittal cerebral lesion (anterior cerebral artery ischemic lesion, parasagittal meningioma, or frontal hematoma). If there is asymmetric motor or sensory disturbance in one arm or one leg without UMN signs, consider radiculopathy, plexopathy, or mononeuropathy. The location of these three depends on the precise pattern of motor, sensory, and reflex abnormalities. If there is symmetric sensory and motor involvement with distal stocking-glove distribution, consider peripheral neuropathy (see p 206). Sphincter disturbance is rare in peripheral neuropathies but may occur in those due to diabetes mellitus or amyloid. In peripheral neuropathy, the

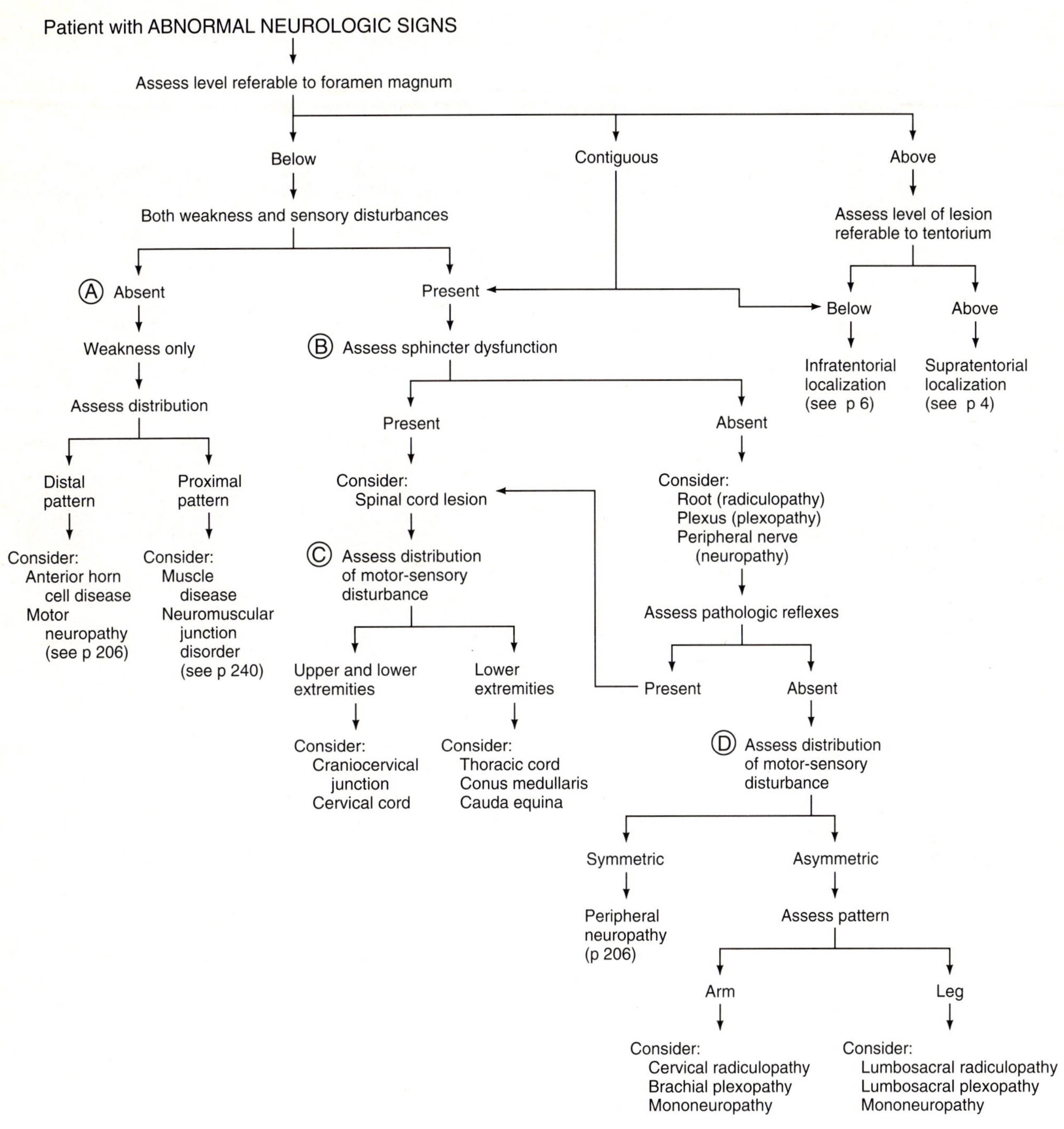

sensory disturbances initially involve the longest nerves; therefore, the short nerves supplying the sacral saddle (rectal) region are spared, in contrast to early involvement of this region with spinal cord lesions.

References

Brazis PW, Masduv JC, Biller J. Localization in clinical neurology. Boston: Little, Brown, 1985.
DeJong RN. The neurologic examination. New York: Hoeber, 1970.

ONSET OF NEUROLOGIC DISORDERS

Leon A. Weisberg, M.D.

If the onset of neurologic symptoms is sudden, consider electrical (seizures with paroxysmal neural discharge, demyelinating disorders with conduction block, migraine with spreading cortical depression) or vascular (ischemia, hemorrhage) conditions. If the onset is insidious or gradual, consider atrophic (degenerative) disorders, a mass lesion (intracranial, intraspinal), or intracranial hypertension. Mass lesions usually cause symptoms by direct neural compression or local tissue infiltration, and rarely by vascular mechanisms (peritumoral hemorrhage, ischemia due to blood vessel compression by tumor). When a tumor causes vascular effects, the onset of neurologic symptoms may be sudden.

A. The presence of "warning" or prodromal symptoms is important. In cases of syncope, these may be nonfocal prodromal symptoms (dizziness, weakness, visual blurring); focal symptoms (motor, sensory, visual) occur in migraine, TIAs, demyelinating disease, or partial seizures. In TIAs, focal symptoms are maximal at the onset, usually with no spread or progression; complete resolution usually occurs within 30 minutes, but symptoms may persist for 24 hours by virtue of the accepted definition of the term TIA. In TIA, neurologic symptoms are usually negative, characterized by loss or impairment of function (e.g., weakness, numbness, visual loss, aphasia). In migraine and seizures, they may be positive, characterized by hyperactivity of tissue function (e.g., scintillation, visual sparkles, clonic jerks, paresthesias). In partial (focal) seizures, there may be jacksonian march, an orderly progressive movement of neurologic symptoms. This represents a rapid march of motor or sensory abnormalities over the extremities, trunk, or face within several minutes. This is caused by excitatory electrical activity that rapidly spreads. There may also be subsequent Todd's postictal paralysis, which may persist for several hours or as long as 24 to 48 hours, and is caused by inhibitory cortical activity. In migraine, neurologic disturbances may evolve or "march" during a 10- to 30-minute interval. The characteristic visual disturbances of migraine spread from the periphery to the center of visual fixation; visual symptoms are followed by contralateral throbbing headache. The evolution of symptoms is *slower* in migraine (owing to the mechanism of spreading cortical depressive activity) than is the spread of seizures. In some migraine disorders, visual symptoms are *not* followed by headache (acephalic migraine), and in some focal seizures (especially the focal occipital variety), headache may be quite marked.

B. If focal signs develop suddenly, consider vascular or demyelinating disease. In patients with suspected vascular disease, a focal deficit without a warning TIA or subsequent deterioration suggests intracerebral hemorrhage. In cerebral infarction, warning TIAs commonly occur in more than half of cases; deterioration may occur after the onset (progressing stroke). Certain types of migraine equivalents that occur in elderly patients may simulate stroke syndromes, and these may occur *without* headache. Onset of neurologic deficit (optic neuritis, transverse myelitis) may be sudden in multiple sclerosis (MS), which is a demyelinating disorder. This is caused by an electrical disturbance referred to as conduction block. In MS, rapid stabilization is often followed by spontaneous gradual improvement. Less commonly in MS, the onset is slow and the course characterized by progressive deterioration; this may simulate the onset usually seen in patients harboring a mass lesion. Diagnostic studies (CT/MRI scan, CSF examination, angiography) may be required to differentiate demyelinating from vascular disease.

C. Paroxysmal disorders in which symptoms resolve rapidly and the patient returns to baseline condition (e.g., TIA, seizure, migraine, narcolepsy, transient global amnesia, vertigo, drop attacks, syncope) may present diagnostic difficulties. A carefully obtained history may provide treatment diagnostic clues. Determine whether consciousness is impaired, as may occur in seizure, syncope, or narcolepsy. In narcolepsy, recurrent and excessive brief sleep episodes occur; differentiation from seizures is established by EEG and sleep studies. In seizures, motor disturbances and postictal abnormalities are common (see p 156). In patients who suddenly lose consciousness without abnormal motor activity, consider Stokes-Adams attacks or hypoglycemia (especially in diabetic patients using insulin). Episodes of sudden mental confusion in which memory is impaired but consciousness is normal suggest transient global amnesia (TGA). The mechanism of TGA is not established, but it does not appear to be a form of vascular (TIA) or electrical seizure disorder. Certain disorders impair equilibrium. Most vertigo episodes are due to vestibular (labyrinthine or inner ear) disorders. If episodic vertigo is associated with hearing loss and tinnitus, consider Meniere's disease. In drop attacks, patients suddenly fall to the ground; these attacks may occur in children with seizures. EEG is abnormal in these cases. In older patients who develop drop attacks without loss of consciousness, consider vertebrobasilar TIA or electrolyte disturbances. In vertigo due to vestibular dysfunction, there are sudden attacks of "spinning" and feelings of dysequilibrium; absence of other brain stem or cerebellar symptoms differentiates vestibular dysfunction from vertebrobasilar TIA (see p 120).

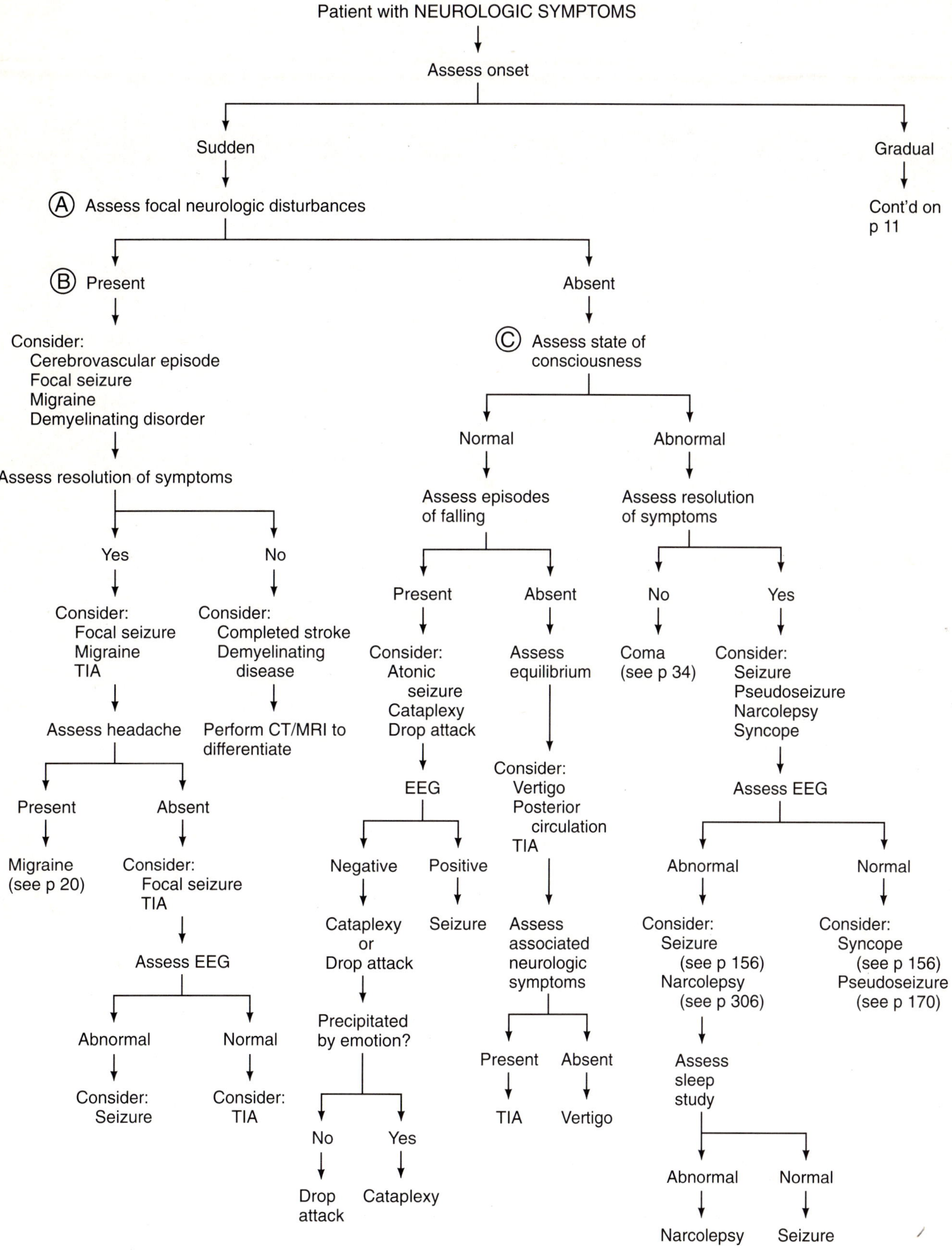

Patient with NEUROLOGIC SYMPTOMS
Assess onset
Sudden
Gradual
Cont'd on p 11
A Assess focal neurologic disturbances
B Present
Absent
Consider:
Cerebrovascular episode
Focal seizure
Migraine
Demyelinating disorder
Assess resolution of symptoms
Yes
No
Consider:
Focal seizure
Migraine
TIA
Consider:
Completed stroke
Demyelinating disease
Assess headache
Perform CT/MRI to differentiate
Present
Absent
Migraine (see p 20)
Consider:
Focal seizure
TIA
Assess EEG
Abnormal
Normal
Consider:
Seizure
Consider:
TIA
C Assess state of consciousness
Normal
Abnormal
Assess episodes of falling
Assess resolution of symptoms
Present
Absent
No
Yes
Consider:
Atonic seizure
Cataplexy
Drop attack
Assess equilibrium
Coma (see p 34)
Consider:
Seizure
Pseudoseizure
Narcolepsy
Syncope
EEG
Consider:
Vertigo
Posterior circulation
TIA
Assess EEG
Negative
Positive
Assess associated neurologic symptoms
Abnormal
Normal
Cataplexy or Drop attack
Seizure
Present
Absent
Consider:
Seizure (see p 156)
Narcolepsy (see p 306)
Consider:
Syncope (see p 156)
Pseudoseizure (see p 170)
Precipitated by emotion?
TIA
Vertigo
Assess sleep study
No
Yes
Abnormal
Normal
Drop attack
Cataplexy
Narcolepsy
Seizure

D. In patients with neurologic symptoms of gradual onset, it is important to ascertain the presence or absence of abnormal findings on neurologic examination. If the examination is negative and symptoms are present for a prolonged time (several years), consider a functional psychiatric disorder. In patients with abnormal neurologic findings, consider an atrophic-degenerative disorder or a mass lesion. With degenerative disorders, the course of subsequent deterioration is slowly progressive. If there is a mass lesion, the course may be characterized by rapid progression; however, some patients with low-grade gliomas, thrombosed (occult) vascular malformations, or meningiomas may show very slow progression over many years. In some patients with neoplasms, seizures may be the only clinical manifestation for many years, and other patterns of neurologic deterioration may only later begin to develop.

References

Eisen A. Neurophysiology in multiple sclerosis. Neurol Clin North Am 1983; 1:615.

Fisher CM. Late life migraine accompaniments. Stroke 1986; 17:1033.

Lauritzen M, Skyhoj OT, Lassen NA, et al. Changes in regional cerebral blood flow during the course of classic migraine attacks. Ann Neurol 1983; 13:633.

Lea AAP, Morrison RS. Propagation of spreading cortical depression. J Neurophysiol 1945; 8:33.

Poser C. Exacerbations, activity, and progression of multiple sclerosis. Arch Neurol 1980; 37:471.

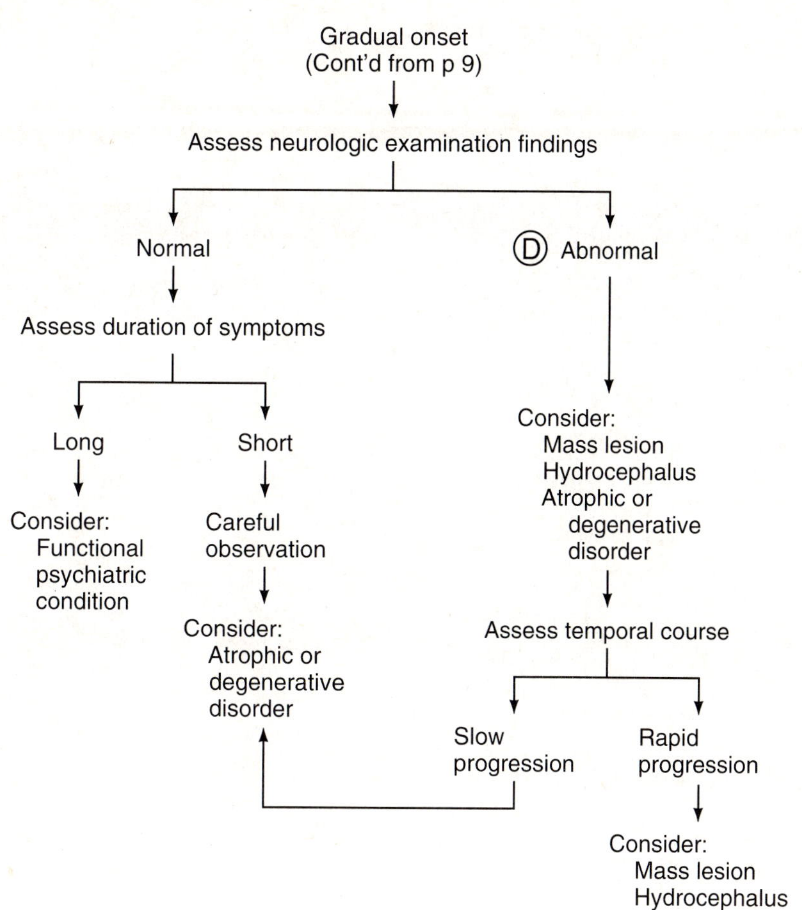

Gradual onset
(Cont'd from p 9)

Assess neurologic examination findings

Normal

(D) Abnormal

Assess duration of symptoms

Long

Short

Consider:
Functional
psychiatric
condition

Careful
observation

Consider:
Atrophic or
degenerative
disorder

Consider:
Mass lesion
Hydrocephalus
Atrophic or
degenerative
disorder

Assess temporal course

Slow
progression

Rapid
progression

Consider:
Mass lesion
Hydrocephalus

COURSE OF NEUROLOGIC ILLNESS

Leon A. Weisberg, M.D.

On the basis of a knowledge of the precise pattern of onset of a neurologic disorder and its subsequent temporal course, the underlying mechanism may be ascertained. Spontaneous neurologic improvement of a monophasic neurologic illness suggests one of these mechanisms: (1) vascular—cerebral infarction, intracerebral hemorrhage; (2) demyelinating disease—if the CNS is involved, consider multiple sclerosis (MS), but a biphasic relapsing-remitting course is much more likely; if the peripheral nervous system is involved, consider Guillain-Barré syndrome (inflammatory demyelinating polyneuropathy); (3) viral disorder—aseptic meningoencephalitis, myelitis, radiculitis, plexitis, neuritis.

A. Stroke may be defined by the temporal profile: (1) TIA, in which episodes usually last 10 to 30 minutes, but it may be 24 hours before the neurologic deficit resolves completely; (2) reversible ischemic neurologic deficit (RIND), in which the focal deficit persists >24 hours but resolves completely within several days or weeks; (3) minor stroke, in which significant (80%) functional recovery occurs within 1 month; (4) major stroke, in which recovery is less complete and slower, so that the patient has persistent neurologic impairment that usually impairs independent functional capability. Some patients in whom TIA is clinically diagnosed actually have cerebral infarction as documented by CT/MRI, despite complete clinical neurologic recovery within the first 24 hours. This condition is defined as cerebral infarction with transient signs (CITS). Rapid stabilization and spontaneous improvement after the onset of focal deficit are consistent with cerebrovascular disorders (infarction, hemorrhage), but this course may also occur in demyelinating disorders. After the initial deficit develops in stroke, subsequent progression is *not* the expected course, although progressing or deteriorating stroke may occur over 24 to 72 hours. The concept of a "slow stroke" is not consistent with our understanding of cerebrovascular pathophysiology. After the initial stroke deficit occurs, clinical improvement is most rapid within 6 months; this improvement may then slow but may continue for several years. Patients with spontaneous or hypertensive intracerebral hematomas do not usually develop recurrent hemorrhage. Intracranial hemorrhage caused by aneurysms or angiomas may recur or be associated with later deterioration after the initial bleeding episode; these occur as a result of (1) ischemia produced by vasospasm, (2) hydrocephalus due to obstruction of CSF pathways by blood, or (3) recurrent hemorrhage.

B. Sudden onset of neurologic signs with subsequent improvement is most consistent with cerebrovascular or demyelinating disease. Certain intracranial mass lesions may cause sudden onset with transient spontaneous improvement to simulate stroke syndrome. A "triphasic" course is characterized by sudden onset of neurologic deficit, followed by a period of stabilization and improvement, and later progressive deterioration. This course is seen with metastases, or less commonly with glioblastoma multiforme or brain abscess. In patients with metastases, hematogenous dissemination of tumor embolus initially causes infarction; this results in sudden onset and subsequent stabilization. Later, as tumor cells multiply, enlargement of the tumor mass and surrounding edema result in delayed neurologic deterioration. In patients with glioblastoma, a triphasic course may be caused by peritumoral hemorrhage, whereas in brain abscess the mechanism of triphasic illness may be related to hematogenous dissemination and embolism of infected material or particles to the brain.

C. Fluctuation or exacerbation of the deficit after initial onset may occur in several conditions. In myasthenia gravis, periods of neurologic worsening are observed throughout the day; between these periods, the patient may appear neurologically normal. In patients whose deficit is caused by MS, there may be episodes of fluctuating neurologic worsening lasting days to weeks. During these episodes, patients may develop exacerbation of a preexisting deficit or new patterns of neurologic deficit. Exacerbations may be interspersed between periods of clinical remission. Some patients with MS report worsening of neurologic impairment toward the end of each day; this is described as "fatigue." These symptoms may be caused by a physiologic conduction block. The history of fluctuating severity of neurologic symptoms in MS may be similar to that reported by patients with myasthenia gravis.

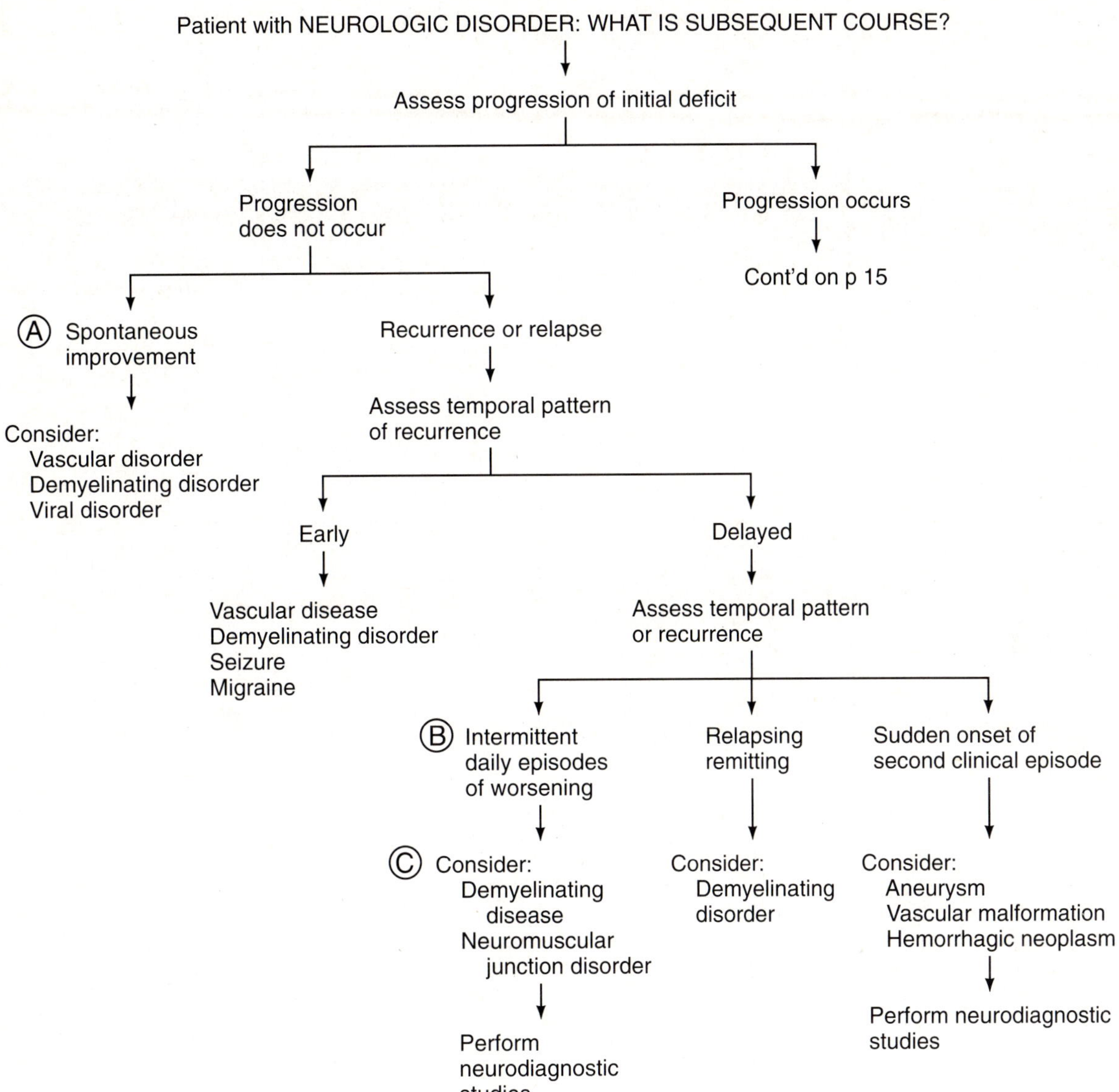

Patient with NEUROLOGIC DISORDER: WHAT IS SUBSEQUENT COURSE?
Assess progression of initial deficit
Progression does not occur
Progression occurs
Cont'd on p 15
A Spontaneous improvement
Recurrence or relapse
Consider:
Vascular disorder
Demyelinating disorder
Viral disorder
Assess temporal pattern of recurrence
Early
Delayed
Vascular disease
Demyelinating disorder
Seizure
Migraine
Assess temporal pattern or recurrence
B Intermittent daily episodes of worsening
Relapsing remitting
Sudden onset of second clinical episode
C Consider:
Demyelinating disease
Neuromuscular junction disorder
Consider:
Demyelinating disorder
Consider:
Aneurysm
Vascular malformation
Hemorrhagic neoplasm
Perform neurodiagnostic studies
Perform neurodiagnostic studies

D. Patients may show progressive worsening after initial recognition of the neurologic deficit. If progression is slow and examination shows positive neurologic signs, consider an atrophic-degenerative disorder. If more rapid deterioration occurs, consider a mass lesion. Some patients with mass lesion (gliomas, arteriovenous malformations, meningiomas) initially present with seizures without neurologic deficit. As the lesion enlarges, a focal deficit may develop. In patients with headache or other neurologic symptoms lasting longer than 1 year and no abnormal neurologic signs, neurodiagnostic studies are unlikely to show an underlying structural lesion, even if the patient reports that these symptoms have intensified.

E. If there is waxing and waning of diffuse neurologic function (e.g., confusion alternating with normal consciousness) throughout the day, consider subdural hematoma (especially if bilateral) or other mass lesions. Suspect a mass lesion if focal signs develop in patients with fluctuating neurologic deficit. These changes in neurologic condition probably relate to shifts in intracranial pressure elevations. The development of confusional episodes at night is seen in Alzheimer's dementia (sundown effect). If there is a change of the location of the focal deficit (e.g., shift from a left- to a right-sided hemiparesis), consider bilateral subdural hematomas, basilar artery occlusion, or recurrent cerebral embolism.

F. If the course is biphasic (initial illness characterized by full recovery followed by a second phase of neurologic deterioration), consider parainfectious conditions (possibly autoimmune mediated), e.g., those involving the peripheral nervous system (inflammatory demyelination of peripheral nerves as in Guillain-Barré syndrome) or the CNS (demyelination as in multiple sclerosis or encephalomyelitis). These may follow viral illness or vaccination and appear to result from an inflammatory response of the cell-mediated type against peripheral or central myelin. If there is neurologic improvement, observe the patient. If there is continued neurologic worsening, repeated neurodiagnostic studies are necessary. The initial neurodiagnostic evaluation may be negative, but if the neurologic condition deteriorates or new signs develop, periodic reassessment is warranted, and repeat evaluation may define the cause of the neurologic disorder.

References

Goldstein LB, Davis, JN. Restorative neurology: Drugs and recovery following stroke. Stroke 1990; 21:1636.

Pallais JE, Pellet W. Brain metastases. In Vinken PJ, Bruyn GW, eds. Handbook of clinical neurology. Vol 18. Amsterdam: North Holland Publishing, 1975:201.

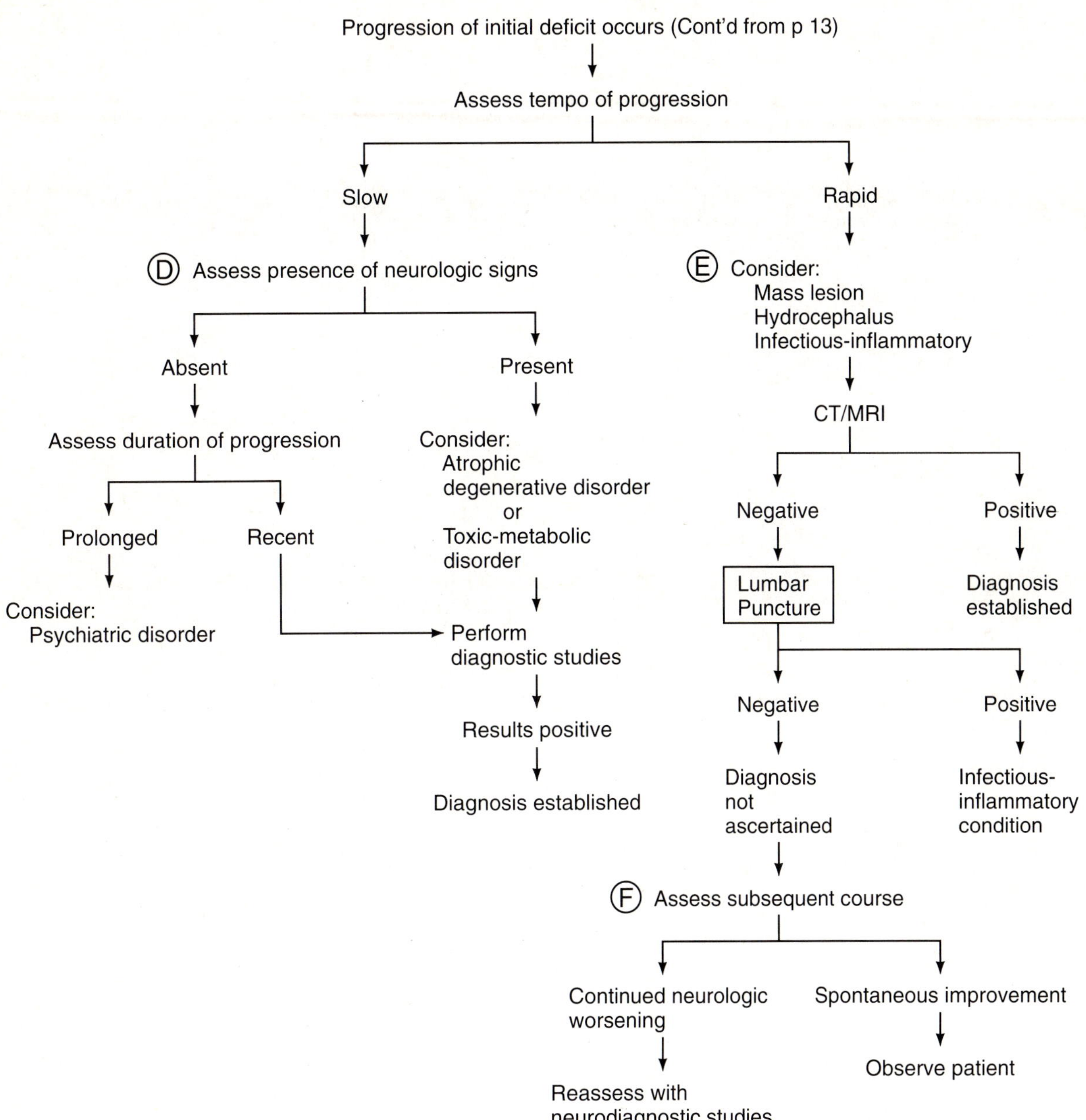

Progression of initial deficit occurs (Cont'd from p 13)
Assess tempo of progression
Slow
Rapid
D Assess presence of neurologic signs
E Consider:
Mass lesion
Hydrocephalus
Infectious-inflammatory
Absent
Present
CT/MRI
Assess duration of progression
Consider:
Atrophic
degenerative disorder
or
Toxic-metabolic
disorder
Negative
Positive
Prolonged
Recent
Lumbar
Puncture
Diagnosis
established
Consider:
Psychiatric disorder
Perform
diagnostic studies
Negative
Positive
Results positive
Diagnosis
not
ascertained
Infectious-
inflammatory
condition
Diagnosis established
F Assess subsequent course
Continued neurologic
worsening
Spontaneous improvement
Observe patient
Reassess with
neurodiagnostic studies

INITIAL HEADACHE

Richard L. Strub, M.D.

Headache is the most common medical symptom. Although usually benign, at times it can represent the first symptom of a serious neurologic disorder. The physician must distinguish the serious from the benign and then define the specific type of headache and its cause. The history is the most important part of the evaluation of patients with headache; care must be taken to elucidate not only the character of the pain but also the course of the headache. In addition to the profile of the presenting headache, it is important to distinguish the chronic recurrent headache, which is rarely life threatening, from the first-time headache that may reflect serious disease.

A. Patients with first-time headache and positive neurologic findings very likely have intracranial disease, possibly hemorrhage, meningitis, or acute hydrocephalus. A full neurologic evaluation is indicated.

B. Patients with sudden headache and completely normal findings on evaluation must be watched carefully. Most neurologists obtain a brain scan (CT or MRI) and many perform a spinal puncture. If no clear benign etiology is present, it is prudent to rule out serious disease (e.g., subarachnoid or intraparenchymal hemorrhage, acute hydrocephalus). If the patient is young and the headache is accompanied by a classic migraine aura, unilateral throbbing pain, and vomiting, a full evaluation may not be necessary.

C. Many medical illnesses are accompanied by headache (e.g., hypertension, infection, pulmonary failure). A headache can also be a side effect of medications. Physical strain and psychological stress can also cause sudden headache.

D. Every headache patient has a first tension, migraine, or cluster headache. Often it is prudent to evaluate the first vascular headache extensively, particularly in those who have neurologic symptoms at the onset. In young females, systemic lupus erythematosus may be heralded by a migraine-type headache. Vascular malformations may also present initially with unilateral headache.

E. The temporomandibular joint syndrome is one cause of headache, usually in the temporal region. It is frequently seen after recent dental work or in patients who grit their teeth at night. The joint itself is usually tender to palpation.

References

Appenzellar O, Feldman RG, Friedman AP. Migraine, headache, and related conditions. Arch Neurol 1979; 36:784.

Dalessio DJ. Wolff's headache and other head pain. New York: Oxford University Press, 1972.

Raskin NH. Headache. 2nd ed. New York: Churchill Livingstone, 1988.

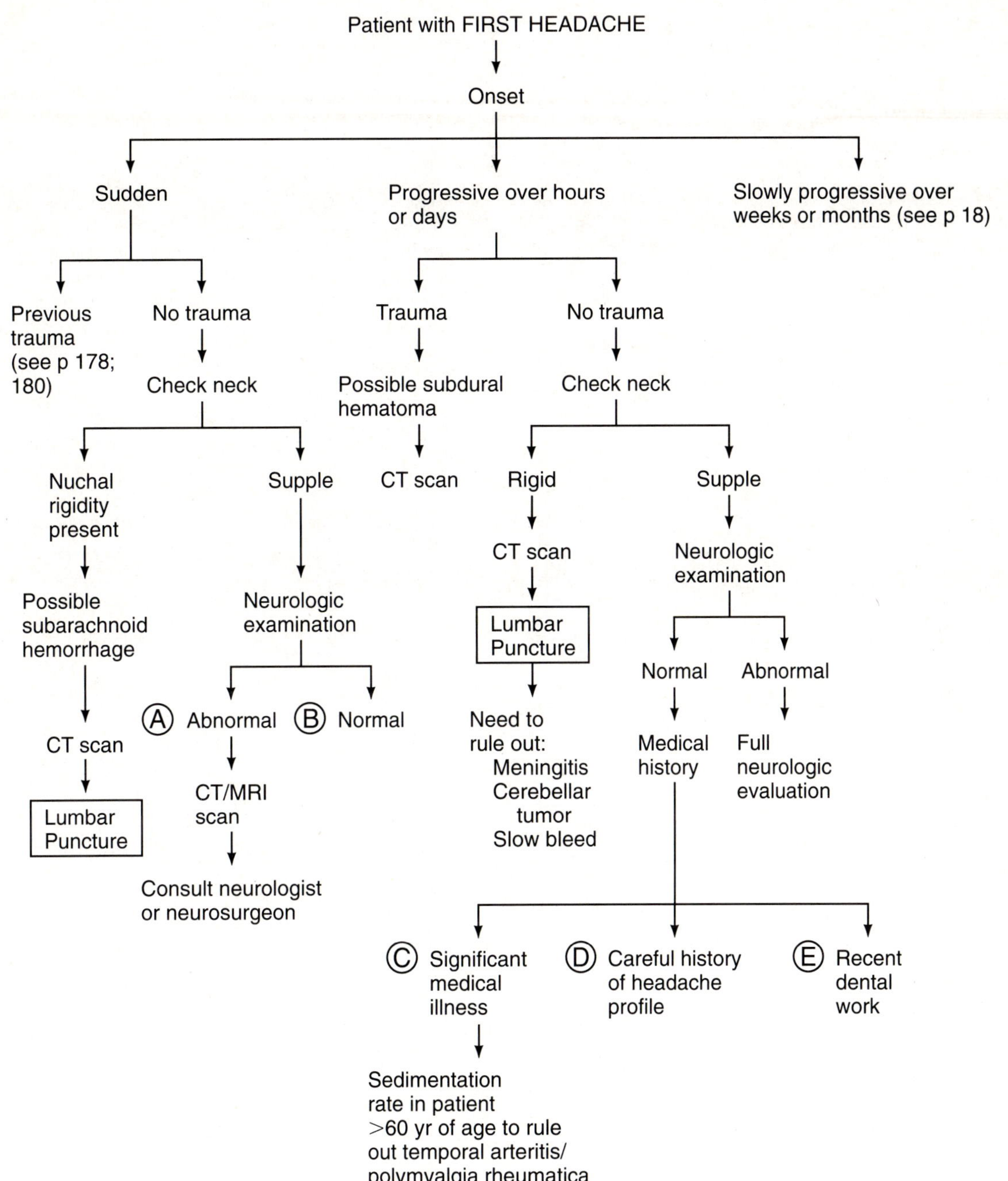

Patient with FIRST HEADACHE
Onset
Sudden
Progressive over hours or days
Slowly progressive over weeks or months (see p 18)
Previous trauma (see p 178; 180)
No trauma
Check neck
Trauma
Possible subdural hematoma
CT scan
No trauma
Check neck
Nuchal rigidity present
Supple
Rigid
CT scan
Supple
Neurologic examination
Possible subarachnoid hemorrhage
Neurologic examination
Lumbar Puncture
CT scan
A Abnormal
B Normal
Need to rule out:
Meningitis
Cerebellar tumor
Slow bleed
Normal
Abnormal
Lumbar Puncture
CT/MRI scan
Medical history
Full neurologic evaluation
Consult neurologist or neurosurgeon
C Significant medical illness
D Careful history of headache profile
E Recent dental work
Sedimentation rate in patient >60 yr of age to rule out temporal arteritis/ polymyalgia rheumatica

CHRONIC HEADACHE

Richard L. Strub, M.D.

A. A chronic progressive headache suggests some type of specific progressive pathologic process (brain tumor, uncontrolled hypertension, sinusitis, pseudotumor cerebri). Recurrent headache is more likely to have a benign cause (migraine, muscle contraction, cervical spondylosis).

B. Ask about blurred vision (an indication of either papilledema or optic nerve inflammation), focal weakness, and diplopia.

C. If the patient has pain and tenderness over the perinasal sinuses even in the absence of other symptoms of sinusitis, obtain sinus x-ray films or a CT scan of the sinuses.

D. Headache is common in patients with hypertension, but be careful not to ascribe all headaches in hypertensives to high blood pressure. If the pressure is well controlled, look elsewhere for the cause of the headache.

E. In elderly patients the new onset of a progressive (particularly unilateral) headache may indicate temporal arteritis. This is a potentially dangerous disease because involvement of the ophthalmic artery can lead to blindness. The sedimentation rate is usually increased and the temporal artery may be tender. Temporal artery biopsy frequently can indicate a definite diagnosis.

F. Patients with significant neurologic symptoms and signs require extensive neurologic evaluation.

G. It is important to characterize carefully the nature, location, and course of the headache; the history alone will suggest the diagnosis. There are no specific neurodiagnostic tests for migraine, tension, or cluster headaches. A neurologic examination should be performed in all these patients, but the findings almost always are normal. If there are focal neurologic findings, the diagnosis of simple chronic recurrent headache is in question and a full evaluation is warranted.

H. The cluster headache is always on one side, usually occurs in males, is triggered by alcohol, frequently starts at night, and is intense. The patient must pace the floor, eyes tearing and nose stuffy. The headache lasts 1 to 2 hours and occurs in clusters (e.g., nightly for several months). Prophylactic medication yields the best results. There is a variant in women that involves more predominantly temporal pain that responds to indomethacin.

I. Classic migraine occurs more frequently in women, is unilateral (usually a preferred side but occasionally on the opposite side), and is preceded by an aura that is usually visual (e.g., streaks of light, scotomata, field defects, sparkling dots). The headache lasts 1 to 3 hours, is often accompanied by nausea and vomiting, may occur more often during or after stress, and tends to be familial.

J. Common migraines or tension vascular headaches may or may not be related to classic migraine. In these, there is no aura, the headache builds bilaterally with throbbing but usually no vomiting, and the pain lasts for many hours. Pain is usually frontotemporal. Treatment as for classic migraine is usually not successful. In general, migraine headaches have a distinct onset and termination, may be preceded by nausea, and may respond to ergots.

K. Tension or muscle contraction headaches may occur in emotionally stressed individuals or in those who are somewhat perfectionistic and whose life involves juggling many factors to keep everything running smoothly. Treatment consists of helping them to understand the cause and to make cautious use of non-narcotic analgesics, relaxation, biofeedback, small doses of antidepressant medication, or mild tranquilization (whenever necessary but not daily).

References

Appenzellar O, Feldman RG, Friedman AP. Migraine, headache, and related conditions. Arch Neurol 1979; 36:784.

Raskin NH. Headache. 2nd ed. New York, Churchill Livingstone, 1988.

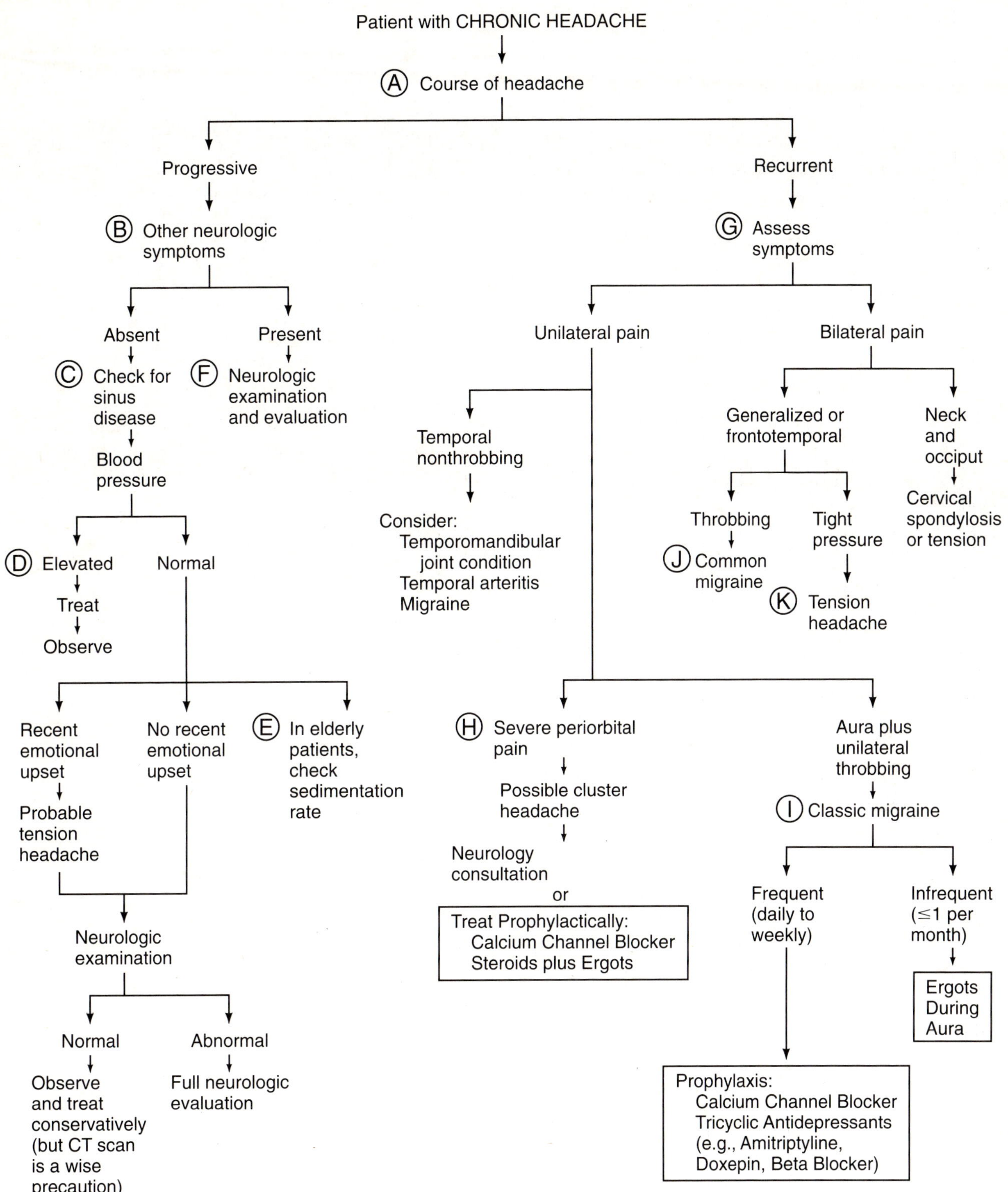

Patient with CHRONIC HEADACHE
A Course of headache
Progressive
Recurrent
B Other neurologic symptoms
G Assess symptoms
Absent
Present
C Check for sinus disease
F Neurologic examination and evaluation
Blood pressure
D Elevated
Normal
Treat
Observe
Recent emotional upset
No recent emotional upset
E In elderly patients, check sedimentation rate
Probable tension headache
Neurologic examination
Normal
Abnormal
Observe and treat conservatively (but CT scan is a wise precaution)
Full neurologic evaluation
Unilateral pain
Bilateral pain
Temporal nonthrobbing
Generalized or frontotemporal
Neck and occiput
Consider:
Temporomandibular joint condition
Temporal arteritis
Migraine
Throbbing
Tight pressure
Cervical spondylosis or tension
J Common migraine
K Tension headache
H Severe periorbital pain
Aura plus unilateral throbbing
Possible cluster headache
I Classic migraine
Neurology consultation
or
Frequent (daily to weekly)
Infrequent (≤1 per month)
Treat Prophylactically:
Calcium Channel Blocker
Steroids plus Ergots
Ergots During Aura
Prophylaxis:
Calcium Channel Blocker
Tricyclic Antidepressants
(e.g., Amitriptyline,
Doxepin, Beta Blocker)

ACUTE MIGRAINE HEADACHE

Richard L. Strub, M.D.

Migraine headache is one of the most painful yet benign conditions that the physician is called on to treat. Migraine sufferers should be taken seriously, since prompt treatment is usually very effective and they can return to a normal routine with minimal pain and disruption of their life. Migraine is treated in three settings: home, office/emergency room, and (in intractable cases) inpatient hospital.

A. In classic migraine headache an aura, usually visual, is present, and prompt treatment will abort the attack before the headache appears. Patients with nocturnal migraine may not be aware of the aura and may be awakened by the pain, thereby missing the opportunity to abort the attack.

B. There are a variety of oral ergotamine preparations that can be swallowed or placed under the tongue. Many ergot medications contain caffeine, a weak vasoconstrictor, that can cause nervousness and insomnia in patients; in such patients the sublingual preparations may be preferable. The most common side effect of ergots is nausea; this may be dose related in some patients. If nausea occurs despite successful headache treatment, reduce the ergot dose or use concomitant antinausea medication. Give 2 mg oral ergotamine at onset, and then 1 mg q 45 to 60 min to a maximum of 6 mg/24 hr. *Do not use this agent in patients with ischemic vascular disease.*

C. In some patients there is no aura or the oral ergot fails to prevent the headache.

D. Injectable ergots (DHE-dihydroergotamine or sumatriptan) are very effective in arresting a migraine headache in progress. Many patients are able to give themselves subcutaneous or intramuscular injections at home; others prefer to come to the office or emergency room. Tailor treatment to the patient, depending on the amount of nausea produced (this is more of a problem with DHE than with sumatriptan). The initial dose of DHE should be 0.5 to 1 mg; this may be given with an antinausea medication such as metoclopramide, 5 to 10 mg. This dose can be repeated every hour until successful or until a total dose of 3 mg is given.

E. Management of the ergot-resistant intractable migraine varies. Some physicians admit the patient after 3 hours of unsuccessful treatment; others give initial sedative/analgesic treatment before admitting the patient. This author prefers to have patients either take at home, or be given by the nurse or ER staff, narcotic or nonsteroid (Toradol) analgesia, and sedation (usually a benzodiazepine such as diazepam) to help them sleep. Sleep itself is an excellent treatment for migraine. Steroids (prednisone, 40 mg daily for 2 to 3 days, or dexamethasone, 8 to 12 mg daily for 2 days) have a role in controlling the sterile, chemically induced vascular inflammation that accompanies an intractable migraine. These can be started anytime after the 3 hours of failed treatment with ergots. These anti-inflammatory medications definitely shorten the course of a serious prolonged migraine attack.

F. When patients require admission for intractable migraine, the mainstays of treatment are (1) IV DHE, 0.5 to 1.0 mg q8h, (2) IV metoclopramide, 5 to 10 mg q8h or similar antinausea preparation, (3) IV dexamethasone, 8 to 16 mg, (4) sedation, and (5) possible analgesic-narcotic agents.

References

Mondell BE. Office management of acute headache. Headache Q 1992; 3:4.

Raskin NH. Headache. 2nd ed. New York: Churchill Livingstone, 1988.

Silberstein SD. Intractable headache: Inpatient and outpatient treatment strategies. Neurology 1992; 42(Suppl 2):1.

Subcutaneous Sumatriptan International Study Group. Treatment of migraine attacks with sumatriptan. N Engl J Med 1991; 325:316.

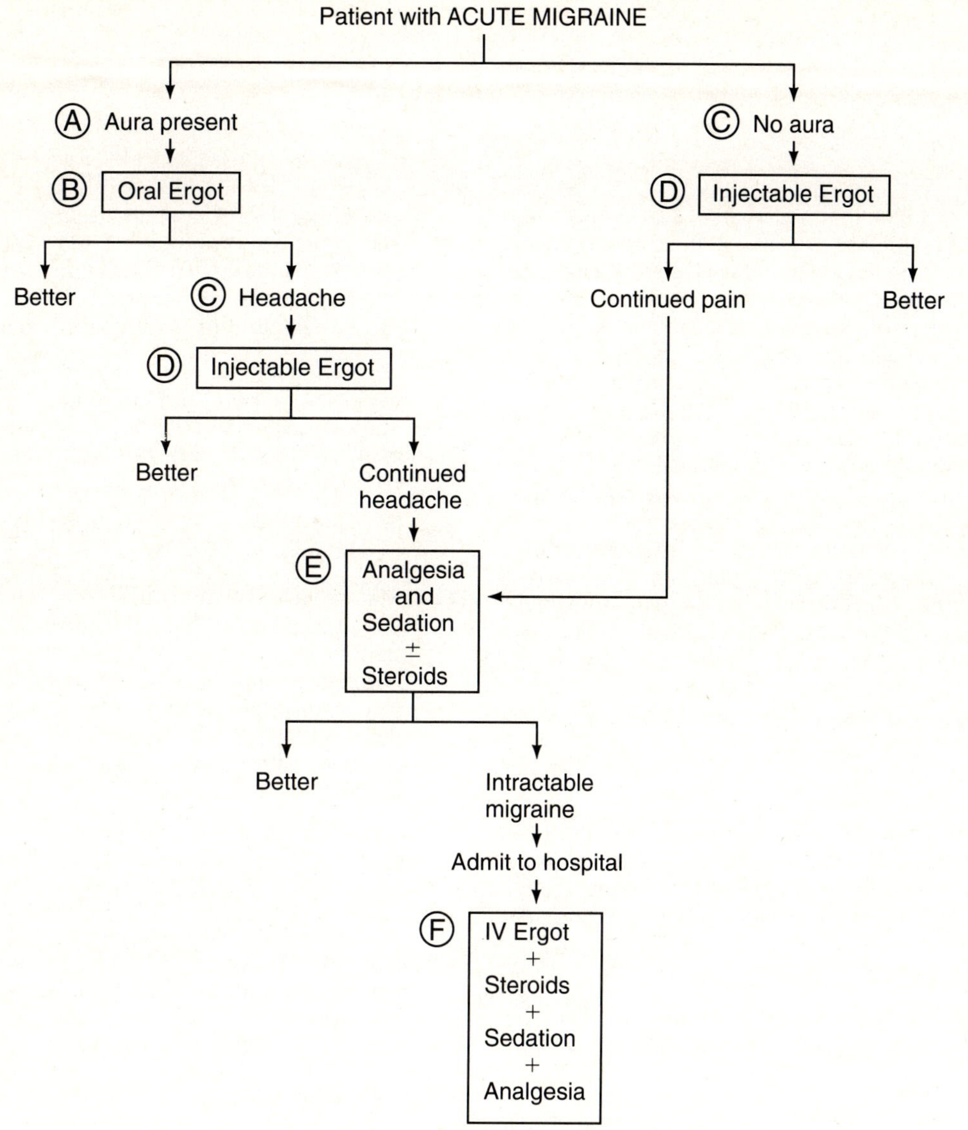

Patient with ACUTE MIGRAINE
A Aura present
C No aura
B Oral Ergot
D Injectable Ergot
Better
C Headache
Continued pain
Better
D Injectable Ergot
Better
Continued headache
E Analgesia and Sedation ± Steroids
Better
Intractable migraine
Admit to hospital
F IV Ergot + Steroids + Sedation + Analgesia

FACIAL PAIN

Richard L. Strub, M.D.

A. The onset of trigeminal neuralgia or tic douloureux is usually in late middle age. Be cautious about making this diagnosis in younger patients unless they have multiple sclerosis. The pain in tic douloureux is lancinating or shock-like. It lasts momentarily and makes the patient cringe. Pains can occur in a repetitive fashion. Trigger zones in the mouth or on the lips are common; cold or hot food also triggers pain. The pain is usually in the mandibular and maxillary divisions of the trigeminal nerve but is possible in any combination of the three roots. Ophthalmic pain alone is rare; in such cases, consider eye disease. A full neurologic evaluation is rarely useful. On occasion, dental pain secondary to an apical abscess can present with sudden strong face pain. Dental pain usually lasts for several minutes after it starts, but can mimic trigeminal neuralgia. In any atypical case it is wise to consult a dentist before embarking on long-term medical treatment.

B. Persistent pain suggests a destructive or inflammatory lesion.

C. Temporomandibular joint (TMJ) dysfunction can cause face pain. The jaw often clicks, the joint is often tender, and pain is most frequently in the temple region. Treat with indomethacin (Indocin), 25 mg four times a day.

D. Temporal arteritis is one feature of the collagen disorder polymyalgia rheumatica. The condition presents with migratory arthritis, unilateral head pain, and visual loss. It appears in individuals over age 60 and must be promptly treated with steroids (e.g., prednisone, 60 mg daily). Follow the sedimentation rate and reduce the steroid level to an every-other-day dose; maintain this treatment for years.

E. Atypical facial pain is a poorly understood entity of uncertain cause. The pain tends to be chronic, dull, and nonlancinating. It is also widespread over the side of the head and neck. It can be treated successfully with antidepressant medication or mild tranquilizers.

F. In many patients with persistent face pain, a dental condition is responsible.

G. Many diseases that occur in or around the brain stem can produce facial pain (infection of the petrous bone, tumors of the pons, tumors around the brain stem, chronic meningitis, vascular malformation). It is best to consult a neurologist or neurosurgeon to evaluate these complicated cases. The best single test to evaluate a lesion in this area of the nervous system is the MRI scan.

References

Couch JR. Face pain. Semin Neurol 1988; 8(4):298.

Goodman BW. Temporal arteritis. Am J Med 1972; 67:839.

Penman J. Trigeminal neuralgia. In Vinken PJ, Bruyn AW, eds. Handbook of clinical neurology. Vol 5. Amsterdam: Elsevier, 1968:296.

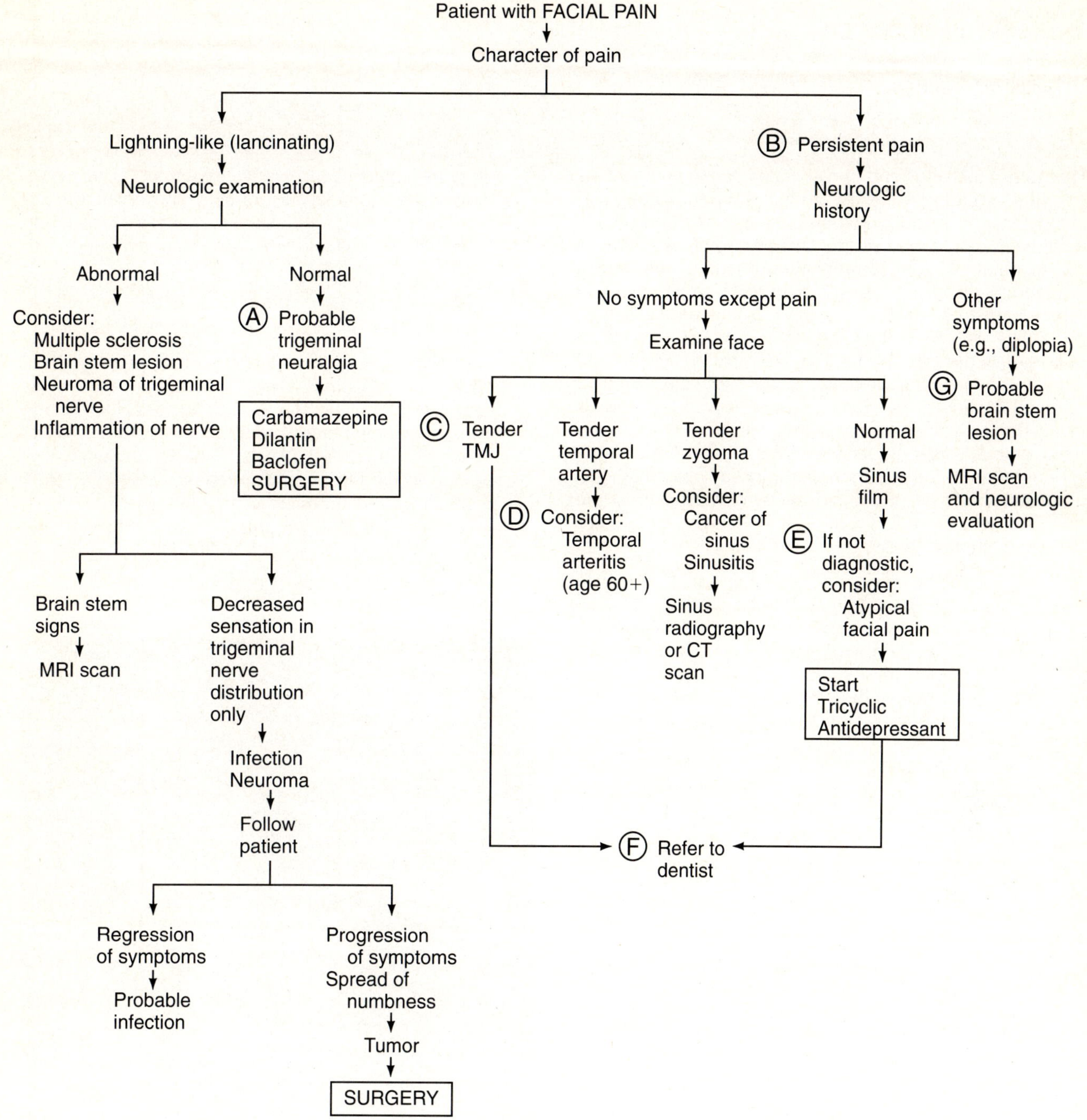

Patient with FACIAL PAIN
Character of pain
Lightning-like (lancinating)
Neurologic examination
Abnormal
Consider:
Multiple sclerosis
Brain stem lesion
Neuroma of trigeminal nerve
Inflammation of nerve
Normal
(A) Probable trigeminal neuralgia
Carbamazepine
Dilantin
Baclofen
SURGERY
Brain stem signs
MRI scan
Decreased sensation in trigeminal nerve distribution only
Infection
Neuroma
Follow patient
Regression of symptoms
Probable infection
Progression of symptoms
Spread of numbness
Tumor
SURGERY
(B) Persistent pain
Neurologic history
No symptoms except pain
Examine face
(C) Tender TMJ
Tender temporal artery
(D) Consider:
Temporal arteritis (age 60+)
Tender zygoma
Consider:
Cancer of sinus
Sinusitis
Sinus radiography or CT scan
Normal
Sinus film
(E) If not diagnostic, consider:
Atypical facial pain
Start Tricyclic Antidepressant
(F) Refer to dentist
Other symptoms (e.g., diplopia)
(G) Probable brain stem lesion
MRI scan and neurologic evaluation

NECK PAIN

Richard L. Strub, M.D.

Diseases of the spine and its associated neural components (spinal cord and nerve roots) produce several different and characteristic clinical symptoms or symptom clusters (back pain, weakness in the legs and arms, sensory complaints in the extremities, gait abnormalities, bladder and bowel symptoms). Because back pain syndromes are discussed in other chapters, the discussion here centers on the patient presenting with neurologic dysfunction related to damage or disease in the neural structures. Neck pain is approached clinically in much the same way as low back pain. The pain may occur suddenly or develop progressively. Trauma is often the cause of acute symptoms. Spontaneous nontraumatic pain is usually more significant, as it can indicate a serious nonmusculotendinous etiology. A neurologic examination must be performed to identify damage to the neural structures in the neck, specifically the spinal cord and cervical nerve roots.

A. The goal of the history and examination is to elucidate signs and symptoms of root or spinal cord disease. The symptoms of root involvement are weakness in the arm, radiating pain, and paresthesias. The symptoms of spinal cord dysfunction are stiff (spastic) legs, altered sensation in the trunk and legs, and autonomic dysfunction (bowel, bladder, and sexual dysfunction). One of the most common causes of neck pain is cervical spondylosis in which cervical discs have degenerated and facet joints hypertrophied. This usually occurs in middle-aged men who have done physical labor. This degenerative process narrows both the spinal canal, producing myelopathy (spinal cord damage), and the neural foramina, resulting in radiculopathy (nerve root damage).

B. The signs of root dysfunction are loss of a single reflex, sensory loss in a root distribution, or muscle weakness in a muscle or muscle group supplied by a single nerve root. Spinal cord dysfunction is determined by spasticity in the legs (increased tone, hyperreflexia, positive Babinski sign) and signs of bowel and bladder dysfunction. Mechanical signs (muscle spasm, restricted movement, tenderness, pain on neck movement) indicating musculoskeletal disease should also be sought on examination.

C. Patients with normal findings on neurologic examination frequently demonstrate mechanical signs, which often respond to conservative treatment. If the symptoms arose secondary to trauma, conservative treatment is indicated; if the pain arose spontaneously and is progressive, more intensive evaluation is suggested.

D. Conservative treatment includes rest, heat, nonsteroidal anti-inflammatory drugs, mild analgesics, muscle relaxants, and (in more severe cases) neck traction.

E. The choice of tests is related to the particular details of each case. Trauma resulting in spinal cord signs requires immediate neurosurgical consultation and immobilization but no additional tests. In cases of suspected vertebral collapse (metastatic cancer, myeloma, osteoporosis, inflammatory disease), plain x-ray views and an MRI scan are obtained first (Fig. 1). In suspected multiple sclerosis, an MRI scan and spinal fluid examination are indicated.

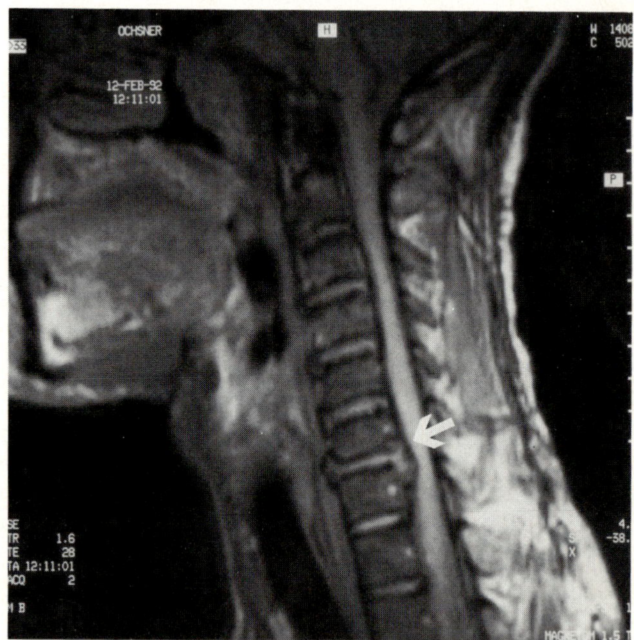

Figure 1 Sagittal MRI view of the cervical spine, showing herniated nucleus pulposus with pressure on the spinal cord *(arrow)*.

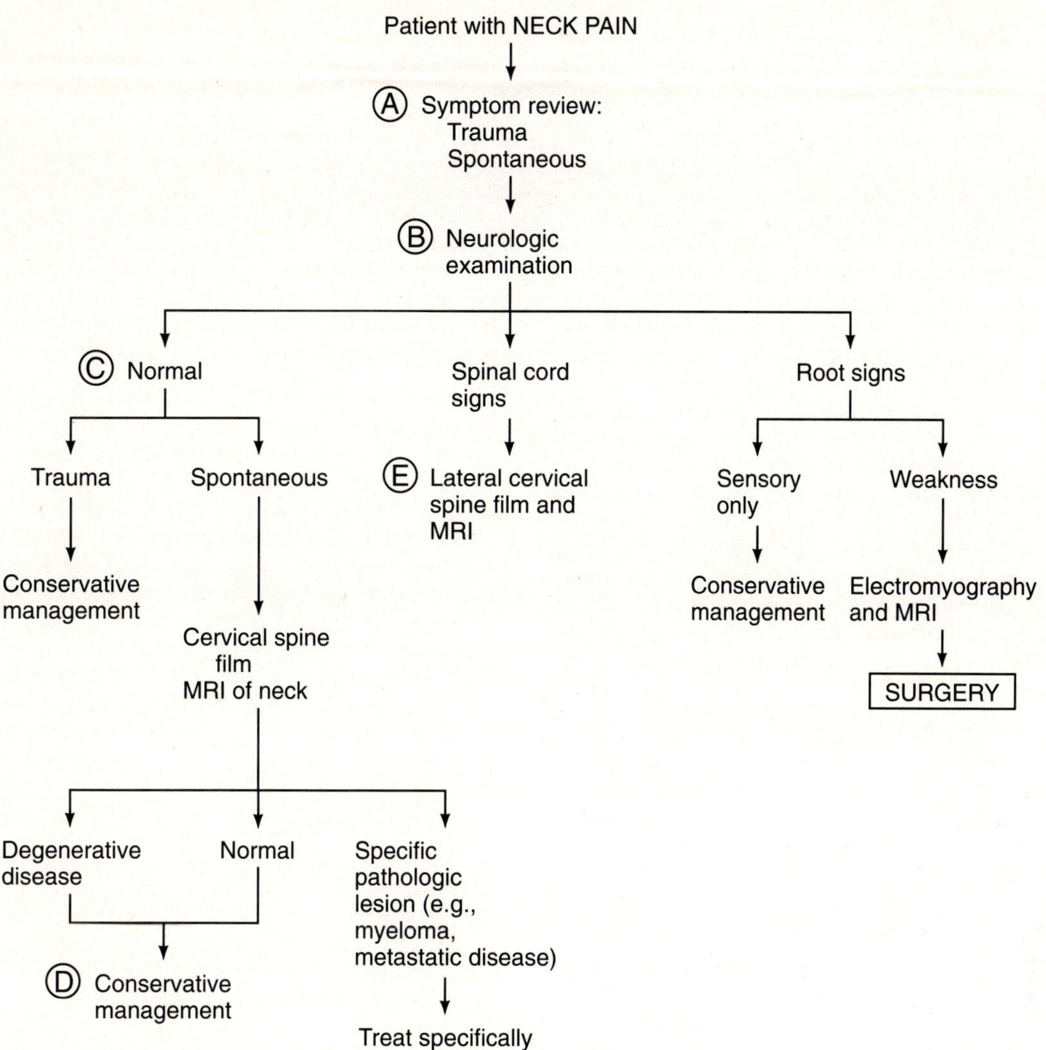

Patient with NECK PAIN
A Symptom review:
Trauma
Spontaneous
B Neurologic examination
C Normal
Spinal cord signs
Root signs
Trauma
Spontaneous
E Lateral cervical spine film and MRI
Sensory only
Weakness
Conservative management
Cervical spine film MRI of neck
Conservative management
Electromyography and MRI
SURGERY
Degenerative disease
Normal
Specific pathologic lesion (e.g., myeloma, metastatic disease)
D Conservative management
Treat specifically

HAND AND ARM PAIN

Leon A. Weisberg, M.D.

A. If hand and arm pain do not radiate to the forearm, shoulder, or neck, assess whether pain is localized to the median or the ulnar nerve distribution. Patients with carpal tunnel syndrome (CTS) usually complain of wrist or hand pain, but pain may also radiate to the forearm (see p 218). Pain due to CTS is usually dull and aching but may be sharp or burning. In patients with vague and poorly described arm pain, always consider CTS. In CTS, paresthesias are typically present in median nerve distribution; this includes the thumb, index, and middle fingers and the radial surface of the ring finger. Sensory symptoms are most severe at night, are worsened by activities causing repetitive wrist flexion, and are relieved by hand shaking or discontinuing the activity that precipitated the symptoms. Motor symptoms are less common than sensory symptoms, but patients with CTS may have difficulty removing tops of jars or cans.

B. In CTS, symptoms are reproduced by tapping over the wrist (Tinel sign) or causing forced wrist flexion (Phalen sign). Sensory loss is present in a median-innervated pattern, and the motor defect may involve the abductor pollicis or opponens pollicis.

C. Electromyography (EMG) and nerve conduction velocity (NCV) tests should confirm the location of median nerve compressive neuropathy. In rare cases of CTS, EMG/NCV tests may be normal. Some musculoskeletal diseases cause hand and arm pain, including those resulting from inflammation of the synovial bursae (rheumatoid arthritis, gout, trauma). In these conditions, there is local hand and arm pain and tenderness; these are increased by limb movement, in contrast to CTS, in which symptoms are relieved by limb movement. Tenosynovitis of the abductor and extensor pollicis brevis (de Quervain's disease) may simulate CTS; however, ulnar deviation of the hand with the thumb flexed into the palm exacerbates pain in this condition.

D. Hand and arm pain develop in patients with Raynaud's phenomenon, which may simulate CTS, but in this condition *all* fingers are affected and symptoms are precipitated by cold exposure. In reflex sympathetic dystrophy (RSD), pain and paresthesias involving the hand are prominent. In RSD, movement invariably intensifies pain, whereas in CTS shaking the hand relieves pain. In both RSD and CTS, there may be sympathetic vasomotor abnormalities (changes in sweating, temperature, color of skin) and trophic changes (skin atrophy, reduced nail and hair pattern). The diagnosis of RSD is established by response to nerve block, and EMG shows no abnormality, as compared with the characteristic abnormality in CTS.

E. The ulnar nerve may be entrapped at the elbow or wrist. With elbow compression, sharp shooting pain may develop in the hand and fifth digit. These symptoms often occur at night or as the elbow is repetitively flexed (see p 220). With cervical radiculopathy due to C8 nerve root compression, neck pain is usually present and paresthesias extend to the forearm and shoulder. Rarely, spinal cord lesions (syringomyelia, glioma) cause deep aching arm and hand pain; however, neurologic examination shows motor, sensory, and reflex abnormalities indicating a spinal cord lesion.

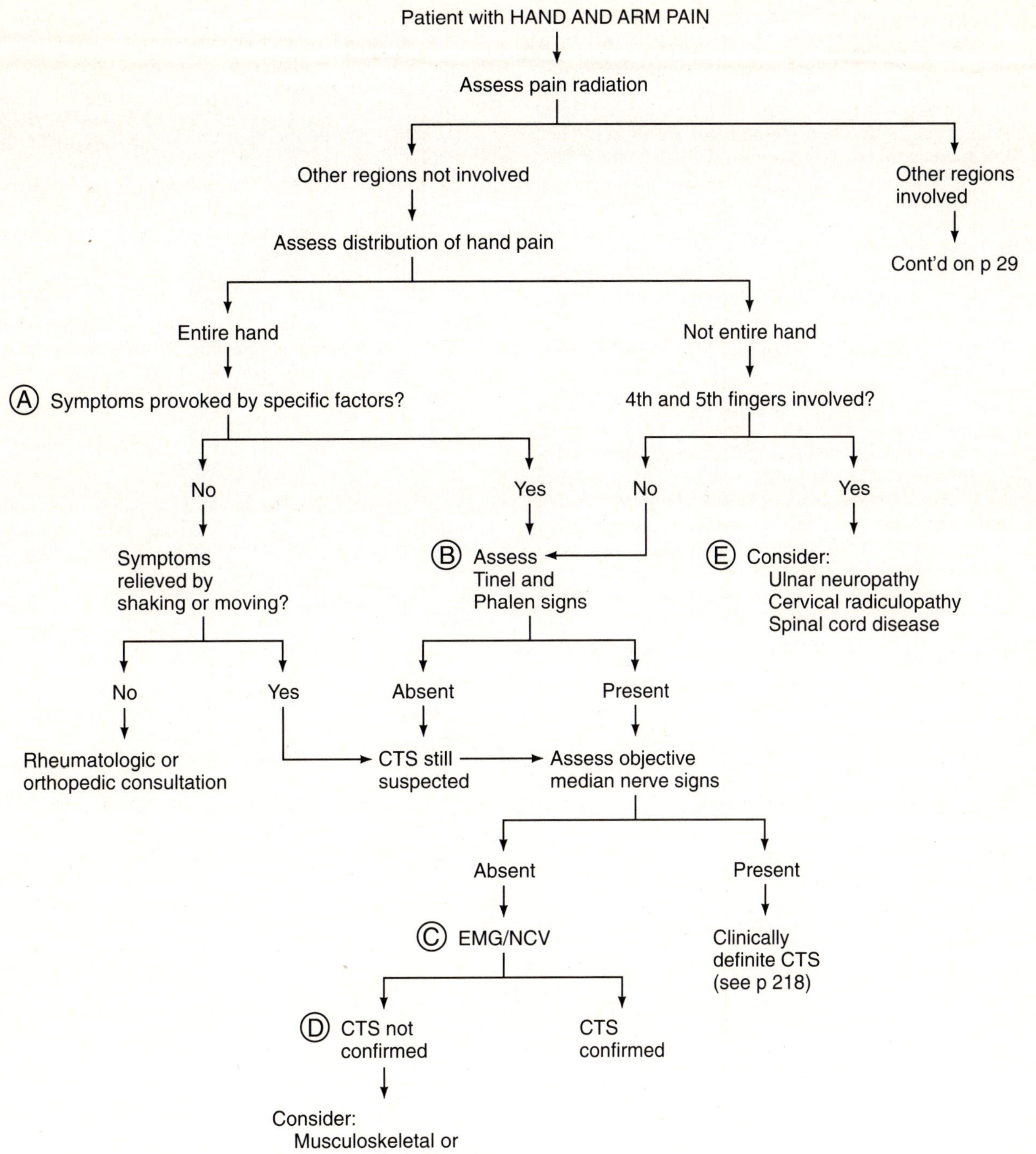

Patient with HAND AND ARM PAIN
Assess pain radiation
Other regions not involved
Other regions involved
Cont'd on p 29
Assess distribution of hand pain
Entire hand
Not entire hand
A Symptoms provoked by specific factors?
4th and 5th fingers involved?
No
Yes
No
Yes
Symptoms relieved by shaking or moving?
B Assess Tinel and Phalen signs
E Consider:
Ulnar neuropathy
Cervical radiculopathy
Spinal cord disease
No
Yes
Absent
Present
Rheumatologic or orthopedic consultation
CTS still suspected
Assess objective median nerve signs
Absent
Present
C EMG/NCV
Clinically definite CTS (see p 218)
D CTS not confirmed
CTS confirmed
Consider:
Musculoskeletal or rheumatologic disorder

F. The median nerve may rarely be entrapped at the level of the shoulder, proximal humerus, or elbow. With median nerve compression at the shoulder or humerus, forearm pronation (weakness of the pronator teres and quadratus) and flexion of the interphalangeal joint of the thumb and index finger are weak. When the median nerve is compressed at the elbow, the initial symptom is aching pain in the proximal forearm, which is intensified by repetitive elbow movement. When the examiner applies pressure over the pronator teres, the patient reports tenderness, whereas Tinel and Phalen signs are negative. In proximal median neuropathy, EMG shows abnormalities in those muscles above the wrist, as contrasted with CTS, in which abnormal findings are only abnormal distal to the wrist.

G. Cervical radiculopathy affecting the C6 or C7 roots causes forearm pain and tenderness, but there is usually neck pain as well as motor, sensory, and reflex (biceps due to C6 and triceps due to C7) signs. Neck pain, reflex abnormalities, and lack of reproduction of hand symptoms are indicative of C7 radiculopathy and should permit differentiation from CTS; however, both conditions may be present at the same time. In brachial plexus lesions, the pattern of weakness is different from that in median nerve lesions. In thoracic outlet syndrome, there is arm pain and heaviness in the arm that is exacerbated by arm exercise; however, pain usually radiates to the ulnar arm region. In thoracic outlet syndrome, clinical findings are confined to a C8 and T1 distribution. There may be vascular-autonomic changes in the hand. The radial pulse may be obliterated with arm elevation and turning the head to the opposite shoulder (Adson's maneuver). A bruit may be heard over the clavicle or in the axilla. Chest radiography may show a cervical rib. Symptoms of thoracic outlet syndrome are of either a vascular (compression of the subclavian artery) or a neural (compression of the lower or medial trunk of the brachial plexus) origin. In RSD, sympathetic autonomic and trophic changes are present but usually no motor or sensory disturbances.

References

Dawson DM, Hallett M, Millender LH. Entrapment neuropathies. 2nd ed. Boston: Little, Brown, 1990:5–105.

Schwartzman RJ, McLellan TL. Reflex sympathetic dystrophy. Arch Neurol 1987; 33:556.

Spinner RJ, Bachman JW, Amadio RJ. The many faces of carpal tunnel syndrome. Mayo Clin Proc 1989; 64:829.

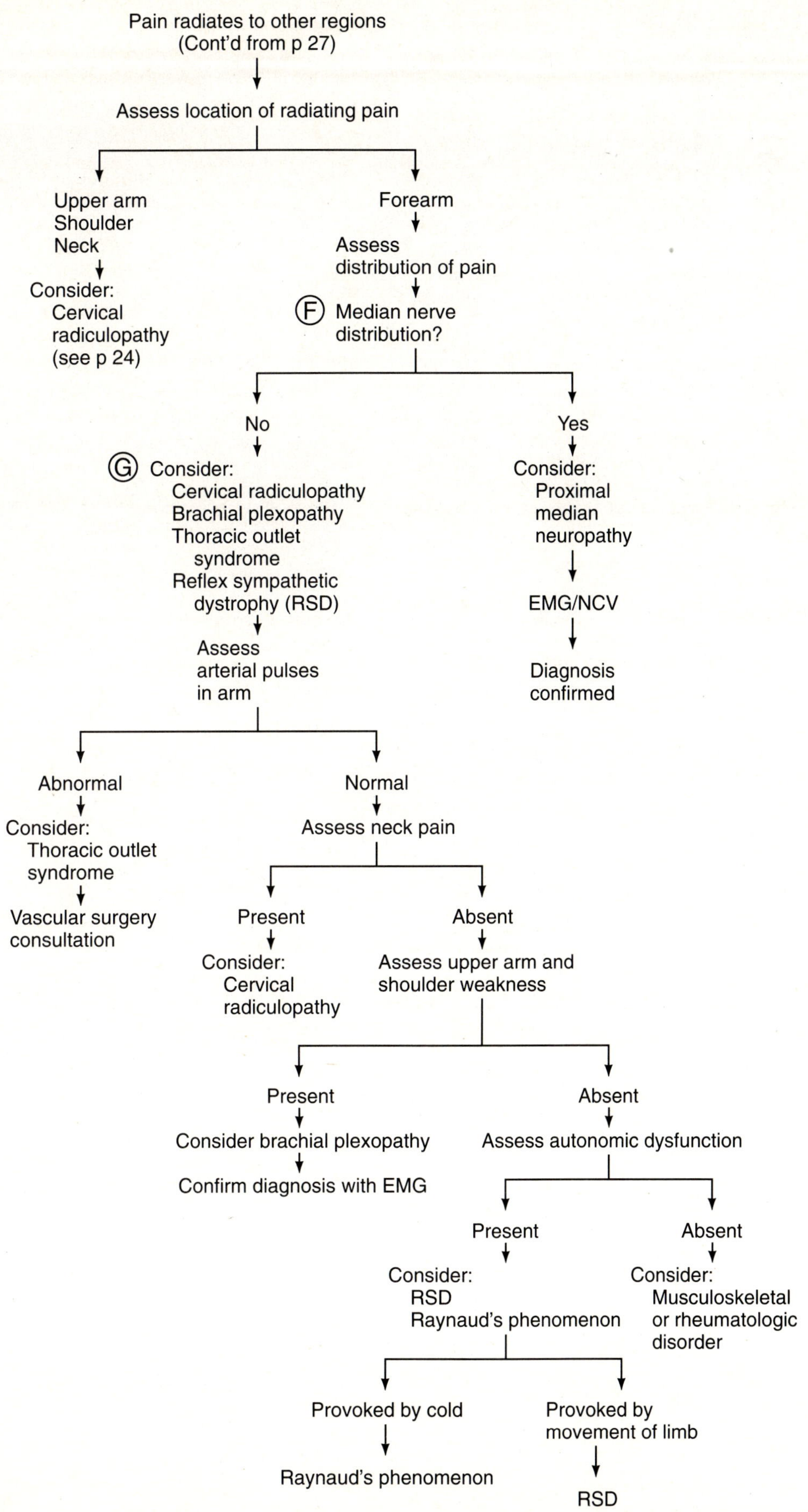

Pain radiates to other regions
(Cont'd from p 27)

Assess location of radiating pain

Upper arm
Shoulder
Neck

Consider:
Cervical
radiculopathy
(see p 24)

Forearm

Assess
distribution of pain

F Median nerve
distribution?

No

G Consider:
Cervical radiculopathy
Brachial plexopathy
Thoracic outlet
syndrome
Reflex sympathetic
dystrophy (RSD)

Assess
arterial pulses
in arm

Yes

Consider:
Proximal
median
neuropathy

EMG/NCV

Diagnosis
confirmed

Abnormal

Consider:
Thoracic outlet
syndrome

Vascular surgery
consultation

Normal

Assess neck pain

Present

Consider:
Cervical
radiculopathy

Absent

Assess upper arm and
shoulder weakness

Present

Consider brachial plexopathy

Confirm diagnosis with EMG

Absent

Assess autonomic dysfunction

Present

Consider:
RSD
Raynaud's phenomenon

Absent

Consider:
Musculoskeletal
or rheumatologic
disorder

Provoked by cold

Raynaud's phenomenon

Provoked by
movement of limb

RSD

LOW BACK PAIN

Richard L. Strub, M.D.

Low back pain is a very common, usually benign (though no less important) complaint. Trauma is an important cause of acute pain but is also frequently the basic cause of chronic intermittent back pain. Spontaneously appearing back pain has a more ominous import; this suggests that the disease is not musculotendinous as in trauma, but rather involves vertebrae, neural structures, and intrapelvic or intra-abdominal structures. The general diagnostic approach to all low back problems, be they post-traumatic or spontaneous, acute or chronic, is similar. The major emphasis of the evaluation is a search for neurologic dysfunction. If a significant neurologic deficit is found, prompt neurosurgical or orthopedic consultation is indicated, and surgical decompression of the spine is often required. In patients with nontraumatic back pain, a full evaluation is required.

A. The important factors to investigate in lumbar pain are leg weakness, a positive straight leg test, shooting or steady pain in the legs, bowel and bladder dysfunction, and areas of numbness or paresthesia (these are characteristic of nerve root impingement). Slowly progressive pain unrelieved by a change in position suggests a significant destructive or infectious process. On the other hand, pain exacerbated by activity and relieved by rest is usually mechanical back pain. In general, back pain without radiating leg pain indicates musculotendinous or arthritic disease, not disc rupture.

B. The most significant neurologic signs are weakness and bowel or bladder dysfunction. Reflex hypofunction and sensory loss, although indicative of nerve root compression, do not require emergency intervention.

C. At this point, patients who have sustained trauma are treated differently from those with spontaneous back pain. In the case of trauma, it can be fairly safely assumed that the back pain was the result of the trauma, and treatment can proceed without further diagnostic evaluation.

D. Conservative management includes bed rest, heat, attention to lifting, the avoidance of sitting, analgesics, muscle relaxants, possibly anti-inflammatory medications if there is considerable root pain, and sedation.

E. The patient with spontaneous back pain must be investigated for intra-abdominal conditions, primary bone disease (e.g., osteomyelitis, tumor, multiple myeloma), or less common conditions, such as spinal arteriovenous malformation. MRI scan, bone scan, serum electrophoresis, abdominal and pelvic examinations (or rectal examinations in males), and possibly spinal puncture are carried out if the foregoing are nondiagnostic.

References

Cailliet R. Low back pain syndrome. Philadelphia: FA Davis, 1981.

Macnab I, McCulloch JA. Backache. 2nd ed. Baltimore: Williams & Wilkins, 1989.

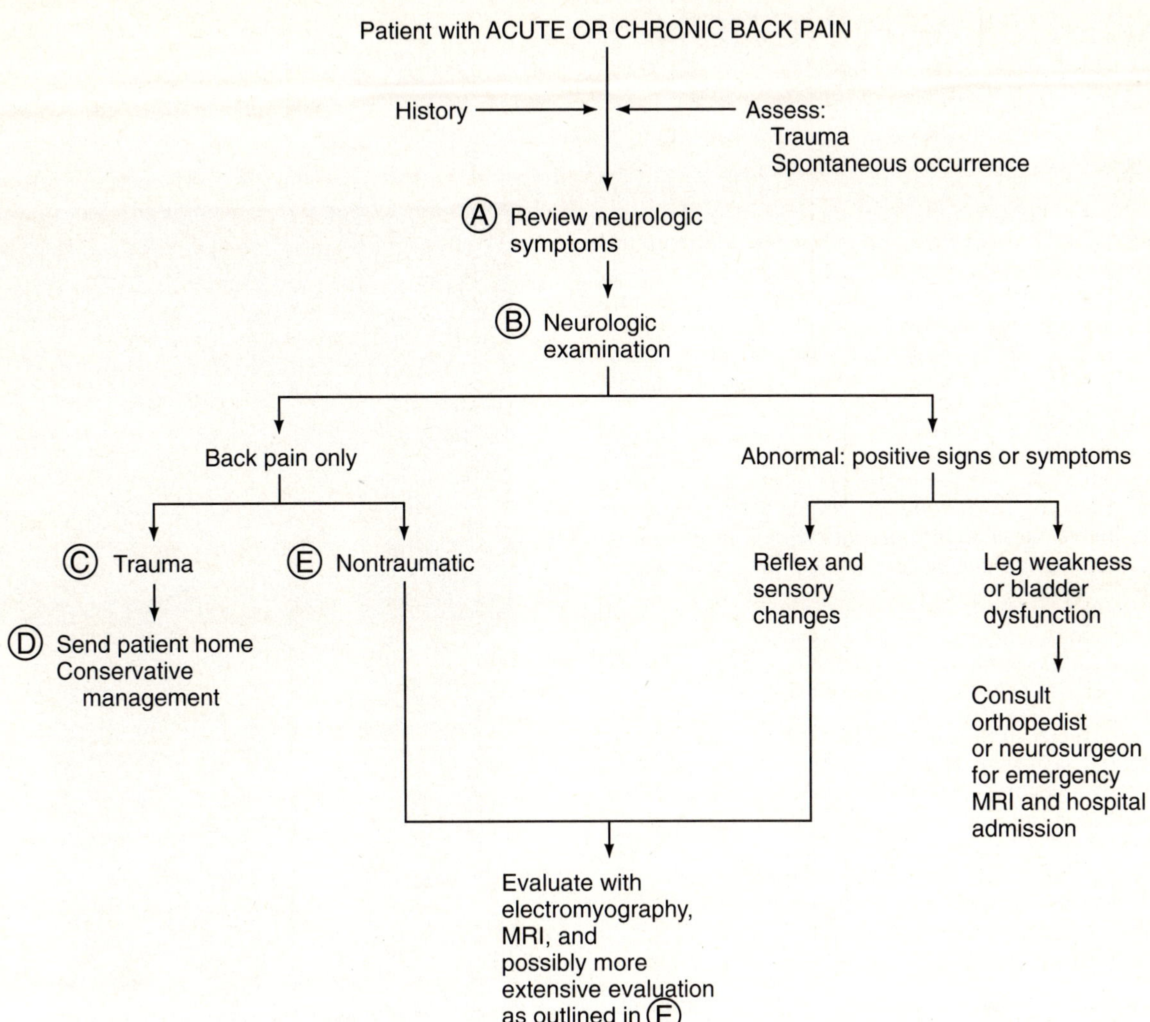

Patient with ACUTE OR CHRONIC BACK PAIN
History
Assess:
Trauma
Spontaneous occurrence
A Review neurologic symptoms
B Neurologic examination
Back pain only
Abnormal: positive signs or symptoms
C Trauma
E Nontraumatic
Reflex and sensory changes
Leg weakness or bladder dysfunction
D Send patient home Conservative management
Consult orthopedist or neurosurgeon for emergency MRI and hospital admission
Evaluate with electromyography, MRI, and possibly more extensive evaluation as outlined in E

BLADDER DYSFUNCTION

Richard L. Strub, M.D.

A. When a patient complains of incontinence, difficulty in passing urine, or frequent and urgent urination, the cause may be either urologic or neurologic. If it is neurologic, the disease can be in the CNS (brain or spinal cord), producing a small volume, spastic bladder, or in the nerve roots of the lower sacral segments (S3, S4, S5), producing a flaccid, large-capacity bladder.

B. Incontinence, mental symptoms, and ataxia are the three characteristic symptoms of communicating (normal-pressure) hydrocephalus, but frontal tumors or multiple strokes can also produce this clinical picture. Bladder incontinence is far more common than bowel incontinence.

C. At this point a neurologic lesion is strongly suspected, and a full neurologic examination is performed to establish the location or level of the lesion.

D. When rectal and bladder tone is decreased and perianal sensation is also diminished (S3, S4, S5), there is a lesion either in the conus medullaris of the spinal cord or in the cauda equina (intradural or extradural). If there is considerable pelvic pain, consider pelvic cancer; if the process is painless, the differential diagnosis includes ependymomas and lipomas (intradural), L1–L2 disc disorder, or inflammation (viral or syphilitic).

E. Bowel or bladder dysfunction with spasticity in the legs suggests spinal cord disease. Look carefully for the level of involvement (sensory level, arm reflexes). Possible diagnoses include cord tumor, multiple sclerosis, low cervical disc disease, inflammatory or vascular disease of the cord, and other rarer possibilities.

F. If findings on urologic evaluation are normal or cystometrography indicates a neurogenic bladder, further neurodiagnostic tests such as CT or MRI of the lumbar area, a myelography (Fig. 1), and spinal fluid analysis are indicated.

G. With bilateral upper motor neuron signs and specific brain stem signs (e.g., diplopia, vertigo, facial numbness, Horner's syndrome), consider tumor (if slowly progressive), stroke, or multiple sclerosis (if abrupt in onset).

H. Absence of brain stem signs indicates bilateral cerebral disease: multiple strokes, large frontal tumors, bilateral tumors (metastatic), hydrocephalus, chronic

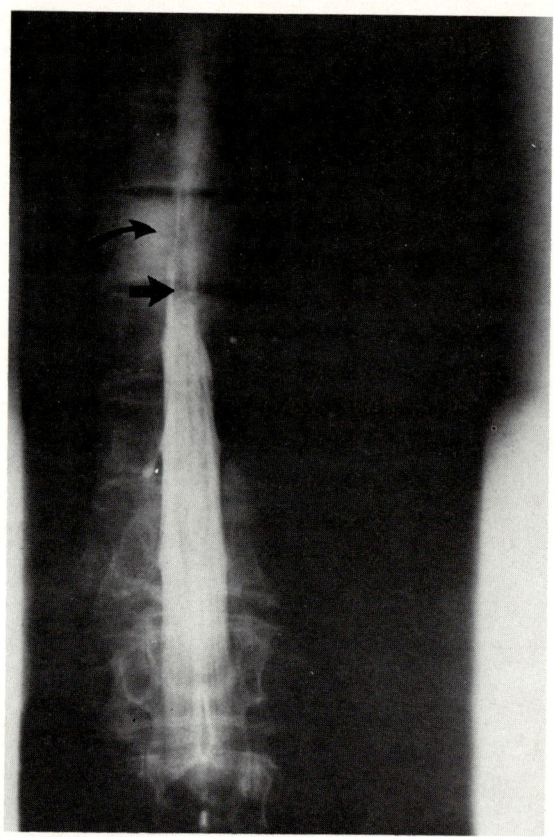

Figure 1 Myelogram shows complete blockade of dye column in the thoracic region *(black arrow).* This was due to a metastatic neoplasm that shows bone erosion *(curved arrow).*

infection (e.g., syphilis, toxoplasmosis, cryptococcosis, progressive multifocal leukoencephalopathy), a rare leukodystrophy, or degenerative disease.

I. Bilateral motor findings, including control of swallowing and speech, are frequently seen in patients with a multi-infarct state secondary to hypertension, diabetes, and other small vessel disease. This condition, called pseudobulbar palsy, is a common cause of bladder control problems.

Reference

Sotolongo JR Jr. Urogenital problems in neurology. Semin Neurol 1988; 8(2)..

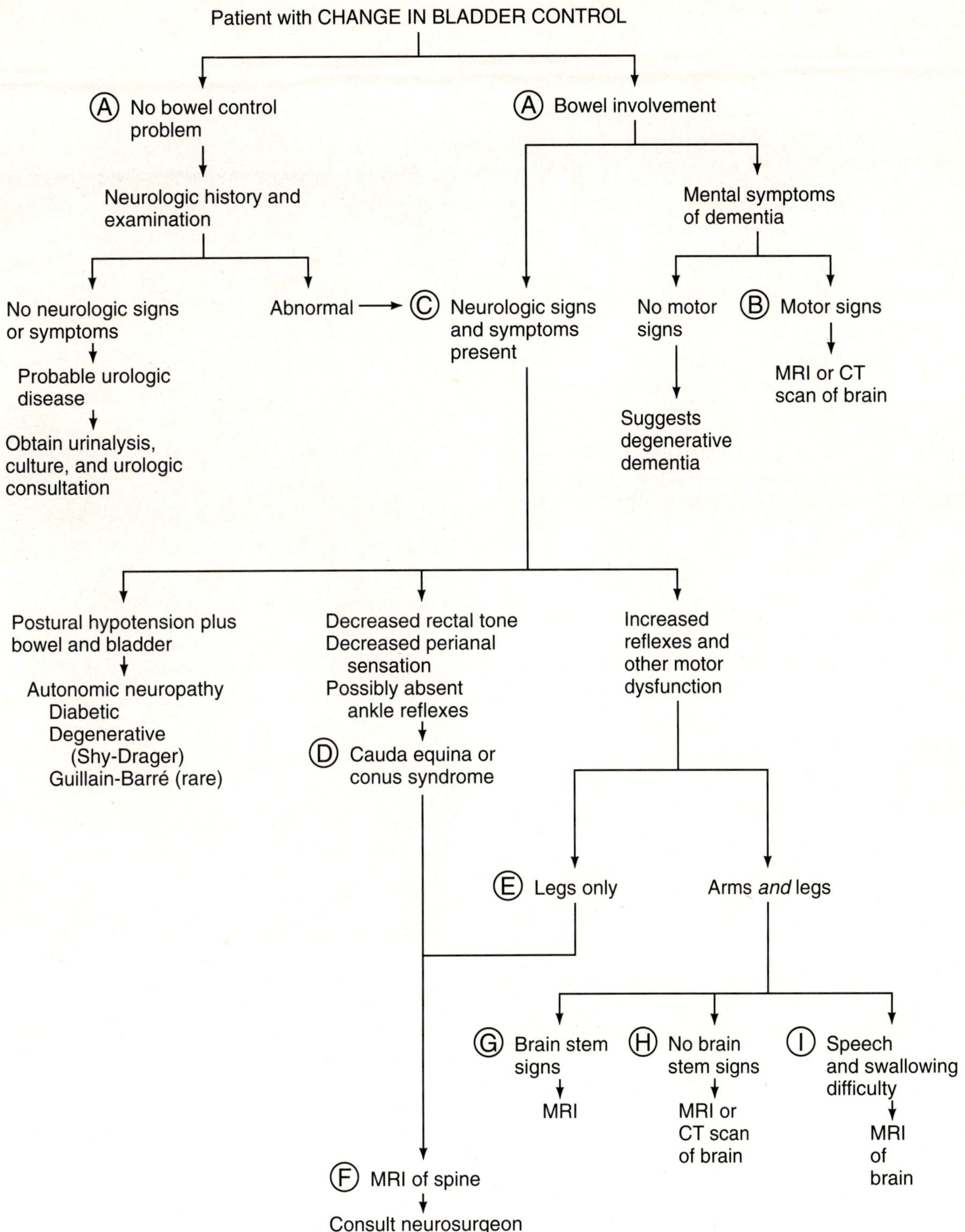

Patient with CHANGE IN BLADDER CONTROL

A No bowel control problem

A Bowel involvement

Neurologic history and examination

Mental symptoms of dementia

No neurologic signs or symptoms

Abnormal

C Neurologic signs and symptoms present

No motor signs

B Motor signs

Probable urologic disease

Suggests degenerative dementia

MRI or CT scan of brain

Obtain urinalysis, culture, and urologic consultation

Postural hypotension plus bowel and bladder

Decreased rectal tone
Decreased perianal sensation
Possibly absent ankle reflexes

Increased reflexes and other motor dysfunction

Autonomic neuropathy
Diabetic
Degenerative
(Shy-Drager)
Guillain-Barré (rare)

D Cauda equina or conus syndrome

E Legs only

Arms and legs

G Brain stem signs

H No brain stem signs

I Speech and swallowing difficulty

MRI

MRI or CT scan of brain

MRI of brain

F MRI of spine

Consult neurosurgeon

COMA

Richard L. Strub, M.D.

Evaluation of the comatose patient requires a direct and expeditious approach. The first step is to establish basic life support; the second is to determine the cause.

A. Neurologic examination of the comatose patient is important and does not take long. The principal aspects of the examination are (1) a description of the level of consciousness (e.g., a painful stimulus causes purposeful movement, groaning, and eye opening)—always describe movement, vocalization, and ocular response; (2) the respiration pattern; (3) the pupillary response; and (4) the response of eye movement to head turning (doll's eye maneuver)—with an intact brain stem the eyes move, and with a damaged brain stem the eyes stay in the plane of the head and do not move relative to the head. The main goal is to separate the medical (toxic or metabolic) cases (two-thirds) from the neurologic cases. In metabolic cases the pupils are reactive, brain stem reflexes are present (e.g., doll's eyes, caloric responses, and corneal reflexes), and muscle stretch reflexes are symmetric. Note that patients in metabolic coma may have a positive Babinski sign bilaterally and even exhibit decerebrate posturing.

B. "Normal" means that brain stem reflexes are intact and there is no asymmetry in motor and sensory reflexes.

C. In supratentorial lesions, there is usually asymmetry of reflexes and a unilateral dilated pupil, but a normal doll's eye response (unless there is massive herniation). In infratentorial lesions, bilateral motor signs and brain stem signs are commonly seen (Fig. 1).

D. Patients with abnormal neurologic findings and normal scans often have sustained a cerebral infarction. If the history is not clear, a medical evaluation is indicated.

E. If the CT scan clearly shows subarachnoid hemorrhage, a lumbar puncture is not necessary.

F. In trauma patients, do not manipulate the neck. Assess brain stem reflexes using the cold caloric test, not the doll's head maneuver.

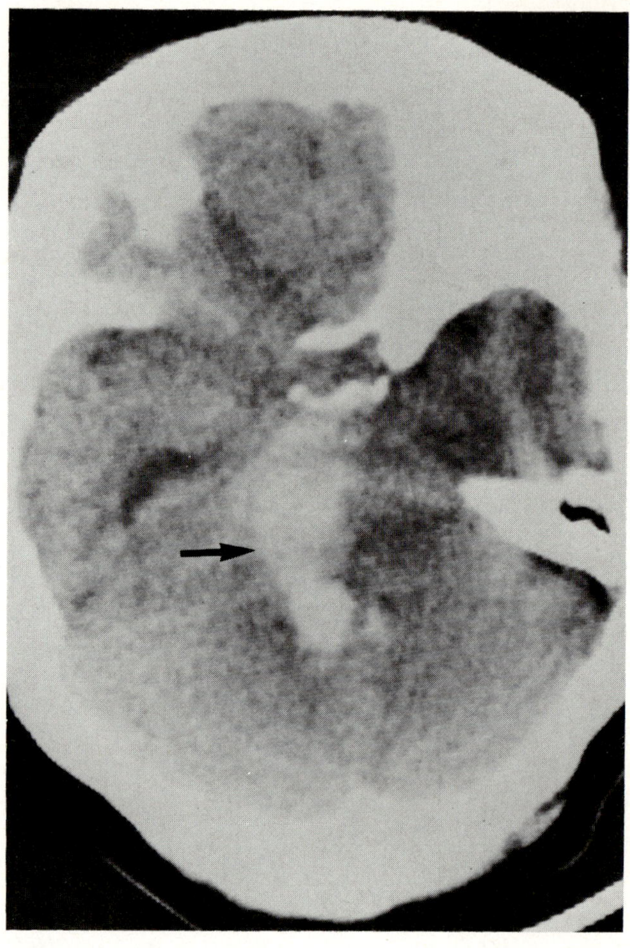

Figure 1 CT scan shows a large pontine hemorrhage *(arrow).*

Reference

Plum F, Posner G. The diagnosis of stupor and coma. 3rd ed. Philadelphia: FA Davis, 1980.

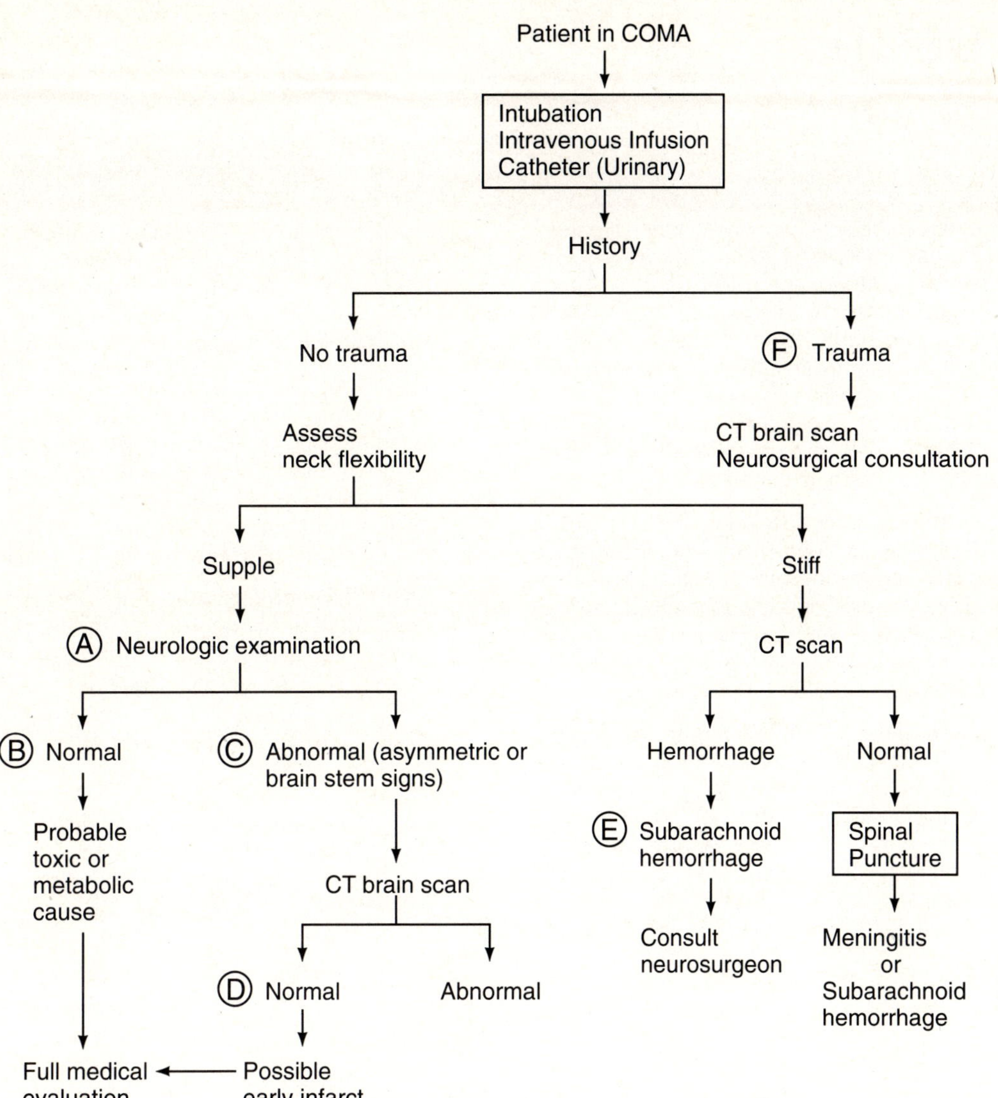

Patient in COMA
Intubation
Intravenous Infusion
Catheter (Urinary)
History
No trauma
F Trauma
Assess
neck flexibility
CT brain scan
Neurosurgical consultation
Supple
Stiff
A Neurologic examination
CT scan
B Normal
C Abnormal (asymmetric or
brain stem signs)
Hemorrhage
Normal
Probable
toxic or
metabolic
cause
CT brain scan
E Subarachnoid
hemorrhage
Spinal
Puncture
D Normal
Abnormal
Consult
neurosurgeon
Meningitis
or
Subarachnoid
hemorrhage
Full medical
evaluation
Possible
early infarct

BRAIN DEATH

Richard L. Strub, M.D.

In most states, death can be legally declared when a patient is brain dead yet has continuing cardiac function. This determination has been important in the field of organ transplantation, particularly heart transplantation. Even though the diagnosis of brain death is usually made by either a neurologist or a neurosurgeon, it is important that all physicians understand the accepted criteria for the establishment of brain death. Electroencephalography is no longer considered critical to the diagnosis; if it is used, there should not be any brain activity $>2\mu v$.

A. The cause of the coma is important. Patients with a toxic overdose, anoxic coma, or metabolic disease can recover after appearing brain dead on examination. Currently, there is not enough information to decide when such a coma is irreversible. Patients with demonstrable structural brain lesions are the only ones in whom brain death should be considered.

B. On examination, if the patient exhibits any purposeful movement, opens the eyes, makes spontaneous eye movement with the eyes held open, or emits any vocal response, there is viable brain function. The presence of reflexes in the limbs does not necessarily indicate a viable brain; reflex responses may reflect a spinal cord response alone.

C. Brain stem reflexes include pupillary response (the pupils must be dilated and fixed), eye movements either with head turning (oculocephalic or doll's eye reflex), or cold caloric test (50 ml of ice water in each ear), corneal, and gag reflexes must be absent.

D. Hyperventilate the patient for 10 minutes with 100% oxygen and then take him or her off the respirator for 10 minutes. The P_{O_2} level will remain high; the P_{CO_2} level will rise (>50 mm) and trigger respiration if the brain stem respiratory centers are still viable. To prevent hypoxia during the test, 100% O_2 at 15 L/min should be delivered by tracheal catheter.

E. After determining that the criteria for brain death have been fulfilled, the neurologist should consult with the attending physician and family. If all agree, life support systems can be removed.

References

Marks SJ, Zisfein J. Apneic oxygenation in apnea tests for brain death. Arch Neurol 1990; 47:1066.

Plum F, Posner G. The diagnosis of stupor and coma. 3rd ed. Philadelphia: FA Davis, 1980.

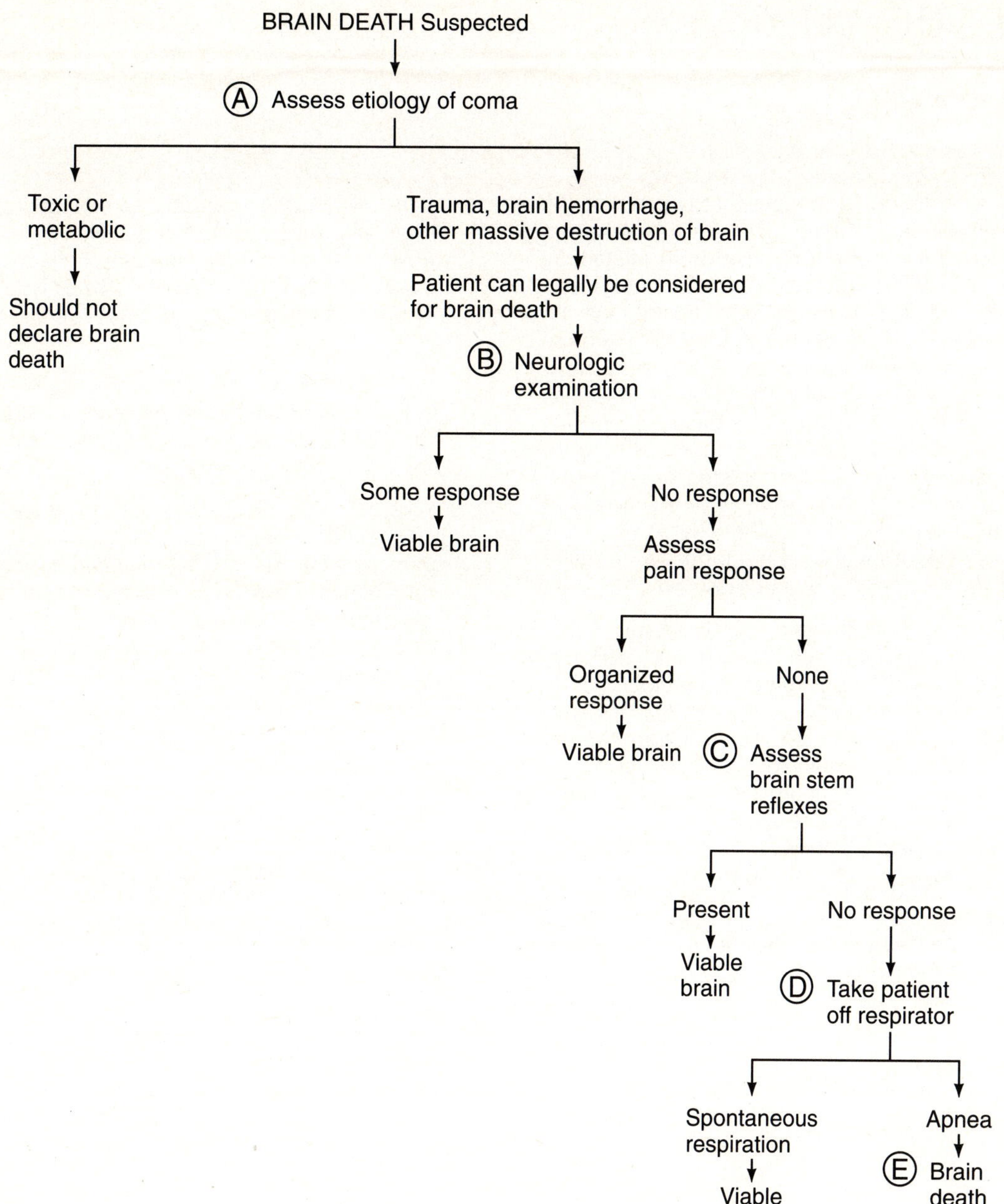

BRAIN DEATH Suspected
A Assess etiology of coma
Toxic or metabolic
Trauma, brain hemorrhage, other massive destruction of brain
Should not declare brain death
Patient can legally be considered for brain death
B Neurologic examination
Some response
No response
Viable brain
Assess pain response
Organized response
None
Viable brain
C Assess brain stem reflexes
Present
No response
Viable brain
D Take patient off respirator
Spontaneous respiration
Apnea
Viable brain
E Brain death

SYMMETRIC WEAKNESS

Carlos A. Garcia, M.D.

Weakness is a diminution of strength that is noted at the onset of movement and should be differentiated from fatigability or weariness during exercise. Both fatigability and weakness should be differentiated from numbness, stiffness, lack of balance, and incoordination. Once the presence of true weakness is established, try to determine the site of the lesion: corticospinal tract, anterior horn cells, peripheral nerves, neuromuscular junction, or muscles. Observations that help include (1) the mode of onset—whether weakness came on suddenly or in an insidious or slowly progressive manner; (2) the location of the weakness, distal or proximal; (3) the symmetry or asymmetry of the muscles involved; and (4) whether the weakness is segmental or whether it involves one muscle, an isolated group of muscles, or a large group of muscles.

A. When weakness is symmetric, starts distally in the extremities, is associated with flaccidity and areflexia, is of acute onset, and progresses rapidly in an ascending manner, check for sensory deficit. If sensation is normal, perform a rectal examination. Normal sphincter tone usually indicates an acute ascending polyneuropathy (see p 206). However, an acute polyneuropathy may also present with weakness that starts proximally and descends.

B. Weakness that is distal, has a slow insidious onset, remains localized to the legs or arms, and may or may not be associated with sensory deficit in a stocking and glove distribution represents a polyneuropathy, and diagnostic studies are necessary to determine the cause. Diabetes mellitus and alcoholism are the most frequent causes. The diagnosis of polyneuropathy is confirmed by a prolonged nerve conduction velocity study.

C. When weakness is of slow onset, is symmetric and proximal, and affects the hip and shoulder muscles, and when there is no sensory deficit, suspect a limb girdle syndrome (see p 42).

D. When weakness is symmetric and acute and affects proximal and distal muscles, with involvement of sphincters, check for rectal tone and urinary retention. Finding the sensory level to pricking pain localizes the level of the lesion in the spinal cord. Check for spine deformities or tenderness. Involvement of only the legs indicates paraplegia; involvement of both arms and legs indicates quadriplegia. MRI of the spine or myelography is required.

References

Brooke MH. A clinician's view of neuromuscular diseases. 2nd ed. Baltimore: Williams & Wilkins, 1986.

Haerer AF. DeJong's the neurologic examination. 5th ed. Philadelphia: JB Lippincott, 1992.

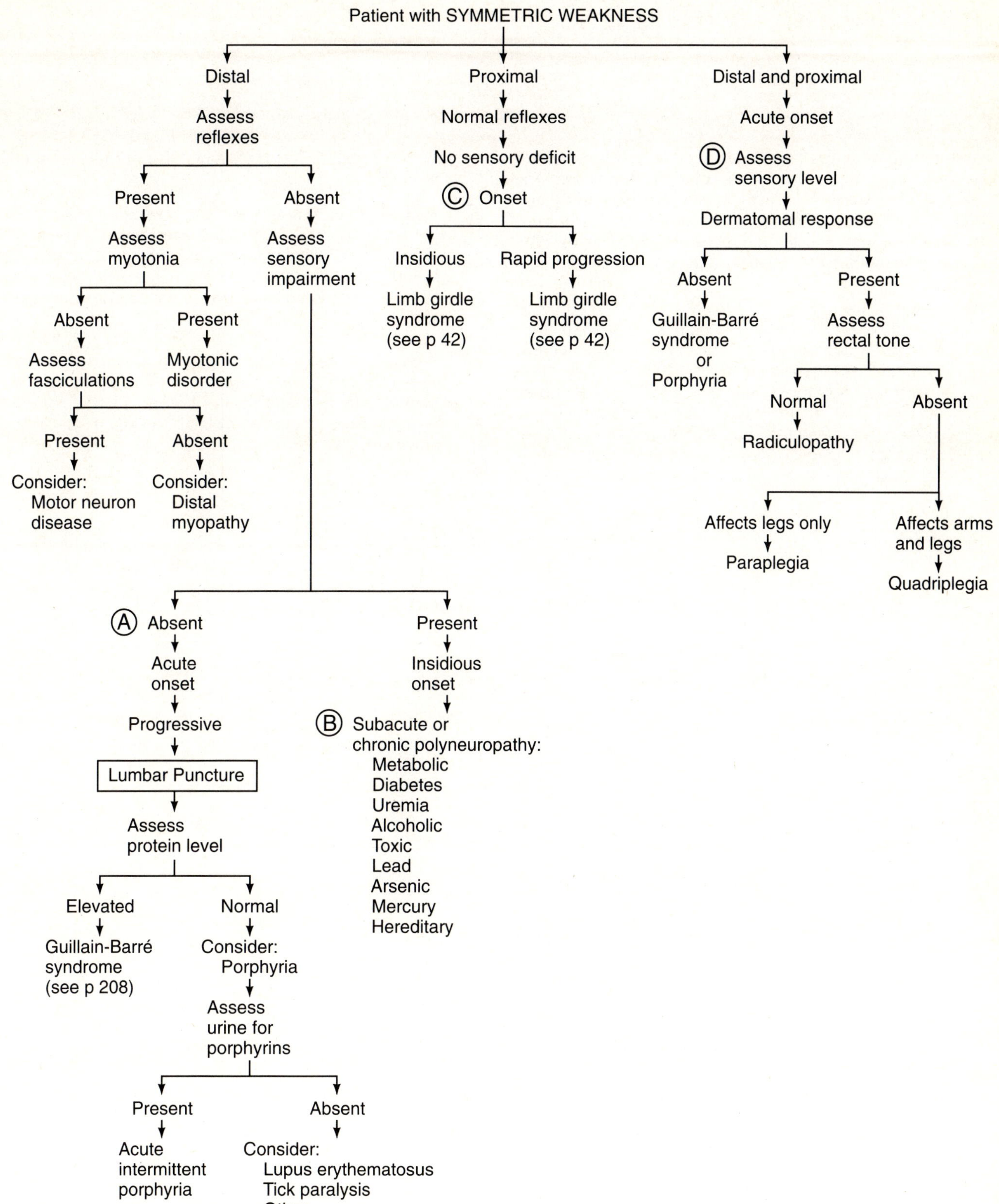

Patient with SYMMETRIC WEAKNESS

Distal
Assess reflexes

Present
Assess myotonia

Absent
Assess fasciculations

Present
Consider:
Motor neuron disease

Absent
Consider:
Distal myopathy

Present
Myotonic disorder

Absent
Assess sensory impairment

A Absent
Acute onset
Progressive
Lumbar Puncture
Assess protein level

Elevated
Guillain-Barré syndrome (see p 208)

Normal
Consider: Porphyria
Assess urine for porphyrins

Present
Acute intermittent porphyria

Absent
Consider:
Lupus erythematosus
Tick paralysis
Other

Present
Insidious onset
B Subacute or chronic polyneuropathy:
Metabolic
Diabetes
Uremia
Alcoholic
Toxic
Lead
Arsenic
Mercury
Hereditary

Proximal
Normal reflexes
No sensory deficit
C Onset

Insidious
Limb girdle syndrome (see p 42)

Rapid progression
Limb girdle syndrome (see p 42)

Distal and proximal
Acute onset
D Assess sensory level
Dermatomal response

Absent
Guillain-Barré syndrome or Porphyria

Present
Assess rectal tone

Normal
Radiculopathy

Affects legs only
Paraplegia

Absent
Affects arms and legs
Quadriplegia

ASYMMETRIC WEAKNESS

Carlos A. Garcia, M.D.

Asymmetric weakness may be acute or subacute in onset or may begin slowly and insidiously. Acute asymmetric weakness is frequently associated with flaccidity and areflexia regardless of the site of the lesion. In CNS lesions, the tone becomes spastic and the stretch reflexes become hyperactive within 3 to 6 weeks after the onset.

A. When acute asymmetric weakness is seen in one extremity, check for the strength of individual muscles. If a group of muscles innervated by one nerve is affected, a mononeuropathy is likely. External compression of the nerve during sleep or anesthesia may be the cause of the weakness. Vascular lesions of some nerves (femoral, third cranial nerve) may occur in diabetic patients. If the weak muscles are innervated by several adjacent nerves, look for root or plexus injuries.

B. When acute weakness affects the entire extremity, suspect a root lesion or CNS involvement. When one of the upper extremities is affected, consider a stretch brachial plexus injury or other plexopathy.

CNS vascular lesions may also produce acute monoplegia.

C. When both extremities and the lower part of the face are affected on the same side, consider a contralateral CNS lesion. Dysphasias are seen in hemispheric lesions affecting the dominant hemisphere. Remember that the tone and reflexes change with time (see above).

D. Weakness of slow onset and insidious progression usually affects large groups of muscles and produces hemiplegia or monoplegia. If long tract signs are present, a degenerative or mass lesion is the likely diagnosis.

References

Brooke MH. A clinician's view of neuromuscular diseases. 2nd ed. Baltimore: Williams & Wilkins, 1986.
Haerer AF. DeJong's the neurological examination. 5th ed. Philadelphia: JB Lippincott, 1992.

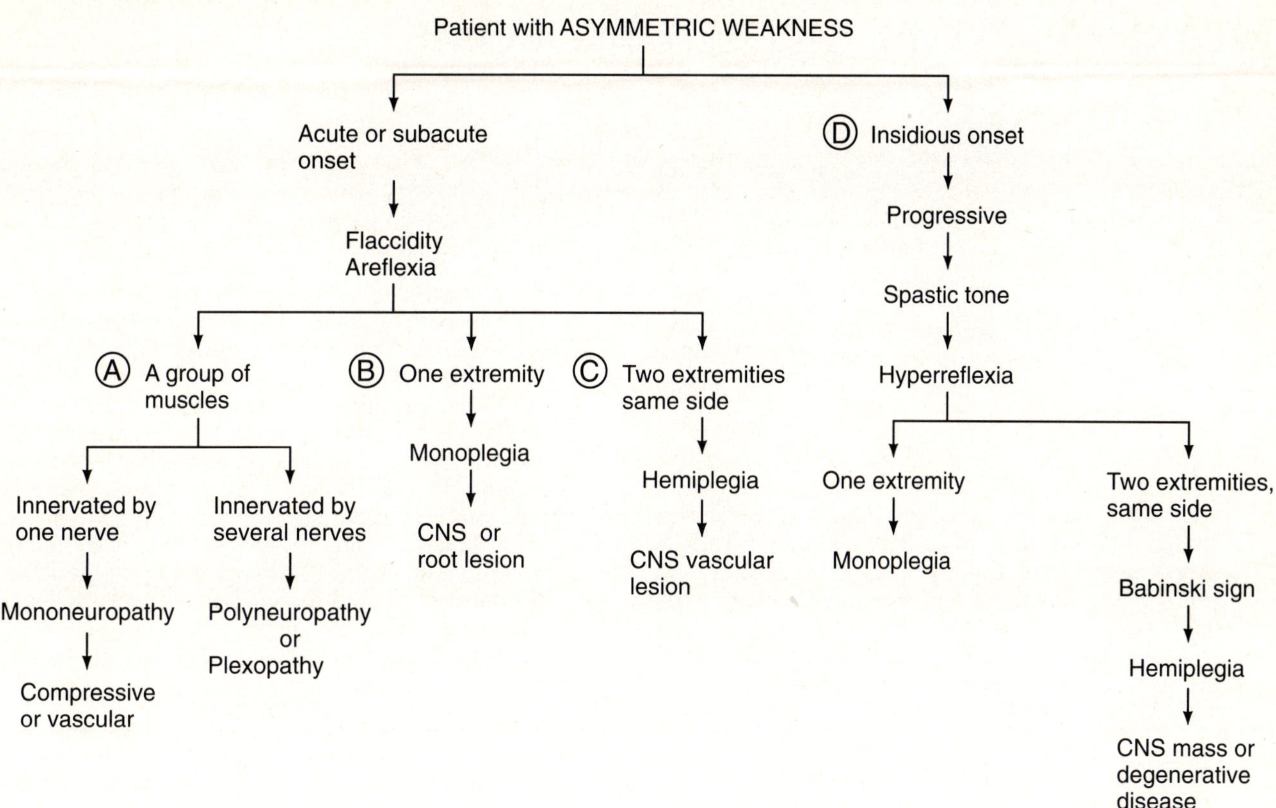

Patient with ASYMMETRIC WEAKNESS
Acute or subacute onset
D Insidious onset
Flaccidity Areflexia
Progressive
Spastic tone
Hyperreflexia
A A group of muscles
B One extremity
C Two extremities same side
Monoplegia
Hemiplegia
CNS or root lesion
CNS vascular lesion
Innervated by one nerve
Innervated by several nerves
Mononeuropathy
Polyneuropathy or Plexopathy
Compressive or vascular
One extremity
Two extremities, same side
Monoplegia
Babinski sign
Hemiplegia
CNS mass or degenerative disease

WEAKNESS: LIMB GIRDLE SYNDROME

Carlos A. Garcia, M.D.

Proximal weakness of the shoulders and hip muscles usually presents in a slow and insidious way and may have different causes according to the age at onset, family history, and associated neurologic features. A complete evaluation, including a complete history and neurologic examination, muscle enzyme determinations, electrophysiologic tests, and a muscle biopsy, is usually required to diagnose these conditions.

A. Metabolic muscle diseases are rare. The glycogen type II disorder (Pompe's disease) is one of the most common metabolic myopathies and may present in infancy, childhood, or adulthood. Children and adults may present with proximal muscle weakness, and adults often with respiratory impairment. Electromyography (EMG) shows a pseudomyotonic response, and muscle biopsy shows a vacuolar myopathy. Biochemistry is necessary to identify the enzyme defect (acid maltase deficiency).

B. Spinal muscular atrophy varies in onset but may present in infancy (Werdnig-Hoffmann), childhood, adolescence, or adulthood (Kugelberg-Welander disease). The reflexes are usually absent. There may be fasciculations of the tongue in infants and children. Electrophysiologic studies show chronic denervation, and fascicular atrophy in the muscle biopsy specimen is diagnostic of denervation.

C. A group of congenital myopathies (e.g., central core, centronuclear, and nemaline myopathy) are slowly progressive, usually benign, and frequently familial. The work-up is usually negative except for muscle biopsy findings that are diagnostic of the disease.

D. Myasthenia gravis (MG) may present as proximal muscle weakness. The Tensilon test, electrophysiologic studies, and acetylcholine receptor (AChR) antibodies are diagnostic of this disease (see p 240).

E. Proximal muscle weakness with an onset in adolescence or early adulthood, and a slow but relentless progression, is seen in limb girdle muscular dystrophy. The neck muscles are affected very late in the disease. There is no swallowing difficulty, and the reflexes remain normal until the muscles become atrophic. The creatine kinase (CK) level is elevated early in the disease, and the electromyogram shows myopathic features. The muscle biopsy specimens show dystrophic changes. Testing for the presence of dystrophin by immunofluorescent staining of the muscle biopsy will differentiate dystrophinopathies such as Duchenne, Becker, and manifesting carrier of Duchenne or Becker dystrophy from other dystrophies (see p 228).

F. An adult onset of limb girdle weakness with early neck muscle weakness and dysphagia is highly suggestive of polymyositis. Tenderness of the muscles may be seen in acute cases. The reflexes are normal. The CK is usually elevated. EMG shows irritability of the muscles upon needle insertion and myopathic features. The muscle biopsy shows inflammatory changes in most cases but may be normal or show minimal changes (see p 230).

References

Brooke MH. A clinician's view of neuromuscular diseases. 2nd ed. Baltimore: Williams & Wilkins, 1986.

Haerer AF. DeJong's the neurological examination. 5th ed. Philadelphia: JB Lippincott, 1992.

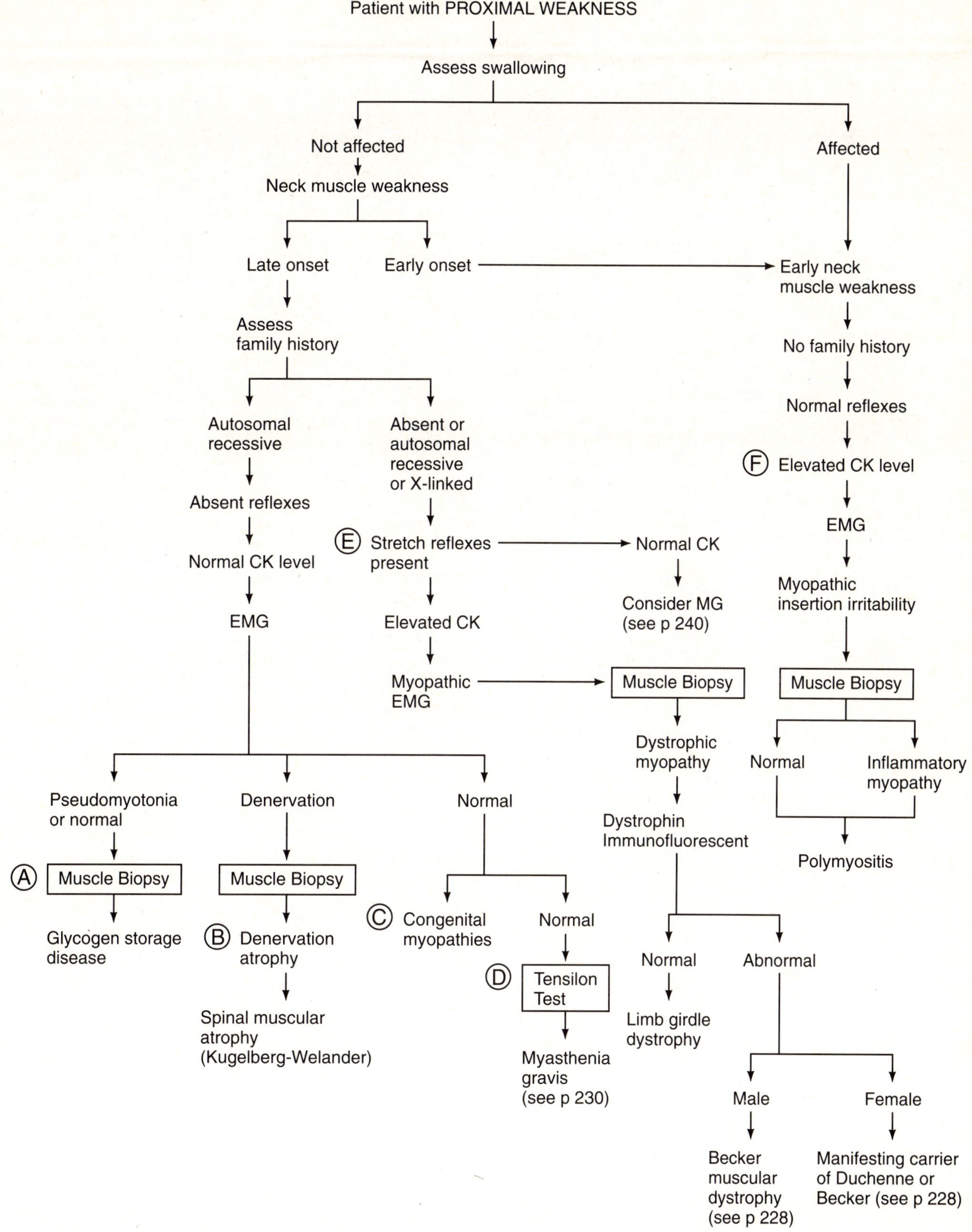

Patient with PROXIMAL WEAKNESS
Assess swallowing
Not affected
Affected
Neck muscle weakness
Late onset
Early onset
Early neck muscle weakness
Assess family history
No family history
Normal reflexes
Autosomal recessive
Absent or autosomal recessive or X-linked
F Elevated CK level
Absent reflexes
EMG
Normal CK level
E Stretch reflexes present
Normal CK
Myopathic insertion irritability
EMG
Consider MG (see p 240)
Elevated CK
Muscle Biopsy
Muscle Biopsy
Myopathic EMG
Dystrophic myopathy
Normal
Inflammatory myopathy
Pseudomyotonia or normal
Denervation
Normal
Dystrophin Immunofluorescent
Polymyositis
A Muscle Biopsy
Muscle Biopsy
Glycogen storage disease
B Denervation atrophy
C Congenital myopathies
Normal
Normal
Abnormal
Spinal muscular atrophy (Kugelberg-Welander)
D Tensilon Test
Limb girdle dystrophy
Myasthenia gravis (see p 230)
Male
Female
Becker muscular dystrophy (see p 228)
Manifesting carrier of Duchenne or Becker (see p 228)

FATIGABILITY

Carlos A. Garcia, M.D.

Fatigability or weariness during exercise with dramatic improvement of strength after rest should be differentiated from weakness, numbness, stiffness, lack of balance, and incoordination.

A. When the weakness is more subjective, being worse in the morning or after sleep, or when the patient feels exhausted while lying down but is able to get out of bed and carry on all the daily activities, a conversion reaction or depression is likely. Chronic fatigue syndrome is a poorly understood condition manifested by debilitating fatigue. The fatigue is frequently preceded by a flulike illness. Viral and immunologic studies suggest association with Epstein-Barr virus, enterovirus, retrovirus, and human herpesvirus 6. Some patients respond to tricyclic antidepressants.

B. Fatigability is a normal physiologic response to excessive exercise and may be seen in trained athletes. Rest usually restores strength, and the neurologic examination is normal.

C. When fatigability is seen after mild or minor exercise, is incapacitating, or is easily reproduced and worsens as the day progresses, the patient has a myasthenic disorder (see p 238). The muscles frequently affected are those most commonly used, such as the ocular (ptosis, diplopia) and bulbar (dysphonia, dysphagia) muscles, but the disorder may affect the trunk and extremity muscles. Patients report inability to complete tasks that previously they were able to perform (climbing two flights of stairs, walking several blocks, folding laundry, combing the hair, carrying and lifting grocery bags). If objective weakness is not seen at the time of the examination, try to reproduce fatigability by asking the patient to look up; drooping of the eyelids is seen in myasthenic patients. Ask the patient to sit or squat and get up; myasthenic patients show fatigue. Ask the patient to count to 100; with myasthenic patients the voice becomes nasal. Myasthenia gravis has to be differentiated from neurasthenia and myasthenic syndromes.

References

Brooke MH. A clinician's view of neuromuscular diseases. 2nd ed. Baltimore: Williams & Wilkins, 1986.

Buchwald D, Cheney PR, Peterson DH, et al. A chronic illness characterized by fatigue, neurologic and immunologic disorders and active human herpes virus type 6 infection. Ann Intern Med 1992; 116:103.

Shafran SD. The chronic fatigue syndrome. Am J Med 1991; 90:730.

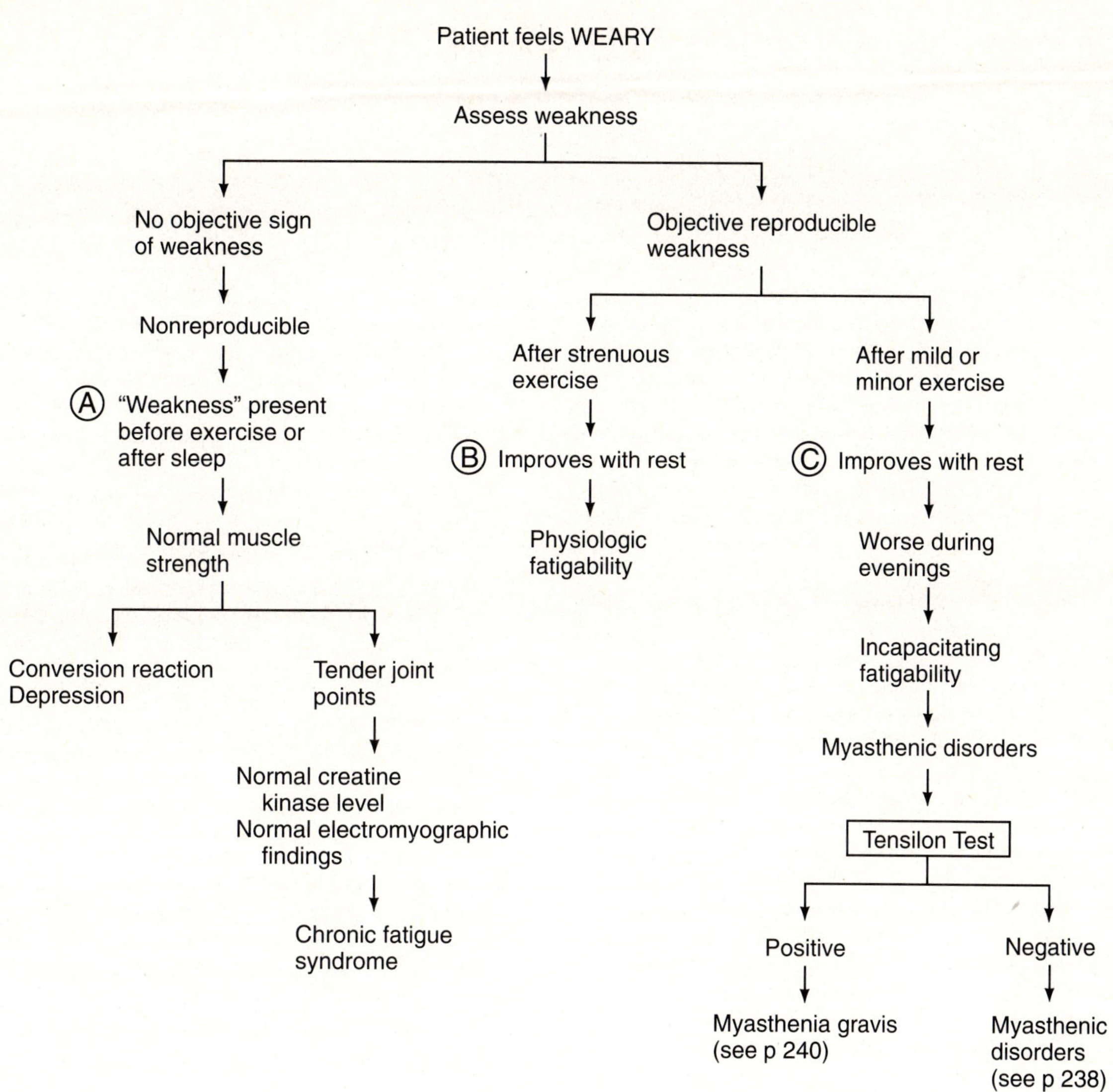

Patient feels WEARY
Assess weakness
No objective sign of weakness
Objective reproducible weakness
Nonreproducible
After strenuous exercise
After mild or minor exercise
A "Weakness" present before exercise or after sleep
B Improves with rest
C Improves with rest
Normal muscle strength
Physiologic fatigability
Worse during evenings
Conversion reaction Depression
Tender joint points
Incapacitating fatigability
Normal creatine kinase level
Normal electromyographic findings
Myasthenic disorders
Chronic fatigue syndrome
Tensilon Test
Positive
Negative
Myasthenia gravis (see p 240)
Myasthenic disorders (see p 238)

CLUMSINESS AND INCOORDINATION (ATAXIA)

Carlos A. Garcia, M.D.

Clumsiness is a lack of dexterity. Incoordination (ataxia) is loss of control in the synergistic performance of movements. Motor activity uses all levels of motor integration, as well as sensory input from the proprioceptive and vestibular systems. Weakness may produce clumsiness, but motor strength is preserved in most patients with disturbances of coordination. Most such disturbances are due to lesions in the cerebellum and its afferent and efferent connections. The following are the deficits most frequently found in ataxia:

Asynergy or dyssynergia. Lack or diminution of coordination between various groups of muscles, producing decomposition of movements. The abnormality is found by testing alternating movements of the hands or tapping on the floor with the feet.

Dysmetria. Loss of ability to measure (judge) the distance, speed, and power of a movement, producing an undershoot or overshoot. The abnormality is found by the finger-to-nose and heel-to-knee-to-toe tests.

Hypotonia. A decrease of muscle tone. The abnormality is found by passively moving the extremities.

Intention (kinetic) tremors. Rhythmic movements produced or intensified when a voluntary movement is attempted. They disappear with rest. They may be observed in the extremities as well as in the head (titubation). The abnormality is found by asking the patient to perform movements against gravity.

Scanning speech. Slow, slurred, jerky speech. The abnormality is found by asking patients to count, giving them a difficult word to pronounce (e.g., Massachusetts), or asking them to hold a note for several seconds.

Posture and gait. Patients are unable to stay in an erect position when asked to stand with both feet close together; the trunk sways in all directions, even with the eyes open. The disorder is produced by a midline cerebellar lesion. Patients sway to the side of a cerebellar hemispheric lesion. The ataxic gait is staggering and jerky, with a tendency to fall in any direction.

Pendular reflexes. On eliciting the patellar stretch reflex, the leg continues a to-and-fro movement.

Ocular dysmetria and nystagmus. The eyes lose their smooth pursuit movements, and movements become jerky and saccadic. Rapid involuntary eye movements (saccadic) cause the eyes to miss the targeted object; they either overshoot (go beyond) and have to come back, or undershoot (do not go far enough) and have to move further.

A. In examining the posture and gait, ask the patient to stand with feet close together ("like a soldier"). A normal person stays in an erect posture. When the patient sways in different directions with the eyes open, this is an indication of truncal ataxia of midline or diffuse cerebellar origin. When the patient stays erect but sways or falls when asked to close the eyes (Romberg sign), there is a lack of proprioception. Most likely the vibratory and position senses are absent, owing to posterior column disease, or all forms of sensation are lost in the legs in a stocking distribution, owing to severe sensory polyneuropathy. Sensory ataxia results from both lesions.

B. Sensory neuronopathies are a heterogeneous group of disorders that affect the cell bodies in the dorsal root or trigeminal ganglia. The clinical features are those of dysesthesias or hypesthesias along with severe appendicular and truncal ataxia dependent on visual cues. The onset of neuronopathies may be acute (2 or 3 days), subacute (weeks), or chronic. Neuronopathies may be produced by toxic substances, an excessive amount of vitamin B_6, cisplatin, or the remote effects of cancer or may be hereditary.

C. When truncal ataxia is associated with lack of proprioception, Argyll Robertson pupils (small irregular pupils that fail to react to light but constrict to accommodation), and lancinating leg pains, tabes dorsalis is the most likely diagnosis.

D. An acute pancerebellar syndrome may be due to a toxic reaction, such as phenytoin toxicity.

E. The subacute or chronic pancerebellar syndrome may be due to toxic substances, such as mercury poisoning, or may be a remote effect of cancer and some of the hereditary ataxias.

F. When a pancerebellar syndrome is associated with corticospinal tract disease and there is a family history, the likely disorder is hereditary olivopontocerebellar atrophy. When all these symptoms are seen in young patients and are associated with lack of proprioception, scoliosis, and pes cavus, Friedreich's ataxia is the likely diagnosis.

G. Asymmetric ataxia is usually a hemiataxia and may be associated with head deviation (tilting) toward the side of the lesion. All the symptoms described in ataxia may be found ipsilateral to the lesion.

References

Asbury AK. Sensory neuronopathy. Semin Neurol 1987; 7:58.

Brooke MH. A clinician's view of neuromuscular diseases. 2nd ed. Baltimore: Williams & Wilkins, 1986.

Haerer AF. DeJong's the neurological examination. 5th ed. Philadelphia: JB Lippincott, 1992.

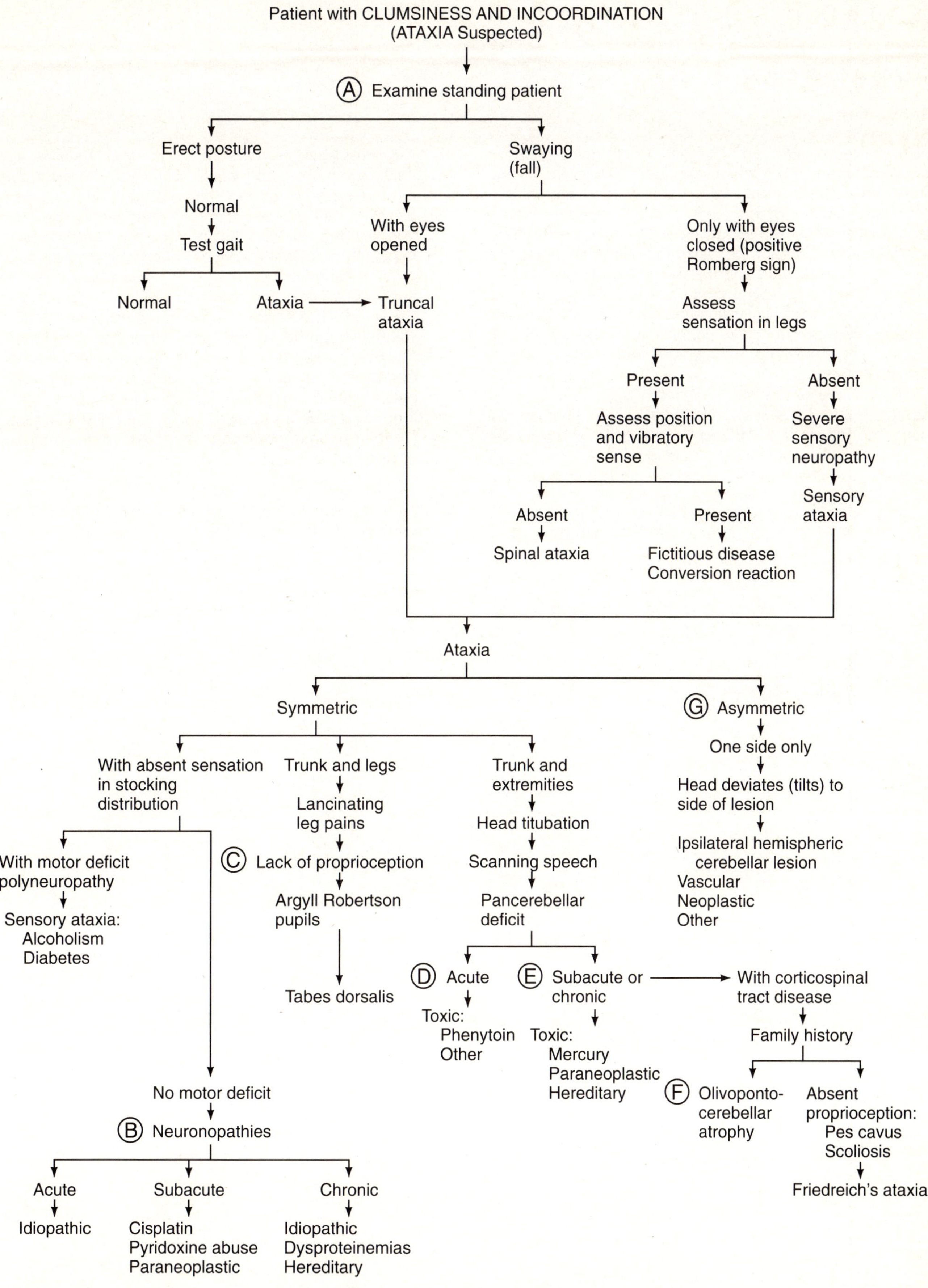

Patient with CLUMSINESS AND INCOORDINATION
(ATAXIA Suspected)
A Examine standing patient
Erect posture
Swaying (fall)
Normal
Test gait
With eyes opened
Only with eyes closed (positive Romberg sign)
Normal
Ataxia
Truncal ataxia
Assess sensation in legs
Present
Absent
Assess position and vibratory sense
Severe sensory neuropathy
Absent
Present
Sensory ataxia
Spinal ataxia
Fictitious disease
Conversion reaction
Ataxia
Symmetric
G Asymmetric
With absent sensation in stocking distribution
Trunk and legs
Trunk and extremities
One side only
Head deviates (tilts) to side of lesion
With motor deficit polyneuropathy
Lancinating leg pains
Head titubation
Ipsilateral hemispheric cerebellar lesion
Vascular
Neoplastic
Other
Sensory ataxia:
Alcoholism
Diabetes
C Lack of proprioception
Scanning speech
Argyll Robertson pupils
Pancerebellar deficit
Tabes dorsalis
D Acute
E Subacute or chronic
With corticospinal tract disease
Toxic:
Phenytoin
Other
Toxic:
Mercury
Paraneoplastic
Hereditary
Family history
No motor deficit
B Neuronopathies
F Olivoponto-cerebellar atrophy
Absent proprioception:
Pes cavus
Scoliosis
Acute
Subacute
Chronic
Friedreich's ataxia
Idiopathic
Cisplatin
Pyridoxine abuse
Paraneoplastic
Idiopathic
Dysproteinemias
Hereditary

WALKING DISTURBANCE

Leon A. Weisberg, M.D.

Examination of gait and station are valuable tests of neurologic function and should be done early in the procedure. Never avoid this part of the examination because the patient feels weak or fatigued. Observe the patient performing the following tasks: rising from chair, standing at rest, heel-to-toe walking, walking on heels and toes, walking sideways and backward, hopping, skipping, crawling, running, stopping and starting walking pattern, balancing on each leg independently for 10 seconds, standing with feet together (initially with eyes open and then with eyes closed [Romberg test]), and walking rapidly around a chair.

Gait is affected by multiple factors (age, gender, body habitus, ground surface). First, determine whether the motor machinery of the lower limbs is intact. Orthopedic conditions (back, hip, knee, leg, ankle), lower extremity vascular insufficiency, arthritis, and leg prostheses all may alter gait patterns. Gait is altered by abnormalities of several systems: weakness (upper or lower motor neuron disturbances); proprioception; cerebellar, basal ganglia, and vestibular systems; loss of gait program or inability to know how to walk (gait apraxia).

A. Proximal weakness suggests myopathy. Patients have difficulty rising from or stepping up onto a chair. Distal weakness suggests neuropathy. Patients have difficulty walking on toes and heels. The foot slaps on the ground because of foot drop; shoe soles are well worn. In monoparesis, patients drag and circumduct one leg. In patients with monoparesis, sensory loss, hyperactive reflexes, and positive Babinski sign suggest a cerebral or spinal cord lesion (anterior cerebral artery infarction, parasagittal lesion). By contrast, unilateral leg weakness without abnormal reflexes or positive Babinski sign suggests a lesion of the lumbosacral plexus, single or multiple peripheral nerves (sciatic, peroneal), or radiculopathy. In paraparesis, patients circumduct both legs, and increased muscle tone (spasticity) causes a scissoring gait pattern. Paraparesis suggests a spinal cord, foramen magnum, or parasagittal lesion.

B. If dizziness and vertigo are present, vestibular or brain stem lesions are likely. Hearing loss or other cranial nerve dysfunction (facial weakness, impaired corneal reflex) may be present with posterior fossa lesions. Exclude otolaryngologic conditions (labyrinthitis, vestibular neuronitis) before performing neurodiagnostic studies (see p 68).

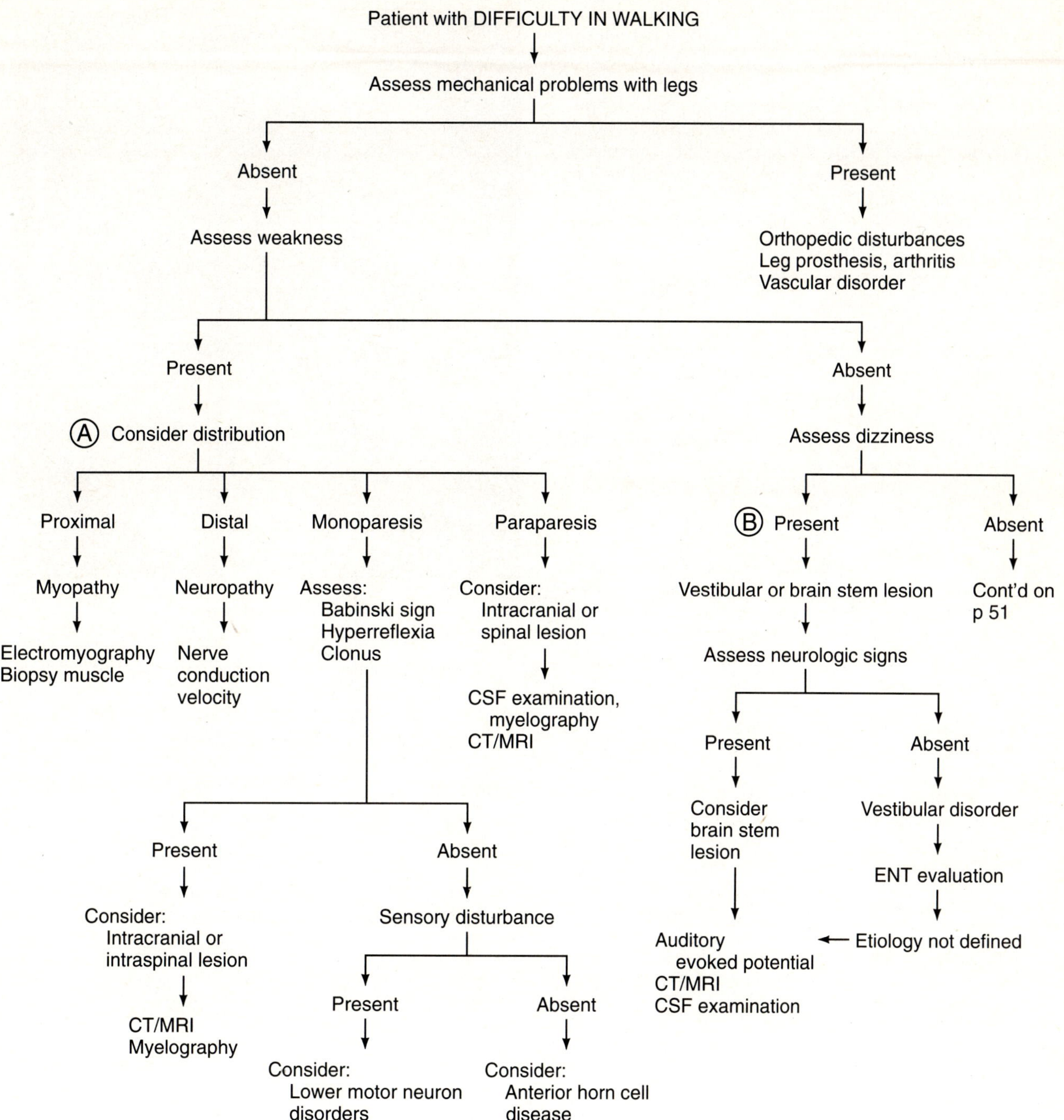

Patient with DIFFICULTY IN WALKING
Assess mechanical problems with legs
Absent
Present
Assess weakness
Orthopedic disturbances
Leg prosthesis, arthritis
Vascular disorder
Present
Absent
A Consider distribution
Assess dizziness
Proximal
Distal
Monoparesis
Paraparesis
B Present
Absent
Myopathy
Neuropathy
Assess:
Babinski sign
Hyperreflexia
Clonus
Consider:
Intracranial or
spinal lesion
Vestibular or brain stem lesion
Cont'd on
p 51
Electromyography
Biopsy muscle
Nerve
conduction
velocity
CSF examination,
myelography
CT/MRI
Assess neurologic signs
Present
Absent
Present
Absent
Consider
brain stem
lesion
Vestibular disorder
Consider:
Intracranial or
intraspinal lesion
Sensory disturbance
ENT evaluation
CT/MRI
Myelography
Present
Absent
Auditory
evoked potential
CT/MRI
CSF examination
Etiology not defined
Consider:
Lower motor neuron
disorders
Consider:
Anterior horn cell
disease

C. If a patient stands with feet together and normal balance but becomes unsteady with eyes closed (positive Romberg sign), consider a proprioceptive abnormality. There is usually decreased position sensation in the legs. Consider a spinal cord (multiple sclerosis, tabes dorsalis, vitamin B_{12} deficiency) or peripheral nerve lesion. If the spinal cord is involved, Babinski signs are present; in neuropathy, ankle jerks are absent.

D. If patients are equally unsteady with the eyes open or closed and there is incoordination and ataxia, consider cerebellar dysfunction. Gait impairment and symptoms of intracranial hypertension suggest a posterior fossa mass lesion; this may be intracerebral (astrocytoma, metastasis) or extracerebellar, in the tentorial or cerebellopontine region. If gait impairment develops suddenly, consider posterior fossa hemorrhage (Fig. 1) or infarction. If progression of gait impairment and ataxia is slow, consider a metabolic or atrophic cerebellar disorder (e.g., spinocerebellar degeneration).

E. If gait is unsteady and cerebellar signs are absent, observe for resting tremor, impaired postural reflexes, and difficulty in initiating gait; this is consistent with basal ganglia dysfunction. If resting tremor is absent, observe for gait apraxia. This condition is defined as inability to use the legs for walking in the absence of sensory or motor impairment. In gait apraxia, the legs have increased tone and do not leave the ground (magnetic gait). Gait apraxia is usually due to normal-pressure hydrocephalus (NPH). These patients also show clinical signs of dementia and urinary incontinence. Establish the diagnosis of NPH by CT or MRI or cisternography (isotope, metrizamide). Some elderly patients show gait impairment that suggests gait apraxia or parkinsonism, even though no other findings of these disorders are noted. This gait pattern is characterized by stooped, flexed posture and short steps and may progress to senile paraplegia. The cause of this senile gait condition is not usually established by diagnostic studies.

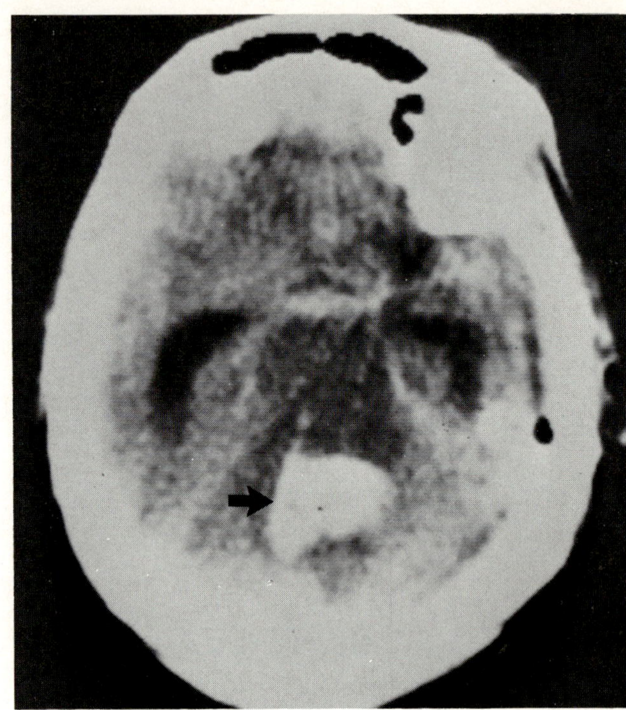

Figure 1 CT scan shows cerebellar hemorrhage.

F. Consider psychiatric disturbances if gait machinery and neurologic systems are normal but the patient has difficulty using the legs for standing (astasia) or walking (abasia). Hysterical gait disorder represents a diagnosis of exclusion and should be made very carefully, usually only after appropriate neuroimaging tests are negative.

References

Fos PJ, McLin CL. The risk of falling in the elderly: A subjective approach. Med Decis Making 1990; 10:195.

Grimm RJ. Disorderly walks. Neurol Clin North Am 1984; 2:615.

Keane JR. Hysterical gait disorders: 60 cases. Neurology 1989; 39:586.

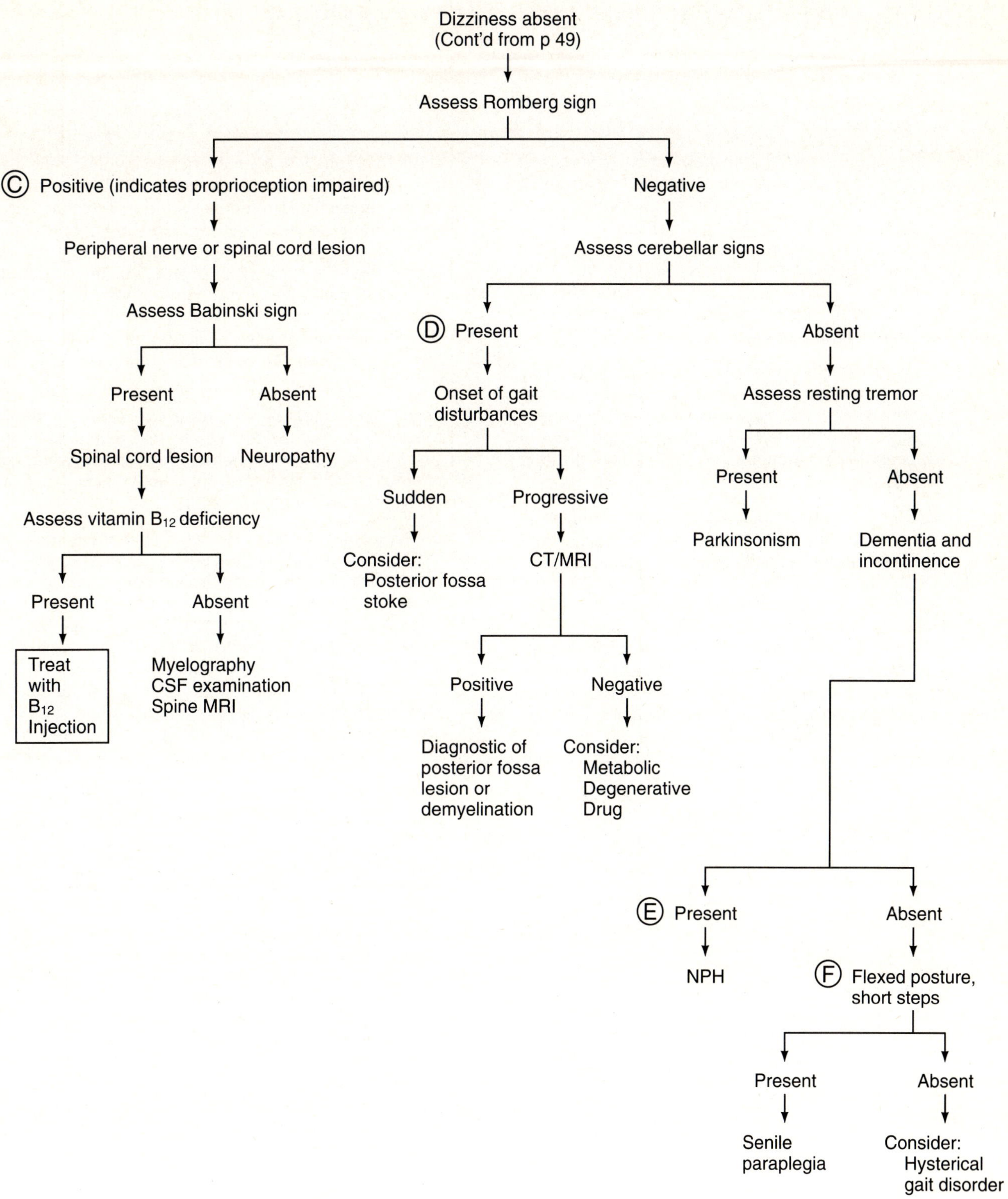

Dizziness absent
(Cont'd from p 49)
Assess Romberg sign
C Positive (indicates proprioception impaired)
Negative
Peripheral nerve or spinal cord lesion
Assess cerebellar signs
Assess Babinski sign
D Present
Absent
Present
Absent
Spinal cord lesion
Neuropathy
Onset of gait disturbances
Assess resting tremor
Assess vitamin B$_{12}$ deficiency
Present
Absent
Sudden
Progressive
Present
Absent
Treat with B$_{12}$ Injection
Myelography
CSF examination
Spine MRI
Consider:
Posterior fossa stoke
CT/MRI
Parkinsonism
Dementia and incontinence
Positive
Negative
Diagnostic of posterior fossa lesion or demyelination
Consider:
Metabolic
Degenerative
Drug
E Present
Absent
NPH
F Flexed posture, short steps
Present
Absent
Senile paraplegia
Consider:
Hysterical gait disorder

ABNORMAL INVOLUNTARY MOVEMENTS

Leon A. Weisberg, M.D.

Observe the patient at rest, during ambulation, in sustained postures, or while carrying out voluntary (purposeful) movements. Direct attention to the head (eyelids, lips, tongue, mouth), trunk (neck, spine, pelvis), arms, and legs. Dyskinesias usually disappear during sleep (except for myoclonus and tics); they reappear and increase with certain emotional states (e.g., anxiety). Describe the dyskinesias (location, speed, amplitude, rhythmicity, duration, interference with purposeful activity).

A. Of dyskinesias most prominent at rest, the pill-rolling parkinsonian hand tremor (three cycles/sec) is most common. This tremor is coarse, and is easily seen as the patient sits with hands placed in the lap. Tremor disappears with voluntary movement and postural maintenance.

B. Fasciculations are undulating, arrhythmic ripples of muscles occurring at rest or after exercise; these movements are not of sufficient force or amplitude to move the limb joint. They may occur in asymptomatic patients (benign fasciculations) as a normal finding. If fasciculations occur in patients with weak and wasted muscles, consider motor neuron disease. The diagnosis of anterior horn cell disease is established clinically and confirmed by electromyography (see p 224). Most fasciculations have no clinical significance, but they are alarming to patients and physicians.

C. Choreiform movements appear as fidgetiness or motor restlessness. Chorea interferes with voluntary activity, creating an impression of clumsiness. Movements of the face, tongue, head, neck, or arms result in bizarre body postures (see p 250). Tics are movements or vocalizations that are brief, rapid, stereotyped, and nonpurposeful. They are constant in morphology and location (eyelid blinks, head twitches, shoulder shrugs, grunting) and occur at irregular frequencies and intervals. They are enhanced by anxiety, are reduced if the patient is distracted, and may persist during sleep. Patients can voluntarily suppress tics for short periods. Simple motor tics are common in the general population and may begin in childhood or young adulthood. They may remit and may be barely noticed. Abnormal vocalizations (grunting, barking, cursing, coughing) are characteristic of tics in Tourette's syndrome (see p 254). In this condition, there are motor tics and verbal utterances that may be socially embarrassing and incapacitating.

D. Chorea may be generalized or focal. These movements may be arrhythmic and asymmetric; they interfere with voluntary activity. Myoclonic jerks are random, rapid jerking movements involving the extremities. These usually involve the distal extremities (wrists, fingers) and interfere with purposeful activity. For example, if myoclonic jerk suddenly occurs while patients are holding an object, loss of control may cause them to drop the object. Akathisia (motor restlessness) may involve the entire body but usually predominantly involves the legs (restless leg syndrome). It is not strictly an abnormal movement but rather represents an urge to remain in constant motion.

E. Postural or intentional tremors are rapid rhythmic movements that occur when the extremities are sustained in an outstretched position or when an attempt is made to carry out a movement, such as touching an object (see p 248).

F. Dystonia may be slow or rapid and there may be sustained muscular contractions (see p 252). It may involve the neck in spasmodic torticollis, hand or arm in writer's cramp, or foot in equinovarus deformity. Athetosis represents a group of disorders characterized by slow, sustained spasms of the fingers, wrists, or feet. In athetosis, there is almost continuous movement with the upper extremity in a characteristic position (forearm pronated, wrist flexed, fingers abducted and hyperextended). Athetoid movements may be slow and simulate dystonia; they may also be rapid, simulating chorea. Myoclonus is a sudden and brief involuntary contraction of a single muscle or group of muscles that causes movement of the involved body part. Myoclonic jerking movements may be single or repetitive, focal or diffuse, rhythmic or arrhythmic, frequent or infrequent. They may occur at rest or with voluntary (intentional) activity. Some forms are stimulus sensitive (e.g., startle myoclonus). Most forms persist during sleep, except for palatal myoclonus, a rhythmic myoclonus due to brain stem dysfunction. Myoclonus may have multiple causes: psychological (nocturnal or sleep), epileptic, and symptomatic. The last-named is usually related to a diffuse (toxic or metabolic) encephalopathic state but may be related to brain (Jakob-Creutzfeldt disease, posthypoxic cerebellar intentional myoclonus), brain stem (palatal myoclonus), or spinal (spinal myoclonus) injury or disease.

Reference

Duvoisin R. Clinical diagnosis of the dyskinesias. Med Clin North Am 1970; 56:1321.

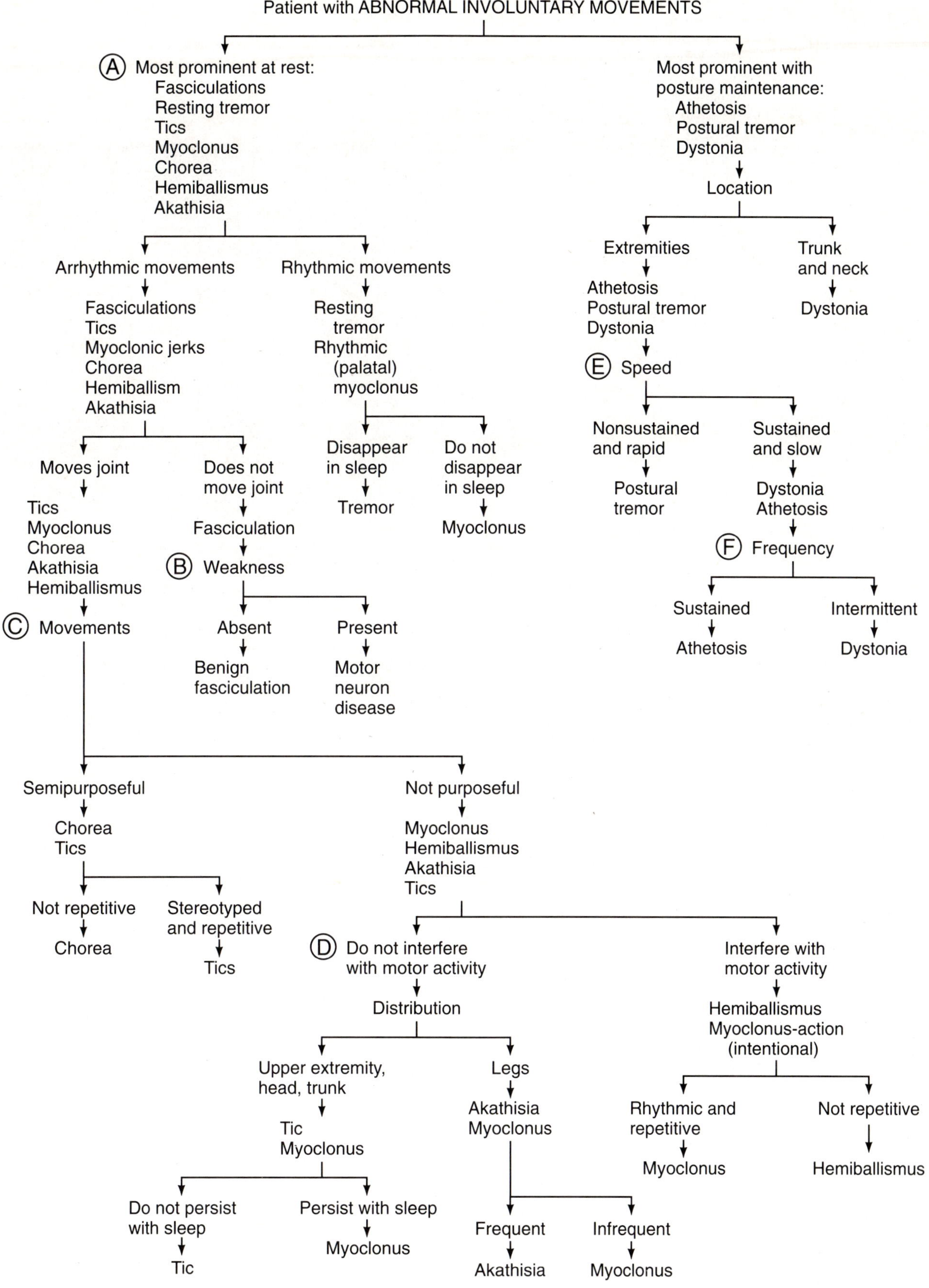

Patient with ABNORMAL INVOLUNTARY MOVEMENTS
A Most prominent at rest:
Fasciculations
Resting tremor
Tics
Myoclonus
Chorea
Hemiballismus
Akathisia
Most prominent with posture maintenance:
Athetosis
Postural tremor
Dystonia
Location
Arrhythmic movements
Rhythmic movements
Fasciculations
Tics
Myoclonic jerks
Chorea
Hemiballism
Akathisia
Resting tremor
Rhythmic (palatal) myoclonus
Extremities
Trunk and neck
Athetosis
Postural tremor
Dystonia
Dystonia
E Speed
Moves joint
Does not move joint
Disappear in sleep
Do not disappear in sleep
Nonsustained and rapid
Sustained and slow
Tics
Myoclonus
Chorea
Akathisia
Hemiballismus
Fasciculation
Tremor
Myoclonus
Postural tremor
Dystonia
Athetosis
C Movements
B Weakness
F Frequency
Absent
Present
Sustained
Intermittent
Benign fasciculation
Motor neuron disease
Athetosis
Dystonia
Semipurposeful
Not purposeful
Chorea
Tics
Myoclonus
Hemiballismus
Akathisia
Tics
Not repetitive
Stereotyped and repetitive
Chorea
Tics
D Do not interfere with motor activity
Interfere with motor activity
Distribution
Hemiballismus
Myoclonus-action (intentional)
Upper extremity, head, trunk
Legs
Rhythmic and repetitive
Not repetitive
Tic
Myoclonus
Akathisia
Myoclonus
Myoclonus
Hemiballismus
Do not persist with sleep
Persist with sleep
Tic
Myoclonus
Frequent
Infrequent
Akathisia
Myoclonus

FASCICULATIONS AND MYOKYMIA

Carlos A. Garcia, M.D.

A. Fasciculations are involuntary, painless, spontaneous, repetitive, irregular twitches of small groups of muscle fibers that may be seen through the skin and mucosa and are not associated with joint movements. In infants (with baby fat) and in obese adults the fasciculations are difficult or impossible to see. The tongue is an accessible and easy site to detect fasciculations. Tongue fasciculations are frequently seen in children with spinal muscular atrophy and in the bulbar form of amyotrophic lateral sclerosis (ALS) in adults. Use electrophysiologic studies to diagnose or confirm clinical findings.

B. Myokymia is an involuntary, painless, spontaneous, repetitive, slow, undulating contraction of bands or strips of muscle fibers.

C. When fasciculations are generalized and associated with muscle atrophy and weakness, they are highly suggestive of degeneration or irritation of the anterior horn cells, as seen in motor neuron disease (see p 224).

D. When the fasciculations are isolated and not associated with atrophy or other neurologic symptoms, look for dysthyroidism and toxic cholinomimetic substances (organic phosphorus and other compounds).

E. Localized fasciculations are usually seen in the upper extremities and may be found in cervical spondylosis (radiculopathy). Look for long tract signs in the legs and neurogenic bladder indicative of spinal cord compression (myelopathy). When the localized fasciculations are associated with atrophy of the hands and sensory dissociation, suspect an intramedullary tumor or syringomyelia. MRI of the spine or myelography will confirm the diagnosis (Fig. 1). Localized fasciculations in the arms associated with areflexia and abnormal nerve conduction velocities (NCV) suggest demyelinating neuropathy.

F. Localized fasciculations not associated with atrophy or other neurologic abnormalities are frequently seen in the calves or hand muscles and are usually benign. Myokymias of the eyelid muscles or lips are usually induced by fatigue and are benign. They may represent benign fasciculations.

G. Constant myokymia associated with contractures of the feet and hands, atrophy of distal muscles, and hyperhidrosis are symptoms of Isaac's syndrome (neu-

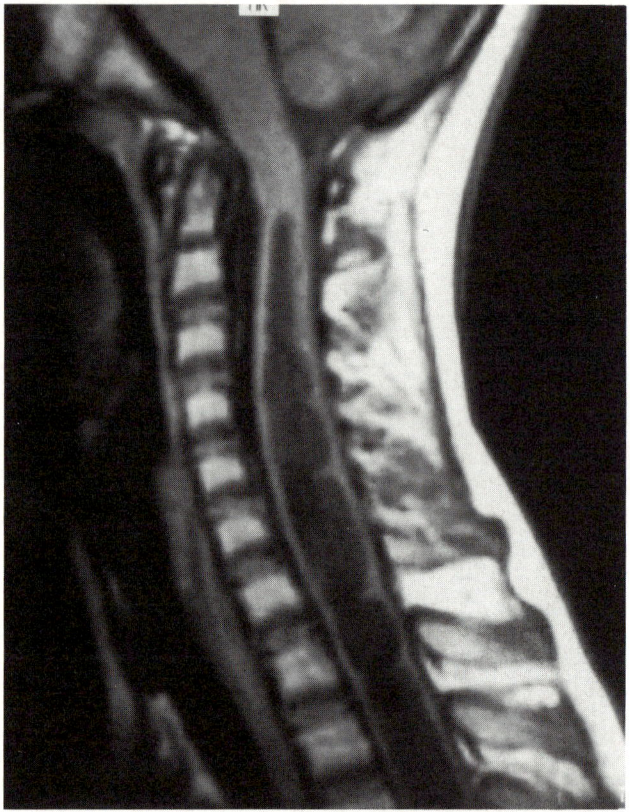

Figure 1 MRI of the cervical spinal cord shows a large hypointense (slightly more hypointense than CSF) intramedullary lesion that begins in the high cervical region and extends downward to the thoracic region. This pattern is characteristic of syringomyelia.

romyotonia) and related disorders. Some patients have myokymia and muscle stiffness (stiff-man syndrome), which is made worse by voluntary activity but persists during rest and sleep. The abnormal activity seems to originate in distal motor nerves. The symptoms may be reduced by treatment with phenytoin or carbamazepine (Tegretol).

References

Brooke MH. A clinician's view of neuromuscular diseases. 2nd ed. Baltimore: Williams & Wilkins, 1986.

Haerer AF. DeJong's the neurological examination. 5th ed. Philadelphia: JB Lippincott, 1992.

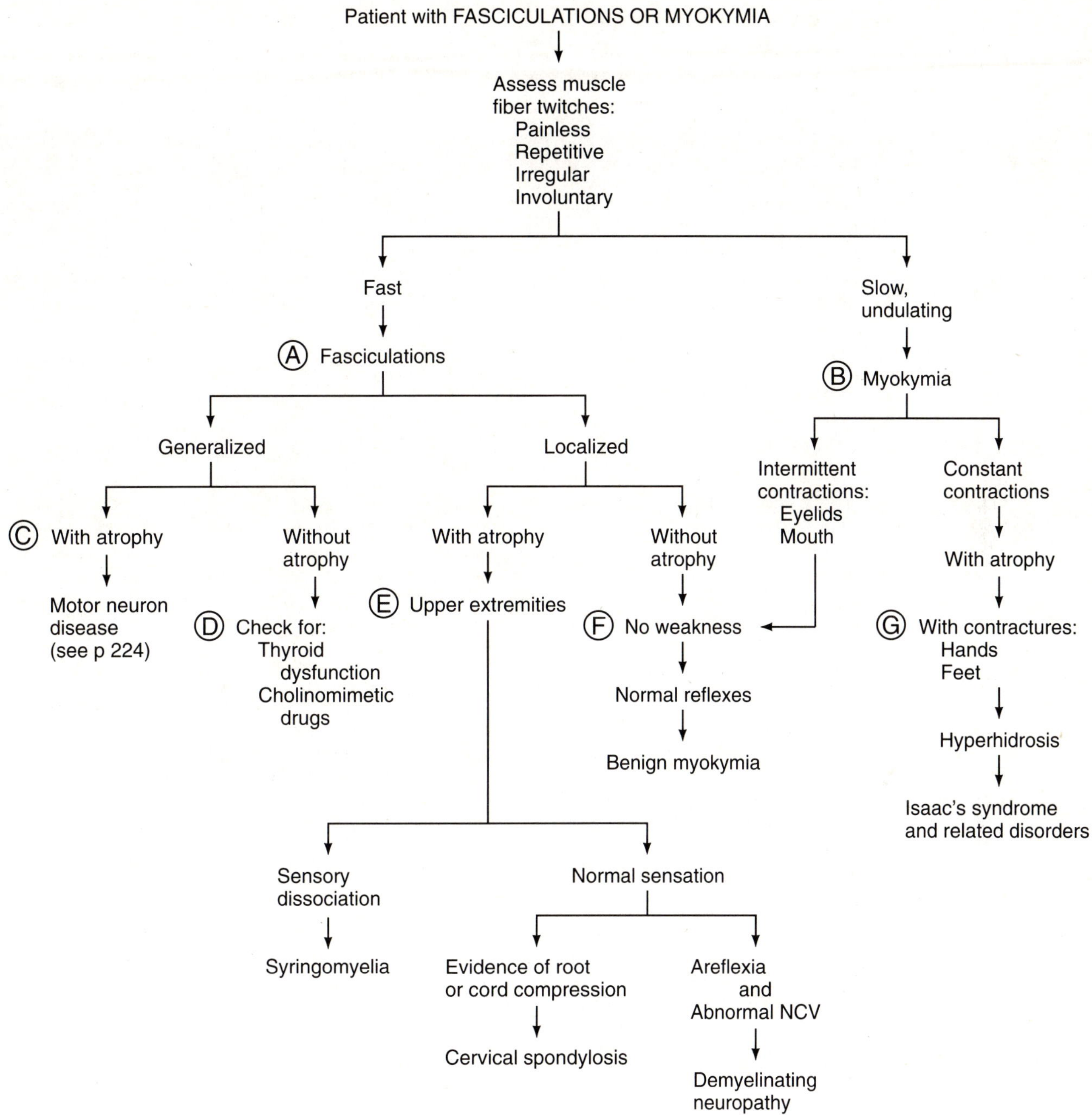

Patient with FASCICULATIONS OR MYOKYMIA
Assess muscle
fiber twitches:
Painless
Repetitive
Irregular
Involuntary
Fast
Slow,
undulating
A Fasciculations
B Myokymia
Generalized
Localized
Intermittent
contractions:
Eyelids
Mouth
Constant
contractions
C With atrophy
Without
atrophy
With atrophy
Without
atrophy
With atrophy
Motor neuron
disease
(see p 224)
D Check for:
Thyroid
dysfunction
Cholinomimetic
drugs
E Upper extremities
F No weakness
G With contractures:
Hands
Feet
Normal reflexes
Hyperhidrosis
Benign myokymia
Isaac's syndrome
and related disorders
Sensory
dissociation
Normal sensation
Syringomyelia
Evidence of root
or cord compression
Areflexia
and
Abnormal NCV
Cervical spondylosis
Demyelinating
neuropathy

MUSCLE CRAMPS AND ACHES

Carlos A. Garcia, M.D.

Cramps are transient, painful, involuntary muscle contractions that may last several seconds or several minutes. Electromyography (EMG) shows brief bursts of high-frequency motor unit potentials. Almost everyone at some time experiences muscle cramps. Transient benign cramps occur frequently in childhood and during pregnancy. In some patients the cramps are precipitated by minor exercise and may be disabling. In many patients the condition remains undiagnosed, even with the help of EMG and muscle biopsy, histochemistry, electron microscopy, and biochemical analysis. When cramps and aches are associated with dark urine, suspect myoglobinuria (see p 234).

A. In young children and in women during pregnancy, cramps usually occur at rest and mainly at night, are of short duration, and recur frequently. Findings on the neurologic examination are normal and there are no abnormalities in the laboratory test results. Most of these cases are handled properly by pediatricians and obstetricians.

B. In young adults when cramps are recurrent and are seen at rest or precipitated by minor exercise, inquire about and investigate for thyroid disease and the use of diuretics (electrolyte disturbance, especially potassium) and hypocholesterolemic drugs (clofibrate). Order electrolyte and serum calcium and magnesium levels. If any abnormality is found, treat accordingly. The prognosis is good.

C. Focal muscle cramps may be precipitated by vigorous and sustained exercise and often respond to muscle stretching. Cramps localized to the hands may be seen in pianists and writers. They probably represent a focal form of dystonia (see p 252). Nocturnal cramps usually cause painful flexion of the feet and toes. These frequently awaken the patient from sleep. Treat with calcium, quinine (200 to 300 mg/day), or diphenhydramine (Benadryl), 50 to 100 mg at bedtime. Diazepam and phenytoin are occasionally effective. Some patients respond well to Tonocard (tocainide HCl).

D. Muscle cramps and leg pains in adults that are precipitated by exercise and resolve after a few minutes of rest are usually due to peripheral vascular disease. Refer the patient to a vascular surgeon. Some patients develop muscle aches and cramps 24 to 48 hours after heavy exercise related to soft tissue injury.

E. Recurrent muscle cramps that are disabling should be investigated in detail. A complete history and neurologic examination, followed by muscle enzyme determinations (creatine kinase, CK), is necessary. Electrophysiologic studies, including an ischemic exercise test, should precede a muscle biopsy for histochemistry, electron microscopy, and biochemical analysis. In many cases, all the test results are normal or borderline abnormal, or show minimal nonspecific changes on the muscle biopsy, and the diagnosis remains undetermined. Quinine, phenytoin, and amitriptyline may decrease the cramps in some patients. Tonocard is usually effective and safe.

F. Some tests may disclose early signs of peripheral neuropathies, motor neuron disease, and some of the myopathies. Muscle aches, cramps, stiffness, exercise intolerance, and peripheral nerve hyperexcitability have been reported to respond to carbamazepine. In rare cases, muscle histochemistry may reveal a vacuolar myopathy that biochemical tests may confirm as a storage disorder due to a defect in glycogen or lipid metabolism.

References

Moxley RT III. Cramps. In: Johnson R, ed. Current therapy in neurologic disease. 3rd ed. Philadelphia: BC Decker, 1990:410.

Tahmoush AJ, Alonso RJ, Tahmoush GP, Heiman-Patterson TD. Cramp-fasciculation syndrome: a treatable hyperexcitable peripheral nerve disorder. Neurol 1991; 41:1021.

Telerman-Toppet N, Bacq M, Khoubesserian P, Coers C. Type 2 fiber predominance in muscle cramp and exercise myalgia. Muscle Nerve 1985; 8:563.

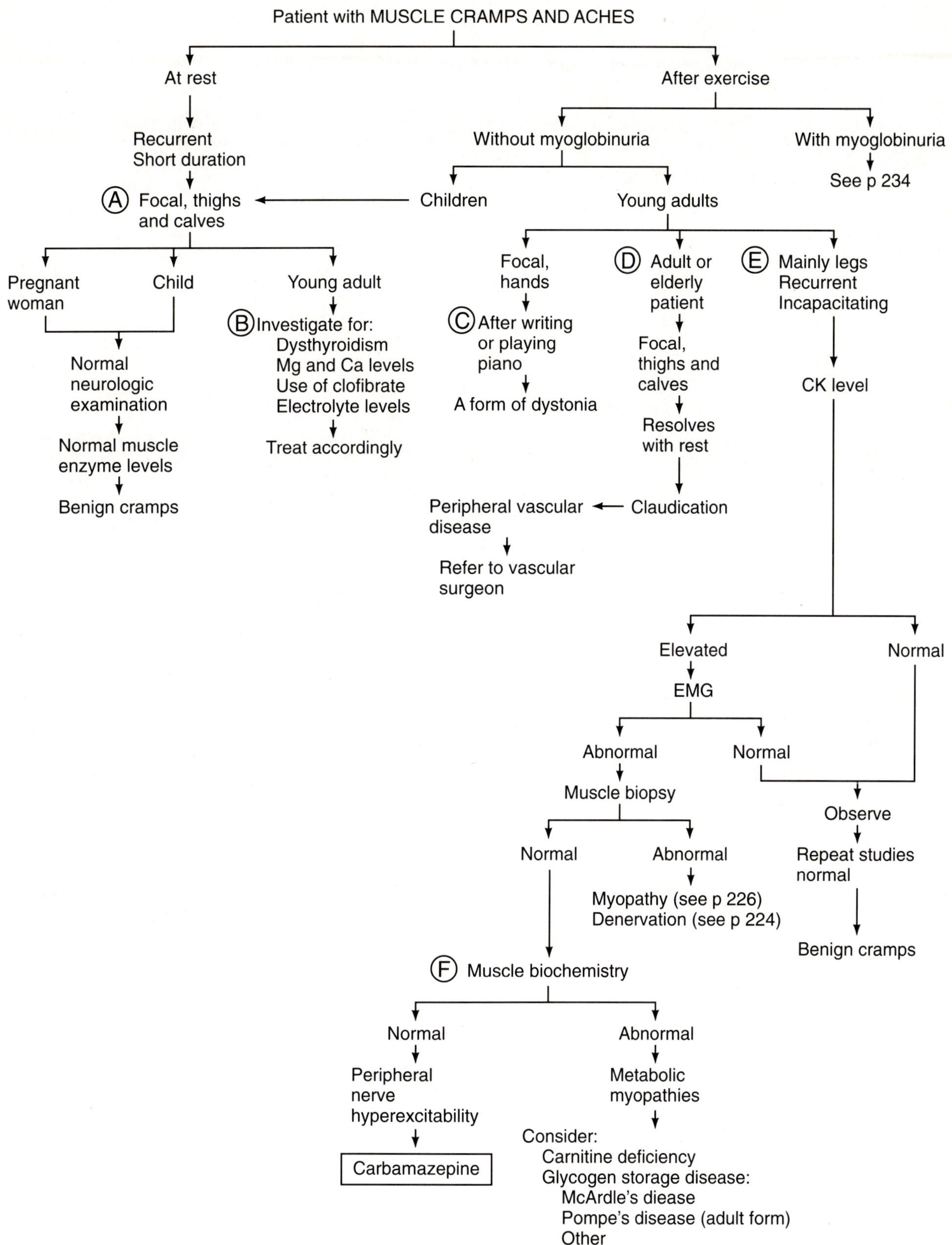

Patient with MUSCLE CRAMPS AND ACHES
At rest
After exercise
Without myoglobinuria
With myoglobinuria
See p 234
Recurrent
Short duration
A Focal, thighs and calves
Children
Young adults
Pregnant woman
Child
Young adult
Focal, hands
D Adult or elderly patient
E Mainly legs Recurrent Incapacitating
Normal neurologic examination
B Investigate for:
Dysthyroidism
Mg and Ca levels
Use of clofibrate
Electrolyte levels
C After writing or playing piano
Focal, thighs and calves
CK level
Normal muscle enzyme levels
Treat accordingly
A form of dystonia
Resolves with rest
Benign cramps
Peripheral vascular disease
Claudication
Refer to vascular surgeon
Elevated
Normal
EMG
Abnormal
Normal
Muscle biopsy
Observe
Normal
Abnormal
Repeat studies normal
Myopathy (see p 226)
Denervation (see p 224)
Benign cramps
F Muscle biochemistry
Normal
Abnormal
Peripheral nerve hyperexcitability
Metabolic myopathies
Carbamazepine
Consider:
Carnitine deficiency
Glycogen storage disease:
McArdle's diease
Pompe's disease (adult form)
Other

TRANSIENT VISUAL LOSS

Leon A. Weisberg, M.D.

Transient visual loss (TVL) that is unilateral, lasts for short intervals (usually <30 min), and occurs without scintillations (bright flashing lights) is called amaurosis fugax. This may be caused by vascular (central retinal artery or posterior ciliary artery ischemia) or ocular disorders. These transient visual obscurations may also occur in papilledema. Amaurosis fugax may be caused by ischemia involving the retinal arterial system in carotid artery disease or cardiogenic cerebral embolism. In amaurosis fugax due to vascular ischemia, patients describe the sensation of a veil or curtain extending over one eye, causing reduced vision; this resolves completely, in the reverse pattern in which visual loss evolved. In some cases, visual loss is less severe; patients describe a similar sequence, but vision becomes hazy or foggy. Bilateral TVL may be due to retinal ischemia (usually systemic arterial hypotension) or, most commonly, bilateral occipital ischemia in vertebrobasilar disease. In TVL, headache and visual scintillations are important features in determining the precise mechanism.

A. If TVL is unilateral, absence of headache suggests a vascular (thromboembolic) mechanism. Remember that acephalic (without headache) migraine may occur in patients with unilateral TVL. In acephalic or retinal migraine, visual disturbance builds slowly over 5 to 20 minutes, moves across the visual field, and rapidly disappears. There is a characteristic scintillating (zigzag lines, sparkles) pattern. In patients with TVL, listen carefully to the neck vessels for carotid bruit. Retinal embolism (cholesterol, platelet-fibrin, calcific) may be seen by funduscopy when vision is impaired and may disappear when vision returns. This indicates a thromboembolic source of visual loss because the retinal vessels provide a mirror for the aortocranial circulation. In patients with unilateral TVL, perform angiography for a potential carotid lesion (stenosis, occlusion, dissection, ulceration) and make a complete investigation for a cardiac embolic source. With carotid disease, there may be central retinal artery occlusion or retinal artery branch occlusion. If a cardiac source is identified, give anticoagulants to prevent a cerebral hemispheric ischemic stroke. If a surgically accessible carotid artery lesion is identified, consider carotid endarterectomy; if the lesion is not surgically accessible, use anticoagulant or antiplatelet drugs. Amaurosis fugax rarely results in permanent visual loss because of the rich collateral circulation to the retina. If funduscopy shows no abnormality, check for postural hypotensive change. If this is negative, investigate for a hyperviscosity condition (multiple myeloma, polycythemia vera, thrombocytosis, macroglobulinemia, sickle cell anemia), hypercoagulable conditions, or vasculitis. Ocular causes of unilateral TVL include drusen, swollen optic nerve, and exercise-induced visual loss secondary to optic neuritis (Uhthoff's sign).

B. If headache accompanies TVL, look for funduscopic evidence of papilledema (Fig. 1), which indicates intracranial hypertension (hydrocephalus, intracranial mass, pseudotumor cerebri). In TVL due to intracranial hypertension, visual loss is usually bilateral. Visual loss usually lasts for only seconds and may occur multiple times, whereas in amaurosis fugax, episodes last longer and are less frequent. In TVL due to hypertensive vascular crisis (see p 154), retinal vessels are abnormal (arteriolar narrowing, hemorrhages, exudates). If TVL is accompanied by headache and scintillation, consider retinal migraine. In elderly patients with unilateral headache and visual loss, consider temporal arteritis (although visual loss is usually not transient). Check visual fields for hemianopic defect (see p 304).

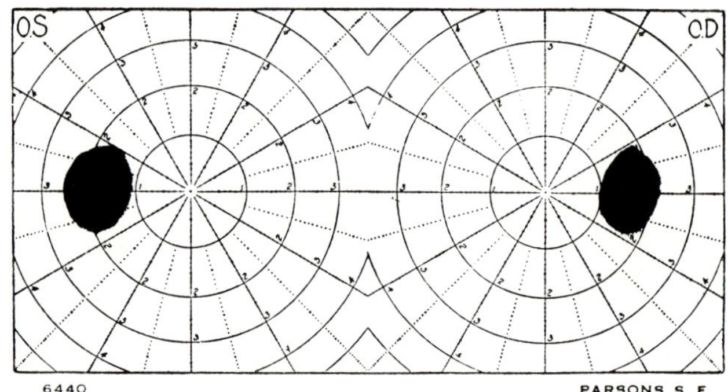

Figure 1 Visual fields show enlarged blind spots due to papilledema.

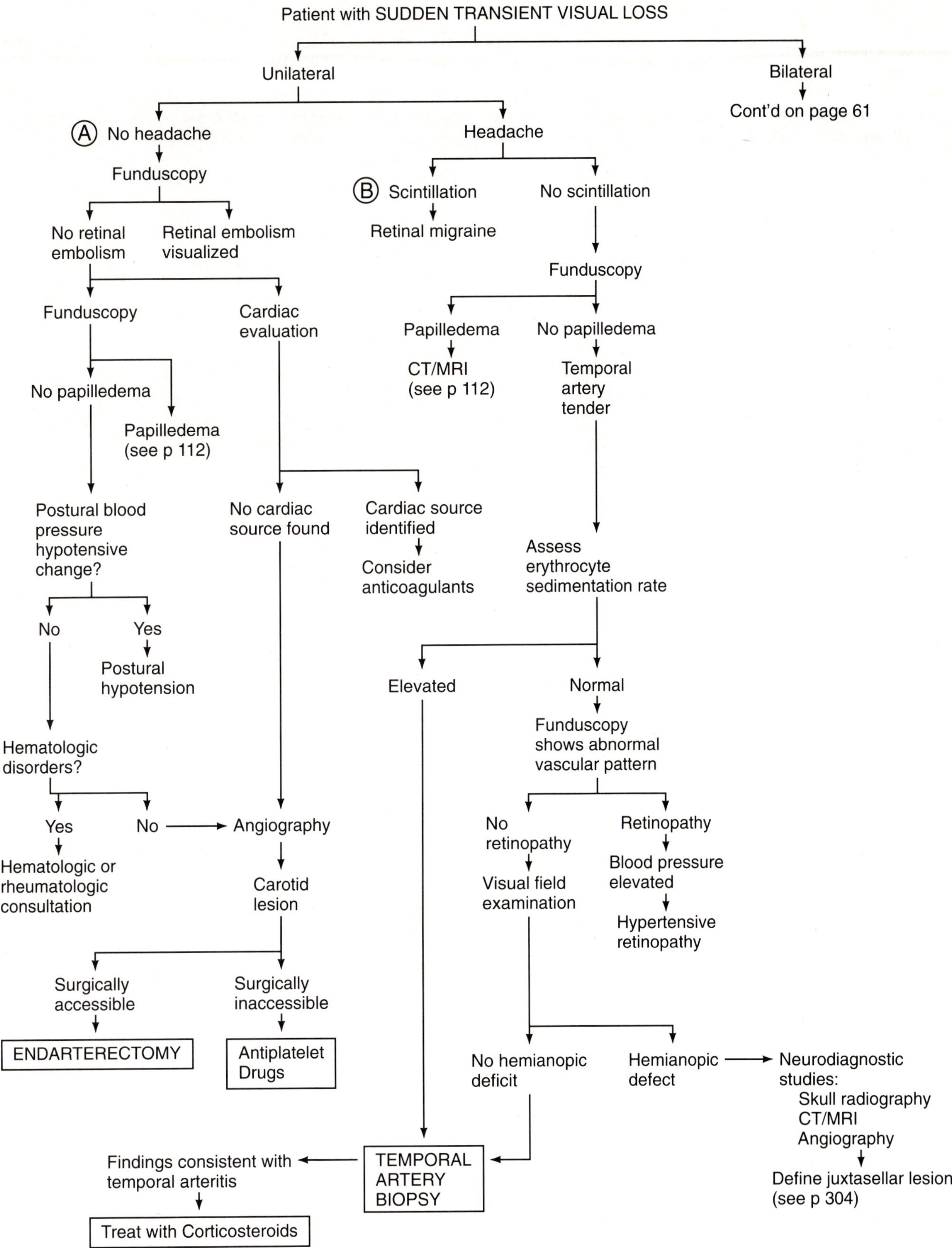

Patient with SUDDEN TRANSIENT VISUAL LOSS
Unilateral
Bilateral
Cont'd on page 61
A No headache
Funduscopy
No retinal embolism
Retinal embolism visualized
Funduscopy
Cardiac evaluation
No papilledema
Papilledema (see p 112)
Postural blood pressure hypotensive change?
No
Yes
Postural hypotension
Hematologic disorders?
Yes
No
Hematologic or rheumatologic consultation
Angiography
Carotid lesion
Surgically accessible
Surgically inaccessible
ENDARTERECTOMY
Antiplatelet Drugs
No cardiac source found
Cardiac source identified
Consider anticoagulants
Headache
B Scintillation
No scintillation
Retinal migraine
Funduscopy
Papilledema
No papilledema
CT/MRI (see p 112)
Temporal artery tender
Assess erythrocyte sedimentation rate
Elevated
Normal
Funduscopy shows abnormal vascular pattern
No retinopathy
Retinopathy
Visual field examination
Blood pressure elevated
Hypertensive retinopathy
No hemianopic deficit
Hemianopic defect
Neurodiagnostic studies:
Skull radiography
CT/MRI
Angiography
Define juxtasellar lesion (see p 304)
TEMPORAL ARTERY BIOPSY
Findings consistent with temporal arteritis
Treat with Corticosteroids

C. If TVL is bilateral and followed by headache, consider classic migraine. There are usually scintillations, which occur at the edge of the visual loss (scintillating scotomata) and extend across visual fields (as a result of spreading cortical depressive electrical activity). During migraine attack, there may be homonymous hemianopia; EEG may show a focal slow wave pattern. Migraine may simulate occipital seizures. During occipital seizures, patients report lights or colors moving rapidly across visual fields. Scintillations are characteristic of migraine and rarely occur with occipital seizures. In patients with occipital seizures, EEG shows focal spike discharges; these EEG patterns are not seen with migraine. On the basis of the clinical features, it is usually possible to differentiate migraine from occipital seizures, but EEG may be required to confirm this diagnosis.

D. If TVL is bilateral and there is no headache, consider decreased flow with ischemia involving the retinal arteries or vertebrobasilar arterial system. Ask the patient about brain stem symptoms (diplopia, vertigo, weakness). With systemic hypotension, visual loss closes in from the periphery to the central visual field. In patients with unilateral or bilateral TVL, exclude primary ophthalmologic disease (glaucoma, uveitis, scleritis). If these are excluded, consider a conversion reaction; this is rare in patients with TVL.

References

Burger SK, Saul RF, Selhorst JB, et al. Transient monocular blindness caused by vasospasm. N Engl J Med 1991; 325:870.

Marshall J, Meadows S. The natural history of amaurosis fugax. Brain 1968; 91:419.

Sandok BA, Troutmann JC, Raminez-Lassepas M, et al. Clinical-angiographic correlations in amaurosis fugax. Am J Ophthalmol 1975; 79:137.

Savino PJ, Glaser JS, Corsody J. Retinal stroke. Arch Ophthalmol 1977; 95:1185.

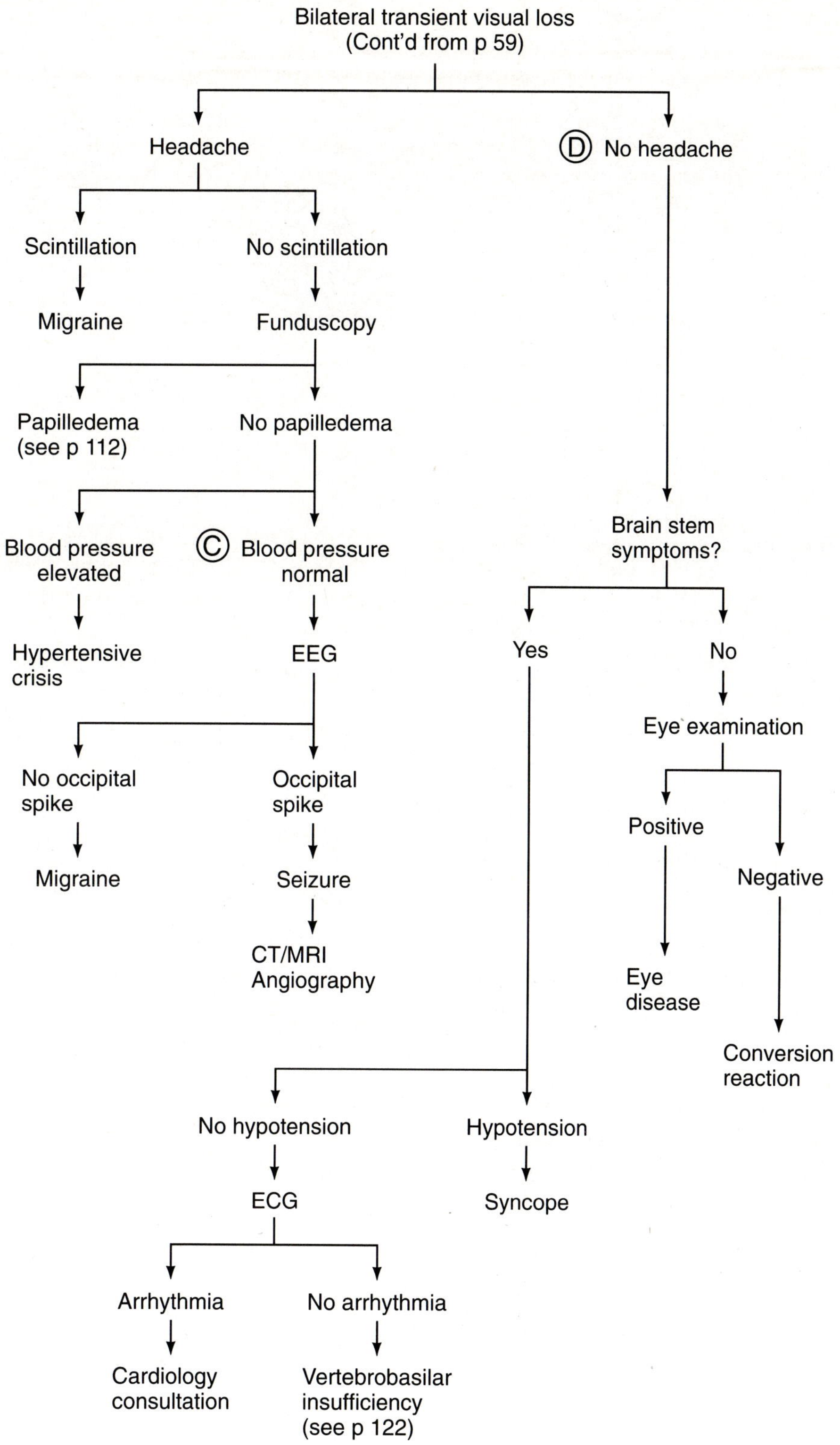

Bilateral transient visual loss
(Cont'd from p 59)

Headache

D No headache

Scintillation

No scintillation

Migraine

Funduscopy

Papilledema
(see p 112)

No papilledema

Blood pressure elevated

C Blood pressure normal

Brain stem symptoms?

Hypertensive crisis

EEG

Yes

No

Eye examination

No occipital spike

Occipital spike

Positive

Negative

Migraine

Seizure

CT/MRI
Angiography

Eye disease

Conversion reaction

No hypotension

Hypotension

ECG

Syncope

Arrhythmia

No arrhythmia

Cardiology consultation

Vertebrobasilar insufficiency
(see p 122)

FIXED VISUAL LOSS

Leon A. Weisberg, M.D.

Potential locations of lesions causing visual loss include the visual apparatus (anterior chamber, rods, cones, retina), optic nerve, optic chiasm, and postchiasmal visual system (optic tracts, optic radiations, occipital cortex).

A. Determine best-corrected acuity using patients' eyeglasses, or have them look through a small pinhole. These methods are usually adequate, but the best method is careful ophthalmologic refraction. If the visual acuity defect can be corrected by refraction, the problem is ophthalmologic. Best-corrected visual acuity is 20/15, not merely 20/20.

B. The swinging flashlight test detects a unilateral relative afferent pupillary defect (Marcus Gunn phenomenon). The examiner shines a bright flashlight into one eye and observes pupillary constriction to light. The light is moved rapidly to the other eye and its reaction is observed. This maneuver is repeated several times. With a relative afferent defect, the affected pupil (with fewer afferent pupilloconstrictor fibers) dilates (rather than constricts) when light is applied. In patients with afferent defect due to unilateral optic nerve dysfunction, pupillary sizes (at rest) are equal (oculomotor nerve efferent lesions cause unequal pupils). The swinging flashlight test is not positive in retinal or macular disease. With bilateral optic nerve dysfunction, pupillary light response may be symmetrically delayed and no pupillary asymmetry is detected.

C. If patients with visual loss have no afferent defect, perform funduscopy to exclude retinal disease. If no evidence of retinal disease is found, examine for strabismus as the cause of visual loss (amblyopia ex anopsia). As the next step, perform a visual field examination. Central scotomata indicate optic nerve lesions; if bilateral, they cause no afferent pupillary defect. Causes of toxic-metabolic optic neuropathy include alcohol, vitamin B_{12} deficiency, drugs, and tobacco. Bitemporal hemianopia indicates a chiasmal lesion. If there is homonymous hemianopia, consider a cerebral lesion (occipital, parietal, temporal). Tunnel vision indicates a nonorganic psychiatric disorder.

D. Visual field examination distinguishes optic nerve lesions from chiasmal lesions. Bitemporal hemianopia results from chiasmal lesions; bitemporal quadrantanopia (Fig. 1) or bitemporal scotoma may also occur with chiasmal lesions. If bitemporal quadrantanopia begins in superior quadrants, consider an initial optic chiasmal compression from an intrasellar lesion extending upward (pituitary adenoma). If there is an inferior temporal quadrant defect, consider compression by a suprasellar lesion such as craniopharyngioma initially compressing superior bitemporal fibers that represent inferior temporal fields. These are best demonstrated using small (2-mm), colored (red, blue) test objects. Nonhemianopic defects such as scotomata (islands of blindness surrounded by normal peripheral vision) are consistent with optic nerve lesions. If a chiasmal defect is suspected, perform neuroimaging to look for a juxtasellar lesion. This includes skull radiography, CT/MRI with special optic nerve and sella views, and angiography (to exclude a vascular lesion such as an aneurysm).

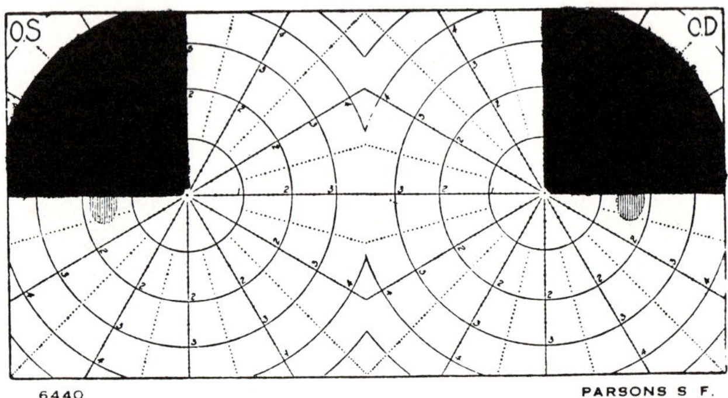

Figure 1 Visual fields show superior bitemporal quadrantanopia due to chiasmal compression by pituitary tumor.

E. If pupillary and visual field findings indicate an optic nerve lesion, progressive visual loss indicates a compressive lesion (e.g., glioma, meningioma). Careful neuroimaging studies are mandatory. Acute onset and a nonprogressive course indicate vascular or demyelinating (optic neuritis) disorders. If optic neuritis is associated with multiple sclerosis (MS), neurologic signs (brain stem, cerebellar, spinal cord) are usually present; however, optic neuritis may be the initial manifestation of MS (see p 300). Funduscopy shows optic pallor in optic neuritis; the optic disc initially may appear normal in retrobulbar neuritis.

F. Ischemic optic neuropathy may result in acute unilateral or bilateral visual loss. There is funduscopic evidence of disc edema, scotomatous field defect, and afferent pupillary defect. There is no effective treatment unless this is caused by arteritis such as temporal arteritis (TA). If the patient has headache, jaw pain, polymyalgia rheumatica, tender temporal artery, or elevated erythrocyte sedimentation rate (ESR), consider TA (see p 304). Retinal artery occlusion causes sudden unilateral visual loss and may be associated with carotid disease (see p 120).

References

Beck RW, Smith CH. The neuro-ophthalmic examination. Neurol Clin North Am 1983; 1:807.

Jamieson M. Loss of vision. Br Med J 1978; 288:1523.

Knight CL, Hoyt WF, Wilson CB. Syndrome of incipient prechiasmal optic nerve compression. Arch Ophthalmol 1972; 87:1.

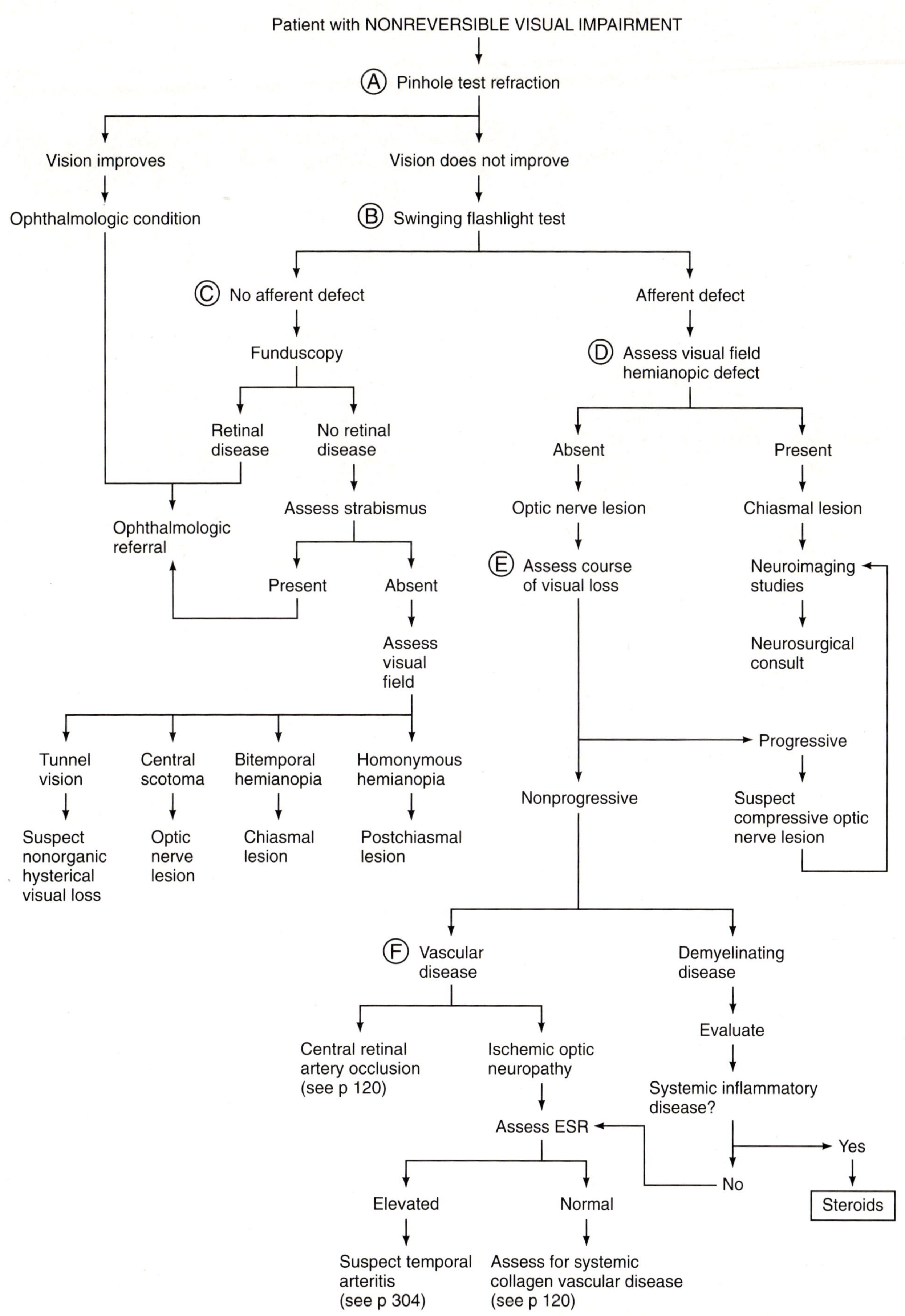

Patient with NONREVERSIBLE VISUAL IMPAIRMENT
A Pinhole test refraction
Vision improves
Vision does not improve
Ophthalmologic condition
B Swinging flashlight test
C No afferent defect
Afferent defect
Funduscopy
D Assess visual field hemianopic defect
Retinal disease
No retinal disease
Absent
Present
Ophthalmologic referral
Assess strabismus
Optic nerve lesion
Chiasmal lesion
Present
Absent
E Assess course of visual loss
Neuroimaging studies
Assess visual field
Neurosurgical consult
Tunnel vision
Central scotoma
Bitemporal hemianopia
Homonymous hemianopia
Progressive
Suspect nonorganic hysterical visual loss
Optic nerve lesion
Chiasmal lesion
Postchiasmal lesion
Nonprogressive
Suspect compressive optic nerve lesion
F Vascular disease
Demyelinating disease
Central retinal artery occlusion (see p 120)
Ischemic optic neuropathy
Evaluate
Systemic inflammatory disease?
Assess ESR
Yes
No
Steroids
Elevated
Normal
Suspect temporal arteritis (see p 304)
Assess for systemic collagen vascular disease (see p 120)

HEARING LOSS

Richard L. Strub, M.D.

The field of neuro-otology is concerned with specific symptoms (e.g., hearing loss, tinnitus, dizziness) in which there is a diagnostic overlap of neurologic and otologic disease. This decision tree and those on tinnitus and dizziness that follow emphasize neurologic conditions. The patient rarely seeks consultation with a neurologist for hearing loss. Rather, it is the otolaryngologist who refers the patient when the deficit is not readily explained by the otologic examination and a neurologic lesion is suspected.

A. Thrombosis or an embolus to the internal auditory artery or its branches can cause sudden unilateral deafness. If the occlusion is proximal or involves the basilar artery, other neurologic signs and symptoms will be present (e.g., dizziness, diplopia, facial weakness or numbness, long tract signs).

B. Acute bilateral hearing loss can be seen in viral infections (e.g., mumps, measles, infectious mononucleosis) as well as in meningitis.

C. The aminoglycoside antibiotics are the drugs that most commonly cause cochlear damage with resultant hearing loss. Furosemide and ethacrynic acid also produce hearing loss that is usually reversible.

D. Slowly progressive bilateral hearing loss is common in elderly patients, in whom sensorineural loss must be differentiated from the surgically correctable conductive loss of otosclerosis. Acoustic trauma resulting from noise is also a common cause of progressive hearing loss. Other rare causes are genetic disease, hypothyroidism, infection, neoplastic disorders, Meniere's disease, and multiple sclerosis.

E. Tumors in the cerebellopontine angle (e.g., schwannoma [acoustic neuroma], meningioma, cholesteatoma, lymphoma) often cause hearing loss as the initial symptom.

References

Meyerhoff WL. Diagnosis and management of hearing loss. Philadelphia: WB Saunders, 1984.

Osguthorpe JD, Melnick W. Clinical audiology. Otolaryngol Clin N Am 1991 24(2).

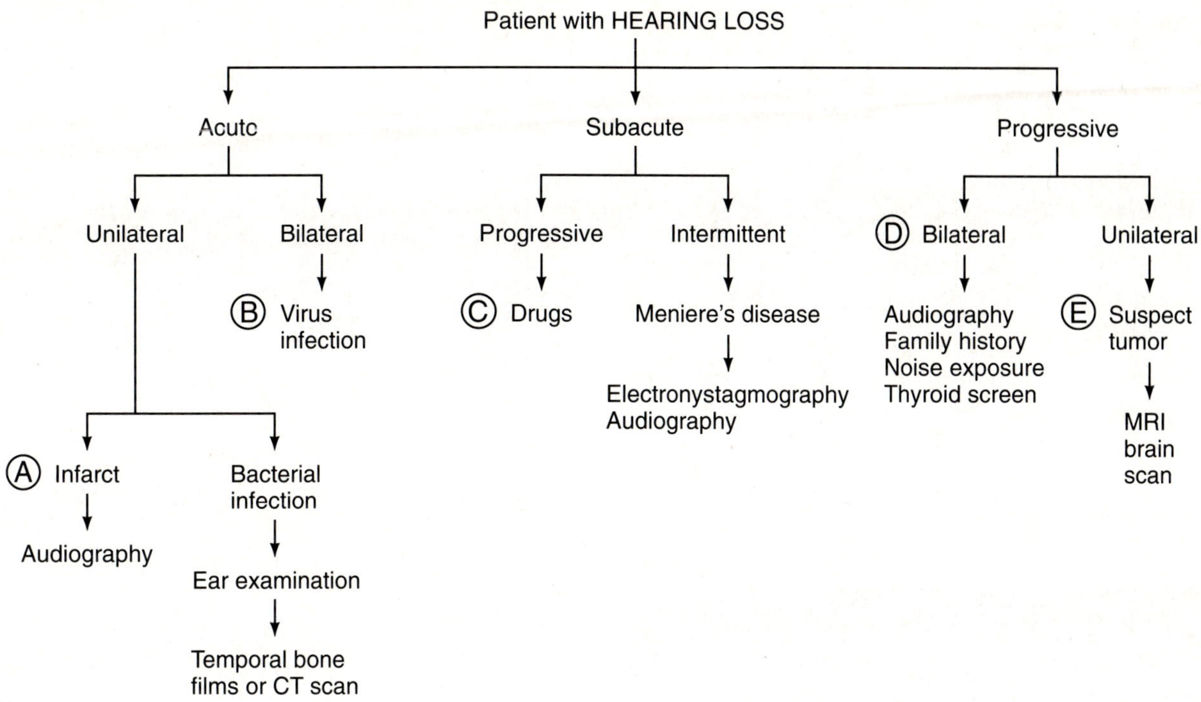

Patient with HEARING LOSS
Acutc
Subacute
Progressive
Unilateral
Bilateral
B Virus infection
Progressive
Intermittent
D Bilateral
Unilateral
C Drugs
Meniere's disease
Audiography
Family history
Noise exposure
Thyroid screen
E Suspect tumor
Electronystagmography
Audiography
MRI brain scan
A Infarct
Bacterial infection
Audiography
Ear examination
Temporal bone films or CT scan

TINNITUS

Richard L. Strub, M.D.

A. Subjective tinnitus is heard only by the patient. It can be caused by lesions in the external canal, tympanic membrane, ossicles, cochlea, cranial nerve VIII, brain stem, and rarely the cortex and is usually associated with some hearing loss.

B. In objective tinnitus the "noise" can be heard by the examiner when placing a stethoscope or his or her own ear over the patient's ear. Objective tinnitus is rare and is due to such uncommon disorders as an arteriovenous malformation, a glomus tumor (chemodectoma—a rare vascular tumor), palatal myoclonus (a rhythmic tremor of the palate), and the noise synchronous with respiration heard in patients with a patent eustachian tube.

C. Quinine, salicylates, aminoglycosides, indomethacin, carbamazepine, and aminophylline can produce tinnitus as a toxic symptom (they affect the cochlea and cranial nerve VIII).

D. When there is a neurologic lesion, such as a tumor of cranial nerve VIII, meningioma, brain stem stroke, or degenerative disease (olivopontocerebellar degeneration), other "neighborhood" signs are usually present (e.g., ataxia, Horner's syndrome, facial weakness or numbness, diplopia).

E. In most patients with mild tinnitus, reassurance alone is sufficient to allay their concern. In some patients, the noise is very loud and extremely stressful; in these, biofeedback, noise masking, or carbamazepine may help. Refer the patient to an otolaryngologist for management.

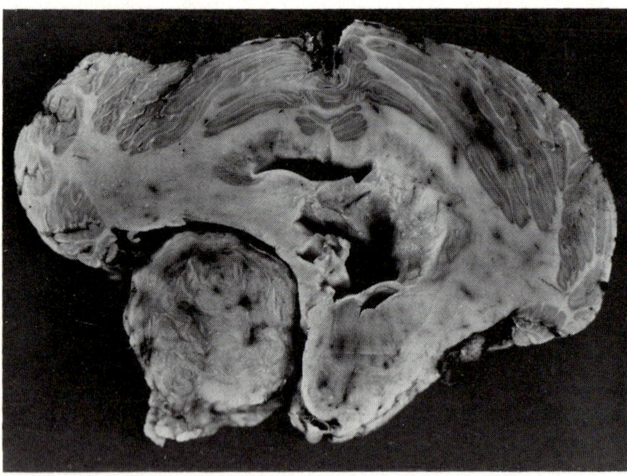

Figure 1 Acoustic nerve sheath tumor (schwannoma) compressing the cerebellopontine area.

References

Baloh RW. Dizziness, hearing loss, and tinnitus: The essentials of neuro-otology. Philadelphia: FA Davis, 1984.

Ciba Foundation Symposium 85. Tinnitus. Summit, NJ: CIBA, 1981.

Lechtenberg R, Shulman A. The neurologic implications of tinnitus. Arch Neurol 1984; 41:718.

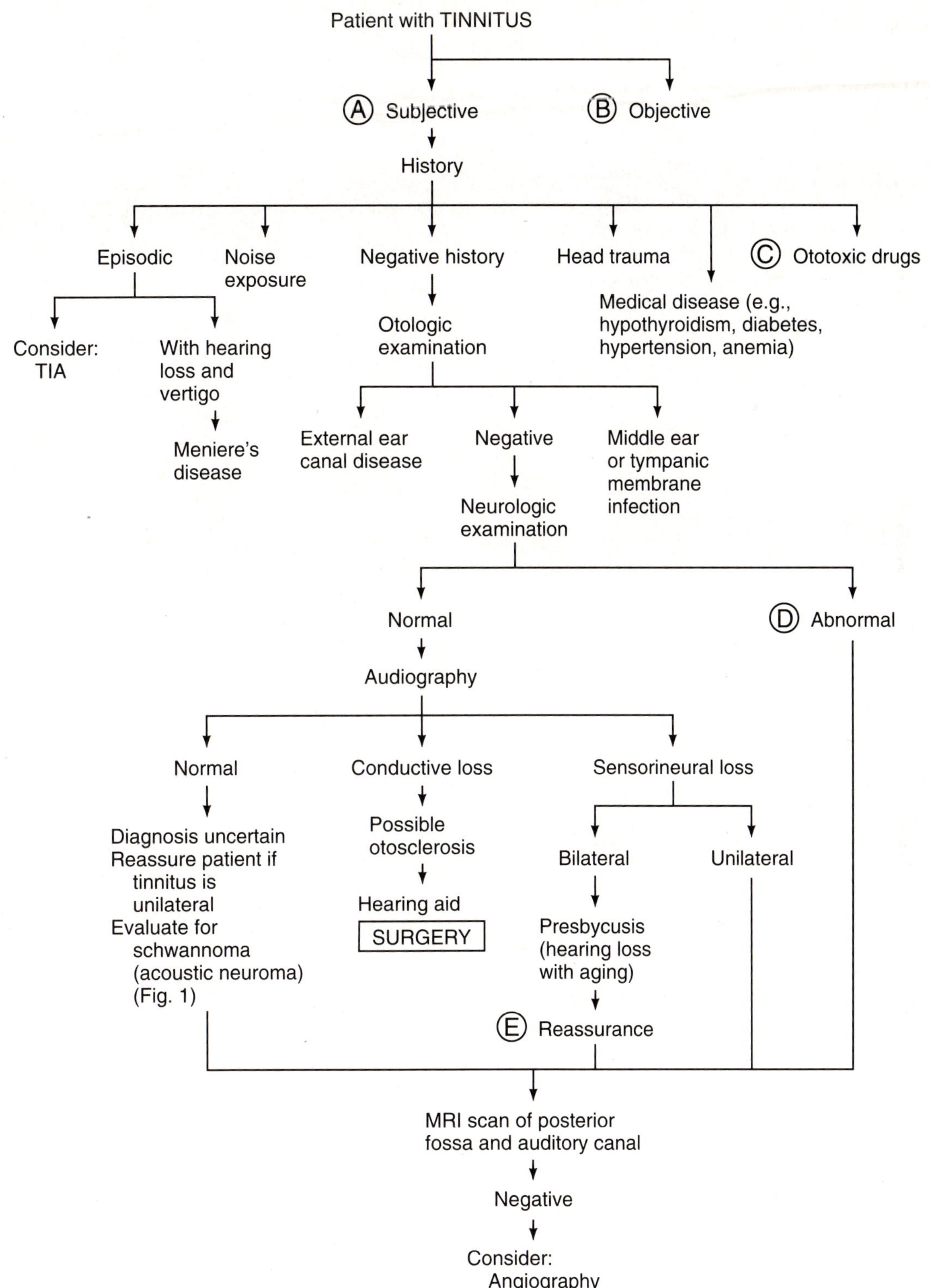

Patient with TINNITUS
A Subjective
B Objective
History
Episodic
Noise exposure
Negative history
Head trauma
C Ototoxic drugs
Consider: TIA
With hearing loss and vertigo
Meniere's disease
Otologic examination
Medical disease (e.g., hypothyroidism, diabetes, hypertension, anemia)
External ear canal disease
Negative
Middle ear or tympanic membrane infection
Neurologic examination
Normal
D Abnormal
Audiography
Normal
Conductive loss
Sensorineural loss
Diagnosis uncertain Reassure patient if tinnitus is unilateral Evaluate for schwannoma (acoustic neuroma) (Fig. 1)
Possible otosclerosis
Hearing aid
SURGERY
Bilateral
Unilateral
Presbycusis (hearing loss with aging)
E Reassurance
MRI scan of posterior fossa and auditory canal
Negative
Consider: Angiography

DIZZINESS

Richard L. Strub, M.D.

The term "dizziness" is used by patients to describe a variety of experiences: vertigo (a rotating or spinning sensation usually associated with disease of the labyrinth or its central connections), faintness or near-syncope, imbalance, or the nonspecific feeling of light-headedness (vague spatial disorientation). It is important when taking the history to establish exactly what the patient is experiencing. All types of dizziness can be psychogenic, but it is best to search diligently for an organic cause rather than conclude that the patient is merely nervous.

A. Light-headedness is a vague term and an equally vague sensation to the patients. They usually describe themselves as being physically somewhat lost in space, feeling as though they had just stepped off an escalator and were unsure of their footing. The feeling can be caused by many factors; presyncope must be considered.

B. Multiple sensory defects (poor vision, hearing, and proprioception) in the elderly make it impossible for them to orient themselves accurately in the spatial environment.

C. There are many sensory nerve endings in the joints and soft tissues of the neck that transmit sensory information to the vestibular nuclei in the brain stem. Some patients with cervical spine disease complain of dizziness with head motion; it is believed that this may be due to irritation of sensory nerve endings.

D. A number of neurologic conditions produce imbalance: cerebellar disease, marked sensory loss in the legs with neuropathy or spinal cord disease, mild hemiparesis or paraparesis, and basal ganglion disorders such as Parkinson's disease.

E. In general, head motion in patients with disease of the semicircular canals (peripheral vestibular system) increases symptoms, whereas it does not appreciably exacerbate symptoms in those with disease in the brain stem—vestibular system, or cerebellum.

F. In some patients, particularly the elderly, head motion itself produces vertigo. The condition is benign (hence, the name benign positional vertigo) but aggravating. On rare occasions, head turning pinches the vertebral arteries, precipitating a basilar TIA.

G. Acute vestibulopathy is a common benign disorder that is very upsetting to the patient. It is often presumed to be due to a viral infection, but this has not been proved. It is important to examine the ears, because bacterial infection (otitis or mastoiditis) also can produce this symptom. If symptoms persist or worsen, obtain an MRI scan. Meclizine and scopolamine are the most effective medications.

H. Some patients with posterior temporal lobe epileptogenic foci have seizures characterized by vertigo alone. In any patient with repeated short (minutes) episodes of vertigo, a seizure evaluation is warranted. TIA in the vertebrobasilar distribution is occasionally characterized by vertigo alone, but this is uncommon.

References

Baloh RW. Dizziness, hearing loss, and tinnitus: The essentials of neuro-otology. Philadelphia: FA Davis, 1984.

Baloh RW, Honrubia V. Clinical neurophysiology of the vestibular system. 2nd ed. Philadelphia: FA Davis, 1990.

Drachman DA, Hart CW. An approach to the dizzy patient. Neurology 1972; 22:323.

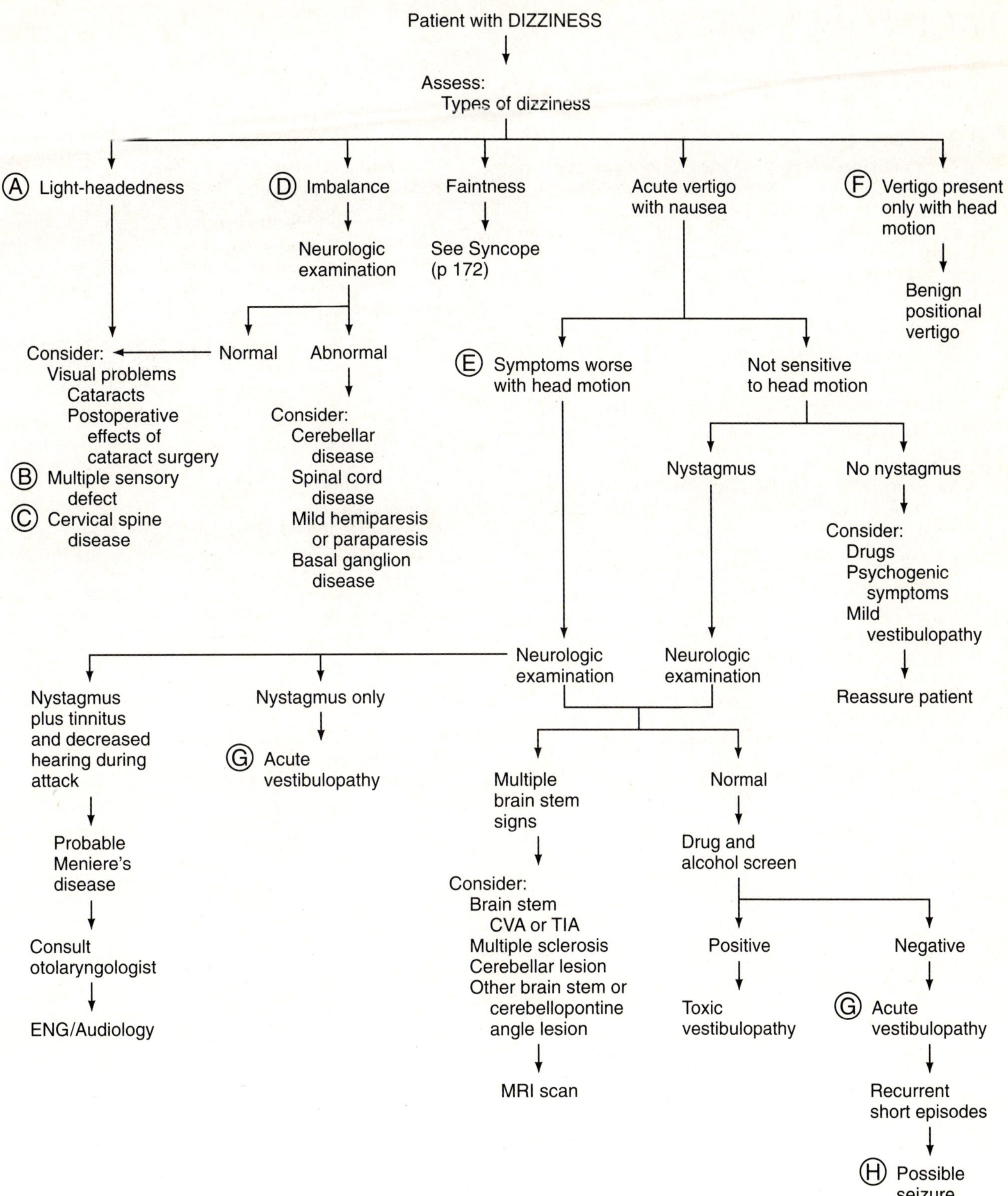

Patient with DIZZINESS

Assess:
Types of dizziness

A Light-headedness

D Imbalance

Faintness

Acute vertigo with nausea

F Vertigo present only with head motion

Neurologic examination

See Syncope (p 172)

Benign positional vertigo

Consider:
Visual problems
Cataracts
Postoperative effects of cataract surgery
B Multiple sensory defect
C Cervical spine disease

Normal

Abnormal

Consider:
Cerebellar disease
Spinal cord disease
Mild hemiparesis or paraparesis
Basal ganglion disease

E Symptoms worse with head motion

Not sensitive to head motion

Nystagmus

No nystagmus

Consider:
Drugs
Psychogenic symptoms
Mild vestibulopathy

Reassure patient

Nystagmus plus tinnitus and decreased hearing during attack

Nystagmus only

G Acute vestibulopathy

Neurologic examination

Neurologic examination

Probable Meniere's disease

Consult otolaryngologist

ENG/Audiology

Multiple brain stem signs

Normal

Consider:
Brain stem CVA or TIA
Multiple sclerosis
Cerebellar lesion
Other brain stem or cerebellopontine angle lesion

Drug and alcohol screen

Positive

Negative

Toxic vestibulopathy

G Acute vestibulopathy

MRI scan

Recurrent short episodes

H Possible seizure

FACIAL WEAKNESS

Richard L. Strub, M.D.

Weakness of the facial musculature may indicate a benign condition (e.g., Bell's palsy) or may be one sign of a significant CNS lesion, (e.g., stroke or brain stem tumor). Because of the seriousness of a diagnostic error, the following diagnostic scheme is designed to help the physician avoid the common pitfalls that lead to misdiagnosis.

A. The patient with bilateral facial weakness usually demonstrates weakness in swallowing and slurred speech.

B. Pseudobulbar palsy is caused by bilateral corticobulbar tract lesions; there are usually other long tract signs.

C. Movement of the forehead on the affected side is a critical factor in the differential diagnosis. If there is no forehead movement, the lesion is either in the facial nucleus of the brain stem (uncommon) or in the peripheral nerve itself (common). If the forehead moves well on the side of the facial weakness, the lesion is likely to be central (upper motor neuron eighth nerve weakness, seen in hemispheric stroke or a mass lesion).

D. Pay particular attention to the neurologic function of the ipsilateral arm and leg; if abnormalities are found there, a hemispheric lesion is strongly suspected.

E. With a peripheral type of facial palsy, the neurologic examination should concentrate on cranial nerve function (e.g., abducens weakness, Horner's syndrome, hearing abnormalities).

F. Idiopathic postinflammatory (Bell's) palsy is common and benign; if the patient lives in an epidemic Lyme disease region, a Lyme titer should be obtained. Facial palsy is one of the most common neurologic signs of Lyme disease.

G. Bell's palsy usually resolves, but it may take weeks to months. If spontaneous resolution does not occur and eye closure is a problem, an ophthalmologist can correct this surgically.

H. The differential diagnosis involves a vast number of possibilities, and most conditions are uncommon, e.g., rare stroke conditions, multiple sclerosis, brain stem glioma, and sarcoidosis. The type of evaluation must be determined by the case; for example, an acute brain stem syndrome in an elderly hypertensive diabetic patient would not occasion the same vigorous search for an etiology as would the same symptoms arising in a 20-year-old.

Reference

Taverner D. The localization of isolated cranial nerve lesions. In: Vinken DJ, Bruyn GW, eds. Handbook of clinical neurology, vol 5. Amsterdam: Elsevier 1969:52.

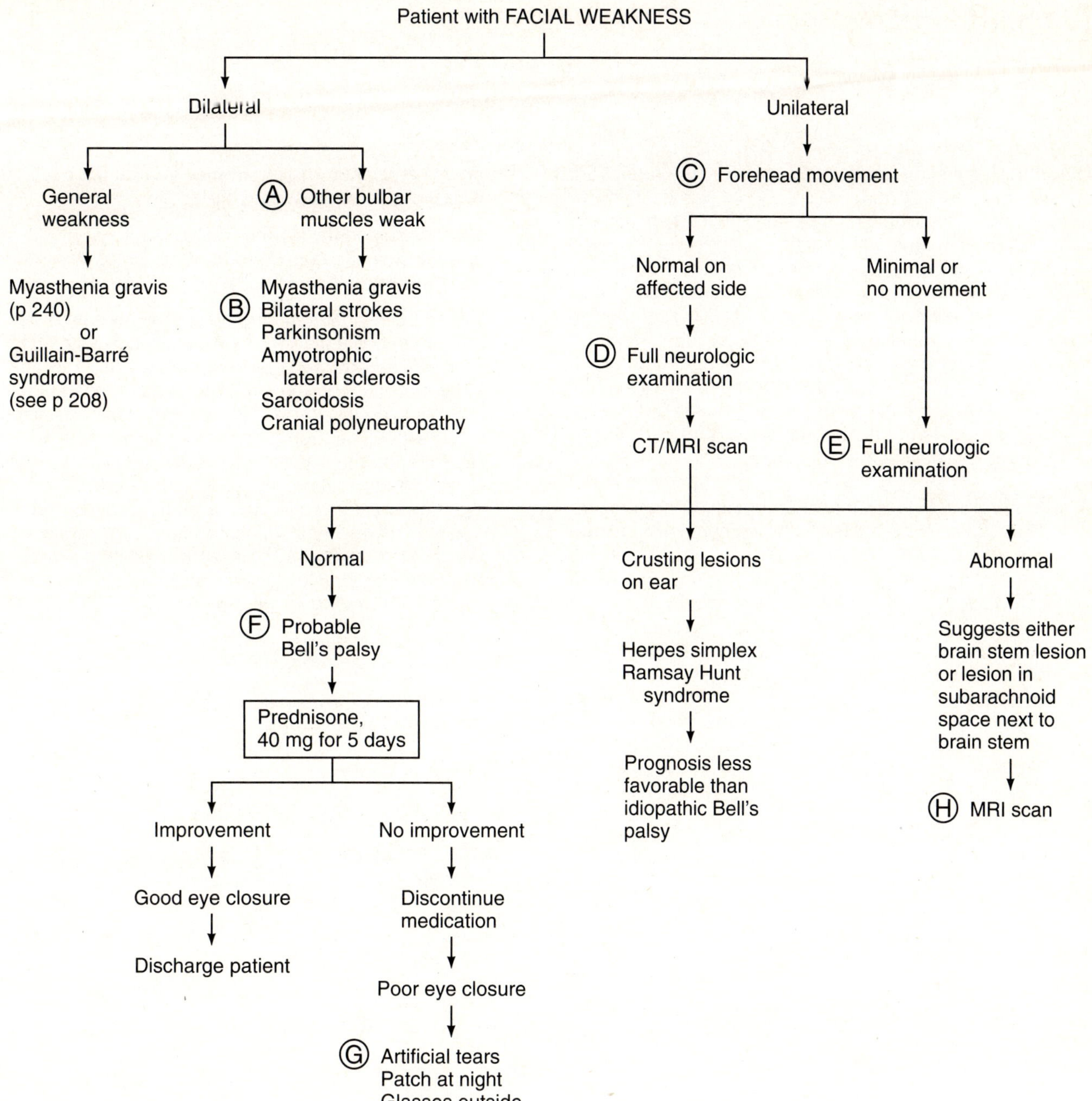

Patient with FACIAL WEAKNESS
Bilateral
Unilateral
General weakness
A Other bulbar muscles weak
C Forehead movement
Myasthenia gravis (p 240)
or
Guillain-Barré syndrome (see p 208)
Myasthenia gravis
B Bilateral strokes
Parkinsonism
Amyotrophic lateral sclerosis
Sarcoidosis
Cranial polyneuropathy
Normal on affected side
Minimal or no movement
D Full neurologic examination
CT/MRI scan
E Full neurologic examination
Normal
Crusting lesions on ear
Abnormal
F Probable Bell's palsy
Herpes simplex Ramsay Hunt syndrome
Suggests either brain stem lesion or lesion in subarachnoid space next to brain stem
Prednisone, 40 mg for 5 days
Prognosis less favorable than idiopathic Bell's palsy
H MRI scan
Improvement
No improvement
Good eye closure
Discontinue medication
Discharge patient
Poor eye closure
G Artificial tears
Patch at night
Glasses outside

DYSARTHRIA

Richard L. Strub, M.D.

Dysarthria refers to a distortion of speech production. Speech may be slurred, nasal, poorly articulated, or dysrhythmic. Dysarthria can be seen in certain aphasic patients in whom innervation of the muscles of articulation is affected along with the language areas of the brain. Many of the muscles used in articulation are also important in swallowing; therefore, many patients with dysarthria also complain of dysphagia. The examiner must learn to recognize the sound of the different types of dysarthria but also must perform a full neurologic examination to identify the particular neurologic structure or structures damaged (e.g., tongue, palate, vocal cords, facial muscles). In this way a more exact diagnosis can be made.

A. A full language examination involves listening to spontaneous speech; assessing comprehension; asking patients to repeat words, phrases, and sentences; and having them name objects, body parts, or parts of objects (e.g., watch crystal, coat lapel).

B. Because drug and alcohol abusers are not always frank about their habits, diligent questioning of both patient and family may be necessary to identify the toxic etiology of the dysarthria. Many prescribed medications, especially psychotropic and anticonvulsant drugs, can also cause dysarthria.

C. Spastic dysphonia is one variety of focal dystonia (e.g., in writer's cramp, torticollis). Botulinum toxin injection is a new and successful treatment.

D. The muscles of articulation are bilaterally innervated. Therefore, bilateral lesions are usually necessary in the corticobulbar tracts to produce dysarthria. The most common cause is the multiple lacunar infarct state seen in hypertension. Often, patients have sustained many small infarctions, each so small that no clinical stroke syndrome occurs with any episode. This results in the gradual, subtle, stuttering course of progressive dysarthria. Patients often have other scattered neurologic signs as well as emotional "incontinence" (laughing or crying at the least provocation), urinary incontinence, and dysphagia. Pseudobulbar palsy is also seen in multiple sclerosis.

Reference

Darley FL, Aronson AE, Brown JR. Motor speech disorders. Philadelphia: WB Saunders, 1975.

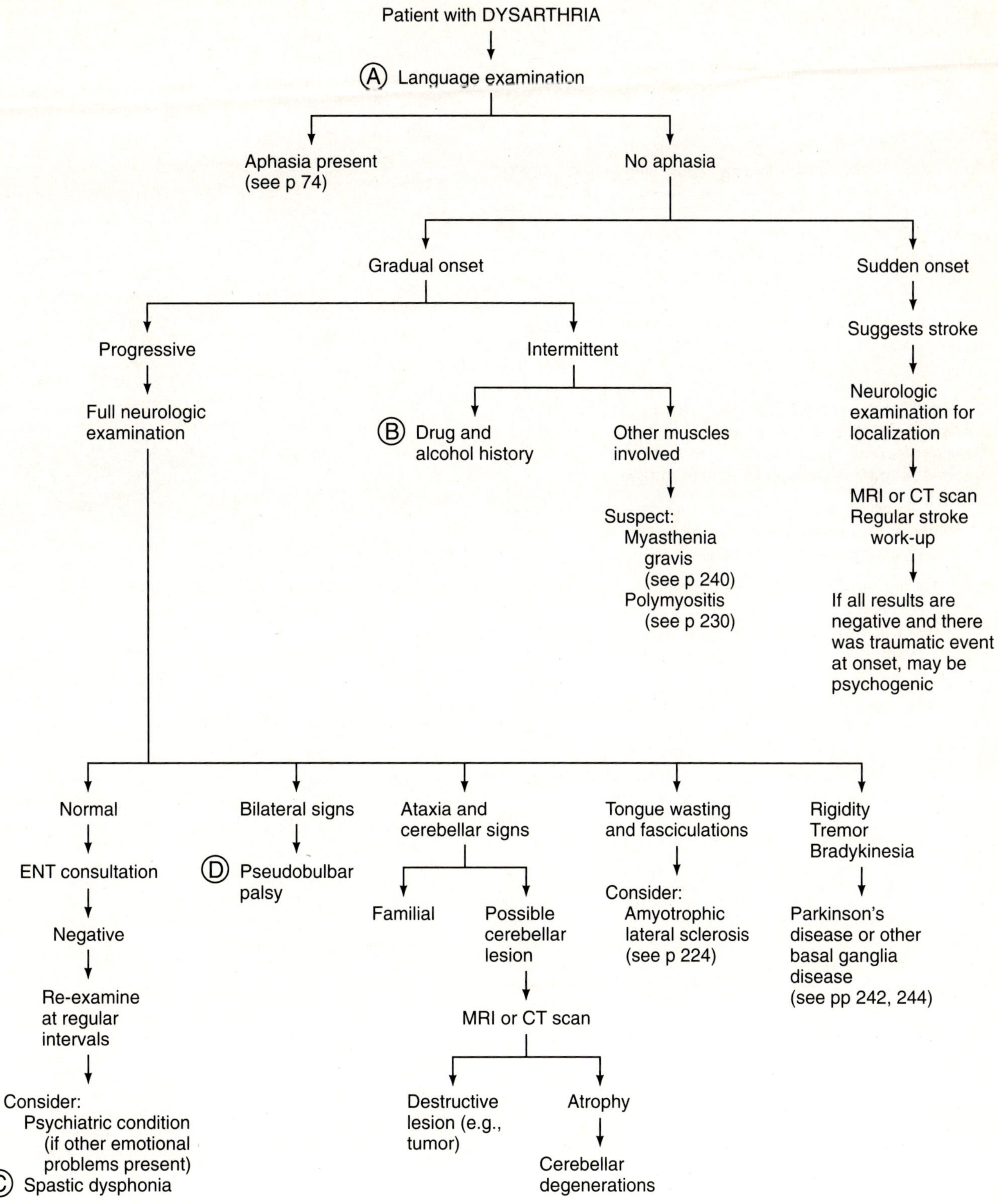

Patient with DYSARTHRIA
A Language examination
Aphasia present
(see p 74)
No aphasia
Gradual onset
Sudden onset
Progressive
Intermittent
Suggests stroke
Full neurologic
examination
B Drug and
alcohol history
Other muscles
involved
Neurologic
examination for
localization
Suspect:
Myasthenia
gravis
(see p 240)
Polymyositis
(see p 230)
MRI or CT scan
Regular stroke
work-up
If all results are
negative and there
was traumatic event
at onset, may be
psychogenic
Normal
Bilateral signs
Ataxia and
cerebellar signs
Tongue wasting
and fasciculations
Rigidity
Tremor
Bradykinesia
ENT consultation
D Pseudobulbar
palsy
Negative
Familial
Possible
cerebellar
lesion
Consider:
Amyotrophic
lateral sclerosis
(see p 224)
Parkinson's
disease or other
basal ganglia
disease
(see pp 242, 244)
Re-examine
at regular
intervals
MRI or CT scan
Consider:
Psychiatric condition
(if other emotional
problems present)
C Spastic dysphonia
Destructive
lesion (e.g.,
tumor)
Atrophy
Cerebellar
degenerations

APHASIA

Richard L. Strub, M.D.

Aphasia is an acquired language disturbance in which the patient makes errors in syntax, word choice, or comprehension. Most cases are due to lesions in the left hemisphere, although right hemisphere lesions can produce some aphasia in many left-handed individuals (rarely in right-handed people). Understanding aphasia is difficult, but learning to perform a simple aphasia examination significantly helps the examiner to categorize the language problem and localize the lesion. One of the main features of language used here is the degree of fluency. Unfortunately, all cases cannot be easily divided in this way and there are many mixed varieties. The classic neurologic aphasic syndromes are presented here. If writing is tested, the examiner will find that all patients with aphasias are agraphic (have difficulty with written language).

A. When assessing spontaneous speech, listen for paraphasias (improper words, such as greel for green), abnormal grammar, and general fluency.

B. Comprehension must be tested in such a way that the patient is not required to give full verbal answers. Ask questions that can be answered by "yes" or "no" or by pointing.

C. Transcortical aphasia is a category in which repetition is good but other language functions are impaired. The lesion is in the "watershed" or border zone of the hemisphere. If the maximal lesion is posterior, comprehension is poor (transcortical sensory aphasia). If the maximal lesion is anterior, spontaneous speech is poor (transcortical motor aphasia). This lesion is seen in patients subjected to hypoperfusion (causes include cardiac arrest, hypotension, carotid occlusion or tight stenosis, and bradycardias) or showers of emboli.

D. Broca's aphasia is seen with lesions in the frontal area and is usually accompanied by right hemiplegia (Fig. 1). Spontaneous speech is halting, effortful, and dysarthric. Patients are agrammatic and use principally nouns and verbs without other grammatical forms.

E. Wernicke's aphasia (poor comprehension yet fluent and often quite paraphasic speech) is usually produced by lesions in the superior temporal lobe and its environs. Hemiplegia is rarely present. This type of aphasia, because of the lack of neurologic findings and rather fluent incoherent speech, is often diag-

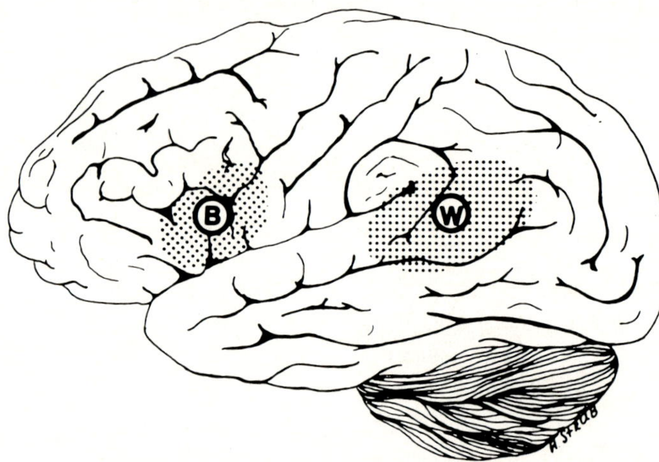

Figure 1 Lateral view of the brain. The stippled area *(B)* indicates the area of damage that can cause Broca's aphasia. *W* shows the area in which damage can produce Wernicke's aphasia.

nosed as a psychosis or confusion. The best single test to differentiate the two is auditory comprehension. Psychotics and confusional patients understand; patients with Wernicke's aphasia do not.

F. In conduction aphasia, the fluent speech is often paraphasic, as is naming. The lesion producing this type of aphasia is usually in the posterior sylvian fissure area, and it extends quite deep into the hemisphere.

G. Anomic aphasia is characterized by fluent, often paraphasic speech with word-finding pauses. Both inferior temporal lesions and parietal or frontal lesions can produce anomic aphasia.

References

Benson DF. Aphasia, alexia, and agraphia. New York: Churchill Livingstone, 1979.

Damasio AR. Aphasia. N Engl J Med 1992; 326:531.

Goodglass H, Kaplan E. The assessment of aphasia and related disorders. 2nd ed. Philadelphia: Lea & Febiger, 1983.

Kertesz A, ed. Localization in neuropsychology. New York: Academic Press, 1983.

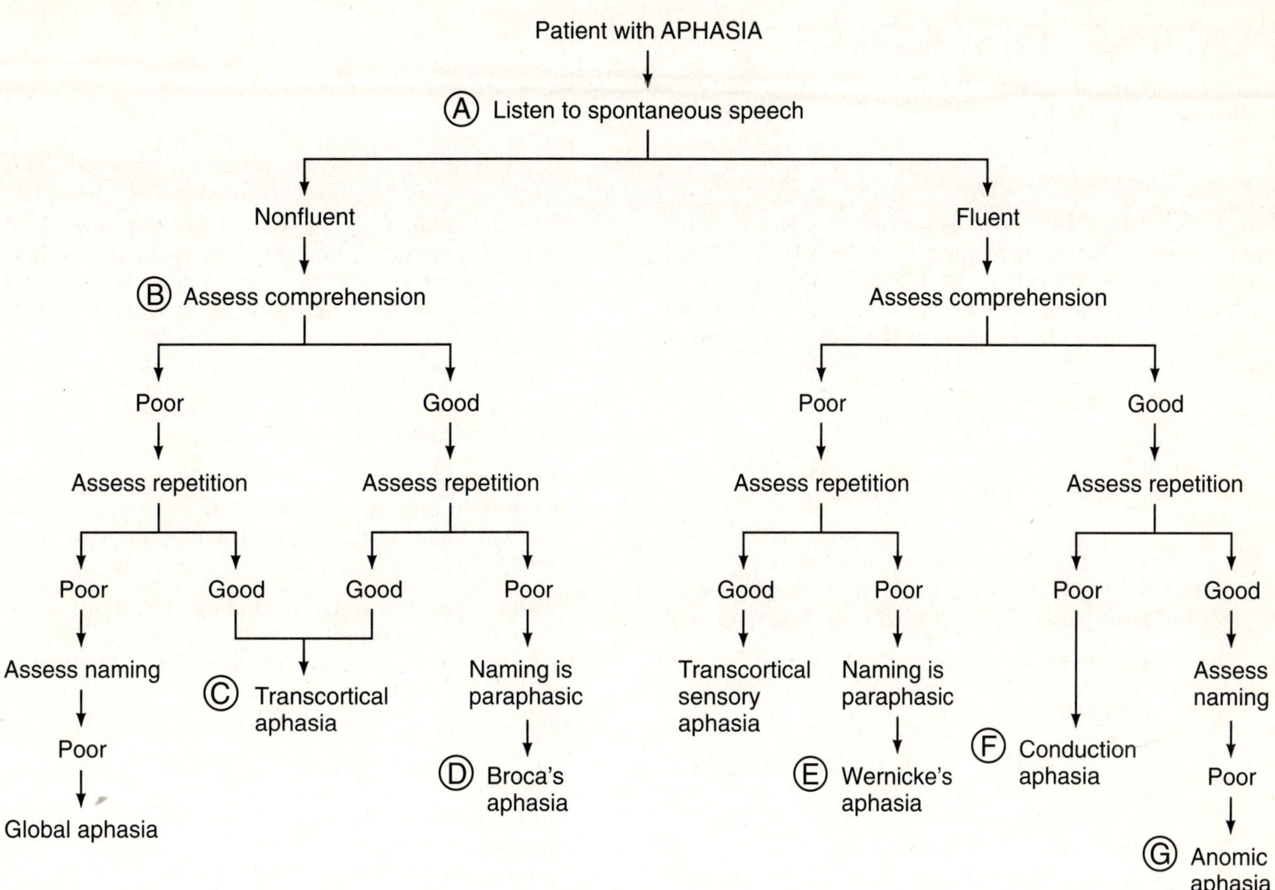

Patient with APHASIA
A Listen to spontaneous speech
Nonfluent
Fluent
B Assess comprehension
Assess comprehension
Poor
Good
Poor
Good
Assess repetition
Assess repetition
Assess repetition
Assess repetition
Poor
Good
Good
Poor
Good
Poor
Poor
Good
Assess naming
C Transcortical aphasia
Naming is paraphasic
Transcortical sensory aphasia
Naming is paraphasic
F Conduction aphasia
Assess naming
Poor
D Broca's aphasia
E Wernicke's aphasia
Poor
Global aphasia
G Anomic aphasia

READING DISORDERS

Richard L. Strub, M.D.

The ability to use a written language system is one of man's higher cortical functions. Since it is such a high-level function, not all individuals in a society are capable of learning to read and write. The various reasons for this are discussed in this section. Because reading is primarily a cortical function, it can be disturbed by damage to the areas of cortex that subserve reading—the left inferior parietal region in right-handed individuals.

A. A developmental reading disorder is one in which the individual was never able to learn to read well as a child.

B. One reason that children do not learn to read is that they have not had an adequate opportunity to go to school or to gain reading instruction at home.

C. Significant psychiatric disease (e.g., autism, childhood schizophrenia) or child abuse may preclude adequate learning.

D. The healthy child who has been to school but is not learning should be fully evaluated for visual and hearing problems and then undergo complete psychological testing. The psychological testing evaluates intelligence, emotional state, and the capacity to acquire specific learning skills.

E. Mild mental retardation is a common cause of reading failure.

F. Learning disabilities are disorders of learning in otherwise normally intelligent children who do not have significant emotional problems and have had an adequate opportunity to learn. Dyslexia is a specific learning disability or aptitude deficit involving reading. Other learning disabled children (probably a majority) have learning problems in various areas. Many also have difficulty in sustaining attention as an additional problem that interferes with learning (attention deficit disorder, minimal brain dysfunction, hyperactive child syndrome).

G. An acquired reading disturbance is called alexia. In all cases of acquired alexia the patient is assumed to have some type of cortical or other distinct brain lesion; because of this, a CT or MRI brain scan is indicated in all cases.

H. When reading is affected by a left hemisphere lesion, there is usually evidence of aphasia, agraphia (difficulty in writing), and other focal signs.

I. Reading problems are rarely the first and only complaint in patients with generalized brain disease. Careful mental status testing usually uncovers widespread cognitive loss.

J. Alexia without agraphia (writing problems) is an uncommon syndrome occurring with left posterior cerebral artery occlusion. There is usually right visual field loss. The lesion damages the corpus callosum and prevents the remaining visual stimuli (left visual field, right occipital lobe) from reaching the written language area in the left parietal lobe.

K. Strokes or other lesions that damage the left parietal area destroy all written language (reading and writing) ability. Aphasia is often present as well.

References

Benson DF. Alexia. In: Frederiks JAM, ed. Handbook of clinical neurology, vol 1. Amsterdam: Elsevier, 1985:433.

Duffy FH, Geschwind N, eds. Dyslexia: A neuroscientific approach to clinical evaluation. Boston: Little, Brown, 1985.

Friedman RB, Albert ML. Alexia. In: Heilman KM, Valenstein E, eds. Clinical neuropsychology. New York: Oxford University Press, 1985:49.

Shaywitz SE, Escobar MD et al. Evidence that dyslexia may represent the lower tail of a normal distribution of reading ability. N Engl J Med 1992, 326:145.

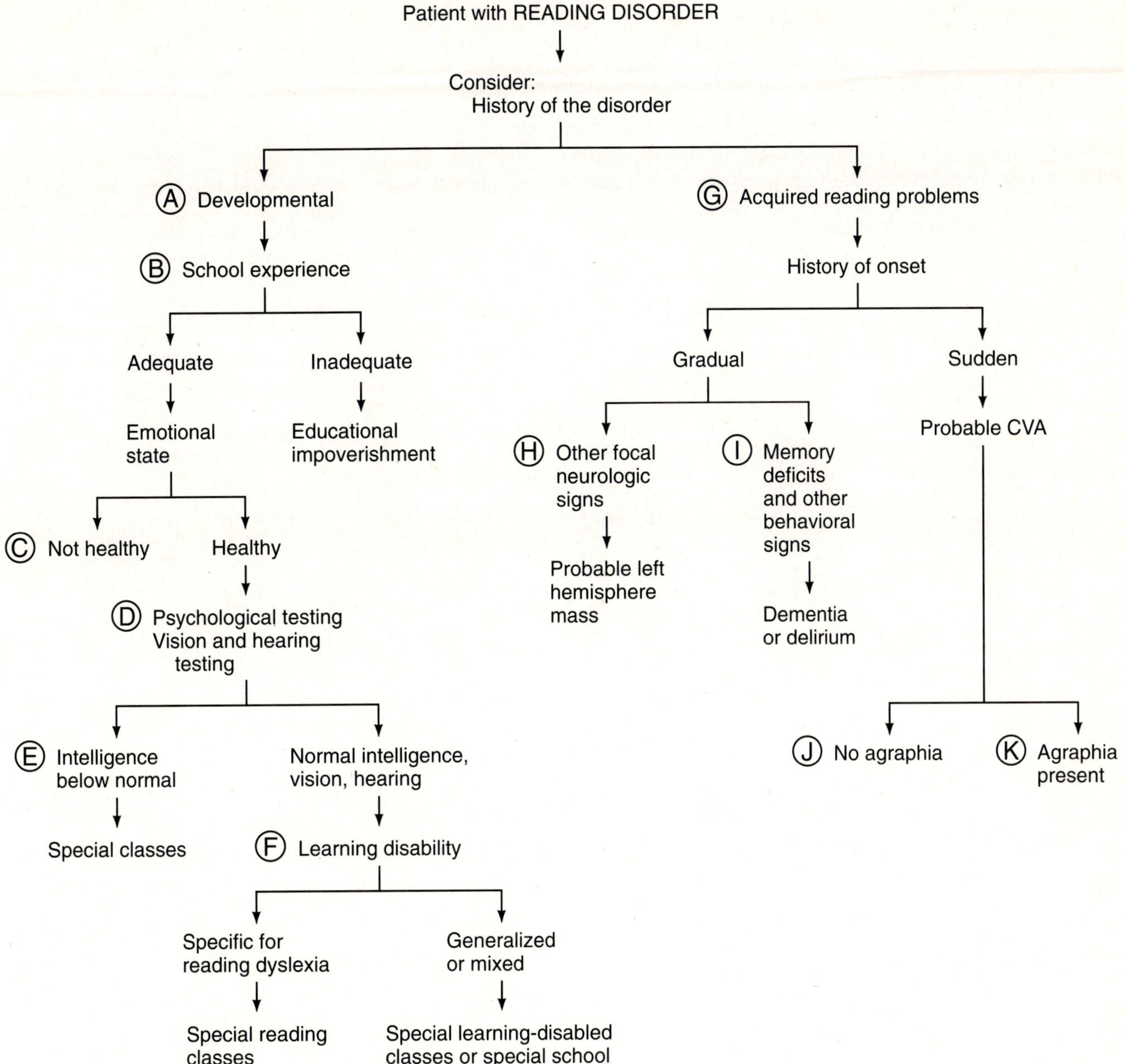

Patient with READING DISORDER
Consider:
History of the disorder
A Developmental
G Acquired reading problems
B School experience
History of onset
Adequate
Inadequate
Gradual
Sudden
Emotional state
Educational impoverishment
Probable CVA
H Other focal neurologic signs
I Memory deficits and other behavioral signs
C Not healthy
Healthy
Probable left hemisphere mass
Dementia or delirium
D Psychological testing Vision and hearing testing
E Intelligence below normal
Normal intelligence, vision, hearing
J No agraphia
K Agraphia present
Special classes
F Learning disability
Specific for reading dyslexia
Generalized or mixed
Special reading classes
Special learning-disabled classes or special school

BEHAVIOR CHANGE

Richard L. Strub, M.D.

Physical disease of the brain often produces a behavior change as the dominant and often only clinical symptom. Memory loss, intellectual decline, personality change, and delirium are all common organically based behavior changes. Such changes can be the manifestations of such diverse conditions as Alzheimer's disease, brain tumors, metabolic derangement, and stroke. The diagnostic problems are to determine whether the behavior change is secondary to physical disease and, if so, the type of organic process responsible. Several important principles or guidelines improve diagnostic accuracy and allow the clinician to develop a more efficient diagnostic strategy. The algorithms in this chapter and the following three chapters outline an approach to diagnosing the cause of behavior change based on the history, speed of onset of symptoms, and nature of the behavior change.

A. Determine whether the patient has experienced previous psychiatric illness. A 40-year-old woman who presents with depression and a history of depression as a teenager and again during her 20s is a prime candidate for a relapse of the depressive illness. She could have a frontal meningioma, myxedema, or cerebral lupus, but these are unlikely.

B. If the patient is elderly, it is highly likely that the behavior change is of organic etiology. Dementia, delirium (acute confusional state or metabolic encephalopathy), and strokes are all common in this age group. In younger patients, chronic drug use, metabolic disease, or brain tumor are more likely.

C. Behavior change in young adults is more likely to be emotional or drug related than due to structural brain disease. The key to diagnosis is skillful history taking, a physical and neurologic examination, and a complete mental status examination.

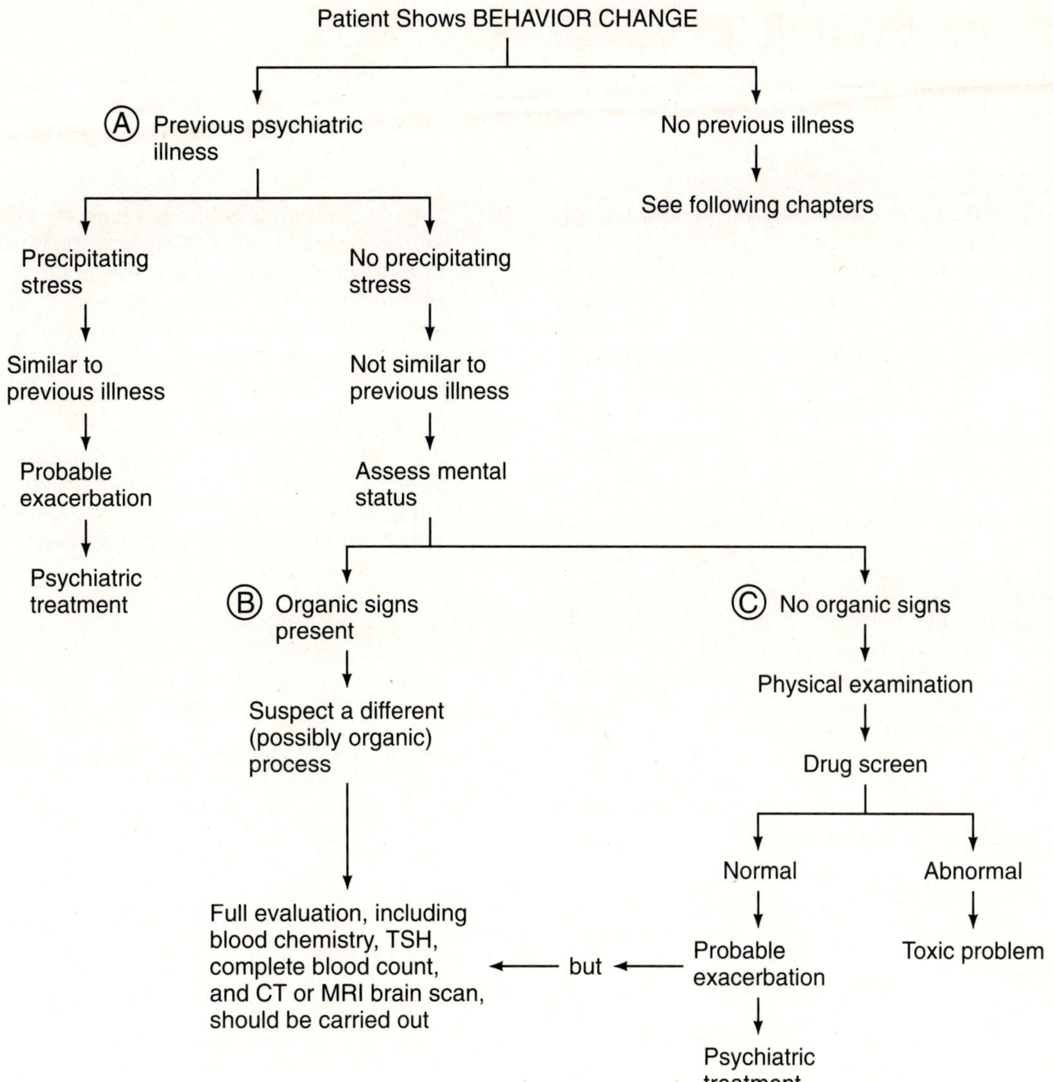

Patient Shows BEHAVIOR CHANGE
A Previous psychiatric illness
No previous illness
See following chapters
Precipitating stress
No precipitating stress
Similar to previous illness
Not similar to previous illness
Probable exacerbation
Assess mental status
Psychiatric treatment
B Organic signs present
C No organic signs
Suspect a different (possibly organic) process
Physical examination
Drug screen
Normal
Abnormal
Full evaluation, including blood chemistry, TSH, complete blood count, and CT or MRI brain scan, should be carried out
but
Probable exacerbation
Toxic problem
Psychiatric treatment

ACUTE BEHAVIOR CHANGE

Richard L. Strub, M.D.

The patient presenting with a new behavioral disorder must be carefully screened for organic disease. The initial diagnostic approach to this group of patient depends on the rapidity of onset of the symptoms: acute (seconds to minutes), subacute (hours to days or longer), or chronic (months to years). A separate decision tree is presented for each. Stroke, head trauma, seizure, and anoxia are the most common causes of sudden changes in behavior. In the elderly the possibility of a stroke should always be considered first. At times, behavior change has been gradual but not noticed by family; when it is recognized, the family often erroneously reports that the change was sudden.

A. A seizure, serious headache, imbalance, or vision difficulties should alert the physician to the possibility of a neurologic basis for the behavior change. A stroke affecting the frontal, parietal, or left temporal lobe often causes behavior change without any motor or sensory neurologic signs or symptoms.

B. The patient may have a history of mild alteration in consciousness, memory loss, and difficulty in doing work and then experience a sudden deterioration.

C. Any patient with a behavior change accompanied by neurologic or organic mental symptoms should be given a careful mental status examination, neurologic examination, and neurodiagnostic evaluation. It is suggested that the evaluation be carried out regardless of the examination findings because of the strong suspicion of organic disease raised by the history.

D. The decision whether to carry out CT or MRI is a major one; both diagnostic procedures are expensive. Because MRI demonstrates ischemic stroke much earlier, it is probably the best test if the patient can hold still during testing. CT is best if hemorrhage is suspected.

References

Strub RL, Black FW. Mental status examination in neurology. 2nd ed. Philadelphia: FA Davis, 1986.
Strub RL, Black FW. Neurobehavioral disorders. Philadelphia: FA Davis, 1988.

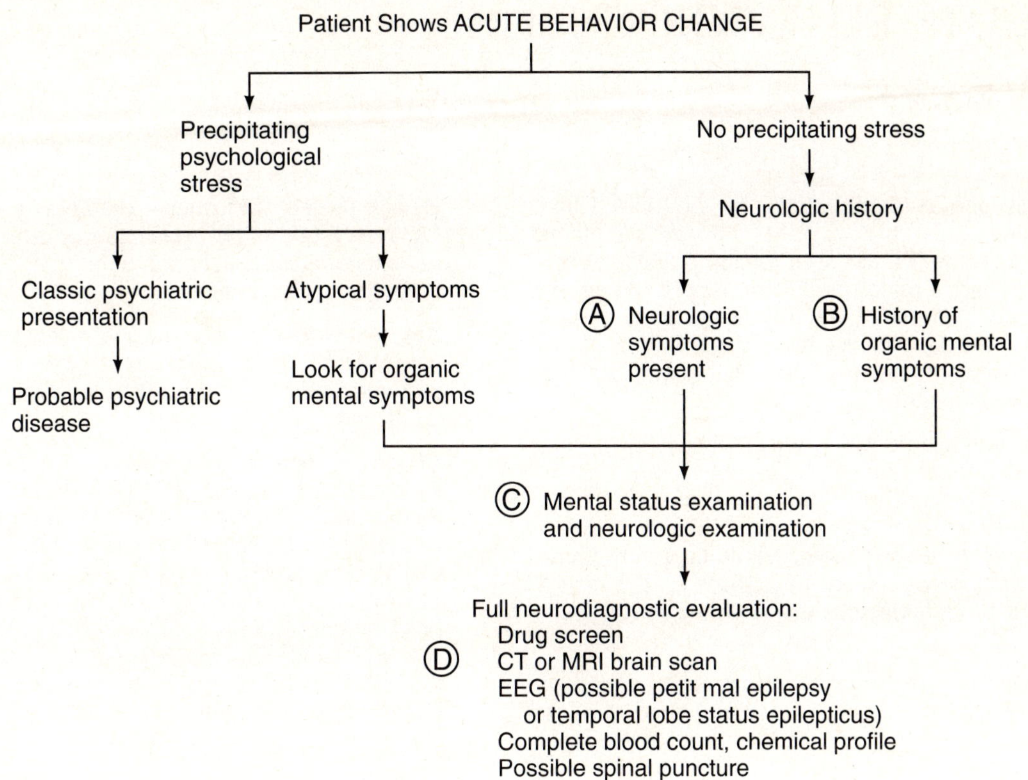

Patient Shows ACUTE BEHAVIOR CHANGE
Precipitating psychological stress
No precipitating stress
Neurologic history
Classic psychiatric presentation
Atypical symptoms
A Neurologic symptoms present
B History of organic mental symptoms
Probable psychiatric disease
Look for organic mental symptoms
C Mental status examination and neurologic examination
Full neurodiagnostic evaluation:
D
Drug screen
CT or MRI brain scan
EEG (possible petit mal epilepsy
or temporal lobe status epilepticus)
Complete blood count, chemical profile
Possible spinal puncture

SUBACUTE BEHAVIOR CHANGE

Richard L. Strub, M.D.

A. Although one is correct 98% of the time when diagnosing a psychiatric disease by its symptoms alone, brain tumors can occasionally produce symptoms that mimic major psychiatric illness. When the history, clinical course, response to medication, and symptoms are not completely consistent with a classic psychiatric syndrome, consider a full neurologic and medical evaluation.

B. Most patients who develop organic behavior change over a period of hours to days present in what is variously called a delirium, an acute confusional state, or metabolic-toxic encephalopathy. This is a common state characterized by lethargy, clouding of consciousness, inattention, incoherent speech, fluctuating course, at times hallucinations, and disorderly behavior.

C. Meningitis is one serious yet treatable cause of subacute behavior change. Fever and headache are usually present, but nuchal rigidity is a pivotal sign. Obtain a CT scan (Fig. 1) first to rule out a mass lesion or extensive subarachnoid hemorrhage before performing a spinal puncture.

D. Any patient with specific neurologic signs (e.g., papilledema, focal weakness, asymmetric reflexes) requires a full neurodiagnostic evaluation including CT or MRI.

E. Dozens of conditions can produce confusional behavior, but the most common are adverse reactions to medication, metabolic or electrolyte imbalance, organ failure (cardiac, pulmonary, hepatic, renal), sepsis, alcohol or drug intoxication, postoperative and intensive care situations, post-trauma confusion, and postictal confusion. Confusional states are commonly seen in patients who are senile or brain damaged, and the effects of the above-mentioned factors are multiplied in this population.

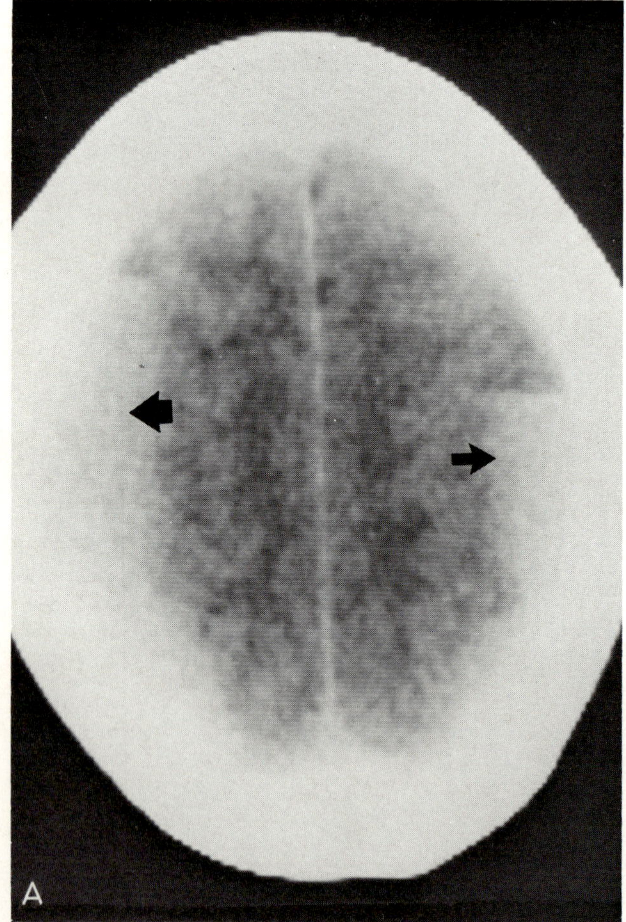
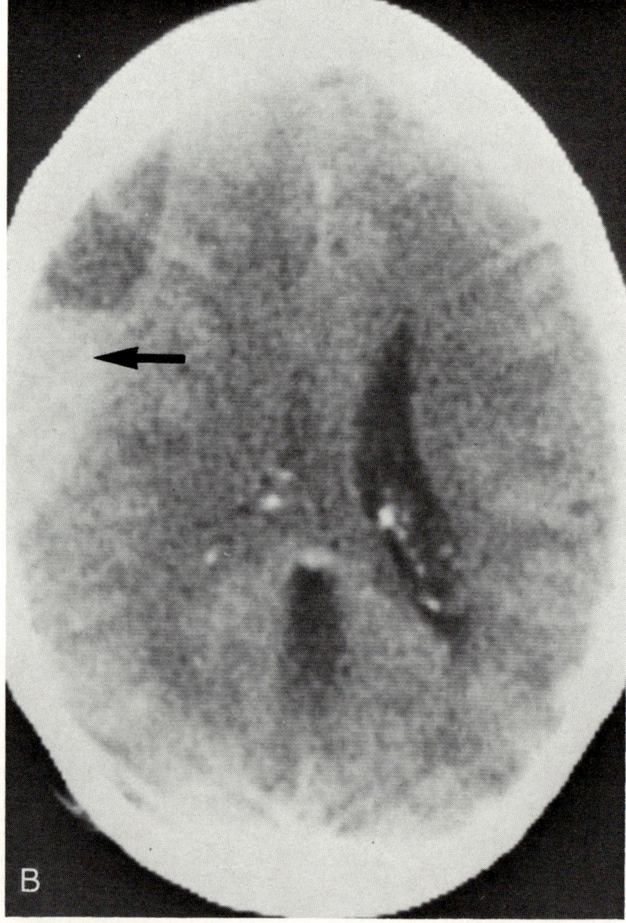

Figure 1   CT scan shows bilateral subacute subdural hematoma *(A)* with left hemisphere mass effect *(B)*.

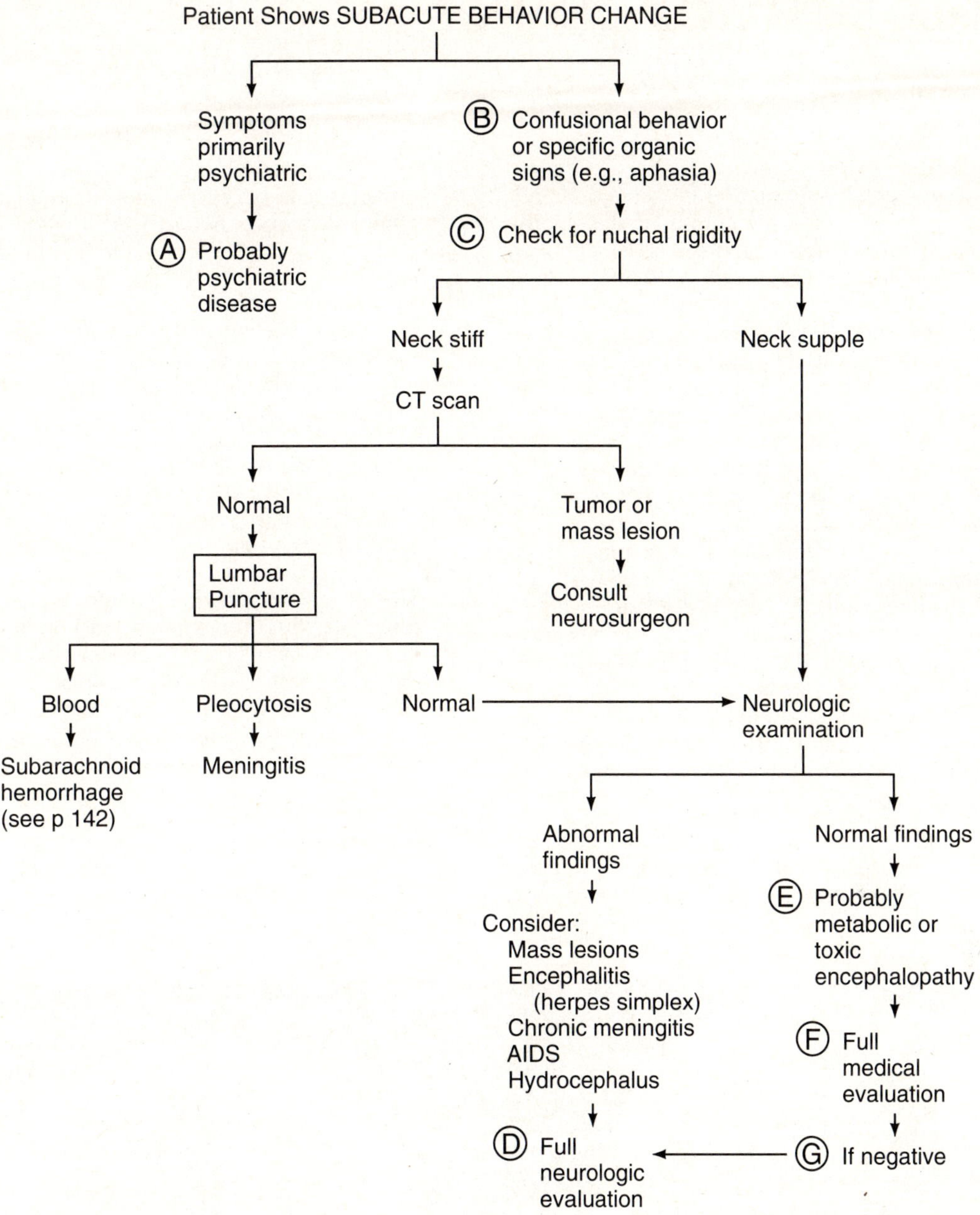

F. The most common causes of delirium are prescription medications, illicit drugs, alcohol, withdrawal of medications, postoperative state, organ failure (renal, hepatic, cardiac, pulmonary), sepsis, and electrolyte imbalance. Frequently a combination of toxic and metabolic factors is present, which is further aggravated by sleep and sensory deprivation.

G. If medical evaluation is normal, a full neurologic evaluation is indicated.

References

Lipowski ZJ. Transient cognitive disorders (delirium, acute and confusional states) in the elderly. Am J Psychiatry 1983; 140:1426.

Strub RL. Acute confusional state. In: Benson DF, Blumer D, eds. Psychiatric aspects of neurologic disease. Vol 2. New York: Grune & Stratton, 1982:1.

CHRONIC BEHAVIOR CHANGE

Richard L. Strub, M.D.

Slowly progressive mental deterioration is a common and important medical problem. It is seen mostly in the elderly and is often due to degenerative brain disease (dementia) of the Alzheimer type. Because dementia or senility is not always secondary to irreversible degeneration, it is critical that physicians view progressive mental change with the same diagnostic enthusiasm as they approach fever or chest pain. Several points need to be emphasized. Depression can mimic dementia and must be considered in the differential diagnosis. Both are characterized by lack of motivation, memory difficulty, and apathy. The depressed patient usually admits to being sad. Depression in the elderly is often quite different from depression in the young: there is less crying, less self-deprecation, more apathy, less suicidal ideation, and less guilt in the older patient. Chronic physical illness and the use of multiple medications can produce a chronic confusional state or encephalopathy that also simulates dementia. The younger the patient with dementia, the greater is the likelihood of finding an unusual nondegenerative cause. Demented patients often develop superimposed secondary depression, confusional states, or stroke; the clinical picture therefore is often complex.

A. Abnormal findings refer to any neurologic findings except snout, grasp, glabellar, and other primitive frontal release signs. A patient with dementia should undergo CT or MRI brain scanning; VDRL test; complete blood chemistry; CBC; and TSH, T_4, and vitamin B_{12} level determinations as a screening evaluation.

B. In communicating hydrocephalus, often called normal-pressure hydrocephalus, the dementia is usually mild. Evaluation includes CT or MRI brain scan and a lumbar puncture for pressure measurement (should be >110 ml CSF). Early Alzheimer's disease in a patient with significant myelopathy from cervical spondylosis can mimic this clinical syndrome. It is a good idea to obtain cervical spine films or an MRI scan of the cervical spine before shunting a patient.

C. The CT or MRI scan differentiates mass lesions such as tumor, subdural hematoma, and brain abscess. Usually, multi-infarction can also be identified, although the scans (especially MRI) can be confusing in the elderly. The history of multi-infarct dementia is usually one of stepwise deterioration with less memory loss than in Alzheimer's disease but multiple neurologic signs.

D. Alzheimer's disease is the most common dementia both in younger patients (45 to 65 years of age) and, particularly, in older patients (Fig. 1). Pick's disease is

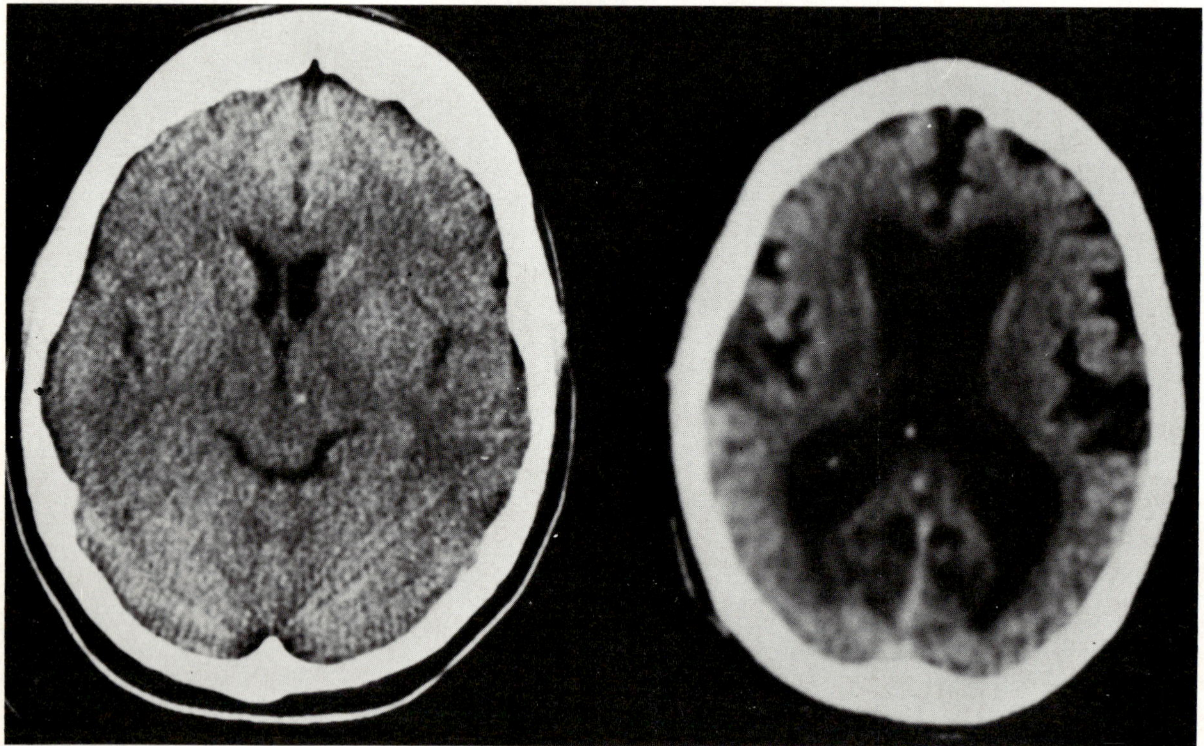

Figure 1 *Left,* CT scan of normal brain. *Right,* CT scan of a patient with Alzheimer's disease.

Patient Shows CHRONIC BEHAVIOR CHANGE
↓
Evaluate for signs of depression

Present → Mental status examination
- No organic signs → Probable primary depression → Psychiatric evaluation
- Organic signs → Possible pseudodementia or dementia plus depression → Trial of Antidepressants → Evaluate for dementia → Dementia

Absent
- No medical illness or medications → Mental status → Organic signs → Dementia / Normal → Probable normal aging or other emotional problem → Psychiatric evaluation
- Significant medical illness or multiple medications → Treat these → Unimproved → Mental status / Improved → Metabolic or toxic encephalopathy (chronic delirium)
- (E) Hypertension, TIAs, or history of CVA → Mental status shows dementia → Possible multi-infarct dementia → MRI scan → Extensive abnormalities → Probable multi-infarct dementia / Insufficient abnormality to account for dementia → (F) Consider: Alzheimer's with incidental CVA; Mixed dementia

(A) Neurologic examination

Abnormal
- Ataxia plus urinary incontinence → (B) Consider: Hydrocephalus → Shunt or Repeated Lumbar Puncture
- Focal neurologic signs → (C) Mass lesion or multi-infarct dementia
- Chorea (family history) → Consider: Huntington's disease
- Myoclonic jerks and parkinsonian features → Consider: Creutzfeldt-Jakob disease → EEG
- Optic atrophy → Consider: General paresis

Normal
- Evidence of meningitis
- Alcohol abuse → Consider: Alcoholic dementia → Yes → Lumbar Puncture → Consider: Syphilis, *Cryptococcus*, Other fungus

Obtain T₃-T₄, TSH, VDRL, B₁₂ ← No
- Positive → Treat accordingly
- Negative → (D) Probable Alzheimer's or Pick's

---

another degenerative dementia but is rare. Elderly patients with degenerative dementia may also sustain small strokes, and the picture of mixed Alzheimer's disease and multi-infarct dementia is not uncommon.

E. Pure multi-infarct dementia is probably not as common as reported. For this diagnosis to be made, the mental status symptoms and signs must initially appear abruptly and progress in a stepwise fashion with each new vascular event. The neurologic examination is usually abnormal and the examiner should be reasonably sure that the mental status changes are due to the cerebrovascular events.

F. Mixed dementia, in which a patient has Alzheimer's disease as well as strokes, is quite common. The strokes must be of sufficient size, multiplicity, or location to be truly considered contributory to the decline in mental status.

Reference

Cummings JL, Benson DF. Dementia: A clinical approach, 2nd ed. Boston: Butterworth-Heinemann, 1992.

MEMORY LOSS

Richard L. Strub, M.D.

There are two main categories of memory loss: an organic memory loss seen in diseases such as Alzheimer's dementia, and the amnesic or dissociative states seen in emotional disease. The organic memory disorder manifests as an inability to learn new material (recent or short-term memory loss); this is due to bilateral disease in certain limbic structures, usually the hippocampi of the temporal lobes (Alzheimer's disease, herpes simplex encephalitis, trauma) or a combination of the mamillary bodies and the dorsal medial thalami (Korsakoff's syndrome). Psychogenic amnesia (hysterical neurosis, dissociative type) is characterized by either a period (hours, days, or longer) that patients do not remember or the more long-term amnesia seen in a fugue state in which patients lose their identity and cannot remember who they are or where they are from. In psychogenic amnesia, patients can learn things during the amnesic period but do not remember them after that period is over.

A. A positive psychiatric history favors psychogenic amnesia, but a careful mental status examination is necessary.

B. Transient global amnesia is usually a type of TIA or migraine phenomenon in which the temporal lobes become ischemic. Postictal confusion or status epilepticus (absence or partial complex) can also present in this fashion. Patients are confusional during the attack and often ask the same question over and over during the episode.

C. After heavy drinking, particularly if preceded by an emotionally upsetting situation, some alcoholics act in a manner similar to a psychogenic amnesic episode. They may travel to a distant city and awake in the morning to wonder how they got there; this has been called a blackout.

D. Korsakoff's syndrome is usually heralded by a period of confusional behavior (Wernicke's encephalopathy) after heavy drinking. Early in Korsakoff's syndrome the recent memory loss is profound and is usually accompanied by confabulation.

References

Hodges JR. Transient amnesia: Clinical and neuropsychological aspects. London: WB Saunders, 1991.

Strub RL, Black FW. Mental status examination in neurology. 2nd ed. Philadelphia: FA Davis, 1985.

Strub RL, Black FW. Neurobehavioral disorders. Philadelphia: FA Davis, 1988.

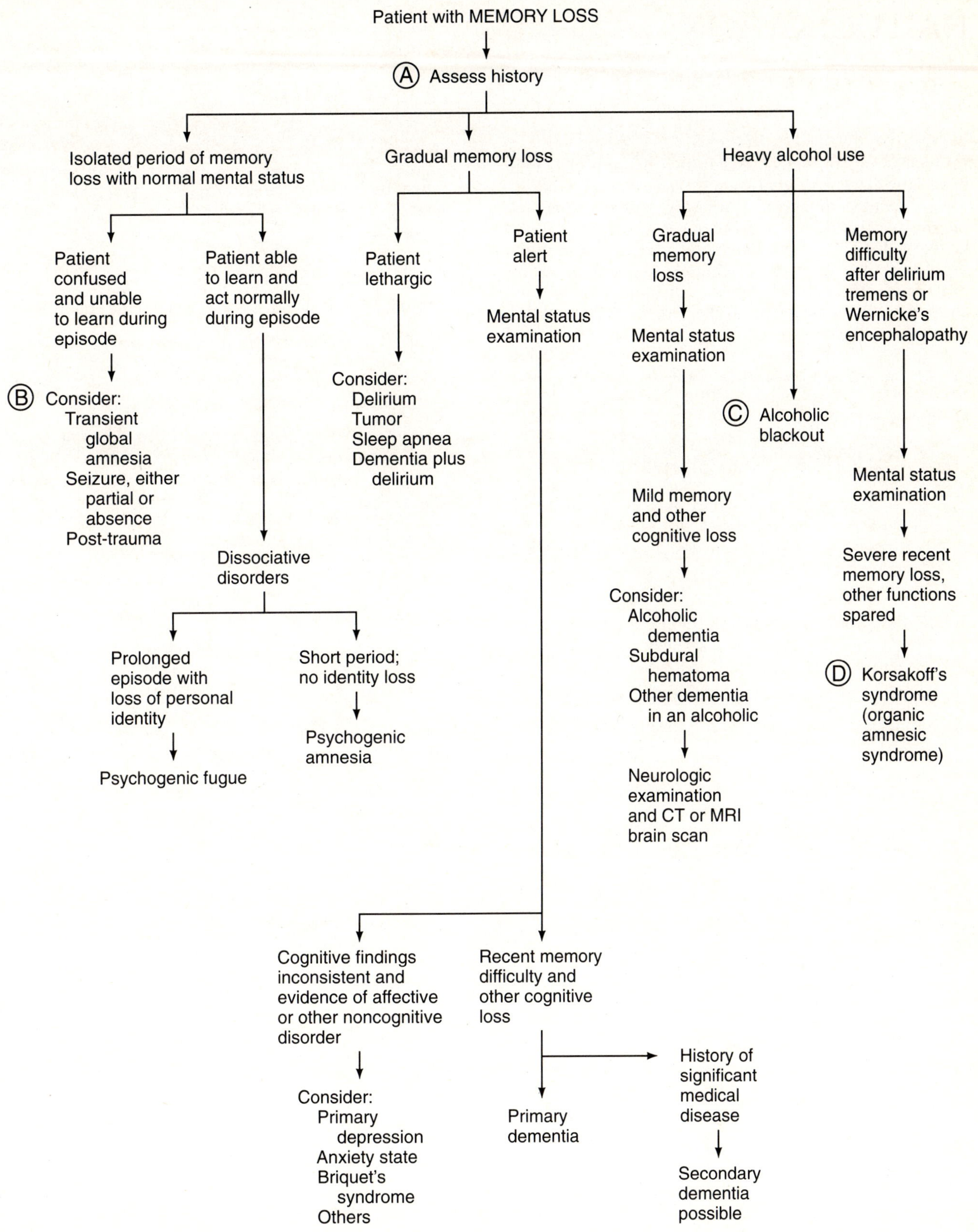

Patient with MEMORY LOSS
A Assess history
Isolated period of memory loss with normal mental status
Gradual memory loss
Heavy alcohol use
Patient confused and unable to learn during episode
Patient able to learn and act normally during episode
Patient lethargic
Patient alert
Gradual memory loss
Memory difficulty after delirium tremens or Wernicke's encephalopathy
B Consider:
Transient global amnesia
Seizure, either partial or absence
Post-trauma
Mental status examination
Consider:
Delirium
Tumor
Sleep apnea
Dementia plus delirium
Mental status examination
C Alcoholic blackout
Dissociative disorders
Mild memory and other cognitive loss
Mental status examination
Prolonged episode with loss of personal identity
Short period; no identity loss
Consider:
Alcoholic dementia
Subdural hematoma
Other dementia in an alcoholic
Severe recent memory loss, other functions spared
Psychogenic fugue
Psychogenic amnesia
Neurologic examination and CT or MRI brain scan
D Korsakoff's syndrome (organic amnesic syndrome)
Cognitive findings inconsistent and evidence of affective or other noncognitive disorder
Recent memory difficulty and other cognitive loss
Consider:
Primary depression
Anxiety state
Briquet's syndrome
Others
Primary dementia
History of significant medical disease
Secondary dementia possible

HALLUCINATIONS

Richard L. Strub, M.D.

Hallucinations are subjective sensory experiences in which there is no environmental source. They can be auditory, visual, tactile, or mixed. Auditory hallucinations are usually associated with schizophrenia, whereas visual and tactile hallucinations are common in patients with acute organic confusional states (delirium). Although this auditory-visual schizophrenia-organic dichotomy is true in great part, it is by no means exclusively so. Hallucinations differ from illusions, which are misperceptions of real things, as in the patient with delirium tremens who thinks that the IV pole is a Masai spear. A delusion, on the other hand, is a false belief and has nothing to do with distortions in sensory perception.

AUDITORY HALLUCINATIONS

A. Since there is some overlap in schizophrenia and alcoholism, it is suggested that such patients be evaluated for other organic lesions, such as partial complex seizure disorder (temporal lobe epilepsy) or brain tumor.

B. Some chronic alcoholics develop chronic hallucinations that sometimes persist through months of abstinence.

C. Schizophrenia can occur in middle-aged and elderly patients. It is best to carry out a full medical and neurologic evaluation.

VISUAL HALLUCINATIONS

A. A seizure beginning in the occipital lobe causes the patient to see colors and light flashes in the opposite visual field. In seizures originating in the posterior temporal area or temporo-occipital junction, formed visual images can be seen and a sense of movement experienced.

B. Demented patients, usually in the later stages of the disease, irrespective of visual acuity, may experience formed hallucinations (e.g., children and people).

C. With diminished vision, some patients may develop vividly formed hallucinations. These are called released hallucinations, for they seem to represent "released" stored visual images.

D. Lesions in the midbrain can produce elaborate visual hallucinations (so-called peduncular hallucinations). Patients may describe faces in every flower in the garden or nonexistent people in the house who seem to interact with them. The exact mechanism of the phenomenon is not known, but it may be associated with the same brain stem system that produces dreams.

References

Surawicz FG. Alcoholic hallucinosis: A missed diagnosis, differential diagnosis and management. Can J Psychiatry 1980; 25:57.

West LJ. A clinical and theoretical overview of hallucinatory phenomena. In: Siegal RK, West LJ, eds. Hallucinations. New York: John Wiley, 1975:299.

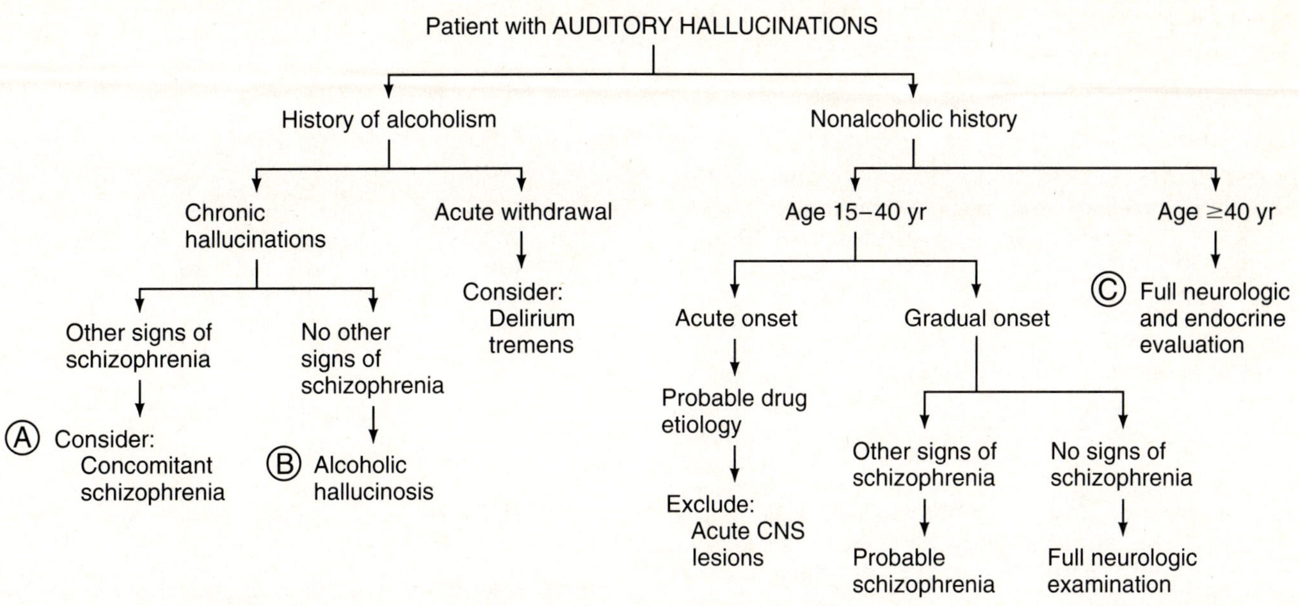

Patient with AUDITORY HALLUCINATIONS
History of alcoholism
Nonalcoholic history
Chronic hallucinations
Acute withdrawal
Age 15–40 yr
Age ≥40 yr
Other signs of schizophrenia
No other signs of schizophrenia
Consider: Delirium tremens
Acute onset
Gradual onset
C Full neurologic and endocrine evaluation
A Consider: Concomitant schizophrenia
B Alcoholic hallucinosis
Probable drug etiology
Other signs of schizophrenia
No signs of schizophrenia
Exclude: Acute CNS lesions
Probable schizophrenia
Full neurologic examination

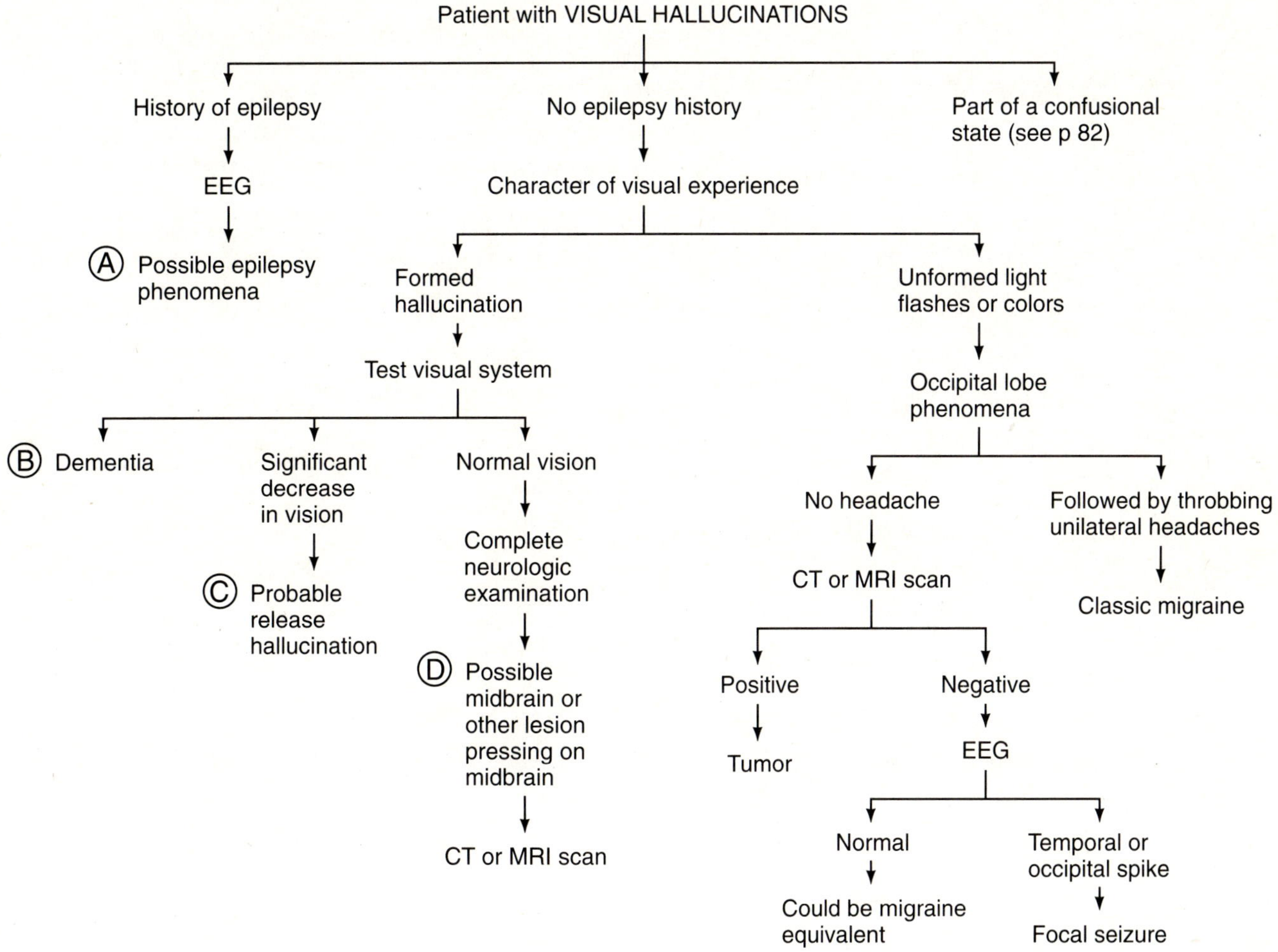

Patient with VISUAL HALLUCINATIONS
History of epilepsy
No epilepsy history
Part of a confusional state (see p 82)
EEG
Character of visual experience
A Possible epilepsy phenomena
Formed hallucination
Unformed light flashes or colors
Test visual system
Occipital lobe phenomena
B Dementia
Significant decrease in vision
Normal vision
No headache
Followed by throbbing unilateral headaches
C Probable release hallucination
Complete neurologic examination
CT or MRI scan
Classic migraine
D Possible midbrain or other lesion pressing on midbrain
Positive
Negative
CT or MRI scan
Tumor
EEG
Normal
Temporal or occipital spike
Could be migraine equivalent
Focal seizure

SMELL AND TASTE DISORDERS

Richard L. Strub, M.D.

Disorders of smell and taste are uncommon but sufficiently interesting to include in this book. Usually resulting from bilateral loss, the disease can present clinically in three ways: a lack of, or decrease in, sensation (anosmia—smell; ageusia—taste); abnormal or perverted sensation (dysosmia-parosmia, dysgeusia); and the perception of a smell when no odor-producing substance is present (olfactory or gustatory hallucination). The causes of decreased sensation are the same as those causing abnormal sensation. Smell sensation is tested with aromatic substances (e.g., spices) and not with strongly irritating substances such as ammonia. Taste is tested by rubbing sugar or salt along one side of the tongue with a cotton applicator. Treatment with zinc sulfate is sometimes helpful in these disorders.

SMELL

A. Temporal lobe disease with an epileptic focus often produces an olfactory aura as part of a partial complex seizure.

B. Congenital anosmia does occur and is regularly seen in albinism.

C. Some influenza and upper respiratory viruses can affect the sense of smell. These usually affect the olfactory system bilaterally. Fortunately, many cases are reversible.

D. Frontal head trauma can cause damage to olfactory nerve endings at the base of the frontal lobes; this mechanism is the most common neurologic cause of anosmia. Frontal craniotomy also often causes anosmia.

E. Any disease that causes inflammation and scarring in the subfrontal subarachnoid space can produce anosmia.

F. Most smell disturbances are due to disease or dysfunction of the nasal mucosa (e.g., membranous rhinitis, atrophic rhinitis, smoking). Sinusitis may cause patients to perceive foul odors (dysosmia, parosmia).

G. Some patients with severe psychiatric disease have the delusion that foul odors are coming from their own bodies or from the environment.

H. A patient with loss of the sense of smell in one nostril usually does not complain of anosmia. If the physician discovers unilateral anosmia, a subfrontal tumor, particularly an olfactory groove meningioma, should be sought.

TASTE

A. Gustatory hallucinations can occur with an epileptic focus in the secondary sensory cortex and insula; they are also seen in severe psychiatric disease.

B. In Bell's palsy, there is often a dysfunction of taste on the posterior third of the tongue on the side of the lesion. The patient may complain of some loss of taste or, more often, an odd taste to food.

C. Viral infections can affect the nerve fibers for taste and cause food to lose its taste or have a very abnormal taste (e.g., very salty or bitter).

D. Many medications produce either a decrease in taste (ageusia) or a distortion of the sense of taste (dysgeusia) (Table 1).

E. The patient with Eaton-Lambert syndrome (myasthenic syndrome, paraneoplastic) often has a dry mouth and complains of a metallic taste.

TABLE 1 Medications That Cause Ageusia and Dysgeusia

Ageusia	Dysgeusia
L-Dopa	Ethambutol
Penicillamine	Vitamin D
Butazolidin	Gold
Amphotericin	Allopurinol
Azulfidine	Flagyl
Azathioprine	Lincomycin
Tegretol-carbamazepine	Aspirin
Baclofen	

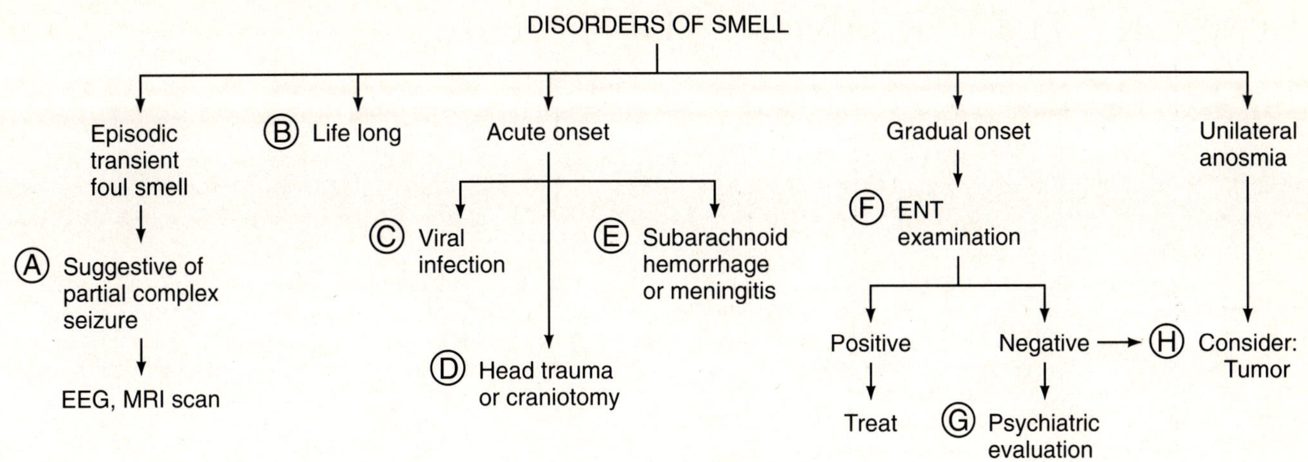

DISORDERS OF SMELL
Episodic transient foul smell
B Life long
Acute onset
Gradual onset
Unilateral anosmia
A Suggestive of partial complex seizure
EEG, MRI scan
C Viral infection
E Subarachnoid hemorrhage or meningitis
D Head trauma or craniotomy
F ENT examination
Positive
Negative
H Consider: Tumor
Treat
G Psychiatric evaluation

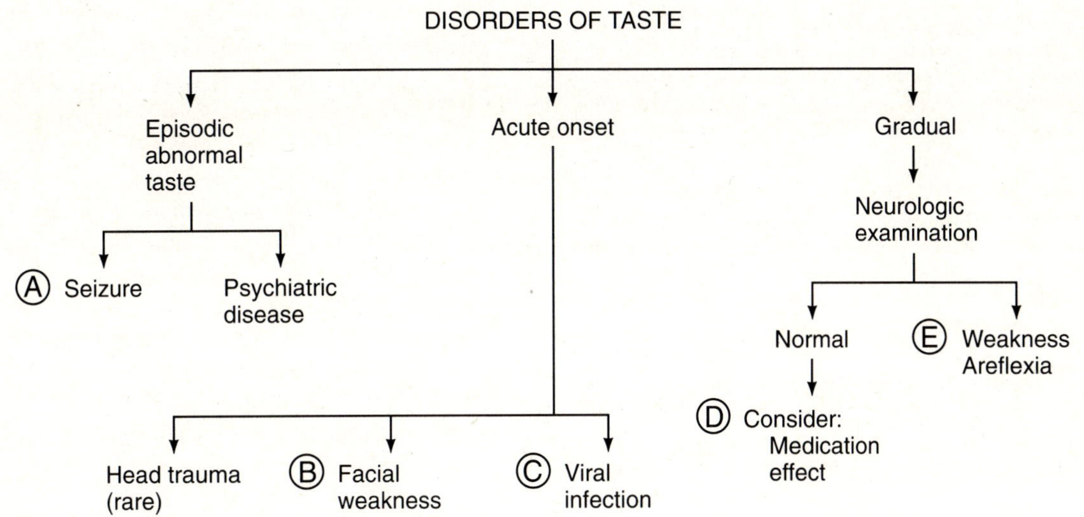

DISORDERS OF TASTE
Episodic abnormal taste
Acute onset
Gradual
A Seizure
Psychiatric disease
Neurologic examination
Head trauma (rare)
B Facial weakness
C Viral infection
Normal
E Weakness Areflexia
D Consider: Medication effect

SENSORY DISTURBANCE: SUPERFICIAL SENSATION

Carlos A. Garcia, M.D.

The sensory examination is a subjective test that requires the full cooperation and concentration of an alert, intelligent, and reliable patient. The testing of sensory modalities should be brief and the patient carefully instructed about the type of response expected. Testing should be done early in the examination before fatigue occurs. Only painful sensations (pricking, deep pain) can be tested in patients who are not fully alert (delirious, demented, lethargic, comatose).

Patients with peripheral neuropathies may complain of numbness, pins and needles, tingling, and crawling sensations. These spontaneous sensations are called paresthesias. If the paresthesias are unusually painful and burning and are precipitated by minor stimuli (e.g., feet touching bed sheets), they are called hyperesthesias or dysesthesias. An unpleasant, explosive, severely painful sensation triggered by painful stimuli is called hyperpathia; this usually indicates a thalamic lesion ("thalamic pain"). Patients with analgesia (loss) or hypalgesia (decreased painful sensations) have no complaints but may show scars (burned hands) or mutilations of fingers or toes.

Disorders of sensation may be due to alterations in superficial sensations, including touch, pricking pain, and temperature; deep sensations or proprioception, including vibratory, position sense, and deep pain; and cortical or combined sensations, including two-point discrimination and stereognosia (ability to recognize an object by its shape when the patient holds it in the hand without seeing it). Loss of cortical sensation or combined sensations indicate a contralateral parietal (cortical lobe) lesion. Touch sensation is preserved in most sensory disturbances because touch fibers travel in several fasciculi of the spinal cord, and sensation is affected only in transverse myelopathies or severe peripheral neuropathies. Pricking pain and temperature fibers travel together and are altered in the same types of lesions. The fibers cross the midline through the ventral commissure adjacent to the central canal of the spinal cord and ascend in the opposite spinothalamic tract; this explains the loss of temperature and pain sensations with preservation of touch in syringomyelia. For practical purposes, the sensory examination should focus on the detection of abnormalities of pricking pain and vibratory and position senses.

A. The decrease in superficial pain sensation may be symmetric and distal in a stocking and glove distribution, as seen in sensory polyneuropathies (e.g., diabetes, paraneoplastic syndromes). If proprioception is impaired in the legs, the patient may have an unsteady gait, especially with the eyes closed (positive Romberg sign); this represents sensory ataxia.

B. When the superficial sensory loss is in a dermatomal distribution and affects only pricking and temperature with preservation of touch (sensory dissociation), there is a central spinal cord lesion, as seen in intramedullary tumors or syringomyelia.

C. When all modalities of sensation are lost in a segmental fashion and a sensory level is discovered, there is a transverse spinal cord lesion (myelopathy).

D. Asymmetric superficial sensory loss may affect only one nerve (mononeuropathy), multiple nerves in different areas (multiple mononeuropathy), or multiple adjacent nerves.

E. Patchy, poorly localized sensory loss associated with corticospinal tract lesions distally is usually seen in intramedullary infiltrative tumors. Isolated patchy superficial sensory loss may be seen in leprosy.

F. When only one side is affected in a segmental fashion associated with contralateral weakness and contralateral loss of proprioception, there is a hemisection of the spinal cord on the side of the weakness (Brown-Séquard syndrome). The lesion may be a traumatic hemisection, or a compressive lesion produced by a laterally protruded disc or an extramedullary tumor.

G. A hemisensory deficit affecting one side of the face and the contralateral trunk and extremities indicates a medullary-pontine lesion, with involvement of the trigeminal sensory nucleus on the side of the lesion and contralateral ascending spinothalamic tracts that decussate in the spinal cord.

References

Haerer AF. DeJong's the neurologic examination. 5th ed. Philadelphia: JB Lippincott, 1992.

Mayo Clinic and Mayo Foundation. Clinical examinations in neurology. 6th ed. St. Louis: Mosby—Year Book, 1991.

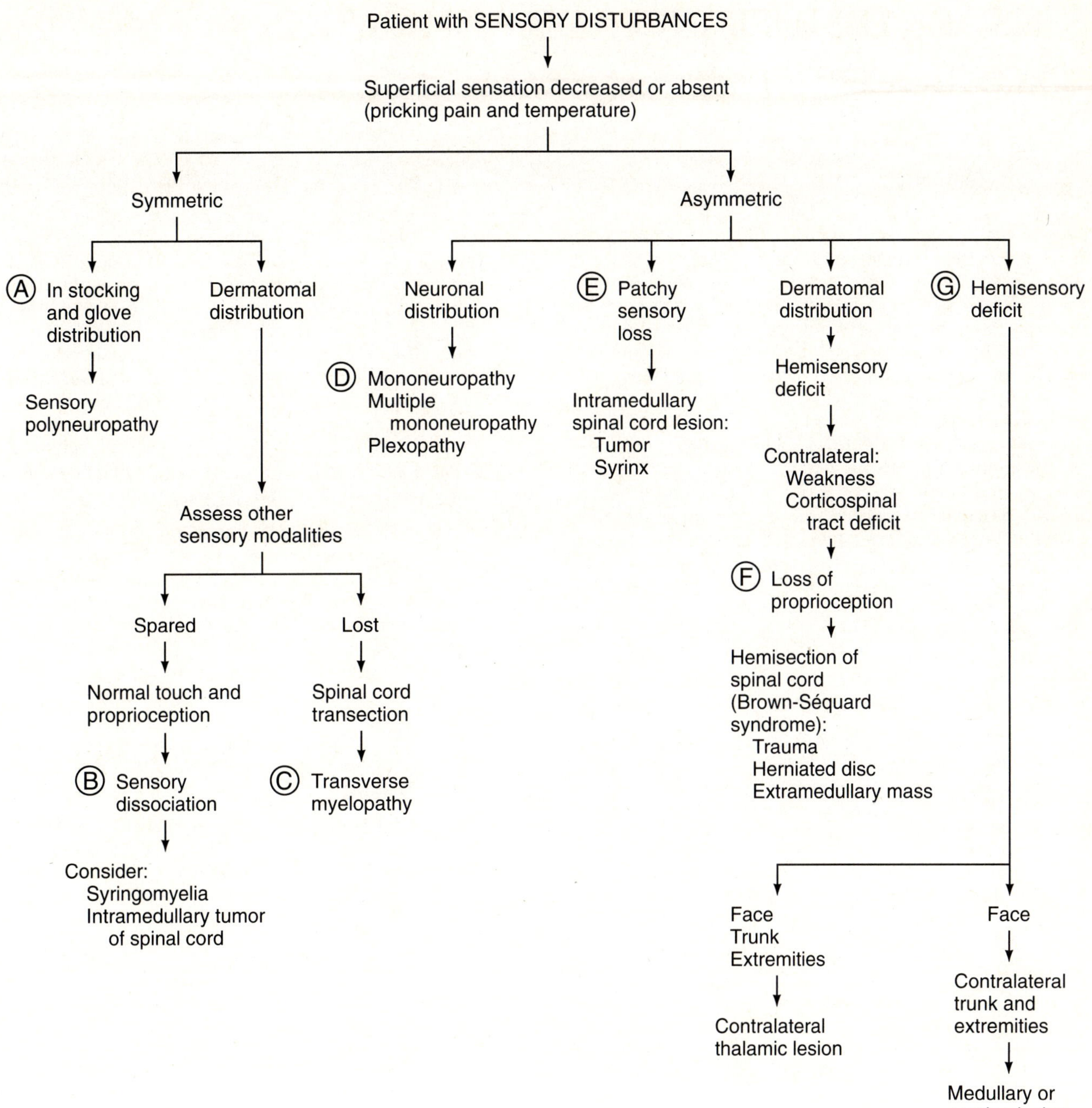

Patient with SENSORY DISTURBANCES
Superficial sensation decreased or absent (pricking pain and temperature)
Symmetric
Asymmetric
A In stocking and glove distribution
Sensory polyneuropathy
Dermatomal distribution
Assess other sensory modalities
Spared
Lost
Normal touch and proprioception
Spinal cord transection
B Sensory dissociation
C Transverse myelopathy
Consider:
Syringomyelia
Intramedullary tumor of spinal cord
Neuronal distribution
D Mononeuropathy
Multiple mononeuropathy
Plexopathy
E Patchy sensory loss
Intramedullary spinal cord lesion:
Tumor
Syrinx
Dermatomal distribution
Hemisensory deficit
Contralateral:
Weakness
Corticospinal tract deficit
F Loss of proprioception
Hemisection of spinal cord (Brown-Séquard syndrome):
Trauma
Herniated disc
Extramedullary mass
Face
Trunk
Extremities
Contralateral thalamic lesion
G Hemisensory deficit
Face
Contralateral trunk and extremities
Medullary or pontine lesion

SENSORY DISTURBANCE: DEEP SENSATION (PROPRIOCEPTION)

Carlos A. Garcia, M.D.

The sensory modality through which a person perceives muscular motion, weight, and position sense is known as proprioception. This is evaluated by testing passive movements of the toes and fingers and the position of the extremities in space (position sense) and by the Romberg test. Ask the patient to stand with feet together, initially with the eyes open and then with them closed. If the patient is equally unsteady with the eyes open or closed, this suggests a cerebellar disorder; however, if the patient is unsteady only with the eyes closed, this indicates a proprioception abnormality. Passive vertical movements of the toes and fingers in most cases are sufficient for testing passive movements and position sense. Most of the fibers carrying these sensations ascend in the posterior column of the spinal cord. Vibratory sense is tested by using a tuning fork of 256 vibrations/sec. The fibers that carry this sensation ascend in the posterior columns and probably in the lateral columns. Deep pain sensation (as contrasted with pricking pain, which is mediated by the lateral spinothalamic tract) is tested by squeezing the Achilles tendon or calves and is lost in patients with tabes dorsalis.

A. Loss of proprioception is seen in a distal symmetric stocking and glove distribution in severe sensorimotor polyneuropathies. In these patients, both superficial and deep sensory modalities are usually abolished.

B. Proprioception can be abolished with preservation of touch, pricking pain, and temperature in tabes dorsalis. The patient usually complains of lancinating leg or abdominal pains, and the examination usually reveals Argyll Robertson pupils.

C. When proprioception is abolished and is associated with corticospinal tract signs, inquire about other family members who may be affected. If the family history is positive, if there are no signs of bladder involvement, and if superficial pain perception is intact, the most likely diagnosis is familial spastic paraparesis. If all these signs are associated with a pancerebellar syndrome (head titubation, speech involvement, nystagmus) and the patient has scoliosis and pes cavus, Friedreich's ataxia is likely. The onset of this disease is usually in childhood or adolescence. If the loss of proprioception is accompanied only by corticospinal tract signs and there is no family history, subacute combined degeneration is a possibility. Obtain a complete blood count with a peripheral smear (look for monocytes and multisegmented polymorphonuclear cells) and test for vitamin B_{12}.

D. When the loss of proprioception is asymmetric, segmental, and on one side of the trunk, the loss is usually due to a hemisection of the spinal cord. There is usually weakness on the same side as the proprioception deficit (side of the lesion), and decreased superficial pain (pricking) and temperature perception on the contralateral side (Brown-Séquard syndrome). The lesions causing this syndrome include traumatic hemisection of the cord, a laterally herniated disc, an extramedullary spinal tumor compressing the cord, vasculitis (systemic lupus erythematosus), and, rarely, demyelinating disease.

E. If superficial sensation is impaired on the contralateral side, consider a spinal cord lesion. If superficial sensation is lost on the same side as the weakness, consider a cerebral lesion.

References

Haerer AF. DeJong's the neurologic examination. 5th ed. Philadelphia: JB Lippincott, 1992.

Mayo Clinic and Mayo Foundation. Clinical examinations in neurology. 6th ed. St. Louis: Mosby–Year Book, 1991.

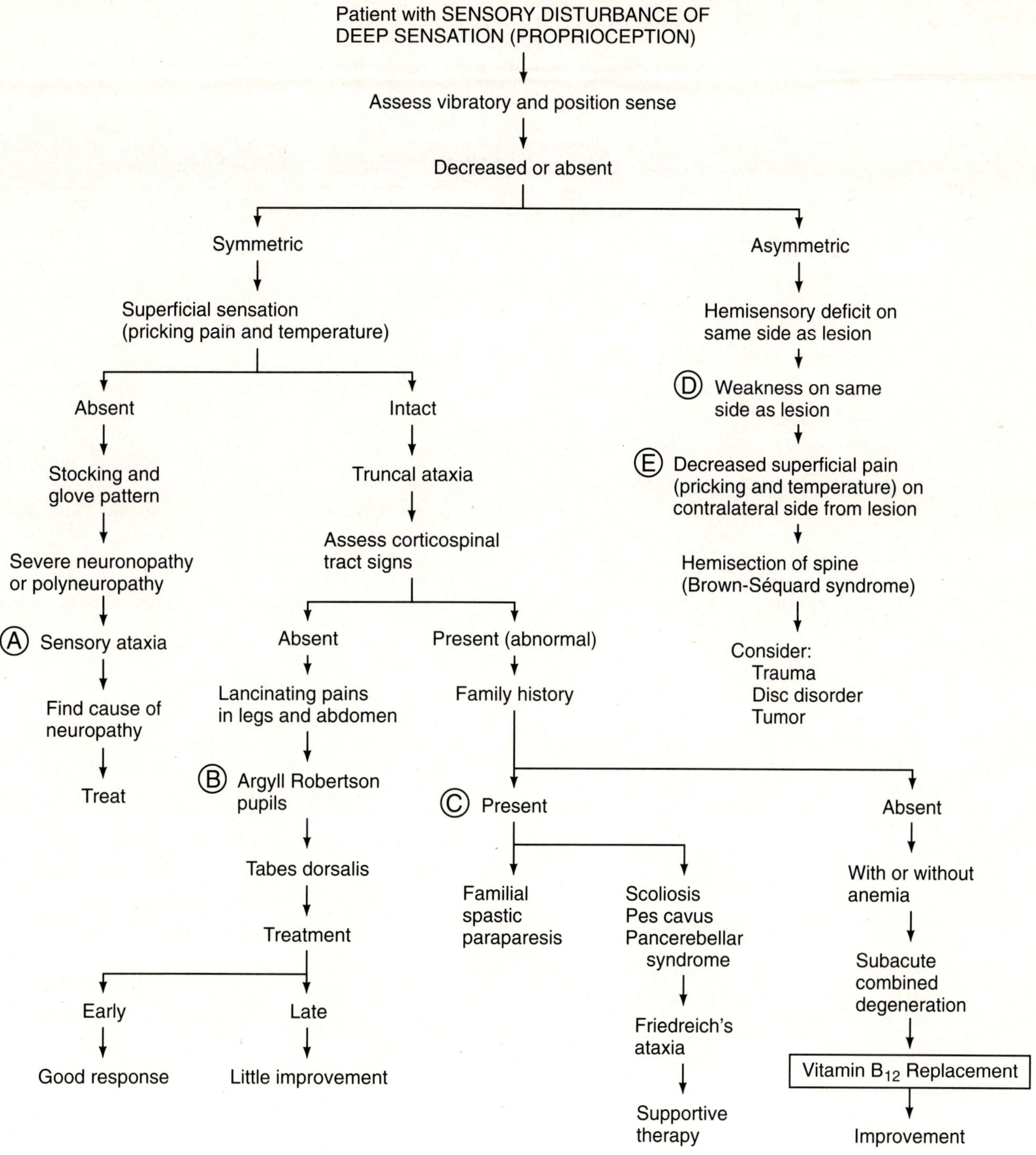

Patient with SENSORY DISTURBANCE OF DEEP SENSATION (PROPRIOCEPTION)
Assess vibratory and position sense
Decreased or absent
Symmetric
Asymmetric
Superficial sensation (pricking pain and temperature)
Hemisensory deficit on same side as lesion
D Weakness on same side as lesion
Absent
Intact
E Decreased superficial pain (pricking and temperature) on contralateral side from lesion
Stocking and glove pattern
Truncal ataxia
Hemisection of spine (Brown-Séquard syndrome)
Severe neuronopathy or polyneuropathy
Assess corticospinal tract signs
Consider:
Trauma
Disc disorder
Tumor
A Sensory ataxia
Absent
Present (abnormal)
Find cause of neuropathy
Lancinating pains in legs and abdomen
Family history
Treat
B Argyll Robertson pupils
C Present
Absent
Tabes dorsalis
Familial spastic paraparesis
Scoliosis
Pes cavus
Pancerebellar syndrome
With or without anemia
Treatment
Early
Late
Friedreich's ataxia
Subacute combined degeneration
Good response
Little improvement
Supportive therapy
Vitamin B$_{12}$ Replacement
Improvement

MUSCLE STRETCH REFLEXES

Carlos A. Garcia, M.D.

The muscle stretch reflex ("myotatic," "tendon," "deep," "periosteal") is an involuntary contraction (jerk) of a muscle in response to sudden stretching by tapping on its tendon. The stretch reflex is a segmental reflex. When eliciting the reflex, the physician is examining the integrity of the reflex arc in the spinal cord or brain stem. (A lesion in the arc abolishes the reflex.) The relationship among reflexes, muscles, and the involved segmental arcs is shown in Table 1. When examining the reflexes, remember the following:

1. The muscle to be tested should be in a relaxed midposition. A totally extended or totally contracted muscle or a severely atrophic muscle does not respond well.
2. Stretch reflexes in the legs are easier to obtain than those in the arms.
3. Asymmetry of the reflexes is more important to the clinician than the intensity of the response (symmetric areflexia or hyperactive reflexes), and the activity of the reflex should be correlated with other neurologic findings. Anxiety may cause hyperactive reflexes as well as unsustained clonus, but this is always symmetric if there is a normal response. Sustained clonus is always abnormal.
4. Clonus is a repetitive reflex response produced by exerting constant pressure on the tested muscle. The clonus can be sustained (response continues indefinitely) or unsustained (response disappears after a few beats). The significance of clonus is the same as that of any hyperactive stretch reflex.
5. Stretch reflexes may change from areflexia seen in an acute CNS lesion (spinal shock) to hyperactivity after 3 to 4 weeks.
6. To obtain a good response, patients must be relaxed. Distract patients by asking questions or asking them to count. If no response is obtained, reinforce the reflex by asking patients to contract muscles other than the ones being tested.
7. Pendular reflexes (on eliciting the reflex, the extremity continues a to-and-fro movement) are seen in cerebellar disease.
8. The examiner must know the segmental arc to be examined.
9. For the purposes of clinical note taking, most physicians grade the reflexes from 0+ to 5+ (Table 2).

A. An isolated finding of symmetric generalized areflexia or hyperactive reflexes has no clinical significance.

B. Areflexia associated with a dilated tonic pupil indicates Adie's syndrome.

C. When areflexia is symmetric and is associated with atrophy and fasciculations, there is anterior horn cell disease. This may be localized to the cervical segments, as in cervical spondylosis or syringomyelia, or may be generalized, as in progressive spinal muscular atrophy (motor neuron disease). When areflexia is associated with a sensory deficit in a glove and stocking distribution, there is a polyneuropathy.

D. If the sensory deficit is found in a segmental (dermatomal) distribution (a sensory level), there is a spinal cord lesion.

E. Asymmetric areflexia is always of clinical significance. If areflexia is found in only one segment, there is a root or nerve lesion.

F. Areflexia seen in several adjacent segments on one extremity indicates a plexus lesion.

TABLE 2   Grading of Muscle Stretch Reflexes

Response	Grade
Absent (areflexia)	0+
Hypoactive	1+
Normal (physiologic)	2+
Hyperactive	3+
Unsustained clonus	4+
Sustained clonus	5+

TABLE 1   Muscles Involved in Segmental Reflexes

Reflex	Muscle Involved	Segmental Arc
Jaw jerk	Masseter muscle	5th cranial nerve
Biceps reflex	Biceps muscle	5th and 6th cervical root
Triceps reflex	Triceps muscle	7th and 8th cervical root
Patellar (knee) reflex	Quadriceps muscle	3rd and 4th lumbar root
Ankle (Achilles) reflex	Gastrocnemius muscle	1st and 2nd sacral root

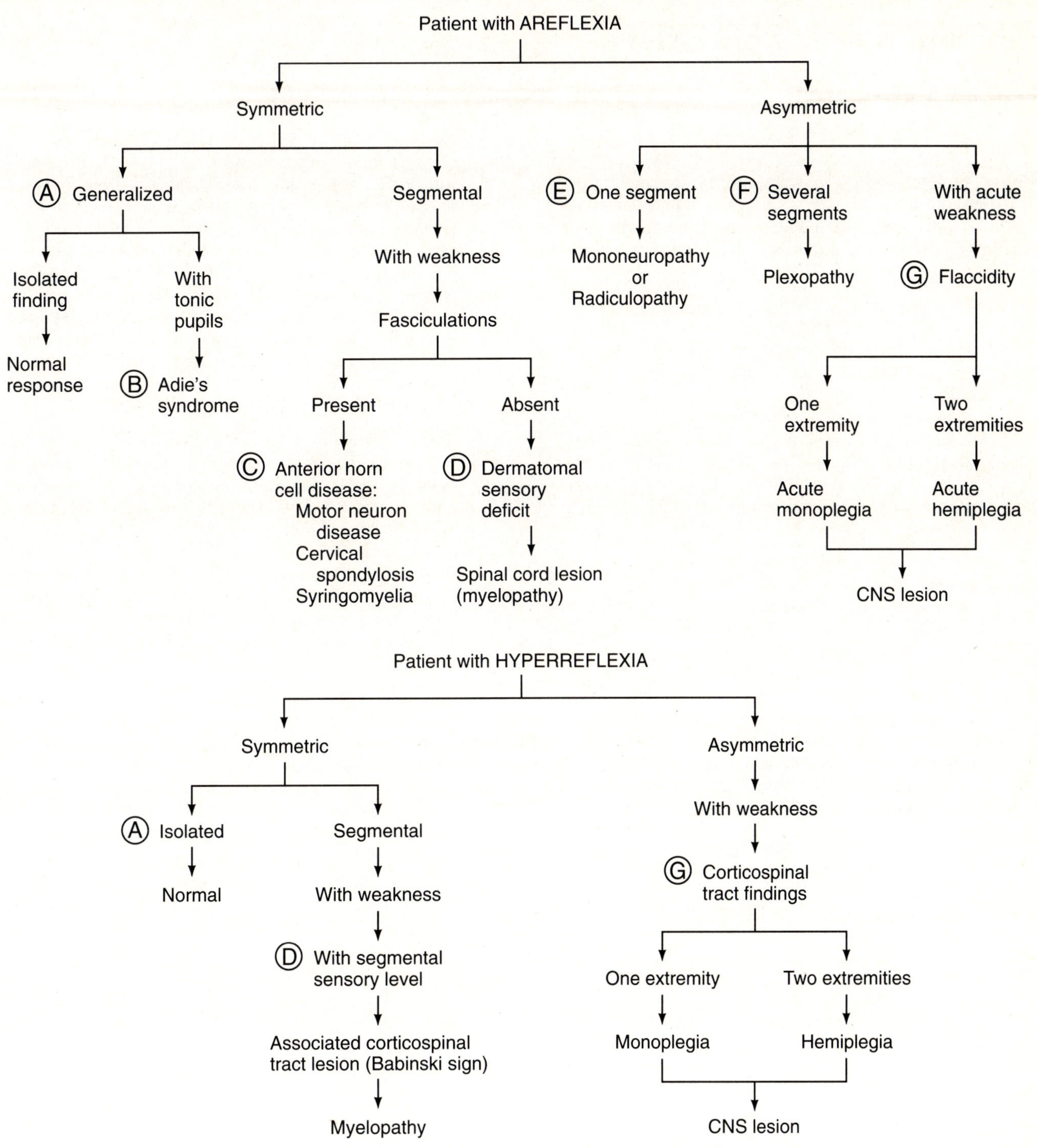

G. Acute CNS lesions, in either the spinal cord or the brain, produce areflexia in the acute (shock) phase. The reflexes change in a few days to become hyperactive. The tone also changes from flaccidity to spasticity.

References

Haerer AF. DeJong's the neurologic examination. 5th ed. Philadelphia; JB Lippincott, 1992.
Mayo Clinic and Mayo Foundation. Clinical examinations in neurology. 6th ed. St. Louis: Mosby—Year Book, 1991.

SUPERFICIAL REFLEXES

Carlos A. Garcia, M.D.

Superficial reflexes are contractions of muscles in response to stimulation of the skin or mucous membranes. These reflexes are slower and fatigue more easily than the muscle stretch reflexes. Only a few are used in clinical practice.

A. The corneal reflex is mediated through the fifth cranial nerve (afferent part) and its thalamic projections and the seventh nerve (efferent part) to the orbicularis oculi muscle. Unilateral loss may be due to a lesion in the fifth cranial nerve, such as a cerebellopontine (CP) angle lesion or any lesion involving the nerve or its projections. Lack of response may be also due to weakness of the orbicularis oculi muscle as a result of a lesion of the seventh cranial nerve (Bell's palsy). In the latter instance the patient blinks in the contralateral eye or withdraws from the stimulus. Absence of both corneal reflexes is seen in brain stem lesions.

B. The plantar reflex is demonstrated when plantar stimulation applied from the heel forward with a blunt object produces plantar flexion of the foot and toes. The reflex is mediated through the L4-S2 roots (tibial nerve). The abnormal response known as the Babinski sign consists of a tonic dorsiflexion of the great toe and separation (fanning) of the other toes. The Babinski sign is found in normal infants and may be found during profound sleep. In comatose patients the sign does not have a localizing value. Otherwise, when present, the Babinski sign indicates a corticospinal tract lesion. The response may be abolished by sensory deficit of the soles. There is frequently no plantar response in acute corticospinal tract lesions. Other less often used superficial reflexes include the pharyngeal (gag) and cremasteric reflexes. The pharyngeal reflex is elicited by touching one side of the pharynx with a tongue blade. The reflex may be absent or exaggerated in normal individuals; the reflex is significant if absent on only one side. The cremasteric reflex is elicited by striking the inner side of the thigh with a blunt object. The cremasteric muscle contracts, elevating the ipsilateral testicle.

C. Abdominal reflexes are mediated through the T7 to T12 roots. The reflexes may be normally absent in obese patients, in multiparous females, and in patients with abdominal scars. The reflex is elicited by striking the skin of the abdomen with a blunt object. In a normal response the underlying abdominal muscles contract. The absence of the reflex associated with hyperreflexia in the lower extremities indicates a lesion of the contralateral corticospinal tract. The reflex is absent on both sides in spinal cord lesions.

References

Haerer AF. DeJong's the neurologic examination. 5th ed. Philadelphia: JB Lippincott, 1992.

Mayo Clinic and Mayo Foundation. Clinical examinations in neurology. 6th ed. St. Louis: Mosby–Year Book, 1991.

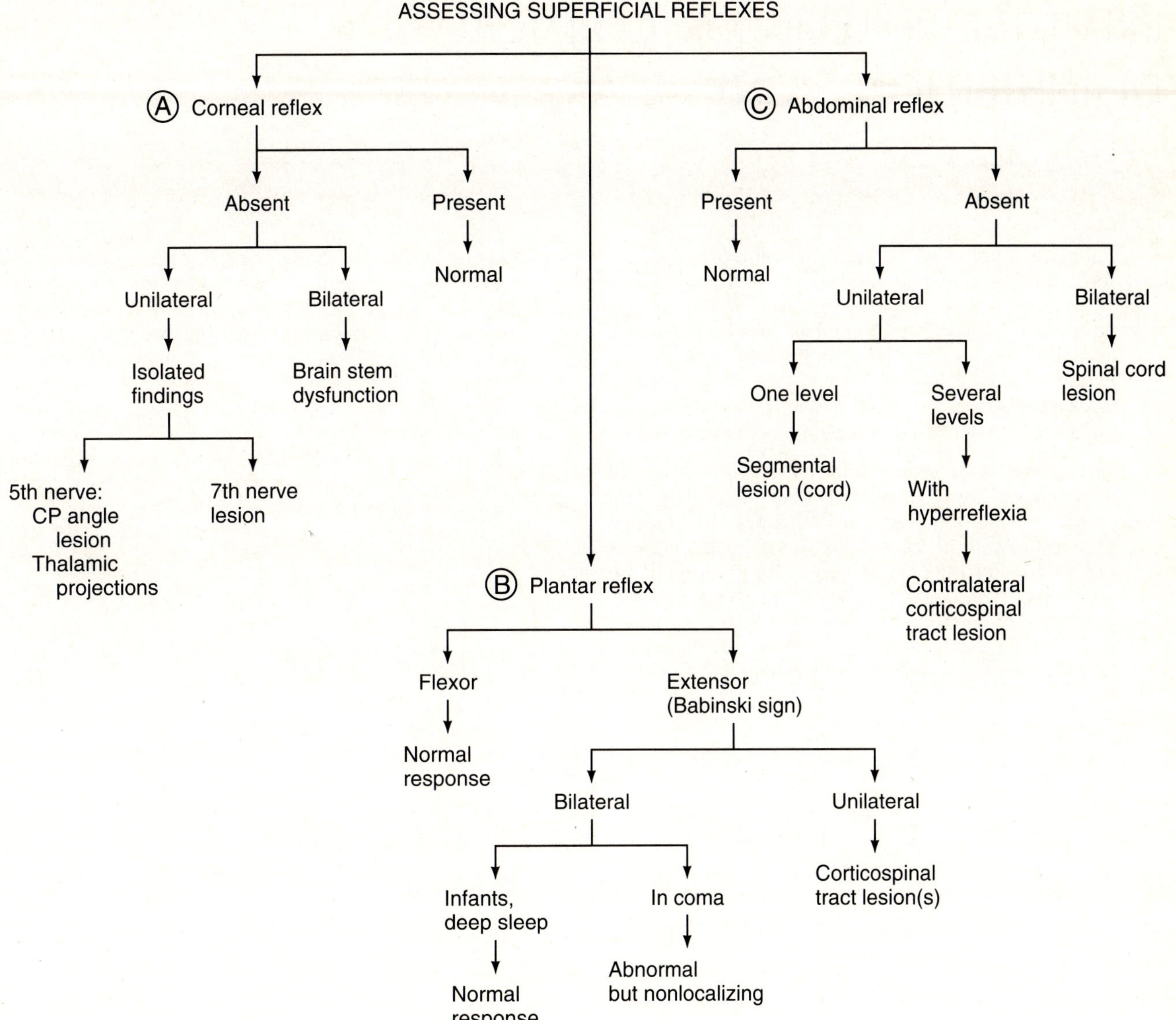

ASSESSING SUPERFICIAL REFLEXES
A Corneal reflex
Absent
Present
Normal
Unilateral
Bilateral
Isolated findings
Brain stem dysfunction
5th nerve: CP angle lesion Thalamic projections
7th nerve lesion
C Abdominal reflex
Present
Normal
Absent
Unilateral
Bilateral
One level
Several levels
Spinal cord lesion
Segmental lesion (cord)
With hyperreflexia
Contralateral corticospinal tract lesion
B Plantar reflex
Flexor
Extensor (Babinski sign)
Normal response
Bilateral
Unilateral
Infants, deep sleep
In coma
Corticospinal tract lesion(s)
Normal response
Abnormal but nonlocalizing

PRIMITIVE REFLEXES OR CORTICAL DISINHIBITION SIGNS

Carlos A. Garcia, M.D.

A. Primitive reflexes or cortical disinhibition signs are seen in normal infants. The reflexes disappear at age 18 months to 2 years and reappear in normal elderly persons and in patients of any age with lesions of the frontal cortex, subcortical frontal white matter, or extrapyramidal system (release effect). The snout and grasp reflexes correlate better with cognitive impairment than the glabellar and palmomental reflexes.

B. These reflexes are seen regularly in the later stages of dementia but are absent in early dementia. All of these reflexes are usually seen in diseases that produce pseudobulbar symptoms. The snout (suck) reflex is elicited by pressing or tapping over the philtrum of the upper lip. The responses consist of a sucking (pursing-pouting) motion of the lips. The grasp reflex is elicited when the patient's palms are scratched by the examiner's fingers or the handle of the reflex hammer. The patient grasps the object and cannot release it, or continues to grasp in response to every consecutive stimulus in spite of a warning by the examiner not to do it. The glabellar reflex is elicited by tapping between the eyebrows, from above to avoid the visual threat and after asking the patient not to blink. The abnormal response consists of continuous blinking after nine consecutive taps. The palmomental reflex is elicited by scratching the patient's palm along the thenar eminence. The response consists of ipsilateral movement of the mentalis (chin) muscle.

Reference

Tweedy J, et al. Significance of cortical disinhibition signs. Neurology 1982; 32:169.

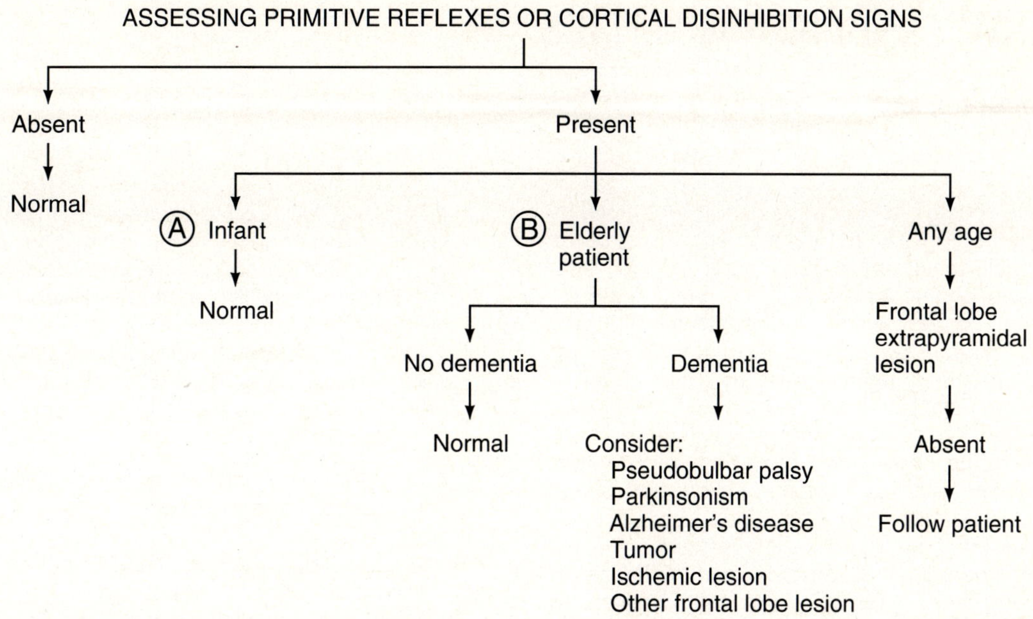

ASSESSING PRIMITIVE REFLEXES OR CORTICAL DISINHIBITION SIGNS
Absent
Normal
Present
A Infant
Normal
B Elderly
patient
No dementia
Normal
Dementia
Consider:
Pseudobulbar palsy
Parkinsonism
Alzheimer's disease
Tumor
Ischemic lesion
Other frontal lobe lesion
Any age
Frontal lobe
extrapyramidal
lesion
Absent
Follow patient

PUPILLARY ABNORMALITIES

Leon A. Weisberg, M.D.

The pupil is the opening in the iris; its size is determined by muscles within the iris. The muscular layer consists of the sphincter pupillae (parasympathetic innervation) and dilator pupillae (sympathetic innervation). Preganglionic parasympathetic neurons originate from the Edinger-Westphal nucleus in the midbrain and travel in the oculomotor nerve. Postganglionic neurons originate from the ciliary ganglion in the orbital apex and travel via ciliary nerves. Preganglionic sympathetic neurons originate in the hypothalamus and descend in the brain stem; postganglionic neurons originate from the superior cervical ganglion and ascend around the carotid artery to enter the orbit with the ophthalmic branch of the trigeminal nerve. Examine shape and size (e.g., miosis or constriction and mydriasis or dilation) of the pupils. Assess the rate and symmetry of pupil response to bright flashlight and the response to fixation on near target. Attention to associated neurologic signs (extraocular and trigeminal nerves, corticospinal and cerebellar findings) is necessary to exclude brain stem, parasellar, and base of skull lesions or tentorial herniation syndromes as the cause of the pupillary abnormalities.

A. Episodic anisocoria depends on activity within sympathetic or parasympathetic neurons. With uncal herniation, unilateral mydriasis and impaired light response may occur ipsilateral to the mass lesion. There may be contralateral hemiparesis. Unilateral mydriasis may occur as a postictal seizure manifestation. Unilateral miosis with ptosis (Horner's syndromes) occurs in cluster or migraine headaches. Determine whether there are any neurologic abnormalities, which would suggest a brachial plexus or spinal cord lesion. If there are no neurologic abnormalities, evaluate (chest radiography, CT, MRI) for a thyroid or mediastinal lesion.

B. In patients with anisocoria, assess light response. If this is normal, consider physiologic anisocoria or Horner's syndrome. In physiologic anisocoria, the difference in pupil size is always <1.5 mm. Horner's syndrome is due to a pre- or postganglionic lesion. If a miotic pupil dilates in response to ocular instillation of the weak adrenergic drug hydroxyamphetamine (Paredrine), the lesion is preganglionic; if it does not dilate, the lesion is postganglionic. (Hydroxyamphetamine causes release of norepinephrine from synaptic vesicles; thus in a preganglionic lesion in which the synaptic supply of norepinephrine is intact, the pupil dilates as the drug is locally instilled. In postganglionic lesions, epinephrine is depleted and there is no pupillary dilation.) For preganglionic lesions, consider hypothalamic and brain stem, spinal cord, neck, or mediastinal lesions. For postganglionic lesions, consider carotid artery abnormalities (dissections, occlusion, headache syndrome including cluster), and lesions contiguous with the cavernous sinus and orbital region.

C. If the light response is impaired, evaluate near-response. An abnormal pupil is usually larger, but this is not always true. If near-response is normal, light-near dissociation indicates a posterior third ventricular or midbrain lesion. If near-target response is absent, slit lamp examination is necessary to exclude iris abnormalities. Test the dilated pupil with 1% pilocarpine to differentiate pharmacologic blockade due to parasympathetic blocking drugs from oculomotor palsy. In third nerve palsies, constriction occurs in response to ocular application of pilocarpine. Oculomotor palsy with a light-fixed, dilated pupil may be due to a compressive lesion; this may be a parasellar lesion (pituitary adenoma, meningioma, aneurysm).

D. If there is unilateral mydriasis with impaired light response and tonic pupillary constriction to near targets, consider Adie's pupil. Patients with this condition may have visual blurring or may be entirely asymptomatic. In Adie's patients, deep tendon reflexes are usually absent (areflexia). There is pupillary constriction in response to 0.125% pilocarpine, indicating cholinergic supersensitivity. Tonic reaction to near targets differentiates an Adie's pupil from an Argyll Robertson pupil. Argyll Robertson pupils are unequal, miotic, and irregularly shaped pupils that may accommodate but do not react briskly to light; they are most commonly due to neurosyphilis.

References

Cremer SA, Thompson HS, Digre KB. Hydroxyamphetamine mydriasis in Horner's syndrome. Am J Ophthalmol 1990; 110:71.

Nadeau SE, Trobe JD. Pupil sparing in oculomotor palsy: A brief review. Ann Neurol 1983; 13:143.

Selhorst JB. The pupil and its disorders. Neurol Clin North Am 1983; 1:859.

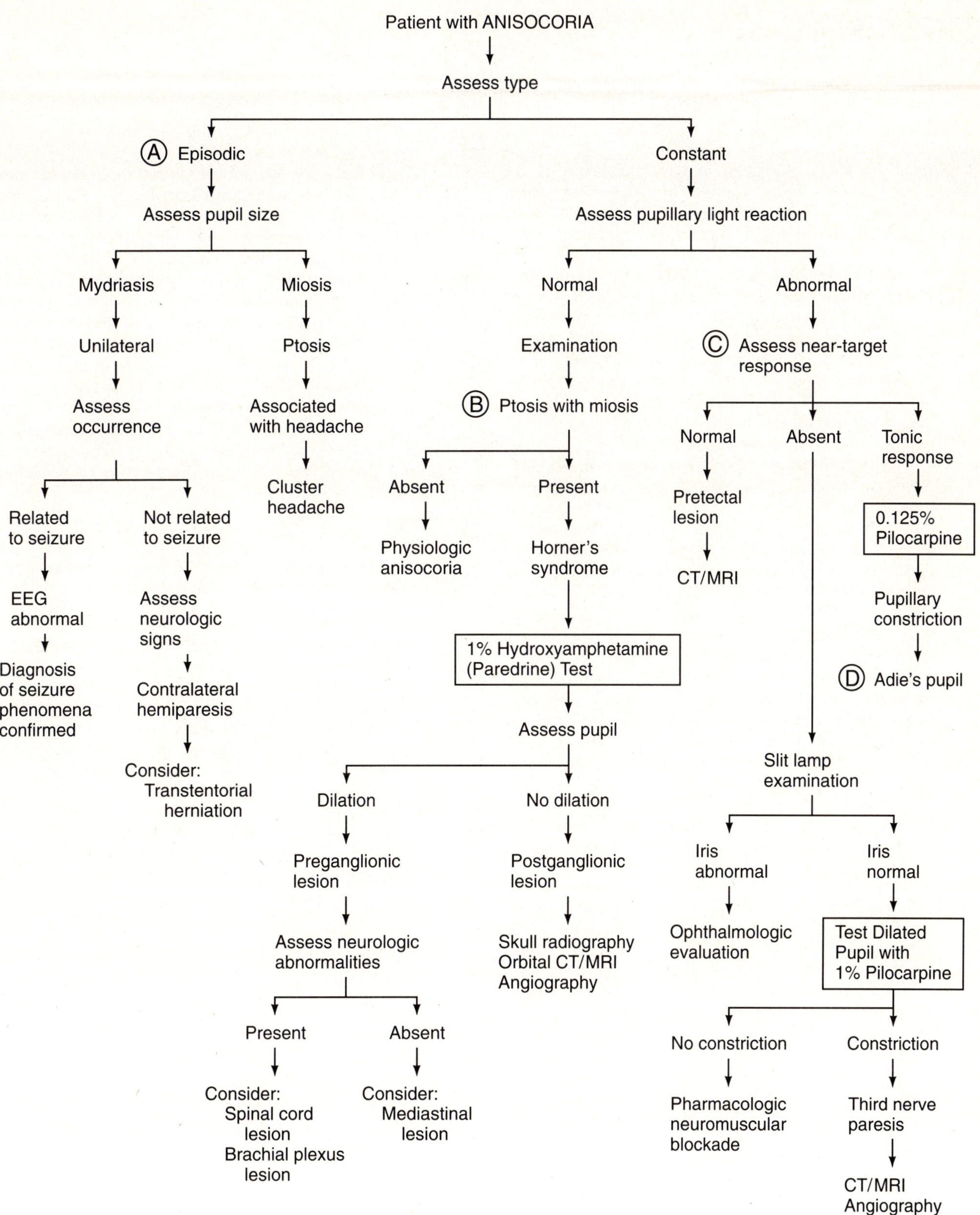

Patient with ANISOCORIA
Assess type
A Episodic
Constant
Assess pupil size
Assess pupillary light reaction
Mydriasis
Miosis
Normal
Abnormal
Unilateral
Ptosis
Examination
C Assess near-target response
Assess occurrence
Associated with headache
B Ptosis with miosis
Normal
Absent
Tonic response
Related to seizure
Not related to seizure
Cluster headache
Absent
Present
Pretectal lesion
0.125% Pilocarpine
EEG abnormal
Assess neurologic signs
Physiologic anisocoria
Horner's syndrome
CT/MRI
Pupillary constriction
Diagnosis of seizure phenomena confirmed
Contralateral hemiparesis
1% Hydroxyamphetamine (Paredrine) Test
D Adie's pupil
Consider: Transtentorial herniation
Assess pupil
Slit lamp examination
Dilation
No dilation
Iris abnormal
Iris normal
Preganglionic lesion
Postganglionic lesion
Ophthalmologic evaluation
Test Dilated Pupil with 1% Pilocarpine
Assess neurologic abnormalities
Skull radiography Orbital CT/MRI Angiography
No constriction
Constriction
Present
Absent
Pharmacologic neuromuscular blockade
Third nerve paresis
Consider: Spinal cord lesion Brachial plexus lesion
Consider: Mediastinal lesion
CT/MRI Angiography

DIPLOPIA

Carlos A. Garcia, M.D.

Diplopia is a visual symptom in which a single object appears as a double image. It has to be differentiated from dim or blurred vision. In true diplopia the patient describes the objects in two different places in space.

A. Ask the patient whether the diplopia persists when one eye is closed. If the answer is yes, there is monocular diplopia, which may be due to optical aberrations in the affected eye, such as keratoconus or subluxation of the lens. Most of these patients have been seen first by an ophthalmologist; if not, they should be referred to one. If there is no ocular disease and the findings on neurologic examination are normal, there is a fictitious disease or a conversion reaction.

  If the diplopia disappears when one eye is closed, there is binocular diplopia. If there is no squint (strabismus) at rest and no misalignment is noticed during rotation of the eyes, the red glass test is performed or the patient is referred to an ophthalmologist. Place a red glass in front of the patient's right eye and ask him or her to look at the small light 3 to 4 feet away; then move the light in the cardinal position of gaze and closer to the patient's eyes. If the patient identifies two images, one red and one white, there is an ocular misalignment. Identify the paretic muscle by remembering that the distance between the two images (true and false) increases in the direction of the paretic muscle and that the false image is usually the more peripheral one. Once you identify the paretic muscle(s), you should try to determine the cause of the lesion. If the patient does not differentiate the two images and the neurologic examinations are normal, there is a fictitious disease or a conversion reaction.

B. When diplopia is binocular, intermittent, and reproducible and disappears after IV injection of Tensilon, the diagnosis is myasthenia gravis. If the Tensilon test is negative, myasthenia gravis is possible, but also consider hyperthyroidism. Remember that myasthenia gravis and hyperthyroidism may involve any or all of the extraocular muscles and that both diseases may occur together or in sequence. Any patient with extraocular muscle weakness should undergo a Tensilon test and thyroid function tests. "Pseudointernuclear ophthalmoplegia" may be seen in myasthenia gravis.

C. When there is diplopia in the presence of strabismus, no proptosis, and a negative Tensilon test, identify the weak muscle(s). If only one muscle is involved and there are no associated neurologic deficits, there may be isolated cranial nerve palsies. If the lateral rectus muscle is affected, there is a sixth cranial nerve palsy. (The most frequent causes are listed in the decision tree.) If the isolated weak muscle is superior oblique, there is most likely a fourth nerve palsy. When any other muscle is affected in isolation or in any combination, there may be a third nerve palsy, usually due to an aneurysm compressing the nerve. The aneurysm is usually at the junction of the internal carotid artery with the posterior communicating cerebral artery. If the pupil is spared, the most likely cause is vascular-diabetic disease.

D. When diplopia is associated with muscle weakness in other areas such as the proximal limb girdle or pharyngeal muscles, there is a myopathy (see pp 226, 236) with ocular muscle involvement.

E. When diplopia is associated with CNS signs, the lesion may be localized by the neurologic findings. When the diplopia is due to vertical gaze palsy mainly in the upward direction (Parinaud's syndrome) and is associated with papilledema, there is most likely a posterior third ventricular mass lesion. Vertical gaze paralysis, mainly on downward gaze, associated with neck rigidity and dementia suggests progressive supranuclear palsy. Medial rectus weakness associated with nystagmus of the abducting eye (internuclear ophthalmoplegia) indicates a lesion in the medial longitudinal fasciculus in the brain stem and on the same side as the paretic medial rectus muscle. In a young patient, this usually indicates a demyelinating lesion; in an elderly patient, it indicates a vascular lesion.

F. Proptosis can produce diplopia and may be due to intraorbital, orbital apex, and cavernous sinus lesions.

References

Haerer AF. DeJong's the neurologic examination. 5th ed. Philadelphia: JB Lippincott, 1992.

Mayo Clinic and Mayo Foundation. Clinical examination in neurology. 6th ed. St. Louis: Mosby–Year Book, 1991.

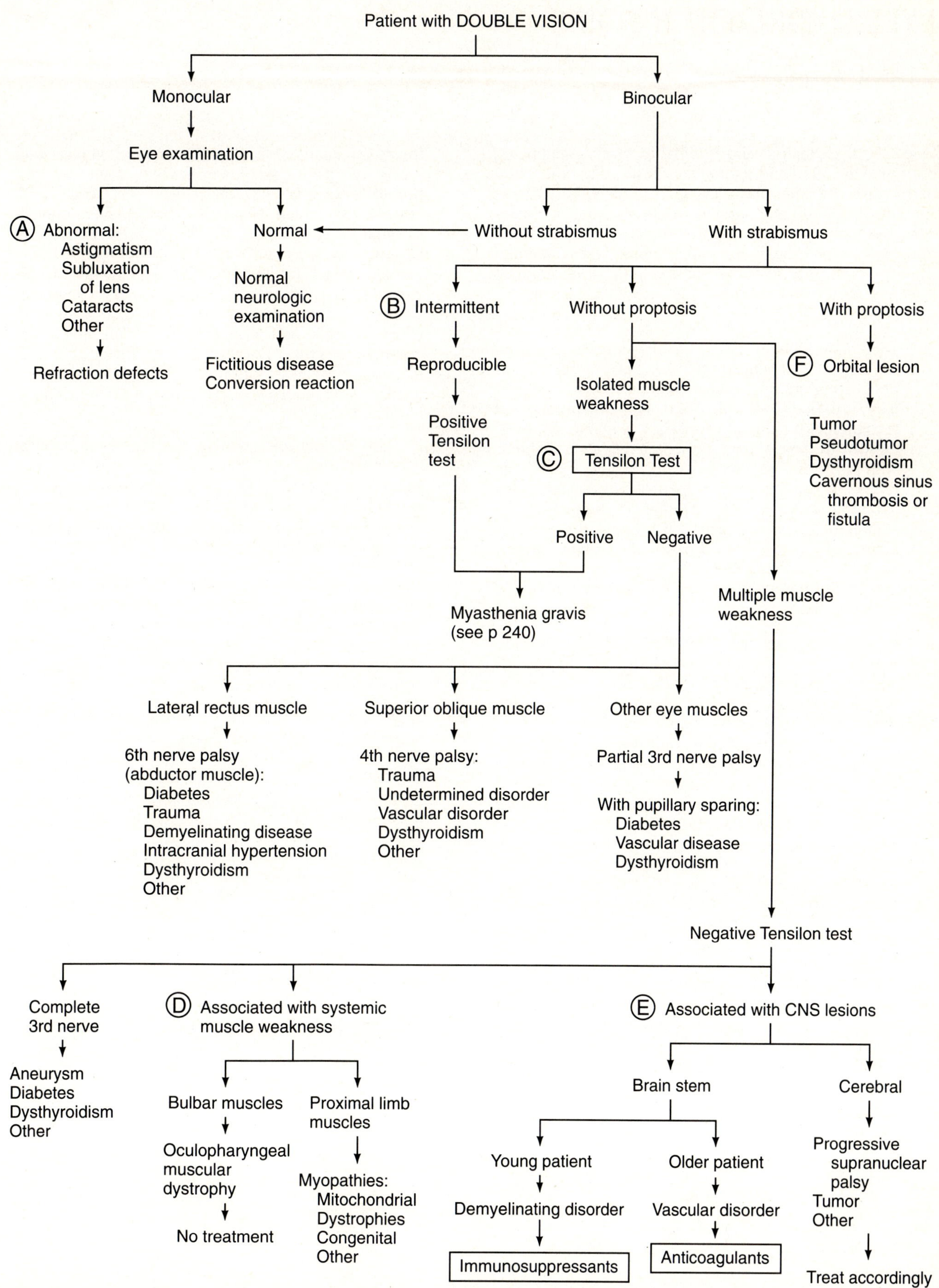

Patient with DOUBLE VISION

Monocular

Binocular

Eye examination

A Abnormal:
Astigmatism
Subluxation
of lens
Cataracts
Other

Refraction defects

Normal

Without strabismus

With strabismus

Normal
neurologic
examination

Fictitious disease
Conversion reaction

B Intermittent

Without proptosis

With proptosis

Reproducible

Isolated muscle
weakness

F Orbital lesion

Positive
Tensilon
test

C Tensilon Test

Tumor
Pseudotumor
Dysthyroidism
Cavernous sinus
thrombosis or
fistula

Positive

Negative

Multiple muscle
weakness

Myasthenia gravis
(see p 240)

Lateral rectus muscle

Superior oblique muscle

Other eye muscles

6th nerve palsy
(abductor muscle):
Diabetes
Trauma
Demyelinating disease
Intracranial hypertension
Dysthyroidism
Other

4th nerve palsy:
Trauma
Undetermined disorder
Vascular disorder
Dysthyroidism
Other

Partial 3rd nerve palsy

With pupillary sparing:
Diabetes
Vascular disease
Dysthyroidism

Negative Tensilon test

Complete
3rd nerve

D Associated with systemic
muscle weakness

E Associated with CNS lesions

Aneurysm
Diabetes
Dysthyroidism
Other

Bulbar muscles

Proximal limb
muscles

Brain stem

Cerebral

Oculopharyngeal
muscular
dystrophy

Myopathies:
Mitochondrial
Dystrophies
Congenital
Other

Young patient

Older patient

Progressive
supranuclear
palsy
Tumor
Other

No treatment

Demyelinating disorder

Vascular disorder

Immunosuppressants

Anticoagulants

Treat accordingly

EYELID DROOP (PTOSIS)

Leon A. Weisberg, M.D.

In ptosis, the upper eyelid droops to cover a significant portion of the pupil and sclera; this causes palpebral fissure narrowing. The latter may also occur in blepharospasm to simulate ptosis. Blepharospasm represents a type of dyskinesia resulting from involuntary orbicularis muscle contraction. Structural eyelid abnormalities (redundant skin on the upper eyelids, eyelid tumor or swelling) may simulate ptosis. True ptosis results from levator palpebral muscle dysfunction.

A. Determine whether ptosis has developed recently or has only recently been noticed. In patients with severe ptosis, this presents no problem; if ptosis is mild, it may be difficult to distinguish recent onset from recent recognition. If old photographs are available, compare these with the patient's present appearance. Patients with ptosis usually have furrowing of the forehead due to excessive contraction of the frontalis muscles. This occurs as these muscles attempt to compensate for levator palpebral weakness. If frontalis furrowing is absent, question the diagnosis of ptosis due to levator palpebral weakness. If onset of ptosis is early in life, congenital ptosis is most common and may be due to birth trauma.

B. If ptosis is recent in onset, check pupillary size and light reactivity. Ocular myasthenia gravis affects skeletal muscles but *always* spares the pupils. Ptosis due to myasthenia may occur without extraocular motility disturbances, but ocular myasthenia is much more likely to be accompanied by diplopia due to impaired extraocular muscle disturbances. Fatigue of the levator muscles in myasthenia may be brought out by having the patient sustain an upward gaze and observing for development of eyelid droop. The diagnosis of suspected ocular myasthenia may be established by clinical improvement after IV Tensilon (edrophonium) injection; however, an initial negative result does not exclude this diagnosis and the test should be repeated. If this test result is negative, make sure that the Tensilon used is pharmacologically active. This is established if patients develop a muscarinic effect of increased lacrimation (tearing) after Tensilon injection. Laboratory study for acetylcholine (ACh) receptor antibody test and repetitive stimulation electromyography (EMG) should be performed in suspected myasthenia patients (see p 238). In older patients with ptosis, eye examination may show lax levator tendons due to levator muscle dehiscence. This condition is corrected by eyelid surgery if ptosis is severe enough to interfere with vision. Ocular myasthenia is more common in young patients, but it may occur in the elderly. Ptosis, swallowing difficulty, and neck muscle weakness may be seen in oculopharyngeal muscular dystrophy. This condition may initially develop in older patients and is inherited as an autosomal dominant disorder. The disorder may involve extraocular muscles; less commonly, there is extremity (proximal distribution), neck, and phonation muscle involvement.

C. If ptosis occurs with ocular motility abnormalities, accommodation impairment, and gastrointestinal (GI) symptoms, consider botulism. In botulism, there is generalized weakness; swallowing and respiratory problems may develop. If ptosis is of sudden onset and unilateral, and if there is impaired ocular motility but normal pupil reactivity, consider diabetic oculomotor paresis. Normal pupil size and reactivity differentiate an ischemic third nerve lesion from extrinsic third nerve compression. If there are ptosis, impaired ocular motility, and normal pupils, consider a variant of Guillain-Barré syndrome, especially if deep tendon reflexes are absent (see p 208).

D. If ptosis is associated with pupillary abnormalities, consider oculomotor paresis due to extrinsic compression (aneurysm, neoplasm, transtentorial herniation) or oculosympathetic dysfunction (Horner's syndrome). In compressive oculomotor lesions, the pupil is dilated and light reactivity is impaired. In Horner's syndrome, miosis and facial anhidrosis occur with ptosis. In ptosis due to Horner's syndrome, the upper lid is elevated (upside-down ptosis).

References

Burde RM, Savino PJ, Trobe JD. Clinical decisions in neuro-ophthalmology. 2nd ed. St. Louis: Mosby—Year Book, 1992:349.

Dortzbach RK, Sutula FC. Involutional blepharoptosis. Arch Ophthalmol 1980; 98:2045.

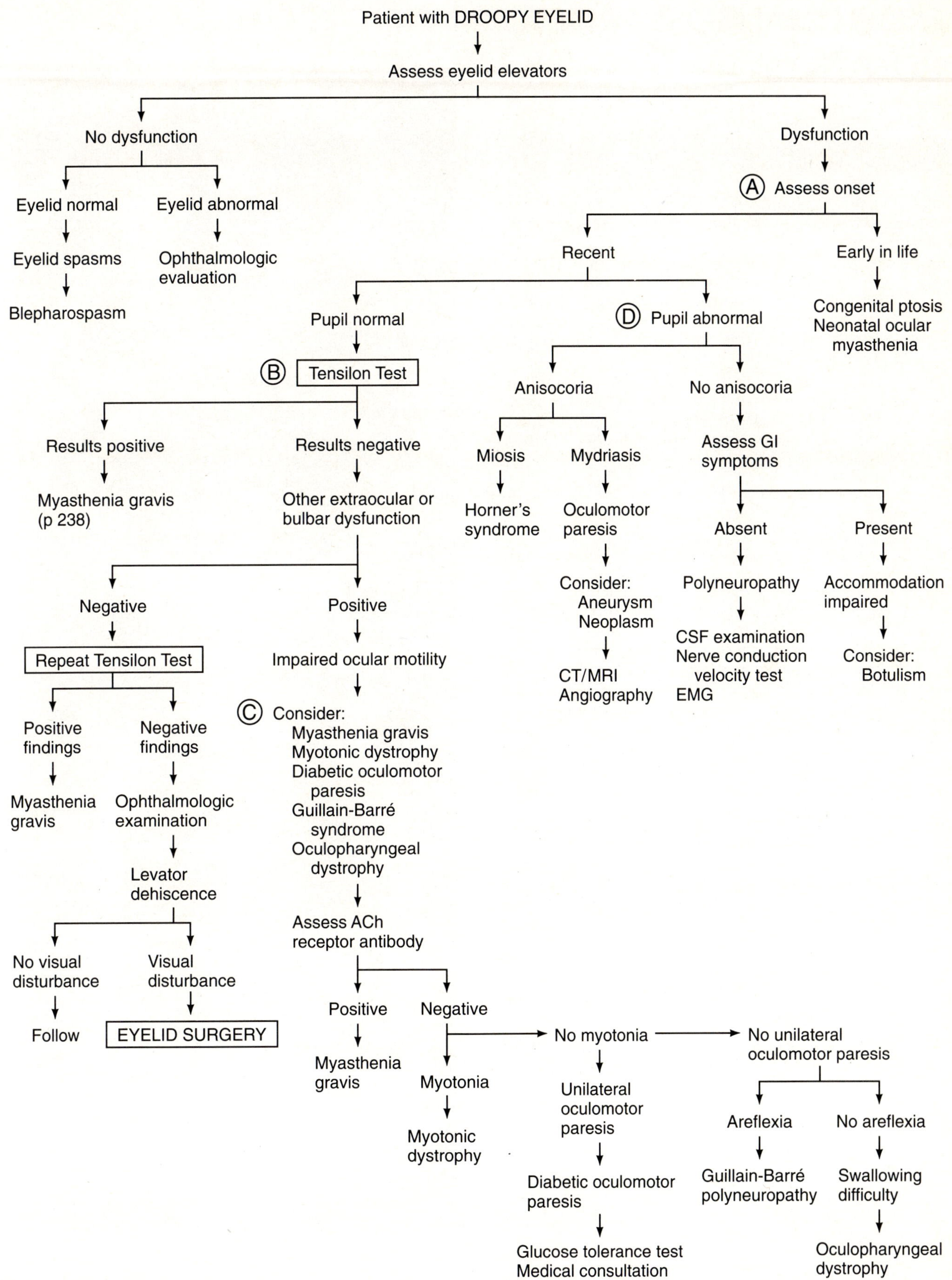

Patient with DROOPY EYELID
Assess eyelid elevators
No dysfunction
Dysfunction
A Assess onset
Eyelid normal
Eyelid abnormal
Eyelid spasms
Ophthalmologic evaluation
Blepharospasm
Recent
Early in life
Congenital ptosis
Neonatal ocular myasthenia
Pupil normal
D Pupil abnormal
B Tensilon Test
Results positive
Results negative
Myasthenia gravis (p 238)
Other extraocular or bulbar dysfunction
Negative
Positive
Repeat Tensilon Test
Impaired ocular motility
Positive findings
Negative findings
C Consider:
Myasthenia gravis
Myotonic dystrophy
Diabetic oculomotor paresis
Guillain-Barré syndrome
Oculopharyngeal dystrophy
Myasthenia gravis
Ophthalmologic examination
Levator dehiscence
Assess ACh receptor antibody
No visual disturbance
Visual disturbance
Follow
EYELID SURGERY
Positive
Negative
Myasthenia gravis
Myotonia
Myotonic dystrophy
No myotonia
No unilateral oculomotor paresis
Unilateral oculomotor paresis
Areflexia
No areflexia
Diabetic oculomotor paresis
Guillain-Barré polyneuropathy
Swallowing difficulty
Glucose tolerance test
Medical consultation
Oculopharyngeal dystrophy
Anisocoria
No anisocoria
Miosis
Mydriasis
Assess GI symptoms
Horner's syndrome
Oculomotor paresis
Consider:
Aneurysm
Neoplasm
CT/MRI
Angiography
Absent
Present
Polyneuropathy
Accommodation impaired
CSF examination
Nerve conduction velocity test
EMG
Consider:
Botulism

EXOPHTHALMOS: PROPTOSIS OF ORBITAL CONTENTS

Leon A. Weisberg, M.D.

Exophthalmos is forward (anterior) globe displacement and is measured with an exophthalmometer. Normal values are 14 to 21 mm. Exophthalmos is usually equal on both sides; an asymmetry of more than 3 mm is abnormal.

A. Dysthyroid ophthalmopathy is the most common cause (uni- or bilateral) of exophthalmos. It is associated with lid retraction so that the upper eyelid is above the sclera; this results in "thyrotoxic stare." There may be reduced eyelid blinking and lid lag (delay in movement of the upper eyelid on downward gaze). These signs are due to sympathetic hyperactivity, not mechanical restriction, and respond to adrenergic blocking drugs.

B. If results of thyroid studies are abnormal, treat the metabolic disorder. If results are normal (including T_3 suppression and thyrotropin-releasing hormone stimulation tests), no other metabolic studies are indicated.

C. In thyroid-related proptosis, extraocular motility is usually impaired. This initially involves the superior and inferior rectus muscles and oblique muscles (less commonly, the medial and lateral rectus muscles). CT and MRI may show individual muscle enlargement; in rare cases, they show proptosis without muscle enlargement. If there is unilateral muscle enlargement, this may simulate an orbital mass. An awareness that unilateral or bilateral apical masses may be due to dysthyroid ophthalmopathy may avoid unnecessary orbital biopsy.

D. Ocular disturbances include diplopia due to impaired extraocular motility, impaired vision due to optic nerve compression, and corneal abnormalities due to severe proptosis. Treat with corticosteroids; if this is unsuccessful, orbital decompression may be needed.

E. If proptosis occurs without lid retraction, consider a mass lesion. Perform CT/MRI. The mass may be intraconal or extraconal. Intraconal masses originate from normal orbital structures. They may be nonneoplastic (vascular malformations) or neoplastic. Neoplasms include primary (optic glioma, meningioma) and secondary (metastases, lymphoma, sarcoma) lesions. The diagnosis is based on surgical biopsy findings.

F. If CT/MRI shows no mass, listen for an orbital bruit. If bruit is present, consider carotid artery–cavernous sinus fistula and perform angiography. CT or MRI may show an enlarged superior ophthalmic vein, enlarged muscles, and an enlarged cavernous sinus.

G. Orbital pseudotumor (Fig. 1) is an inflammatory granulomatous condition of unknown cause. It may

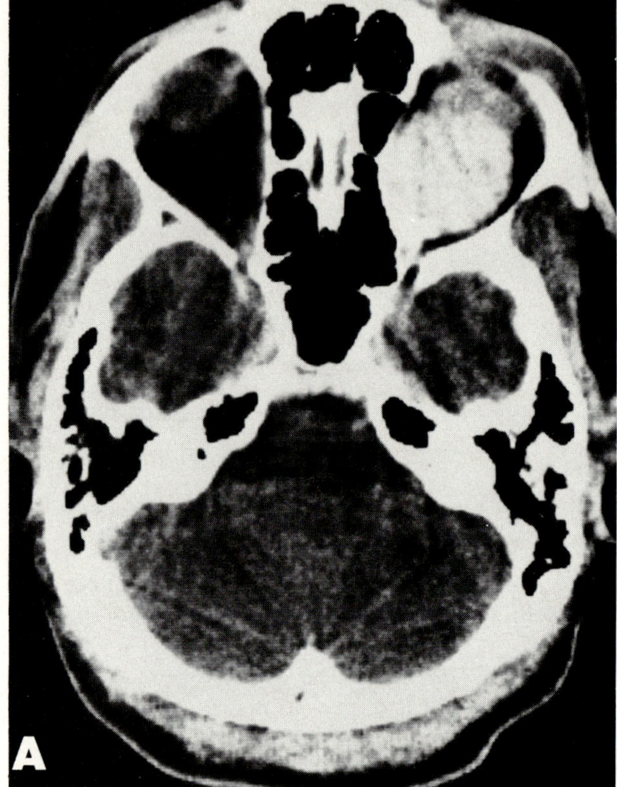

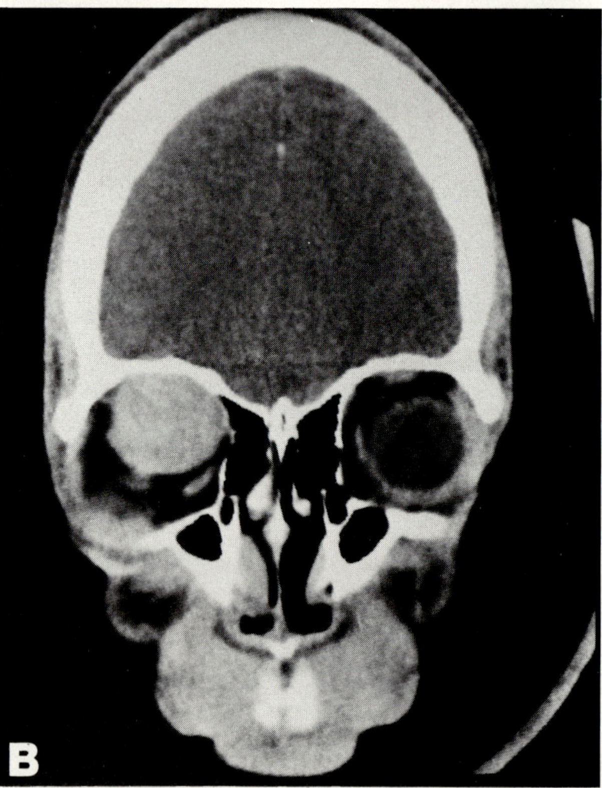

Figure 1 Orbital CT scan shows right retroglobal hyperdense lesion of the axial (*A*) and coronal (*B*) sections. Biopsy findings were consistent with orbital pseudotumor.

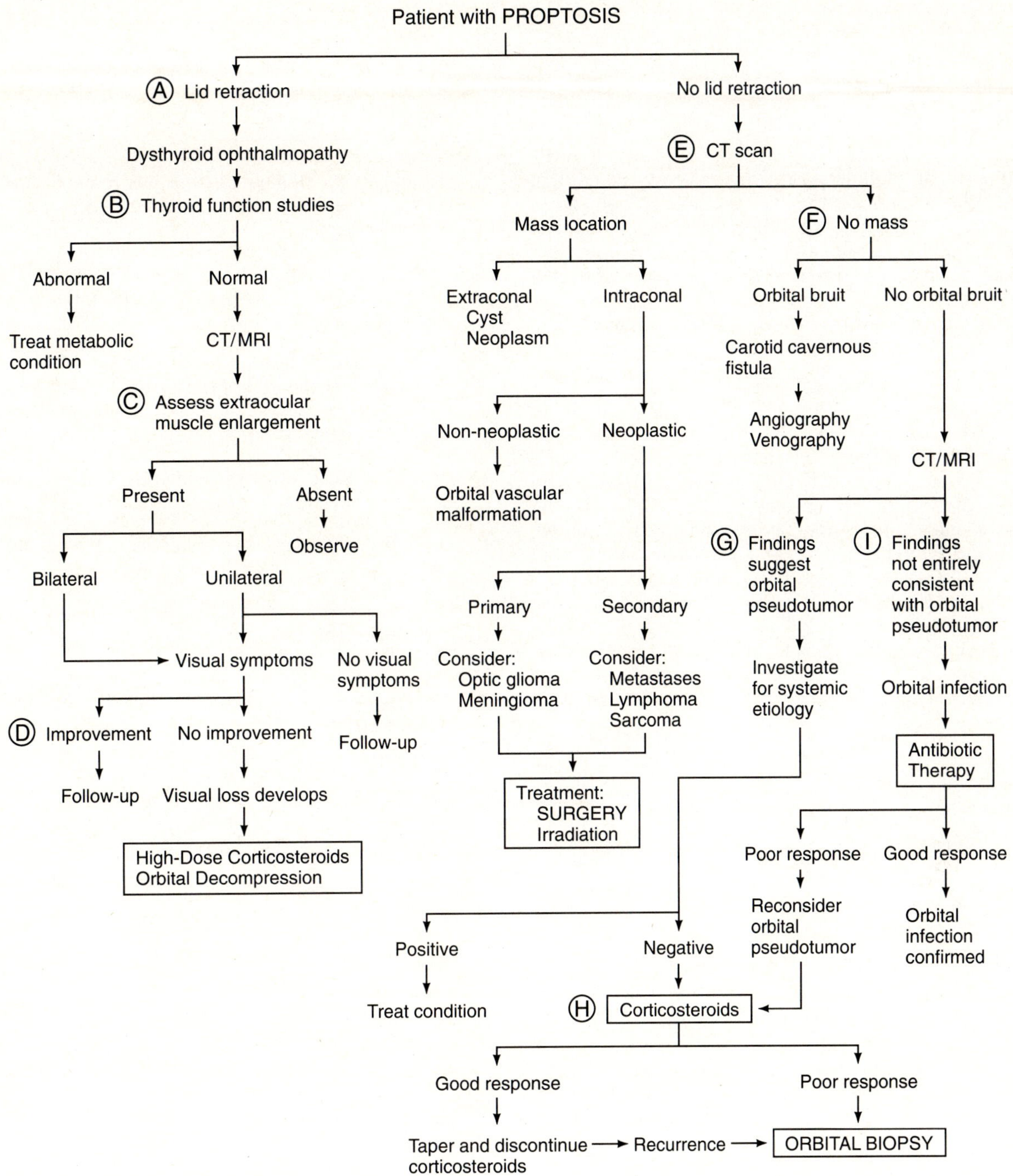

involve the sclera, lacrimal glands, extraocular muscles, optic nerves, cavernous sinus, or superior orbital fissure region. Granulomatous masses may also occur in sarcoidosis, systemic lupus erythematosus, syphilis, Wegener's granulomatosis, and tuberculosis. Diagnostic studies exclude these disorders. In pseudotumor, there are orbital pain and inflammatory signs (conjunctival redness and congestion).

H. If clinical and neuroimaging (CT/MRI) findings are consistent with pseudotumor, treat with corticosteroids; a good clinical response is usually obtained. If there is no response, perform an orbital biopsy. Neoplastic conditions may initially respond to steroids (lymphoma, meningioma); symptoms recur when steroids are withdrawn. Orbital biopsy is necessary if symptoms recur.

I. If CT/MRI findings are inconsistent with pseudotumor, look for evidence of orbital infection. Treat with antibiotics. If there is no response, reconsider the diagnosis of pseudotumor. Biopsy may also be necessary.

Reference

Dresner SC, Kennerdell JS. Dysthyroid orbitopathy. Neurology 1985; 35:1628.

NYSTAGMUS

Richard L. Strub, M.D.

Nystagmus is an involuntary rhythmic eye movement that usually indicates dysfunction in either the peripheral (e.g., semicircular canals) or central (brain stem nuclei or deep cerebellar nuclei) vestibular system. It is a complex but important clinical sign. The discussion here considers only the most common types of acquired nystagmus. If a diagnosis cannot be made easily, refer the patient to a neurologist or neuro-ophthalmologist. Congenital nystagmus also occurs but is not discussed here.

A. Since nystagmus is usually associated with either labyrinth or brain stem dysfunction, the history and examination should concentrate on eliciting other associated signs and symptoms (in the case of brain stem disease, other cranial nerve signs or bilateral long tract signs; in peripheral vestibular (labyrinthine) disease, vertigo, nausea, and imbalance but without other CNS signs). Check visual acuity and carry out a funduscopic examination as well; reduced vision is a common cause of nystagmus. Nystagmus can be horizontal, vertical, rotatory, or pendular. At times, patients actually can see the environment jumping as a subjective representation of the nystagmus (oscillopsia).

B. In an eye (or both eyes) that has markedly reduced vision, spontaneous back-and-forth eye movements are often seen.

C. Vertical dysconjugate (seesaw) nystagmus is sometimes seen when parasellar tumors impinge on the optic chiasm.

D. In patients with lesions around the pineal gland or in the region of the cerebral aqueduct, upward gaze is restricted and produces actual convergence nystagmus (Perinaud's syndrome).

E. Jerk nystagmus refers to nystagmus with a fast component to one side and a slow return movement.

F. In labyrinthine disease, patients demonstrate both horizontal and rotatory nystagmus.

G. Pendular nystagmus is characterized by equal to-and-fro movements.

H. At times a focal motor seizure is manifested primarily by deviated eye movement (conjugate to one side) with nystagmus (fast phase in the direction of gaze).

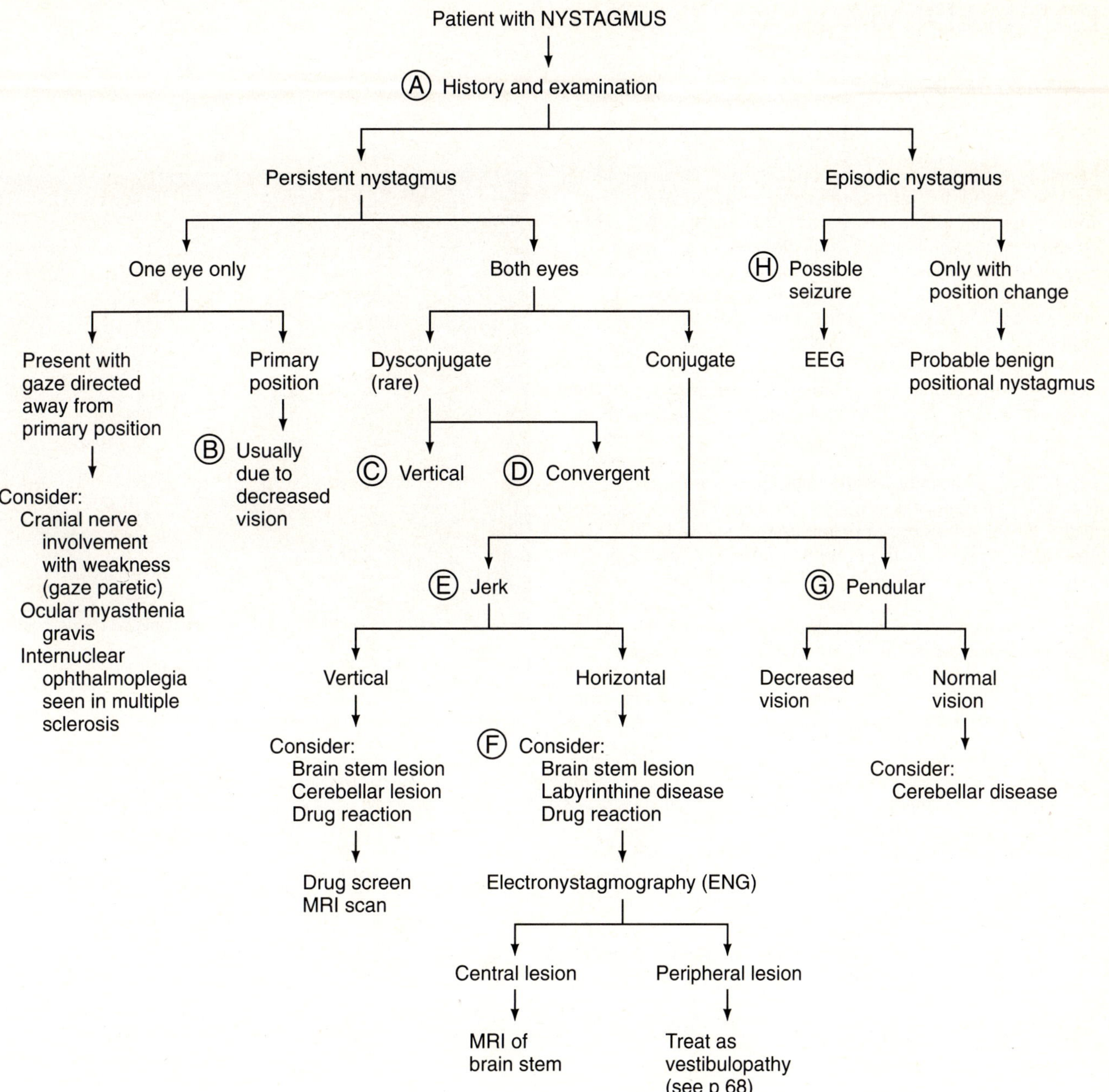

Patient with NYSTAGMUS

A History and examination

Persistent nystagmus

Episodic nystagmus

One eye only

Both eyes

H Possible seizure

Only with position change

Present with gaze directed away from primary position

Primary position

Dysconjugate (rare)

Conjugate

EEG

Probable benign positional nystagmus

Consider:
Cranial nerve involvement with weakness (gaze paretic)
Ocular myasthenia gravis
Internuclear ophthalmoplegia seen in multiple sclerosis

B Usually due to decreased vision

C Vertical

D Convergent

E Jerk

G Pendular

Vertical

Horizontal

Decreased vision

Normal vision

Consider:
Brain stem lesion
Cerebellar lesion
Drug reaction

F Consider:
Brain stem lesion
Labyrinthine disease
Drug reaction

Consider:
Cerebellar disease

Drug screen
MRI scan

Electronystagmography (ENG)

Central lesion

Peripheral lesion

MRI of brain stem

Treat as vestibulopathy (see p 68)

PAPILLEDEMA

Leon A. Weisberg, M.D.

Papilledema is edema of the optic nerve head (papilla), usually caused by increased intracranial pressure (ICP). Edema of the optic nerve may be caused by other conditions in which ICP is not elevated (e.g., papillitis, hypertension, diabetes). Ophthalmoscopic findings in papilledema include loss of spontaneous venous pulsations, optic disc hyperemia (disc pinker than normal), veins appearing dilated, loss of the physiologic cup, blurring of nasal and later temporal disc margins, hemorrhages and exudates surrounding the disc margins, and blurring of the retinal nerve fiber layer (Fig. 1). Visual symptoms, including transient visual obscurations, may be present. Visual acuity is usually preserved until late; pupillary response is normal. Papilledema is usually present bilaterally. If the optic nerve is atrophic, it cannot develop papilledema. This is the case in the Foster-Kennedy syndrome (papilledema in one eye and optic atrophy on the contralateral side). This disorder may be caused by a subfrontal tumor compressing the ipsilateral optic nerve to cause optic atrophy; this tumor also causes ventricular obstruction and intracranial hypertension so that papilledema is visualized on the contralateral side. If papilledema is seen on one side and the opposite optic disc appears normal, this is most likely due to a local orbital condition.

A. In assessing the funduscopic appearance of the optic disc, determine whether venous pulsations are present. The veins are easily recognized because they are slightly larger in diameter and darker than the arteries. Spontaneous venous pulsations almost always indicate that ICP is not elevated. These pulsations are absent in 25% of normal individuals; consider other funduscopic findings in these cases to determine whether papilledema is actually present. Fluorescein intravenous angiography may be useful in diagnosing papilledema. If papilledema is present, fluorescein contrast dye extravasates through vessel walls into the retina. If the optic disc appears elevated but venous pulsations are present, consider certain congenital and acquired disc abnormalities. For example, elevation of the optic nerve head by hyaline bodies (drusen) is commonly misdiagnosed as papilledema (pseudopapilledema). In patients with hypertensive retinopathy, there may be papilledema; however, there are also changes (narrowing) in the caliber of the retinal arteries, usually with hemorrhages and exudates. In hypertensive retinopathy, hemorrhages and exudates extend to the disc periphery and arterioles are narrowed, as contrasted with lack of arterial changes and centrally located hemorrhages and exudates seen in intracranial hypertension. Acute optic disc swelling may occur in young patients with juvenile-onset, insulin-dependent diabetes mellitus. Vision is not impaired and disc edema usually resolves. Disc swelling should be differentiated from diabetic retinopathy associated with visual loss.

B. If spontaneous venous pulsations are absent and there is optic disc edema, the presence of accompanying

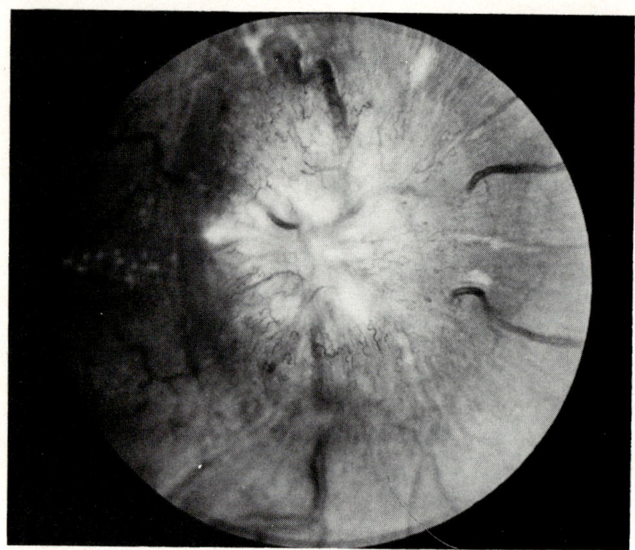

Figure 1 Marked blurring of the disc margins with exudates. This is consistent with papilledema.

neurologic signs indicates that papilledema has resulted from a mass lesion or obstructive hydrocephalus. The finding of papilledema requires full diagnostic evaluation (CT/MRI, angiography, CSF analysis).

C. If neurologic signs are absent in a patient with visual disc edema who also reports visual loss, consider optic neuritis or retinal vascular conditions (central retinal venous or arterial occlusion [CRVO, CRAO]). These conditions usually cause visual impairment. In optic neuritis, the optic disc in the involved eye shows disc edema and there is impaired visual acuity, central scotoma, and impaired pupillary response (unlike papilledema). In CRVO, the disc shows prominent dilated and tortuous veins and retinal hemorrhages. There is loss of vision and central scotoma. Laboratory evaluation includes erythrocyte sedimentation rate, serum electrophoresis, and determination of serum viscosity (hyperviscosity syndromes). Rarely, CRVO may be caused by carotid atherosclerotic disease; noninvasive carotid studies and angiography may be necessary. In CRAO, arterioles are narrowed and embolic fragments may be seen at arterial bifurcations. Initially the disc appears edematous and pale; a cherry-red spot representing retinal infarction may be seen. Pupillary light reaction is impaired in the involved eye. Retinal artery infarction may be central, with complete loss of visual acuity, or it may be segmental, with altitudinal visual loss involving the upper or lower field of vision (altitudinal defect). Such retinal arterial stroke occurs most commonly in patients with atherosclerotic cerebrovascular disease. These patients should be investigated for carotid disease.

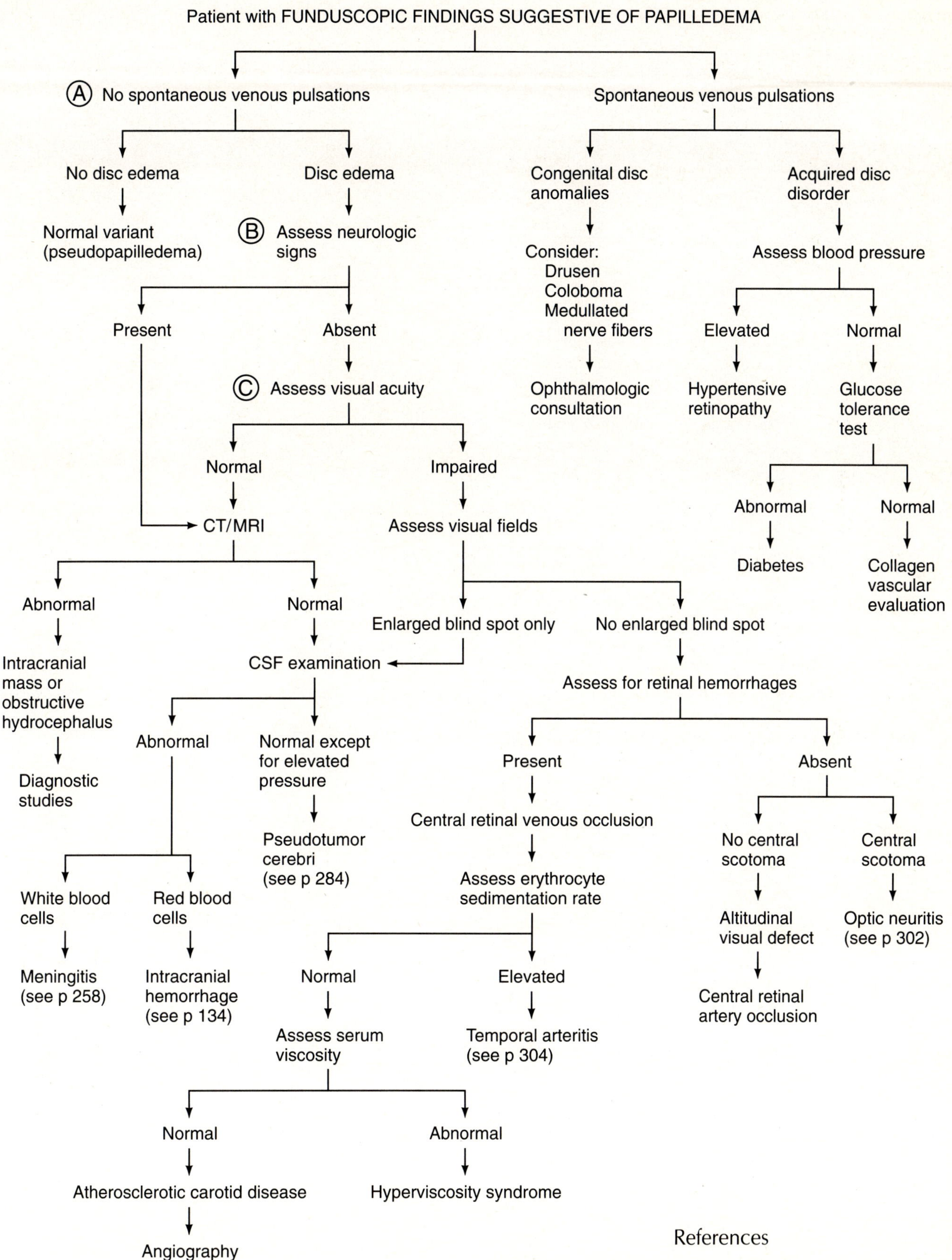

References

Glaser JS. Neuro-ophthalmology. Hagerstown, MD: Harper & Row, 1977:79.

Levin BE. The clinical significance of spontaneous pulsation of the retinal vein. Arch Neurol 1978; 35:37.

SPECIFIC NEUROLOGIC CONDITIONS

VASCULAR DISORDERS

CAROTID BRUIT

Leon A. Weisberg, M.D.

Carotid bruits occur in 2% to 4% of people >45 years of age and in 7% of those >65; they are more common in women than in men. Bruits are most common in hypertensive and diabetic patients. Death from ischemic heart disease and stroke is common in patients with bruits; stroke may occur ipsilateral or contralateral to the bruit, which is a marker of generalized or multifocal vascular disease.

A. To detect a bruit, auscultate the carotid bifurcation below the jaw angle. If flow is laminar, no bruit is heard; if turbulent, a bruit may be heard. Turbulence is due to vessel wall irregularity or increased blood velocity (exercise, fever, anemia, anxiety). Do not compress the artery, as this may artificially induce turbulence, causing an abnormal sound identical to a bruit. Carotid bruits are best detected with the stethoscope bell. Noninvasive imaging shows that bruits may develop with 50% reduction in cross-sectional diameter of the carotid bifurcation. Carotid bruits do not always indicate carotid stenosis but may be due to hemodynamic factors. Loudness of bruit does not correlate with severity of stenosis; carotid occlusion causes no bruit. The point of maximal intensity is an important clue in locating the source of the bruit. If a bruit is heard in the neck but is louder as the stethoscope is moved toward the chest, consider a cardiac source. In patients with a carotid bruit, obtain a detailed history of possible previous transient cerebral or retinal ischemic attacks before concluding that the patient is completely asymptomatic. Earlier stroke symptoms may have occurred but the patient may not have sought medical attention or been aware of the clinical significance of cerebrovascular symptoms. A complete examination is necessary to exclude focal neurologic signs, because a previous stroke may not be recognized in the acute stages. If a history of TIA is elicited or focal neurologic signs suggest a previous stroke, the patient is not asymptomatic. In these cases, neuroimaging (CT/MRI) and cerebral angiography are indicated. The incidence of clinically "silent" strokes is unknown, and it is not known if the finding of "silent" strokes would modify management in otherwise asymptomatic carotid bruit patients. Evidence of a "silent" earlier stroke may be demonstrated by careful neurologic examination or CT/MRI findings.

If a patient with a bruit is asymptomatic, assess for generalized vascular risk factors and perform noninvasive carotid artery studies. At present, there is no evidence to support carotid endarterectomy (CEA) in patients with asymptomatic bruits. Antiplatelet medication is commonly used for high-risk asymptomatic patients, but there are no data supporting therapeutic benefit in preventing a stroke or heart attack in these patients. Patients with asymptomatic bruits are at risk for heart attack, and recognition of a carotid bruit justifies immediate cardiology referral.

B. Noninvasive tests used to evaluate carotid arteries include direct tests (duplex ultrasound [DUS]) and indirect tests (oculoplethysmography, periorbital Doppler ultrasound). Invasive tests include digital subtraction angiography (DSA) and conventional angiography. The role of magnetic resonance angiography is expanding but not clinically defined at this time. DUS identifies hemodynamically significant carotid stenosis. Because of B-mode capability, DUS may detect anatomic abnormalities (ulcers, plaques, plaque hemorrhage). The major vessel wall abnormality that limits ultrasound resolving capability is the presence of calcification within plaques, as this finding degrades image quality. DSA provides direct visualization of carotid and intracranial vessels. Unlike conventional arteriography, DSA does not require arterial catheterization but does require a high volume of contrast agent. Intra-arterial DSA is performed with lower contrast dose and has accuracy equivalent to that of conventional arteriography. Conventional carotid angiography is performed with percutaneous transfemoral catheterization using the Seldinger technique. The examiner employs aortic arch contrast injection to visualize the brachiocephalic vessels and then selectively catheterizes each common carotid artery. Serious complications of angiography may include stroke, myocardial infarction, and death; these occur in 1% of cases. Transient neurologic dysfunction may occur in 5% of cases. Conventional carotid angiography is the most sensitive test to differentiate severe stenosis from complete carotid occlusion. The major limitation of angiography is that it does not detect anatomic vessel wall abnormalities (e.g., ulcerated plaque, intraplaque hemorrhage).

C. If vascular imaging studies show abnormalities in carotid artery contour indicating atheroma, this plaque may cause stenosis, ulceration, or occlusion. Hemorrhage or ulceration may occur within plaques. Ulcers may develop a thrombus formation, which may narrow and occlude the artery. Ulcers may be superficial and regress rather than progress in size. Serial vascular imaging studies may show progression of stenosis even if the patient remains asymptomatic. Noninvasive serial carotid studies may be warranted in patients at high risk for stroke (symptomatic coronary artery or peripheral vascular disease, obese patients, smokers). If a progressing carotid lesion is visualized, options include close observation or angiography. If significant stenosis (>70%) is demonstrated, management choices include follow-up with repeated noninvasive carotid studies, antiplatelet medication, and CEA. The morbidity and mortality rate of CEA is 4%; this procedure should therefore be performed in patients whose stroke risk exceeds this surgical complication rate. In patients with asymptomatic carotid bruit, the risk of ischemic stroke related to

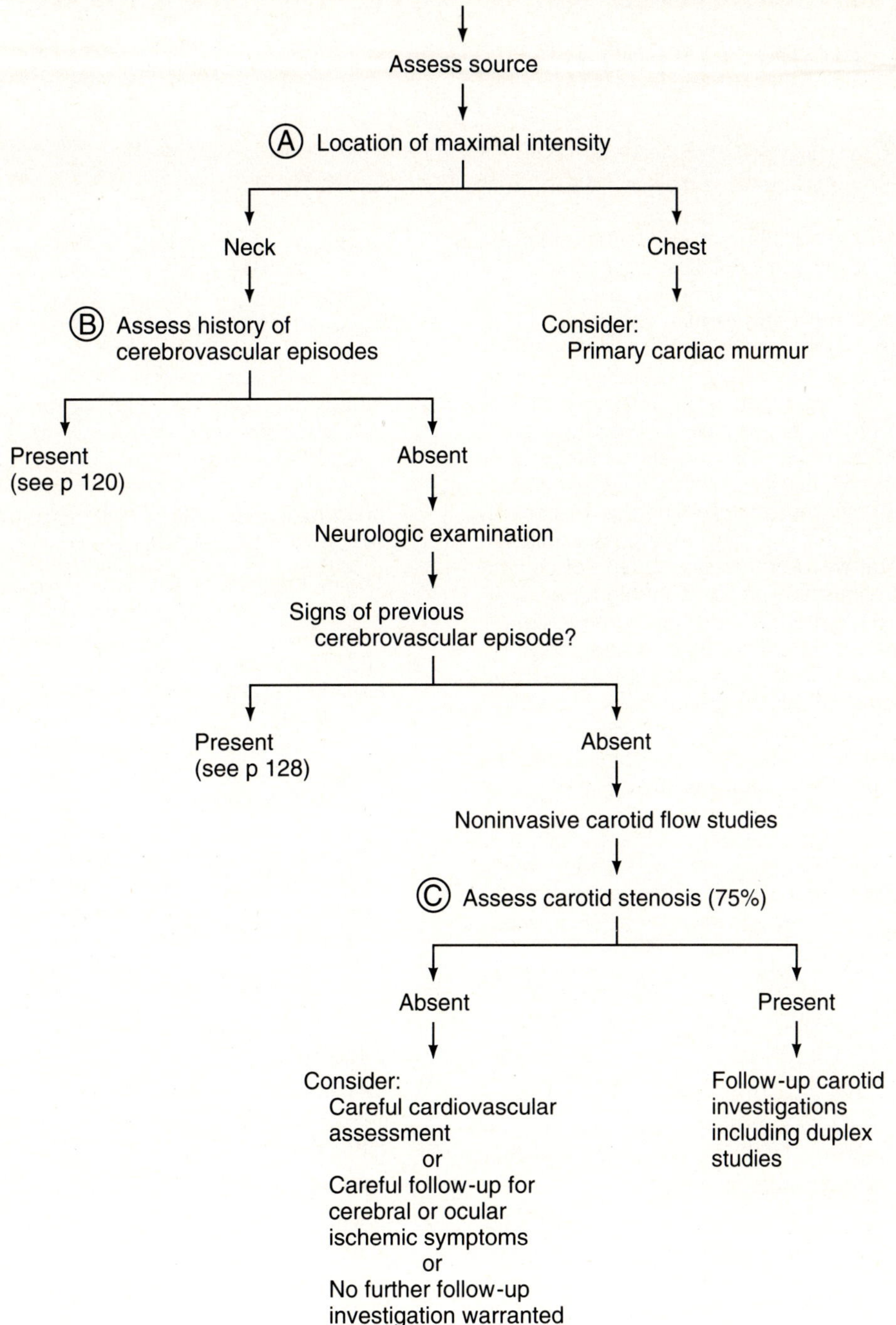

bruit is 0.3% per year. The risk of perioperative stroke is not increased if a patient with an asymptomatic bruit undergoes surgery of any type. It must be emphasized that asymptomatic bruit indicates *generalized* atherosclerotic vascular disease, not focal localized stenotic vessel disease. Patients with asymptomatic bruits are more likely to die of heart attack than of stroke, and evidence that CEA is beneficial in any asymptomatic patient awaits the results of prospective studies.

References

Chambers BR, Norris JW. Outcome in patients with asymptomatic neck bruits. N Engl J Med 1986; 315:860.

Feussner JR, Matchar DB. When and how to study the carotid arteries. Ann Intern Med 1988; 109:805.

Hennerici M, Hulshomer HB, Hefter H, et al. Natural history of asymptomatic extracranial arterial disease. Brain 1987; 110:777.

Wolf PA, Kannel WB, Sorlic P. Asymptomatic carotid bruit. JAMA 1981; 245:1442.

TRANSIENT EPISODES OF FOCAL NEUROLOGIC DYSFUNCTION (TEFND)

Leon A. Weisberg, M.D.

When patients experience TEFND, it is presumed that the mechanism is vascular ischemia and these are diagnosed as transient ischemic attacks (TIAs); however, other neurologic pathophysiologic mechanisms may cause TEFND. In focal seizures, there may be positive clinical phenomena, including clonic motor activity, paresthesias, and flashing lights. These are due to cortical excitatory electrical activity. These seizures spread, march, or progress rapidly across the involved body regions, usually within several minutes. Less commonly, negative clinical features, including weakness, numbness, and visual loss due to cortical negative postical inhibitory activity, may predominate in certain seizure conditions. On the basis of type of clinical characteristics and pattern of spread, it should be possible to differentiate focal seizure activity from ischemic conditions (TIA, migraine). In migraine, focal (visual, sensory, language, or motor impairment) dysfunction may spread across involved visual fields or extremities over a longer time (20 to 60 minutes). This slower progression is due to spreading cortical depression rather than excitatory electrical activity, and along with subsequent development of headache should differentiate migraine from focal seizures or TIA. In unusual cases, intracranial mass lesions (subdural hematoma, abscess, neoplasm) may cause TEFND. This is because of cerebral ischemia or focal seizures related to the intracranial mass lesion. Demyelinating disease may cause TEFND owing to transient conduction block.

A. In patients with TEFND, headache is most consistent with migraine; however, headache may occur in focal seizures, especially those originating in the occipital cortex. EEG spike discharges confirm the diagnosis of focal seizure, but a focal slow wave pattern may be prominent in migraine. Once focal seizures are diagnosed, perform CT/MRI to determine whether there is an underlying structural lesion.

B. Determine the temporal pattern of the episode. TIA is characterized by sudden onset of focal neurologic dysfunction that is confined to a specific vascular arterial distribution. Also, there is usually spread or progression of the neurologic symptoms. By definition, deficit caused by TIA must resolve within 24 hours; however, most TIAs last <30 minutes. If TIA lasts >1 hour, it is unlikely that focal neurologic deficit will resolve within 24 hours. If TIA lasts >1 hour, pathologic ischemic lesions are frequently demonstrated by CT/MRI even though the clinical neurologic deficit completely resolved. In 25% of patients with TIA-like episodes, there is CT or MRI evidence of ischemic lesions despite a normal neurologic examination after the TIA. This occurrence is defined as cerebral infarction with transient signs (CITS). If the episode lasts >24 hours but resolves within several days or weeks, it is defined as reversible ischemic neurologic deficit (RIND). If neurologic deficit persists beyond this period, it is defined as a completed stroke.

C. The mechanism of TIA may be embolism, hypoperfusion, vasospasm, hemodynamic hypotensive crisis, or thrombosis. Hematologic conditions (hemoglobinopathy, polycythemia, leukemia, thrombocytosis), increased blood viscosity (due to macroglobulins or cryoglobulins), or metabolic conditions (hypoglycemia, nonketotic hyperosmolar hyperglycemia) may also cause TEFND but are much less common mechanisms. If vasospasm is present, it should be demonstrated by angiography. If hypotension is a causative factor, symptoms should be induced by the postural blood pressure changes. Laboratory studies should identify these conditions. The precipitating factor must be corrected to prevent recurrence.

D. It is important to accurately diagnose a TIA as the cause of the TEFND, because one third of TIA patients develop a stroke unless adequately treated. If the cause of the TEFND is not one of the vascular ischemic mechanisms, further diagnostic studies are necessary. Be careful not to assume that TEFND is necessarily equivalent to a TIA.

References

Caplan LR. Transient ischemic attacks. Neurology 1988; 38:791.

Levy DE. How transient are transient ischemic attacks? Neurology 1988; 38:674.

Werdelin L, Juhler M. The cause of transient ischemic attacks. Neurology 1988; 38:677.

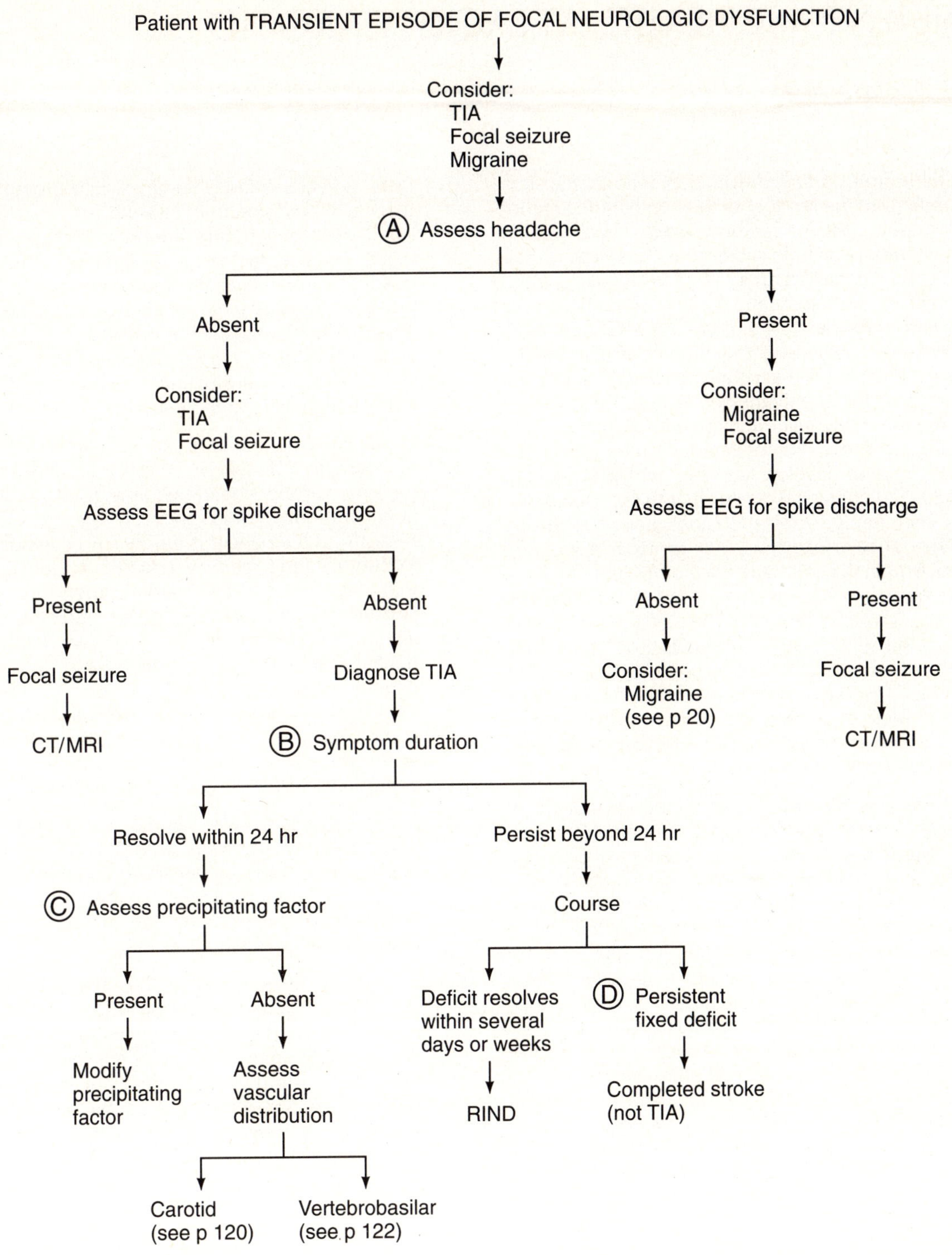

Patient with TRANSIENT EPISODE OF FOCAL NEUROLOGIC DYSFUNCTION
Consider:
TIA
Focal seizure
Migraine
A Assess headache
Absent
Present
Consider:
TIA
Focal seizure
Consider:
Migraine
Focal seizure
Assess EEG for spike discharge
Assess EEG for spike discharge
Present
Absent
Absent
Present
Focal seizure
Diagnose TIA
Consider:
Migraine
(see p 20)
Focal seizure
CT/MRI
B Symptom duration
CT/MRI
Resolve within 24 hr
Persist beyond 24 hr
C Assess precipitating factor
Course
Present
Absent
Deficit resolves
within several
days or weeks
D Persistent
fixed deficit
Modify
precipitating
factor
Assess
vascular
distribution
RIND
Completed stroke
(not TIA)
Carotid
(see p 120)
Vertebrobasilar
(see p 122)

TRANSIENT ISCHEMIC ATTACK: CAROTID

Leon A. Weisberg, M.D.

A TIA in the carotid artery distribution follows transient perfusion deficits in the territory of the ophthalmic anterior (ACA) or middle (MCA) cerebral artery. With ocular ischemia, symptoms include sudden loss of vision ipsilateral to the involved carotid artery (amaurosis fugax, see p 58). Symptoms of ACA ischemia include contralateral leg weakness and numbness; symptoms of MCA ischemia include weakness and sensory impairment usually involving the face and/or arm and generally sparing the leg. If the MCA territory of the dominant hemisphere becomes ischemic, aphasia (language impairment, difficulty with word finding or verbal comprehension) may transiently occur. TIA symptoms develop suddenly, without spread or march; spread is characteristic of migraine or focal seizures. It is uncommon for TIAs to cause mental confusion or headache. They usually last <5 to 15 minutes, are stereotyped, and may occur only once or multiple times. If the deficit does not resolve within 1 hour, it is unlikely to clear completely within 24 hours. The consensus of earlier TIA studies is that 25% to 35% of patients develop cerebral infarction; however, recent studies show that 20% of TIA patients show CT/MRI evidence of cerebral infarction even though the clinical neurologic deficit has resolved within 24 hours. The 5-year mortality rate in TIA patients is 25%; most die of myocardial infarction.

A. The term TIA describes the temporal pattern of ischemia but tells nothing about the underlying vascular mechanism. Without knowing the mechanism, one cannot determine appropriate treatment. For example, TIA due to marked carotid stenosis requires treatment different from that for transient deficit due to sudden blood pressure elevation. On the basis of clinical symptoms, it is possible to classify TIA as subcortical or *lacunar* (e.g., pure motor hemiparesis; pure sensory stroke; or sensorimotor with involvement of face, arm, and leg) or *cortical* (aphasia plus right-sided motor or sensory impairment; sensory or motor disturbance involving the face and arm or leg or incomplete involvement of two regions; aphasia alone). In patients with amaurosis fugax or cortical TIA, angiography is likely to show carotid lesions (stenosis, ulceration, occlusion). Patients with lacunar TIA usually have a negative angiogram, and the mechanism is most likely small vessel disease.

B. Most patients with subcortical TIA are hypertensive; treatment consists of careful blood pressure control. Because the mechanism of lacunar stroke is deep-penetrating arteriolar occlusion due to fibrinoid degeneration and lipohyalinosis, there is no compelling evidence that antiplatelet treatment prevents subcortical lacunar TIA or stroke. Because of the small size of the arterioles involved, angiography is usually negative in these patients.

C. Deep cerebral infarcts (lacunes) in the basal ganglia, thalamus, and internal capsule are *usually* due to small deep-penetrating arteriolar disease; however, when no risk factors are identified, investigate a possible cardiac embolic source (see p 128). When a lacunar infarct is large or giant-sized or has CT/MRI features indicating a hemorrhagic infarct, a cardiogenic embolic source is suggested rather than small vessel disease. Cardiogenic cerebral embolism does not usually cause preceding TIAs.

D. In patients with ocular or cortical carotid TIA, perform angiography. If severe (>75%) carotid stenosis is present, carotid endarterectomy (CEA) is indicated. Surgical mortality and morbidity rates for CEA should be <3%. If the patient is a poor CEA candidate owing to complicating medical conditions, anticoagulation may be used. If the carotid artery is occluded, consider anticoagulation; in this situation, CEA may actually be contraindicated. CEA may cause hemorrhagic infarction due to sudden tissue reperfusion in patients who have complete carotid occlusion. It is important to differentiate the angiographic pattern of complete carotid occlusion from that of severe carotid stenosis (>95%), since CEA may be deleterious in occlusion and life-saving in severe stenosis.

E. If angiography shows stenosis or occlusion of the intracranial carotid artery or MCA, consider anticoagulant or antiplatelet medication. There is no evidence to support the clinical value of a superficial temporal artery–MCA bypass operation in patients in whom these vessels are occluded.

F. If angiography is negative, the TIA may be due to intracranial branch occlusion. These small embolic fragments may disperse before angiography, and thus the angiogram may show no abnormality. An alternative mechanism may be lacunar disease. In some TIA patients who show no angiographic abnormality and are not hypertensive, a full medical and cardiac evaluation should be made (see p 128).

References

Bogousslavsky J, Regli F. Cerebral infarction with transient signs. Stroke 1984; 15:536.

Grotta JC. Current medical and surgical therapy for cerebrovascular disease. N Engl J Med 1987; 317:1505.

Hankey GJ, Warlow CP. Lacunar transient ischaemic attacks: A clinically useful concept. Lancet 1991; 337:335.

Santamaria J, Graus F, Rubio F. Cerebral infarction of the basal ganglia due to embolism from the heart. Stroke 1983; 14:911.

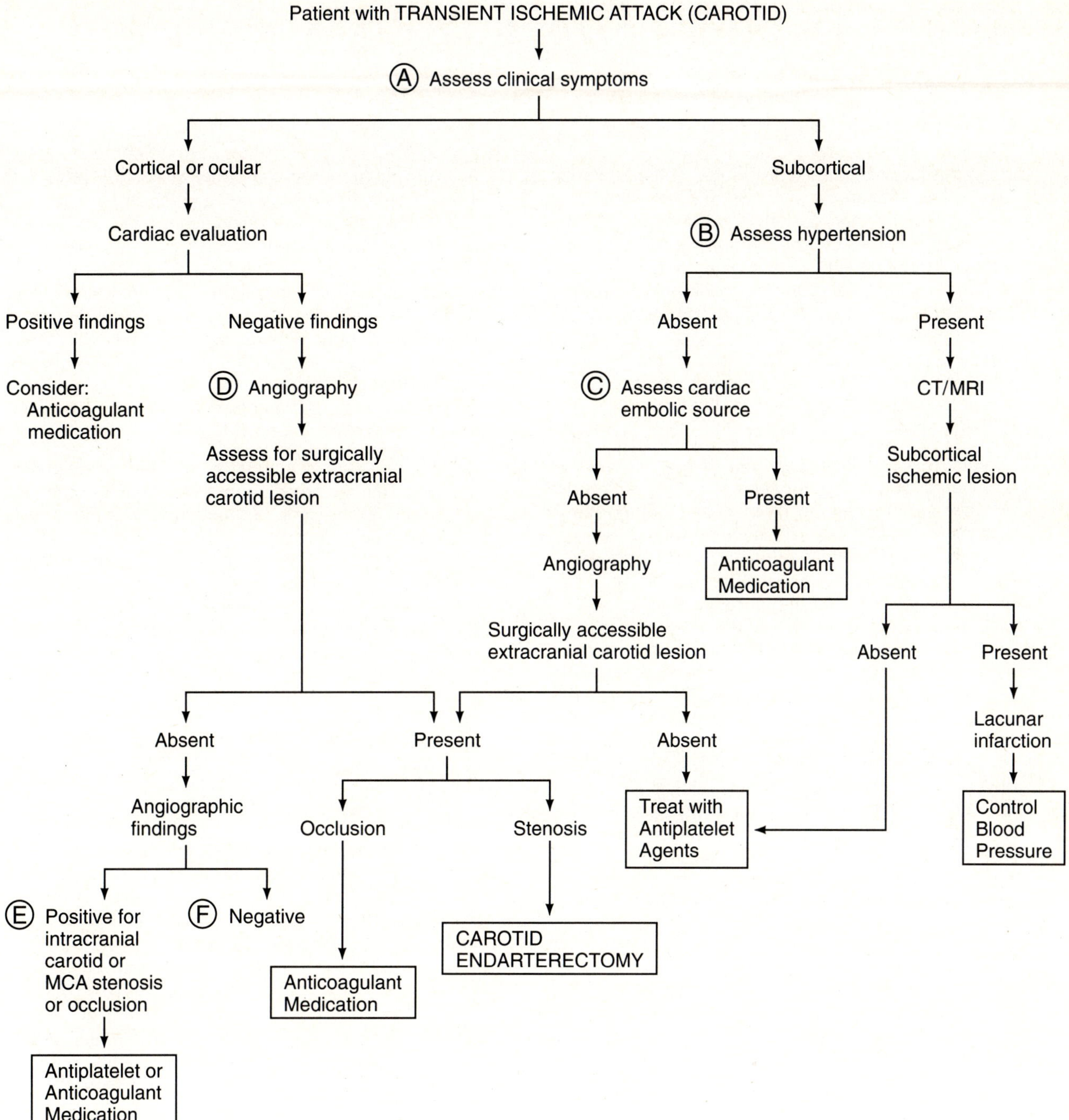

Patient with TRANSIENT ISCHEMIC ATTACK (CAROTID)
A Assess clinical symptoms
Cortical or ocular
Subcortical
Cardiac evaluation
B Assess hypertension
Positive findings
Negative findings
Absent
Present
Consider:
Anticoagulant
medication
D Angiography
C Assess cardiac
embolic source
CT/MRI
Assess for surgically
accessible extracranial
carotid lesion
Absent
Present
Subcortical
ischemic lesion
Angiography
Anticoagulant
Medication
Surgically accessible
extracranial carotid lesion
Absent
Present
Absent
Present
Absent
Present
Absent
Angiographic
findings
Occlusion
Stenosis
Treat with
Antiplatelet
Agents
Lacunar
infarction
E Positive for
intracranial
carotid or
MCA stenosis
or occlusion
F Negative
Anticoagulant
Medication
CAROTID
ENDARTERECTOMY
Control
Blood
Pressure
Antiplatelet or
Anticoagulant
Medication

TRANSIENT ISCHEMIC ATTACK: VERTEBROBASILAR

Leon A. Weisberg, M.D.

The vertebrobasilar (V-B) arterial distribution includes brain stem, cerebellum, thalamus, and occipital and temporal lobes (medial, inferior, and posterior portions). TIA symptoms include bilateral visual loss (homonymous hemianopia, cortical blindness) due to occipital lobe ischemia, weakness (hemiparesis, tetraparesis), cranial nerve disturbances (dysarthria, vertigo, dysphagia, diplopia, facial weakness or numbness), unsteadiness (ataxia), and drop attacks (patient suddenly and briefly falls to the ground, remaining conscious). When any of these symptoms occur alone (vertigo, dysarthria, dysphagia, diplopia), it is unlikely that they represent V-B TIA.

A. TIA pattern is usually stereotyped. V-B TIAs may be precipitated by a change in head or body position. If episodes are induced by rapid change in position (recumbent to standing), consider postural hypotension with reduced cardiac output as the TIA pathogenesis. In patients with syncope, blurring or "graying out" of vision is due to retinal rather than occipital lobe ischemia. It is important to differentiate syncope from V-B TIA. Episodes of vertigo alone are usually due to vestibular or labyrinthine dysfunction, *not* V-B TIA. Hyperventilation episodes cause light-headedness, perioral or extremity paresthesias, and weakness. This occurs during anxiety states and may be associated with cardiac (chest pain, dyspnea, palpitations) symptoms; these may be induced by overbreathing. Hyperventilation attacks should not be confused with V-B TIA, which are not precipitated by overbreathing. Multiple sclerosis may cause transient brain stem and cerebellar symptoms, but the neurologic examination shows abnormalities consistent with this disorder; with TIAs, neurologic findings are normal between attacks. In basilar artery migraine, transient brain stem symptoms are followed by headache and usually vomiting, and migraine usually occurs in younger patients than those with V-B TIA.

B. After TIA symptoms resolve, neurologic findings are normal. If abnormal signs persist after 24 hours, the patient has experienced completed stroke, has nonischemic structural or demyelinating lesion, or shows neurologic evidence of a previous stroke. Perform CT/MRI to exclude a structural or demyelinating lesion.

C. Auscultate for a bruit in the supraclavicular fossa (subclavian artery) or mastoid region (vertebral artery). Check blood pressure in both arms (the difference in systolic pressures of 20 mm Hg is significant) at rest and after exercise. The finding of a bruit and blood pressure difference in the arms in patients with V-B TIA suggests the possibility of subclavian steal syndrome. This results from occlusion or severe stenosis of the subclavian artery, which is proximal to the vertebral artery. In symptomatic subclavian steal syndrome, angiography shows proximal subclavian narrowing with reversal of normal vertebral blood flow pattern. Blood flow reversal in the vertebral artery is a common finding, but most patients with this are asymptomatic. Reconstructive vascular surgery for subclavian steal syndrome is performed only in symptomatic patients.

D. If symptoms are precipitated by head movement, consider craniocervical anomalies (cervical spondylosis, basilar impression); perform cervical spine radiography and MRI. V-B TIA symptoms may be precipitated by vertebral artery compression or stretching. If V-B TIA occurs in a young patient, consider fibromuscular dysplasia. The vertebral artery may undergo spontaneous dissection to cause occlusion or aneurysm formation; the diagnosis of dissection is established by angiography. With vertebral dissection, thrombus formation may occur, requiring anticoagulation therapy, or vertebral artery reconstructive surgery may be indicated.

E. Angiography of the V-B arterial system is indicated to determine the appropriate therapy in TIA patients. Because of the potential risk of angiography, antiplatelet medication may be used first. Evaluate for a potential cardiac embolus of V-B TIA, because anticoagulant therapy is warranted if a cardiac source is demonstrated. If TIAs do not resolve and no cardiac source is found, angiography is indicated. If results are negative, consider a lacunar mechanism and assess the patient for a source of arteriolar lipohyalinosis and fibrinoid degeneration (hypertension, diabetes mellitus). If there is severe vertebral or basilar artery stenosis, treat with oral anticoagulants. If there is V-B arterial occlusion, use heparin for 2 weeks followed by antiplatelet medication.

References

Caplan LR. Vertebro-basilar disease. Current concepts of cerebrovascular disease. Stroke 1980; 15:11.

Henerici M, Klemm C, Rautenberg W. The subclavian steal phenomenon. Neurology 1988; 38:669.

Kubik CS, Adams RD. Occlusion of the basilar artery—clinical and pathological study. Brain 1946; 69:73.

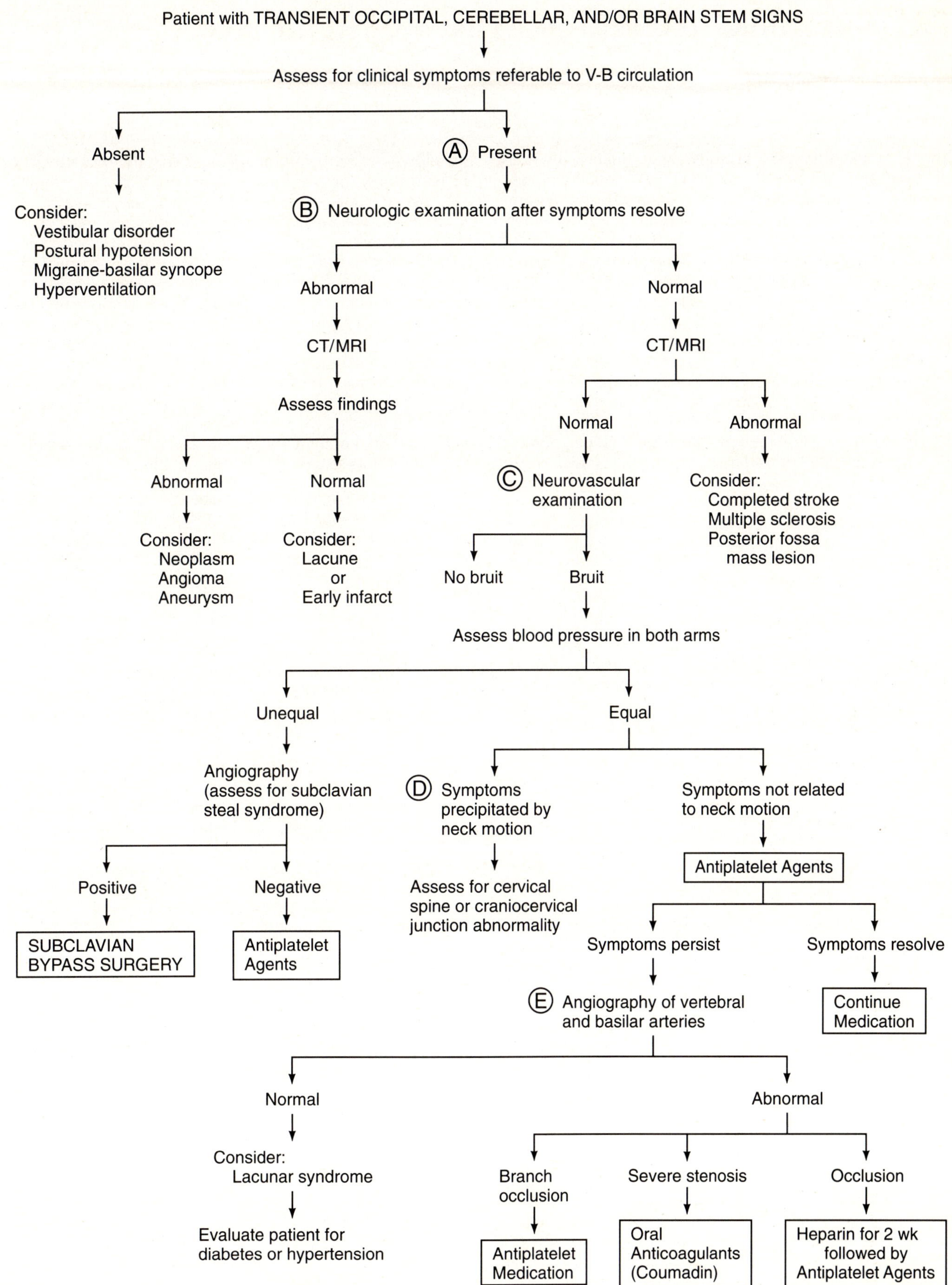

Patient with TRANSIENT OCCIPITAL, CEREBELLAR, AND/OR BRAIN STEM SIGNS
Assess for clinical symptoms referable to V-B circulation
Absent
A Present
Consider:
Vestibular disorder
Postural hypotension
Migraine-basilar syncope
Hyperventilation
B Neurologic examination after symptoms resolve
Abnormal
Normal
CT/MRI
CT/MRI
Assess findings
Normal
Abnormal
Abnormal
Normal
C Neurovascular examination
Consider:
Completed stroke
Multiple sclerosis
Posterior fossa mass lesion
Consider:
Neoplasm
Angioma
Aneurysm
Consider:
Lacune
or
Early infarct
No bruit
Bruit
Assess blood pressure in both arms
Unequal
Equal
Angiography
(assess for subclavian steal syndrome)
D Symptoms precipitated by neck motion
Symptoms not related to neck motion
Positive
Negative
Antiplatelet Agents
SUBCLAVIAN BYPASS SURGERY
Antiplatelet Agents
Assess for cervical spine or craniocervical junction abnormality
Symptoms persist
Symptoms resolve
E Angiography of vertebral and basilar arteries
Continue Medication
Normal
Abnormal
Consider:
Lacunar syndrome
Branch occlusion
Severe stenosis
Occlusion
Evaluate patient for diabetes or hypertension
Antiplatelet Medication
Oral Anticoagulants (Coumadin)
Heparin for 2 wk followed by Antiplatelet Agents

PROGRESSING (DETERIORATING) STROKE

Leon A. Weisberg, M.D.

The term deteriorating or progressing stroke is used to describe stroke in patients whose clinical condition worsens while being observed by a physician. This is presumably due to extension of the cerebral infarction or hemorrhage. Deterioration may also result from systemic or metabolic factors (e.g., hypo- or hyperglycemia, hyponatremia, infection, reduced cardiac output). When initially seen, all patients have the potential for progression; serial examinations should therefore be performed in all stroke patients. The term stroke-in-evolution or progressing (deteriorating) stroke refers to the condition of patients who initially have a partial stable deficit and subsequently experience clinical worsening of the neurologic deficit. Temporal progression may occur over several hours to several days in several patterns: stepwise, gradual, abrupt. Recurrence of stroke within 1 week of the initial stroke strongly indicates a cardiogenic cerebral embolus or large vessel (carotid, vertebrobasilar) distal clot propagation. In carotid ischemic stroke, the deficit should be stable for 24 hours, and in vertebrobasilar stroke for 72 hours, before progression may be regarded as unlikely and a completed stroke can be diagnosed. In some stroke patients, neurologic worsening may be due to intracerebral hemorrhage enlargement or hemorrhagic transformation of an initially ischemic stroke. The natural history of stroke progression has been poorly studied. In one report, 30% worsened, 40% were stable, and 30% improved within the first week. Progression may be more common than clinically reported because onset of stroke often occurs during sleep and progression may not be detected. In other cases, stroke may progress but since the patient is not under medical observation, the deterioration is not recorded by the physician and not reported by the patient. Neurologic change is most likely to be detected when patients are closely monitored.

In ischemic stroke, arterial occlusion results in reduced cerebral blood flow (CBF). CBF is normally 25 to 50 ml/100 g/min. When this falls below 23, reversible ischemic changes may occur. As CBF falls below this critical range, cerebral perfusion protective mechanisms (autoregulation to allow maximal vasodilatation, capillary dilatation to increase flow and volume, hemoglobin-oxygen affinity changes to increase oxygen extraction) are activated. If these protective mechanisms are not effective and collateral blood flow is not adequate, a neurologic deficit occurs. Initial ischemic symptoms are due to neuronal membrane (electrical) failure. If cerebral arterial perfusion is not restored, cerebral infarction occurs. This is complicated by secondary effects of edema, free radical formation, and vascular sludging (increased vascular viscosity) within the cerebral vasculature microcirculation. When cerebral infarction occurs within one arterial distribution, the surrounding brain region may be only marginally perfused (this is referred to as the ischemic penumbra); if perfusion is not restored, cerebral infarction extends to this region, resulting in further neurologic deterioration.

A. Perform CT initially to exclude a hemorrhagic stroke or nonvascular lesion. This lesion may be a primary intracerebral hemorrhage (PIH) or hemorrhagic transformation of an ischemic lesion. The latter condition is usually due to cardiogenic or artery-to-artery embolism. If the initial stroke is due to PIH, neurologic deterioration may be caused by delayed hemorrhage enlargement, vasogenic edema, or hydrocephalus.

B. Cardiac evaluation should be made, especially if there is recurrent stroke. This should suggest the possibility of cardiogenic cerebral embolus. If there is a cardiac embolus, anticoagulant treatment is warranted.

C. If CT/MRI shows edema, it may be either vasogenic or cytotoxic. Both may cause increased intracranial pressure with mass effect and may further reduce CBF. Treatment of edema may be necessary to reduce mass effect and prevent cerebral herniation, which may cause neurologic deterioration. Treatment of vasogenic edema is more effective than that of cytotoxic edema; however, these edema patterns cannot be adequately differentiated on the basis of CT/MRI findings.

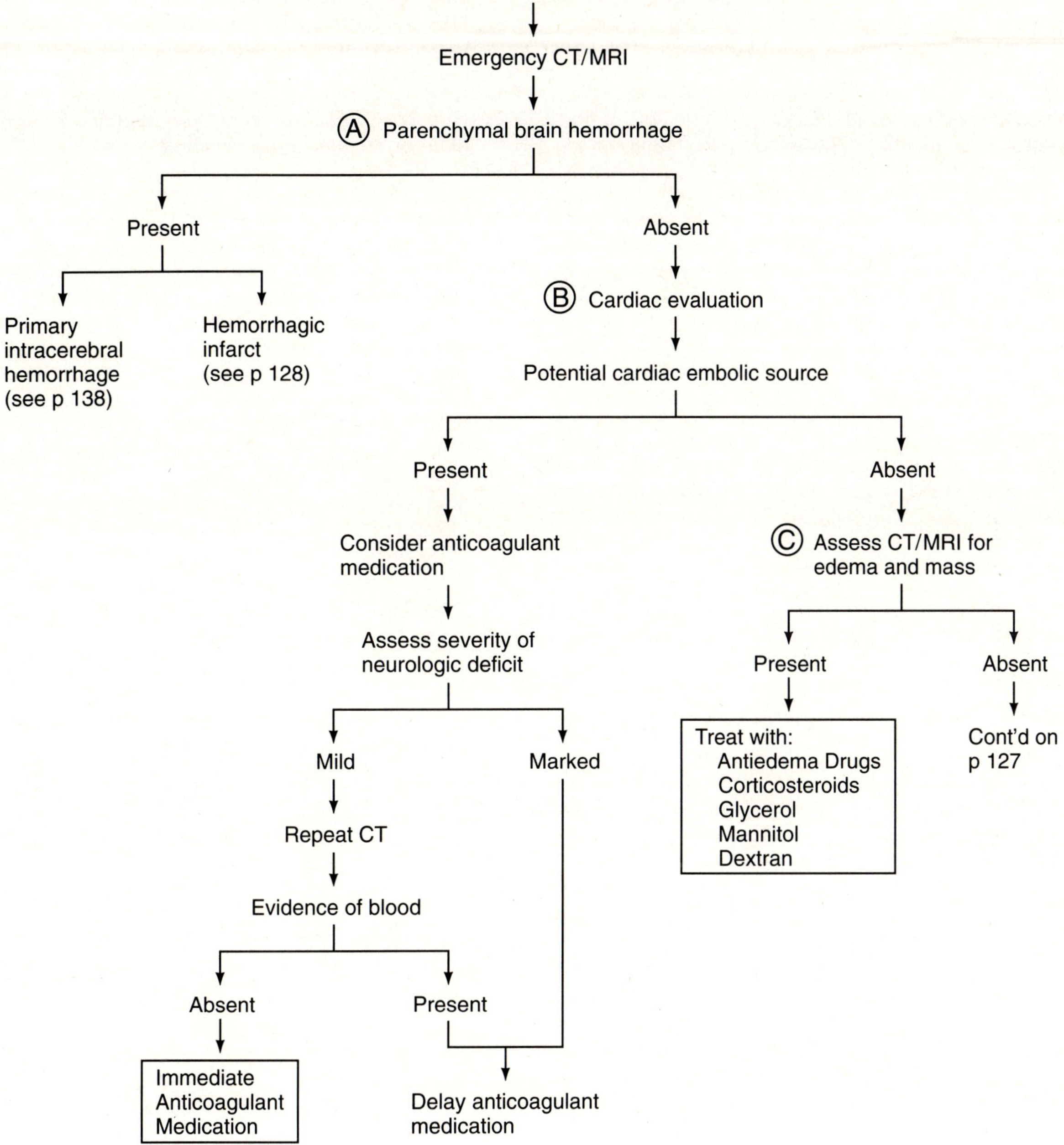

Patient with SUDDEN ONSET OF FOCAL NEUROLOGIC DEFICIT WHO SHOWS SUBSEQUENT NEUROLOGIC DETERIORATION
Emergency CT/MRI
A Parenchymal brain hemorrhage
Present
Absent
Primary intracerebral hemorrhage (see p 138)
Hemorrhagic infarct (see p 128)
B Cardiac evaluation
Potential cardiac embolic source
Present
Absent
Consider anticoagulant medication
C Assess CT/MRI for edema and mass
Assess severity of neurologic deficit
Present
Absent
Mild
Marked
Treat with:
Antiedema Drugs
Corticosteroids
Glycerol
Mannitol
Dextran
Cont'd on p 127
Repeat CT
Evidence of blood
Absent
Present
Immediate Anticoagulant Medication
Delay anticoagulant medication

D. Multiple metabolic derangements may cause neurologic progression in stroke patients. Hypoglycemia should be avoided and rapidly corrected if present; however, hyperglycemia should also be avoided. Several studies indicate neurologic worsening in hyperglycemic patients due to anaerobic glycolysis, which increases tissue lactic acid content. If the syndrome of inappropriate antidiuretic hormone secretion complicates acute stroke, hyponatremia may lead to fluid retention and exacerbate cerebral edema. Certain medications, including antiadrenergics (phenothiazines, antihypertensives), gamma-aminobutyric acid (antiepileptics), and sedatives (phenobarbital, diazepam) may worsen neurologic function. Avoid these drugs in the acute stroke patient if they are not essential medications. Respiratory and cardiac disease may worsen neurologic function owing to reduced cardiac output and carbon dioxide accumulation.

E. Neurologic worsening in the acute stroke patient (hemorrhage, ischemia) may be due to seizures. If spike discharges are seen on EEG, initiate anticonvulsant medication. Prophylactic antiepileptic treatment is not warranted because certain antiepileptic drugs may worsen neurologic function.

F. If the mechanism of stroke progression is not known, angiography may be warranted. If there is major vessel stenosis, anticoagulant medication is given, although there is no randomized prospective study showing this treatment to be effective. Anticoagulants are most likely to be effective when begun immediately after neurologic progression develops; after neurologic deficit has been present and stable for >12 hours, maximal ischemia probably has occurred and anticoagulants are unlikely to be beneficial. The exact mechanism of the potential beneficial effect of anticoagulant medication is not known. It is hypothesized that heparin retards antegrade red thrombus formation. If a major vessel is occluded or intracranial branch occlusion occurs, antiplatelet agents may be effective. If angiography is negative, consider arteriolar disease resulting in lacunar infarction. This small vessel disorder is unlikely to be modified by anticoagulant or antiplatelet medication.

In the acute stroke patient, do not lower blood pressure rapidly: a higher blood pressure may be needed to maintain cerebral perfusion pressure and protect ischemic tissue surrounding the infarction. The role of hemodilution in reducing vascular sludging and viscosity has not been established, but if hematocrit is markedly elevated (e.g., polycythemia), this should be corrected. The role of calcium channel blocking agents in reducing cerebral ischemia is not established. In patients with progressing stroke who have carotid occlusion, carotid endarterectomy (CEA) is not effective. If CEA is performed, immediate tissue reperfusion may result in hemorrhagic infarction, thus increasing the risk of increased neurologic deficit. "Vasospasm" has been reported as the cause of progressing stroke; however, when this pattern is demonstrated by angiography, agents used to reduce vasospasm (e.g., vasodilators) have not been effective.

References

Hachinski V, Norris JW. The acute stroke. Philadelphia: FA Davis, 1985:123.

Millikan CH, McDowell FH. Treatment of progressing stroke. Stroke 1981; 12:397.

Slivka A, Levy D. Natural history of progressive ischemic stroke in populations treated with heparin. Stroke 1990; 21:1657.

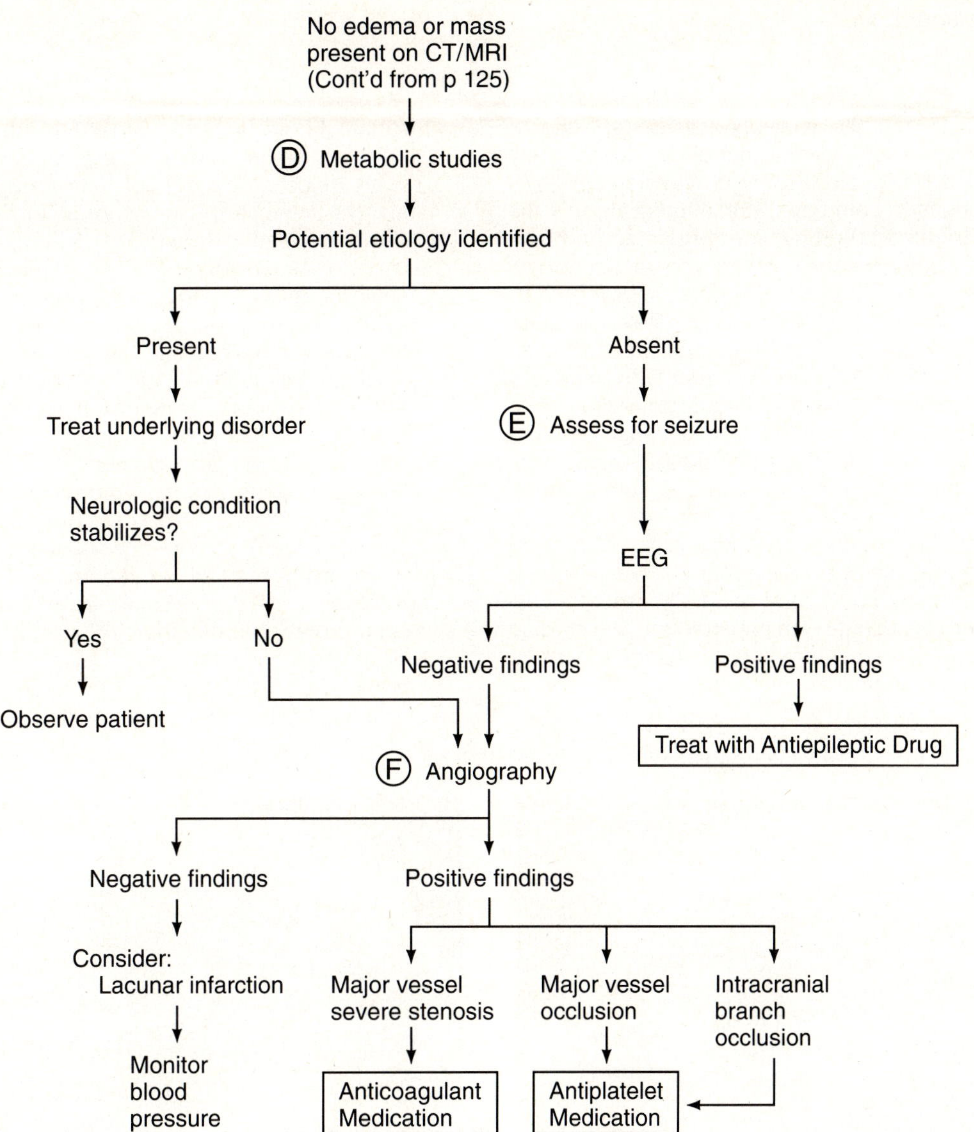

No edema or mass present on CT/MRI (Cont'd from p 125)
D Metabolic studies
Potential etiology identified
Present
Absent
Treat underlying disorder
E Assess for seizure
Neurologic condition stabilizes?
EEG
Yes
No
Negative findings
Positive findings
Observe patient
Treat with Antiepileptic Drug
F Angiography
Negative findings
Positive findings
Consider:
Lacunar infarction
Major vessel severe stenosis
Major vessel occlusion
Intracranial branch occlusion
Monitor blood pressure
Anticoagulant Medication
Antiplatelet Medication

COMPLETED STROKE

Leon A. Weisberg, M.D.

A. The completed stroke is defined as an episode of sudden onset of focal deficit that occurs without any clinical evidence of subsequent progression or deterioration. The term completed stroke indicates only the temporal profile of the vascular episode and nothing about the stroke mechanism or type of neurologic deficit. This may be caused by intracerebral hemorrhage or cerebral infarction (large vessel vascular occlusion). Headache, vomiting, impaired consciousness, and seizures are more common with intracerebral hemorrhage than with cerebral infarction. The initial prognosis of a completed stroke depends on the underlying stroke pathology; the initial mortality rate due to hemorrhage is higher than that with cerebral infarction. In the acute phase of cerebral infarction, stroke mortality depends on infarct size. With large infarcts, immediate death may be 30%, whereas with small infarcts, mortality may be <5%. Stroke recurrence is high in patients with hypertension and cardiac disease, and low in normotensive patients without cardiac abnormalities.

B. CT should be the initial diagnostic study if stroke is suspected. If this shows intracranial blood, suspect subarachnoid hemorrhage (SAH), intracerebral hemorrhage, or hemorrhagic cerebral infarction. CT always detects intracerebral hemorrhage but may not always detect SAH. In cerebral infarction, CT may show hypodense lesions (Fig. 1). CT may be negative if performed before ischemic tissue damage causes electron density changes or blood-brain barrier alteration (this may occur within 7 days), or may be negative if the ischemic lesion is small and less than resolving capability of CT (e.g., brain stem lacunes). MRI is more sensitive than CT in detecting ischemic lesions and may show an abnormality at an earlier stage (within 24 hours) than CT. Perform a lumbar puncture (LP) in patients who have sustained strokes for these reasons: (1) clear uncolored CSF definitively excludes SAH; (2) CSF pleocytosis may occur with stroke syndrome due to inflammatory arteritis; (3) CSF serologic tests are necessary to exclude meningovascular syphilis. LP should not be performed if cerebellar hemorrhage or infarction is suspected, because this procedure may precipitate herniation syndromes and subsequent neurologic deterioration.

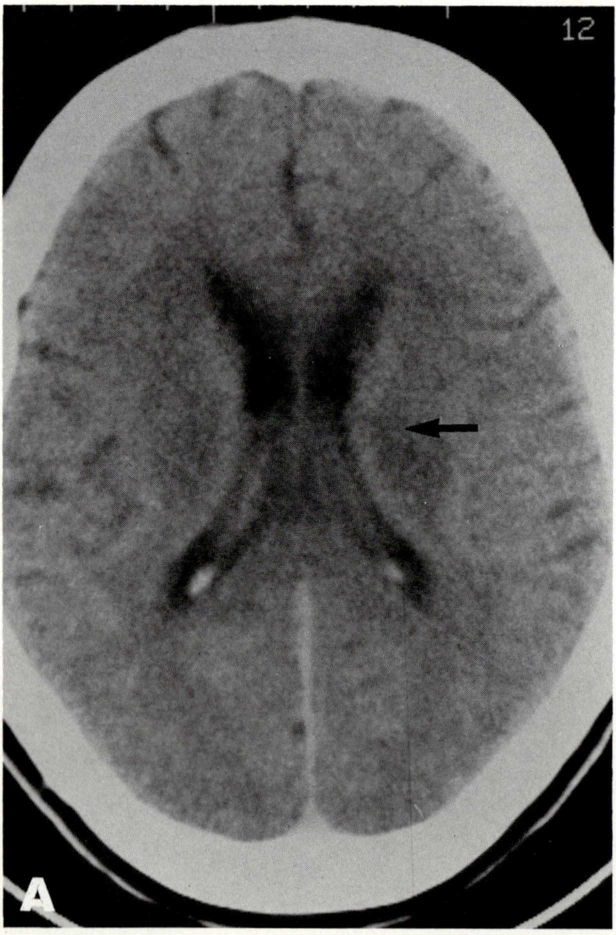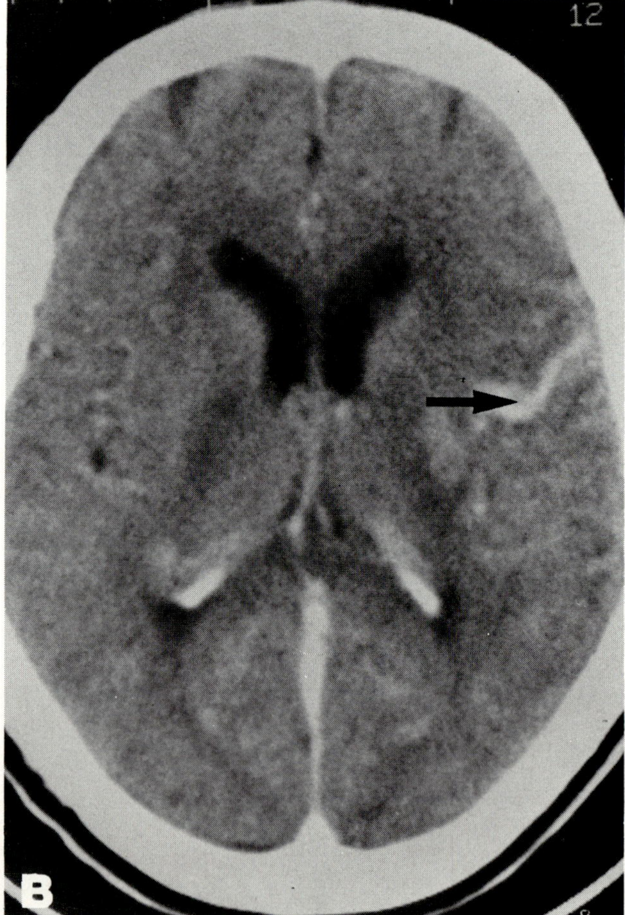

Figure 1 CT scan shows right ganglionic hypodense lesion: *A*, with gyral enhancement; *B*, consistent with cerebral infarction.

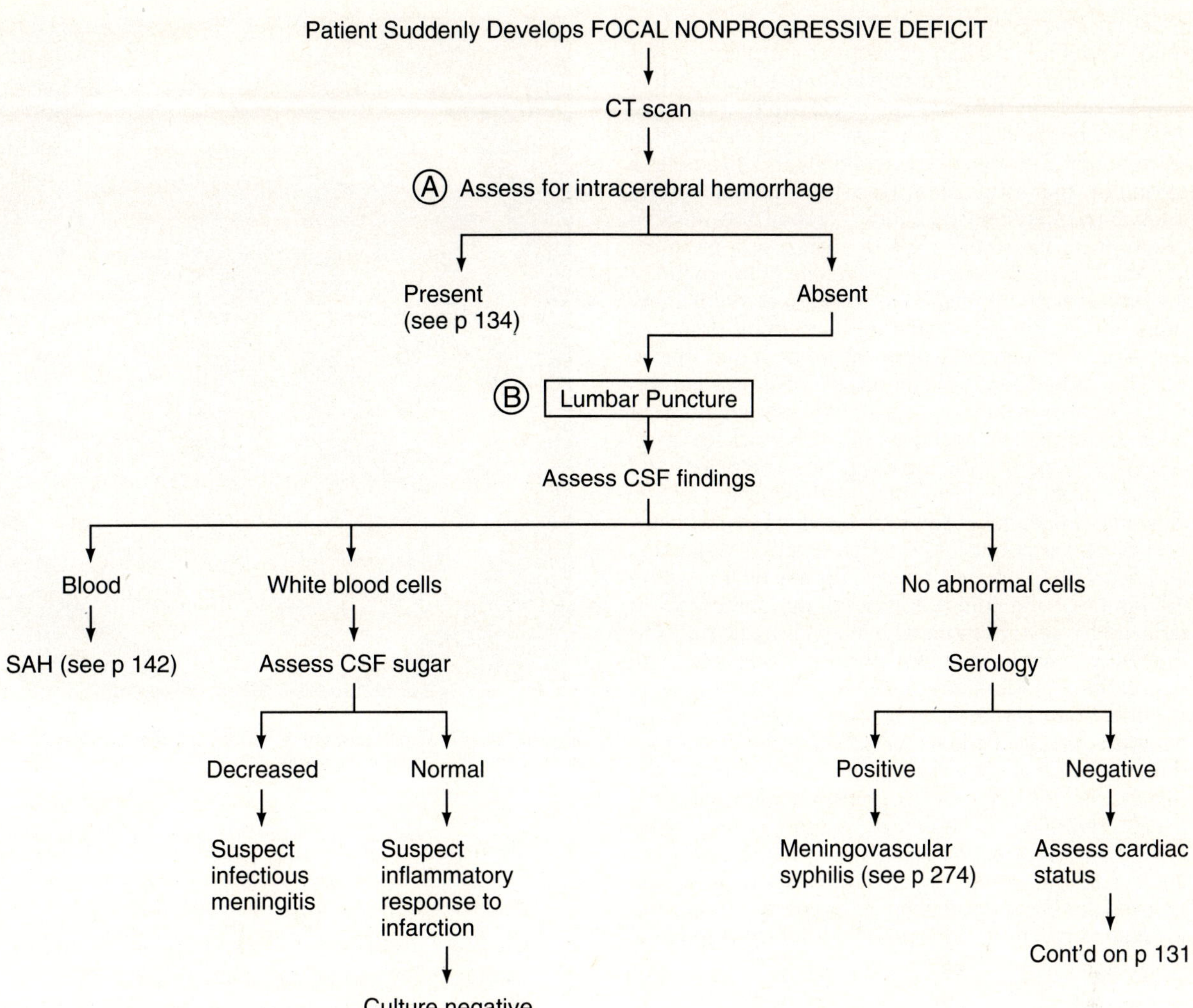

Patient Suddenly Develops FOCAL NONPROGRESSIVE DEFICIT

CT scan

(A) Assess for intracerebral hemorrhage

Present
(see p 134)

Absent

(B) Lumbar Puncture

Assess CSF findings

Blood

White blood cells

No abnormal cells

SAH (see p 142)

Assess CSF sugar

Serology

Decreased

Normal

Positive

Negative

Suspect
infectious
meningitis

Suspect
inflammatory
response to
infarction

Meningovascular
syphilis (see p 274)

Assess cardiac
status

Culture negative

Cont'd on p 131

C. Cerebral infarction may result from large artery (carotid, vertebral, basilar) atherosclerotic plaque. This may contain "white" (platelet-fibrin) thrombus that may secondarily develop antegrade "red" thrombus. This may be the source of a large artery thrombus that subsequently embolizes intracranially. For example, a thrombus that originates from the internal carotid artery may migrate to the middle cerebral artery (MCA) origin or to one of the MCA branches, or a proximal vertebral artery thrombus may migrate to the origin of the basilar artery or one of the posterior cerebral artery branches. Cerebral infarction may result from an embolus that originates from a cardiac mural thrombus. In cardiac cerebral embolism, secondary hemorrhagic transformation of an ischemic lesion may occur after the embolus lodged within the blocked vessel disperses to permit the vessel to become patent and restore blood flow. The enhanced perfusion of the ischemic tissue may result in hemorrhagic transformation of the ischemic tissue. This embolic dispersion and hemorrhagic transformation usually occurs within 72 hours of the initial embolism but sometimes is delayed for several more days. Hemorrhagic transformation is usually, but not always, associated with neurologic deterioration; CT is therefore necessary to exclude brain hemorrhage before anticoagulant medication is begun. Patients with large ischemic lesions due to cardiogenic cerebral embolism are at the highest risk for hemorrhagic transformation, which is usually heralded by neurologic deterioration. If hemorrhagic transformation occurs as a result of cardiogenic cerebral embolism, anticoagulation should be delayed for 3 weeks. When assessing the indication for anticoagulation, consider the risk of precipitating intracranial hemorrhage.

D. Investigate patients with completed stroke for a potential cardiac source if they are young, if they have no vascular risk factors (hypertension, diabetes mellitus, hyperlipidemia), or if CT shows multiple cerebral infarcts. The time of recurrent embolism is variable and depends on the source of the cardiogenic embolism. In patients with acute myocardial infarction, embolism may recur within 3 weeks owing to arrhythmias or the development of a ventricular thrombus. A ventricular aneurysm may develop after myocardial infarction, but this is usually a late complication that may occur many months after the initial myocardial infarction. Post–myocardial infarction patients who develop aneurysms may not require anticoagulants, but cardiac surgery may be needed. Patients who have suffered acute myocardial infarction and have a high risk for developing cerebral embolism should receive anticoagulant therapy for several months. After this time, reassess the situation and weigh continued use of this therapy against the risk of long-term anticoagulation. Cerebral embolism may occur at any time in patients with cardiomyopathies, prosthetic valves, and rheumatic heart disease; these patients should therefore receive anticoagulants indefinitely. Patients with embolism resulting from bacterial endocarditis should not receive anticoagulants because of the high risk of intracerebral hemorrhage due to mycotic aneurysms (see p 148). Mural thrombi occur in atrial

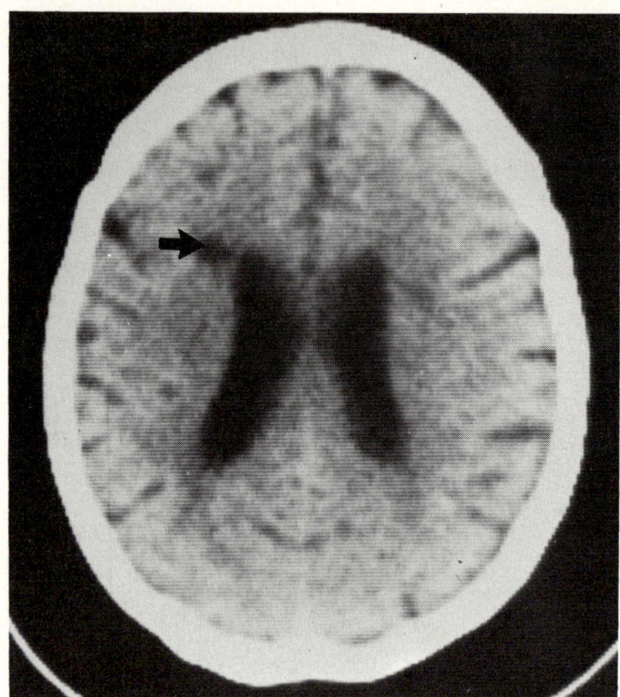

Figure 2 CT scan shows a left hemispheric hypodense lesion consistent with lacunar infarction.

fibrillation of any cause. Stroke risk is 6% per year; anticoagulation is indicated even if an atrial thrombus is not seen on cardiac diagnostic studies.

E. Intracranial hemorrhage develops in 1% of patients receiving anticoagulants. The risk is highest if the embolus disperses and fragments to restore cerebral blood flow to the infarcted tissue. When this occurs, the ischemic "pale" infarction may become hemorrhagic; this hemorrhage may be detected by CT. If clinical deterioration occurs during anticoagulant therapy, perform CT immediately to exclude a brain hemorrhage.

F. Lacunes are small infarcts involving small, deep penetrating arterioles. They may cause lesions in the putamen, thalamus, pons, or internal capsule. These are usually due to hypertension or diabetes mellitus. The small vascular (arteriolar) lesions are not visualized with angiography, but lacunes may be seen on CT/MRI (Fig. 2). Clinical patterns include pure motor hemiparesis (due to internal capsular or pontine infarction), pure sensory syndrome due to thalamic infarction, dysarthria–clumsy hand syndrome due to pontine infarction, and ataxic hemiparesis with pontine or cerebral white matter infarction. Anticoagulation is not indicated with lacunar infarction. If the clinical deficit is more extensive than these lacunar syndromes, or if CT shows a larger lacune (>2 cm), this suggests larger vessel involvement. Investigate these patients for a potential cardiac embolic source and perform angiography. The value of carotid endarterectomy (CEA) in patients with completed stroke who have a surgically accessible extracranial carotid lesion is not established.

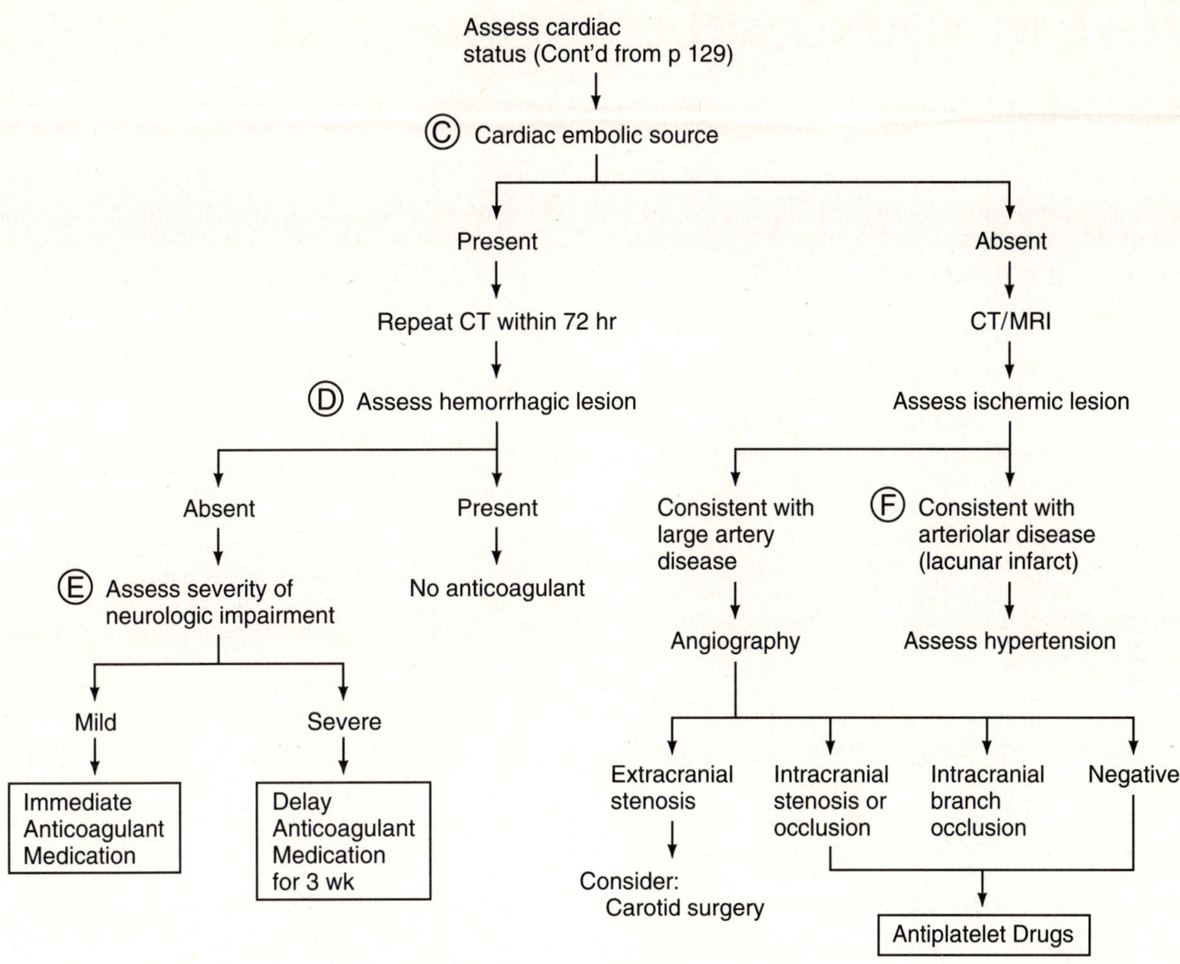

References

Albers GW, Sherman DG. Stroke prevention in nonvalvular atrial fibrillation. Ann Neurol 1991; 30:511.

Barnet HJM. Heart in ischemic stroke. Neurol Clin North Am 1984; 1:291.

Cerebral Embolism Study Group. Immediate anticoagulation of embolic stroke. Stroke 1984; 15:779.

STROKE IN YOUNG ADULTHOOD

Leon A. Weisberg, M.D.

Five percent of strokes affect young adults between the ages of 15 and 45 years. For ischemic stroke, cardiogenic cerebral embolism and premature cerebral atherosclerosis are the most common etiologies; however, laboratory investigations for less common causes are warranted in young patients.

A. Initially determine whether focal neurologic signs are due to stroke. If neurologic signs develop before headache, consider migraine. If demyelinating disease is suspected, MRI or CSF findings may be diagnostic (see p 300). If postictal paralysis is present, EEG may show spike discharges due to focal seizures. A conversion reaction should be considered before extensive neurodiagnostic studies are performed; however, this is a diagnosis of exclusion.

B. CT should be the initial diagnostic study. When CT shows intracranial blood, determine whether this represents primary subarachnoid hemorrhage (SAH) or intracerebral hemorrhage. Perform angiography to delineate any underlying vascular abnormality.

C. If CT shows no blood, perform lumbar puncture to exclude SAH or meningitis. Meningitis may cause inflammatory vasculitis to result in ischemic stroke. CSF serologic tests exclude meningovascular syphilis.

D. Ascertain any history of oral contraceptive use. This is an important stroke risk factor, especially if the patient also smokes cigarettes. Question patients about use of illicit recreational drugs or over-the-counter sympathomimetic agents. Drug use may be a risk factor for 10% of strokes that occur in young adults. Drug-related stroke may be ischemic and hemorrhagic. If headache is a prominent feature, consider migraine-related stroke.

E. Cardiogenic cerebral embolism is the most common cause of stroke in young patients; a complete cardiac evaluation should therefore have high priority even if there are no cardiac manifestations. Certain clinical and diagnostic criteria suggest cardioembolic stroke; however, differentiation of cardiogenic cerebral embolism from other stroke types is difficult unless there is evidence of a cardiac source or CT evidence of hemorrhagic or multiple infarctions. Initial cardiac evaluation includes cardiac examination, ECG, chest radiography, and two-dimensional echocardiography. In selected patients, Holter monitoring, transesophageal and contrast echocardiography, and ultrafast cardiac CT and MRI should be performed. Potential cardiac etiologies include (1) valvular disease (rheumatic heart disease, prosthetic valve replacements, mitral valve prolapse, endocarditis, marasmic endocarditis, congenital heart disease), (2) arrhythmias (atrial fibrillation, sick sinus syndrome), and (3) other cardiac disturbances (ventricular aneurysm, cardiomyopathy, intracardiac defect with paradoxical embolism, myocardial infarction, atrial myxomas).

F. Perform diagnostic investigations to exclude these disorders that may cause stroke: (1) collagen vascular disease (erythrocyte sedimentation rate, lupus erythematosus [LE] preparation, antinuclear antibodies); (2) homocystinuria (urine chromatographic screen for amino acid; (3) amyloidosis (gingival biopsy); (4) hematologic disorders, e.g., sickle cell disease, leukemia, hyperviscosity syndromes, platelet disorders; (5) antiphospholipid antibody disorders (lupus anticoagulant, anticardiolipin antibodies); (6) coagulation disorders (prothrombin and partial thromboplastin times); (7) premature atherosclerosis (lipid profile).

G. Perform angiography if the diagnosis of stroke is not established by any laboratory studies. If a stroke patient has a history of head or neck trauma, consider arterial dissection. Angiography may confirm basal occlusive disease with telangiectasia (moyamoya disease), vasculitis, fibromuscular hyperplasia, or dissection of aortic vessels. Systemic LE causes small vessel vasculitis with occlusions and microinfarction but angiographic lesions may not be seen. Granulomatous (temporal) arteritis involves small blood vessels or large vessels in Takayasu's arteritis (aortic arch pulseless disease); angiography may show a narrowed aortic arch with aneurysmal dilatations. Fibromuscular hyperplasia produces noninflammatory thickening of large blood vessels; this involves extracranial carotid or vertebral arteries and may require surgery on the involved arterial segment.

References

Bevan H, Sharma K, Bradley W. Stroke in young adults. Stroke 1990; 21:382.

Grindal AB, Cohen RJ, Saul RF, Taylor JR. Cerebral infarction in young adults. Stroke 1978; 9:39.

Hart RG, Miller VT. Cerebral infarction in young adults: A practical approach. Stroke 1983; 14:110.

Levine J, Swanson PD. Nonatherosclerotic causes of stroke. Ann Intern Med 1969; 70:807.

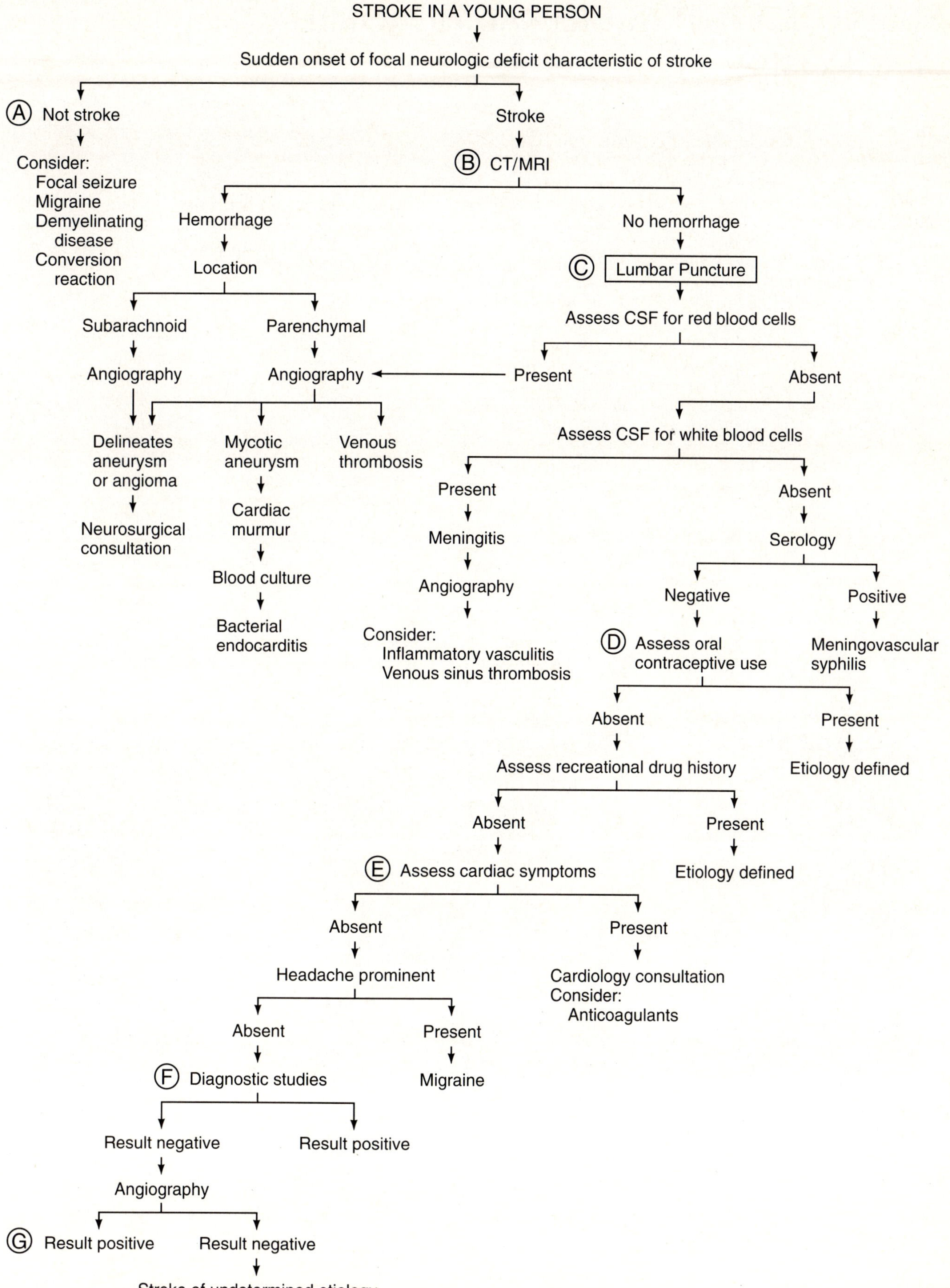

STROKE IN A YOUNG PERSON
Sudden onset of focal neurologic deficit characteristic of stroke
A Not stroke
Stroke
Consider:
Focal seizure
Migraine
Demyelinating disease
Conversion reaction
B CT/MRI
Hemorrhage
No hemorrhage
Location
C Lumbar Puncture
Assess CSF for red blood cells
Subarachnoid
Parenchymal
Angiography
Angiography
Present
Absent
Delineates aneurysm or angioma
Mycotic aneurysm
Venous thrombosis
Assess CSF for white blood cells
Neurosurgical consultation
Cardiac murmur
Present
Absent
Blood culture
Meningitis
Serology
Bacterial endocarditis
Angiography
Negative
Positive
Consider:
Inflammatory vasculitis
Venous sinus thrombosis
D Assess oral contraceptive use
Meningovascular syphilis
Absent
Present
Assess recreational drug history
Etiology defined
Absent
Present
E Assess cardiac symptoms
Etiology defined
Absent
Present
Headache prominent
Cardiology consultation
Consider:
Anticoagulants
Absent
Present
F Diagnostic studies
Migraine
Result negative
Result positive
Angiography
G Result positive
Result negative
Stroke of undetermined etiology

SUSPECTED INTRACEREBRAL HEMORRHAGE: DIAGNOSIS

Leon A. Weisberg, M.D.

Patients present with severe new-onset headache and focal neurologic signs. These clinical symptoms develop rapidly to reach maximal severity within minutes to several hours. In unusual cases of primary intracerebral hemorrhage (PIH), neurologic deterioration progresses more slowly before reaching maximal severity. With PIH, there are focal neurologic signs but usually no meningeal signs. In subarachnoid hemorrhage (SAH), there may be headache and meningeal signs but usually no focal neurologic signs, unless these are due to direct aneurysm compression or a complicating pathologic process (dissection of blood into brain parenchyma, ischemia due to vasospasm). In acute PIH, CT is a 100% sensitive diagnostic tool; it *always* shows a hyperdense lesion (Fig. 1), which represents the blood extravasated into brain parenchyma.

A. If the patient has focal neurologic signs and a stiff neck, SAH is more likely than PIH. In aneurysmal SAH, CT may show blood in one of several characteristic locations: (1) interhemispheric fissure, caval-septal, and frontal lobe regions in an anterior cerebral–anterior communicating artery aneurysm; (2) sylvian cistern and temporal lobe in a middle cerebral artery aneurysm; (3) suprasellar cistern in a carotid artery aneurysm; (4) brain stem cisterns in a basilar artery aneurysm. In aneurysmal SAH, CT may show *no* blood if performed more than 48 hours after an aneurysmal leak or rupture.

B. Lumbar puncture may demonstrate red blood cells (RBCs) and xanthochromia in the CSF in patients with both SAH and PIH. CSF examination is a more sensitive indicator of SAH than CT, because CSF abnormalities indicating intracranial bleeding remain positive longer than on CT. If the CSF shows no RBCs or xanthochromia and is performed within 2 weeks of neurologic ictus, this excludes SAH, but the findings may remain positive for only 48 hours. In the acute phase of SAH, CSF examination is the most sensitive diagnostic study; however, in PIH, CSF examination frequently shows no RBCs, especially if PIH does not extend into the ventricles or break through into the subarachnoid spaces. Certain patients with PIH develop inflammatory CSF polymorphonuclear cell pleocytosis, which may simulate bacterial meningitis. This must be differentiated from infectious meningitis by CSF Gram stain and culture results.

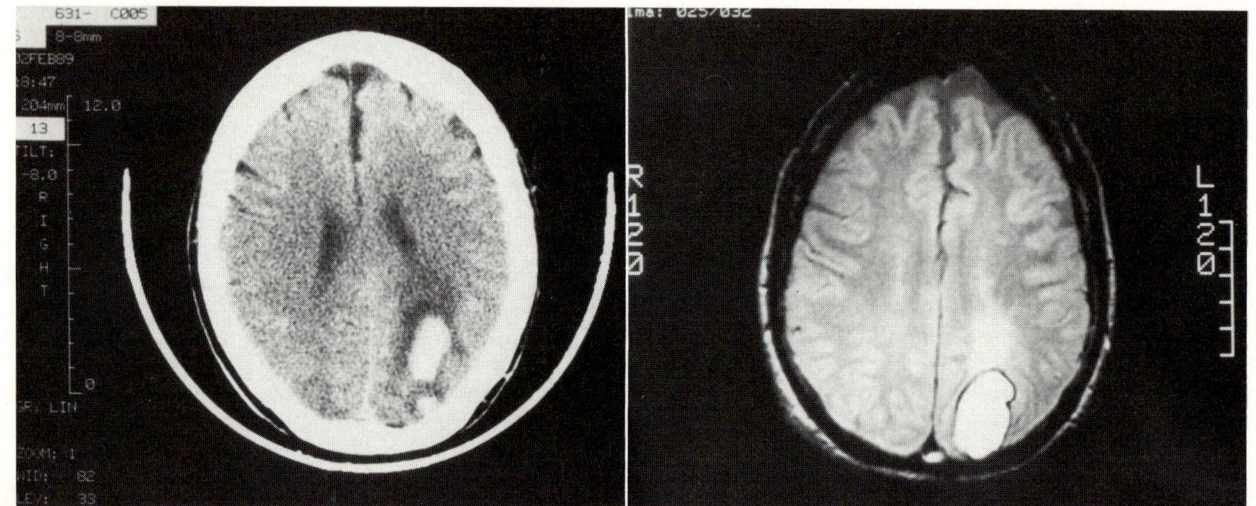

Figure 1 *A,* CT scan shows a hyperdense, nonenhancing, parietal-occipital hemorrhage with a surrounding hypodense region due to edema. *B,* MRI shows a central hyperintense region with a surrounding thin hypointense (black) rim that represents hemosiderin. This is surrounded by a second hyperintense region representing edema. This pattern is consistent with intracerebral hemorrhage.

Patient with SUDDEN ONSET OF HEADACHE AND FOCAL NEUROLOGIC SIGNS

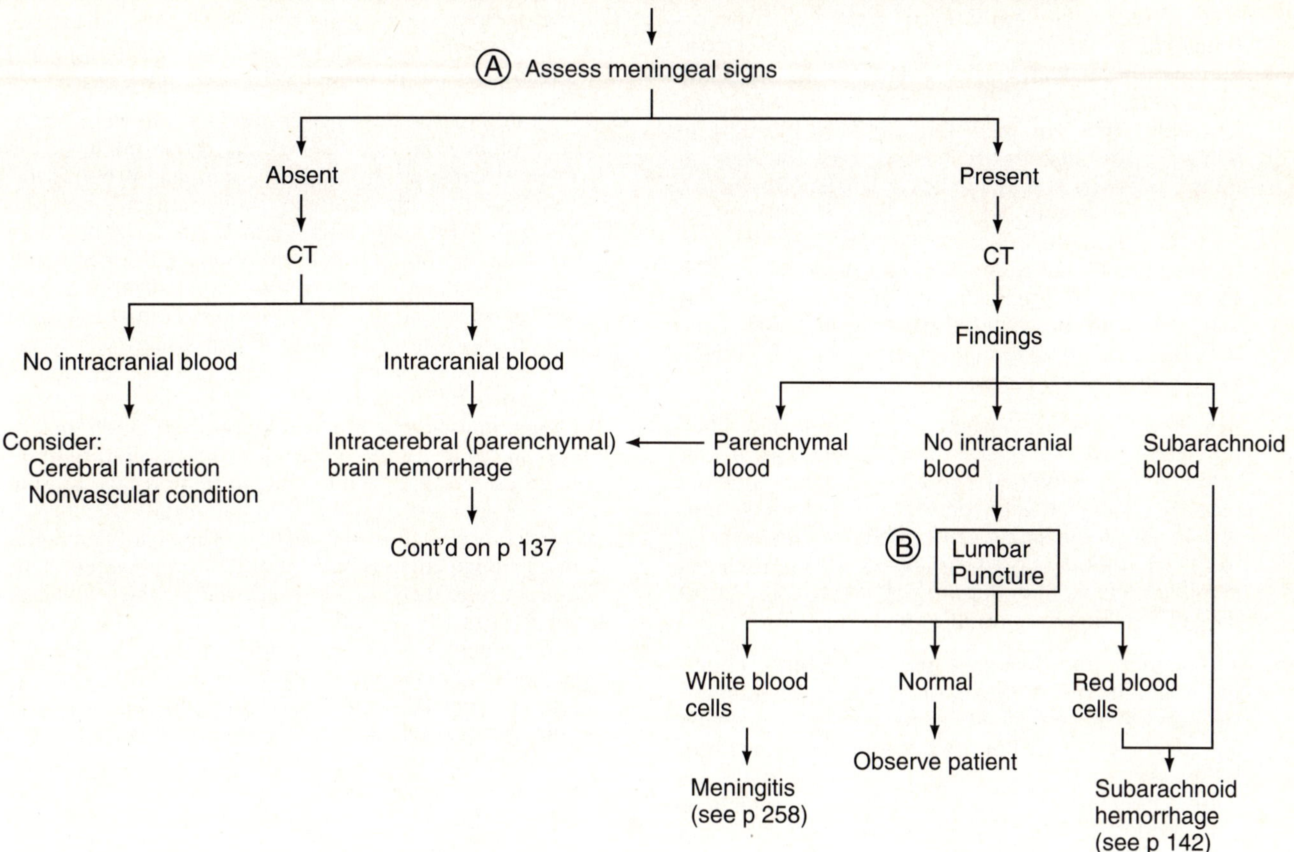

C. Arterial hypertension is the most common cause of PIH. Hemorrhage results from rupture of Charcot-Bouchard arteriolar microaneurysms. These microaneurysms are small and beyond the resolving capability of conventional cerebral angiography; therefore, angiography does not show the source of bleeding in patients with hypertensive hemorrhage. These penetrating arterioles supply the basal ganglia (see Fig. 1), thalamus, brain stem, and cerebellum. If a PIH patient is not hypertensive, consider alternative etiologies. In older patients, consider amyloid angiopathy. The blood vessels are fragile and easily hemorrhage. This diagnosis can be established only by pathologic findings in which abnormal vessels are visualized with Congo red staining techniques.

D. In younger patients, obtain a careful history of illicit drug use (cocaine, phencyclidine), and use of prescription (amphetamines) or over-the-counter (phenylpropanolamine) medications. Urine toxicology tests should be immediately performed in patients who have PIH without known etiology to attempt to detect possible precipitating drugs. Alcohol may cause coagulopathy, which may result in PIH.

E. Coagulation and bleeding studies (platelet count, prothrombin time, partial thromboplastin time) should be performed, especially if patients are receiving anticoagulant or antiplatelet medications. Perform laboratory studies for collagen vascular disease, as these conditions may cause vessel wall abnormalities that produce PIH. Cardiac evaluation and blood cultures exclude bacterial endocarditis; this could result in the development of mycotic aneurysm that might rupture to cause PIH (see p 148).

F. Hemorrhages in the subcortical white matter may be caused by angiomas, aneurysms, or neoplasms (glioblastomas, metastases). Vasculitis and Moyamoya disease (symmetric carotid occlusion associated with an abnormal vascular network in the basal ganglia) may also result in PIH, especially in young adults. In patients with PIH of no known etiology, angiography is necessary to exclude vascular malformation as the cause. In some patients, full evaluation including angiography reveals no cause of PIH. In these, consider amyloid angiopathy or "occult" thrombosed angioma as the possible bleeding source.

G. In putaminal hemorrhage, findings result from extension of hemorrhage through the fiber tracts of the internal capsule; this causes contralateral hemiparesis, usually with hemianesthesia and hemianopia. There may be contralateral conjugate horizontal ocular deviation (in the direction opposite the hemiparesis). In thalamic hemorrhage, hemianesthesia may precede hemiparesis; homonymous hemianopia and impaired upward gaze with forced downward ocular deviation may occur. In pontine hemorrhage, there is sudden onset of coma; other findings include quadriplegia, miotic but reactive pupils, impaired oculocephalic and caloric responses, and respiratory irregularities. Patients with cerebellar hemorrhage present with headache, vomiting, and gait instability (ataxia). Most prominent examination findings in cerebellar hemorrhage include gait ataxia; cranial nerve signs and decreased consciousness develop if the brain stem is subsequently compressed. Subcortical white matter hematomas show findings unique to their location: (1) occipital hematomas cause homonymous hemianopia; (2) parietal hematomas cause hemiparesis and hemisensory deficit, sometimes with spatial neglect for the involved side or aphasia if the dominant hemisphere is involved; (3) temporal hematomas cause aphasia (dominant hemisphere) or confusion (nondominant hemisphere); and (4) frontal hematomas cause leg monoparesis. Seizures may occur with subcortical lobar hematomas, but are unusual with PIH that originates in other locations.

References

Weisberg LA. Subcortical white matter lobar hemorrhages. J Neurol Neurosurg Psychiatry 1985; 48:1078.
Weisberg LA. Nontraumatic parenchymal brain hemorrhages. Medicine 1990; 69:277.

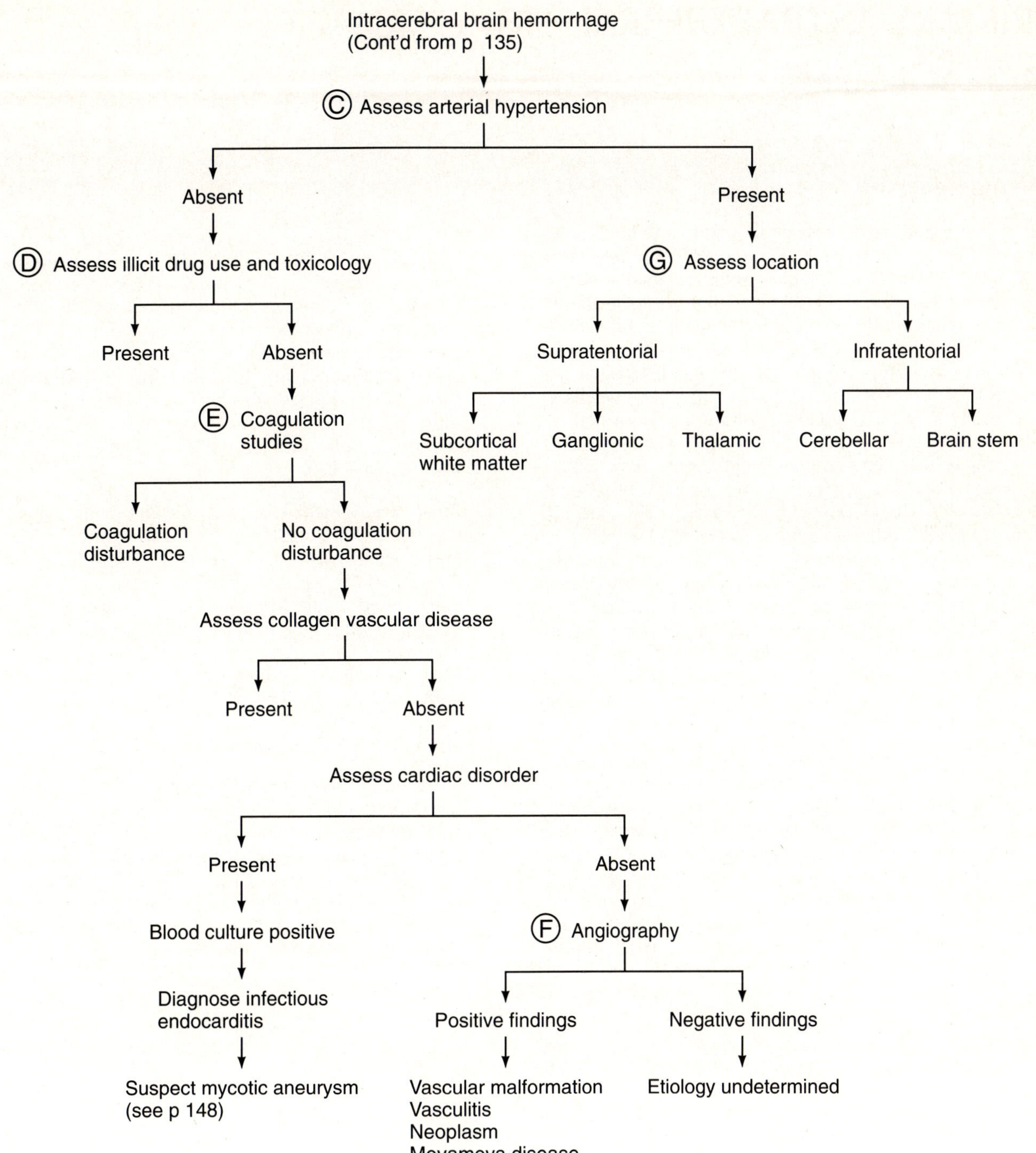

Intracerebral brain hemorrhage
(Cont'd from p 135)
C Assess arterial hypertension
Absent
Present
D Assess illicit drug use and toxicology
G Assess location
Present
Absent
Supratentorial
Infratentorial
E Coagulation studies
Subcortical white matter
Ganglionic
Thalamic
Cerebellar
Brain stem
Coagulation disturbance
No coagulation disturbance
Assess collagen vascular disease
Present
Absent
Assess cardiac disorder
Present
Absent
Blood culture positive
F Angiography
Diagnose infectious endocarditis
Positive findings
Negative findings
Suspect mycotic aneurysm
(see p 148)
Vascular malformation
Vasculitis
Neoplasm
Moyamoya disease
Etiology undetermined

PRIMARY INTRACEREBRAL HEMORRHAGE: MANAGEMENT

Leon A. Weisberg, M.D.

Management options depend on the cause and location of primary intracerebral hemorrhage (PIH). To determine indications for invasive treatments (intracranial pressure [ICP] monitoring, surgical clot evacuation), it is necessary to know the natural history of different types and locations of PIH. Although there is a widespread belief that surgical hematoma evacuation is indicated, there is little evidence to support the value of surgery. For example, if hemorrhage is caused by a ruptured aneurysm or arteriovenous malformation, management includes clot removal and removal of the identified bleeding source. Hypertensive PIH results from rupture of a deeply situated arteriole with subsequent extravasation of blood into brain parenchyma. This usually occurs rapidly, with hematoma reaching maximal size within minutes. In rare instances, a hematoma progressively enlarges over several hours or days; hematoma enlargement has been documented by serial CT studies in unusual cases. The PIH is surrounded by an ischemic and oligemic region; this may compress microcirculation to cause reduced cerebral perfusion pressure (CPP), which may cause surrounding edema. If edema and ischemia are extensive, mass effect and increased ICP develop.

A. The most common cause of PIH is systemic arterial hypertension; therefore, most patients have a history of elevated blood pressure (BP) and take antihypertensive medication. Less commonly, PIH patients are normotensive; however, *reactive* hypertension occurs as a consequence of the expanding brain hemorrhage. This reactive hypertension may represent a compensatory mechanism by which CPP is increased in the presence of the space-occupying hematoma. Monitor the patient's neurologic condition carefully if the elevated BP is lowered, to be sure that adequate cerebral perfusion is achieved. Because maximal hematoma size occurs rapidly, it is unlikely that rapid BP reduction will limit maximal hematoma size or prevent edema. If elevated BP extension is lowered, avoid antihypertensive drugs that lower cerebral blood flow (CBF), depress consciousness, or increase ICP. Nitroprusside and labetalol are used for severe hypertension, despite their vasodilating effect, which may also increase ICP.

B. Treat severe headache due to PIH with analgesic medication. Sympathetic discharge associated with severe head pain may increase BP and elevate ICP. Avoid aspirin because it may exacerbate bleeding. Also, avoid analgesics that depress respiration (morphine, meperidine), because carbon dioxide retention may cause vasodilatation and lead to a secondary increase in ICP. Vomiting may increase ICP; treat it with hydroxyzine (Vistaril). Avoid dehydration by carefully administering IV fluids. Monitor serum sodium to avoid hyponatremia.

C. Impaired consciousness due to PIH usually correlates with increased ICP. An alternative explanation is repetitive seizures; thus, EEG should be monitored. If seizures occur, suppress them with IV phenytoin because they increase CBF and exacerbate intracranial hypertension. Carefully monitor fluid and electrolytes to avoid inappropriate antidiuretic hormone secretion, which may result in hyponatremia.

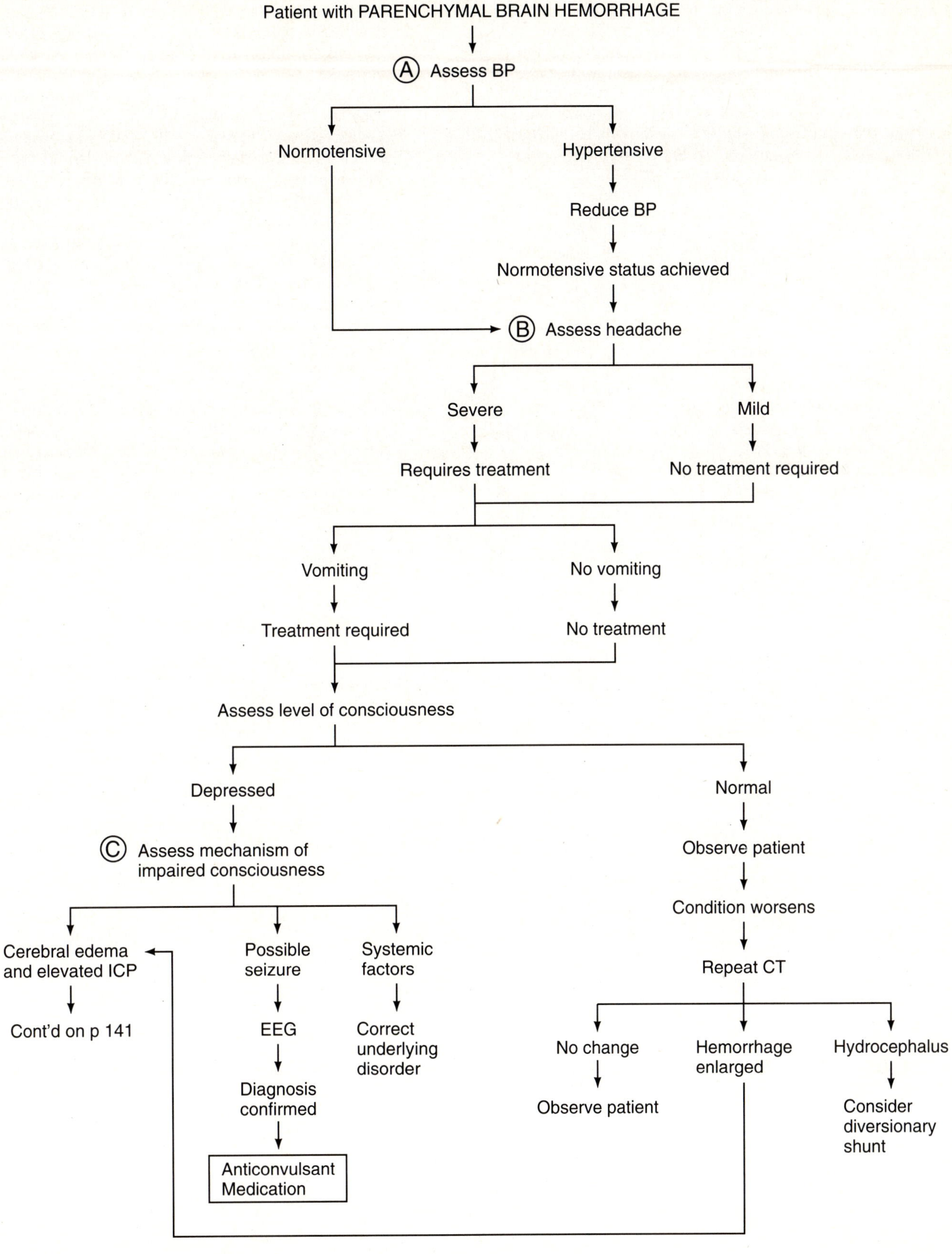

Patient with PARENCHYMAL BRAIN HEMORRHAGE
A Assess BP
Normotensive
Hypertensive
Reduce BP
Normotensive status achieved
B Assess headache
Severe
Mild
Requires treatment
No treatment required
Vomiting
No vomiting
Treatment required
No treatment
Assess level of consciousness
Depressed
Normal
C Assess mechanism of impaired consciousness
Observe patient
Condition worsens
Repeat CT
Cerebral edema and elevated ICP
Possible seizure
Systemic factors
Cont'd on p 141
EEG
Correct underlying disorder
No change
Hemorrhage enlarged
Hydrocephalus
Diagnosis confirmed
Observe patient
Consider diversionary shunt
Anticonvulsant Medication

D. To control elevated ICP due to PIH, first use intubation with hyperventilation (P_{CO_2} should be 30 mm H_2O) and restrict IV fluids to one half of normal maintenance levels. Osmotic agents (mannitol, initial dose of 1 g/kg followed by 0.5 g/kg q4h) extract edematous fluid from brain tissue through an impaired blood-brain barrier. Corticosteroids (dexamethasone, initial bolus of 10 mg followed by 4 mg q6h) reduce vasogenic edema and lower elevated ICP.

E. If the clinical condition does not improve despite these treatments, insert an ICP monitor and consider giving thiopental (Pentothal) to reduce cerebral metabolism, CBF, and increased ICP. Ventricular drainage may reduce increased ICP and prevent the deleterious effects of hydrocephalus.

F. Indications for surgery are controversial. They depend on hematoma size and location and the patient's clinical condition.
   1. Subcortical lobar hematoma. Perform angiography if the cause is unknown. If a neoplasm or vascular malformation is present, it should be evacuated to prevent further bleeding. When no etiology is determined, surgical evacuation is indicated if clinical deterioration occurs after the initial clinical episode.
   2. Putaminal and thalamic hemorrhages usually have a hypertensive etiology. They are deeply situated and occur under the cortical surface. The presence of systemic arterial hypertension and the deep location of the hemorrhage are associated with high morbidity and mortality; surgical evacuation is therefore not warranted. In some thalamic hemorrhages, the parenchymal hemorrhagic component is small but intraventricular hemorrhage is extensive, with resultant obstructive hydrocephalus. In these cases, the patient's clinical condition may improve after ventricular drainage.
   3. Pontine hemorrhages usually have a hypertensive etiology, are surgically inaccessible, and are not associated with elevated ICP. Severe neurologic deficit is due to destruction of the central basal and tegmental pons. Almost all patients with pontine hemorrhage die or have a severe residual neurologic deficit.
   4. Cerebellar hemorrhage. If CT shows hemorrhage >3 cm and there is a posterior fossa mass effect, surgical evacuation is warranted. If the hemorrhage is smaller and/or there is minimal mass effect, nonsurgical management is appropriate. Larger hemorrhages with marked mass effect should be rapidly evacuated before brain stem compression occurs.
   5. Certain hematomas become encapsulated and do not resolve spontaneously. These may undergo delayed progression to cause enlargement in size. CT and MRI findings may simulate an abscess or neoplasm. These should be surgically evacuated to prevent underlying brain tissue compression. In some cases, these are caused by an underlying occult vascular malformation.

References

Mendelow AD. Spontaneous intracerebral hemorrhage. J Neurol Neurosurg Psychiatry 1990; 53:1.

Weisberg LA. How to identify and manage brain hemorrhage. Postgrad Med 1990; 88:169.

Cerebral edema and elevated ICP
(Cont'd from p 139)

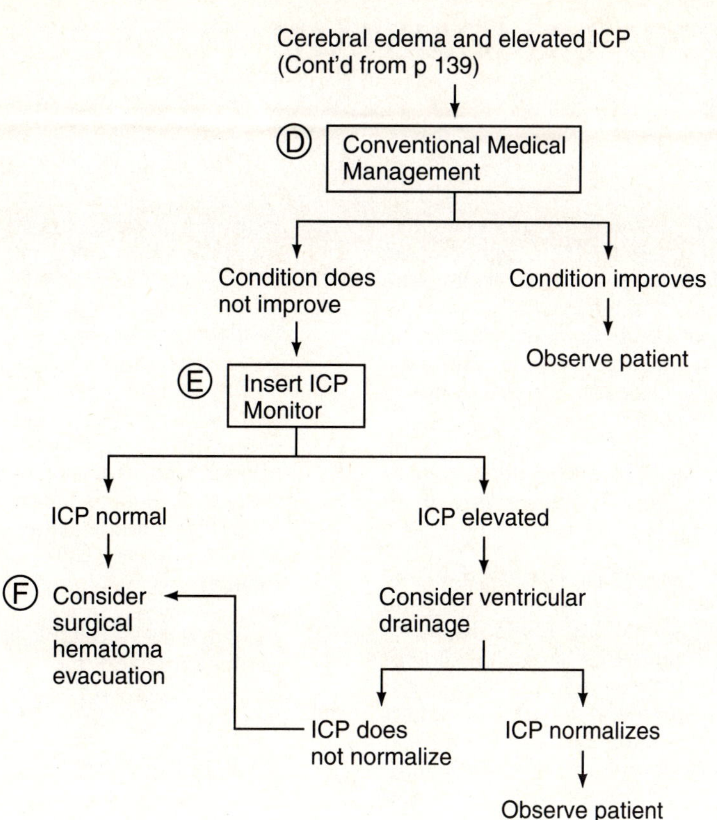

SUBARACHNOID HEMORRHAGE

Carlos A. Garcia, M.D.

The most frequent cause of spontaneous (nontraumatic) primary subarachnoid hemorrhage (SAH) is rupture of an arterial saccular ("berry") aneurysm. In a patient who presents with an acute excruciating headache, it is important to diagnose or rule out SAH. Rebleeding from an aneurysm in a neurologically intact patient may produce a devastating neurologic deficit or death. Early diagnosis is crucial in the treatment of intracranial aneurysms. Remember that a migraine attack may also present as an acute, excruciating headache. A personal or family history of migraine may help in the diagnosis. If there is any doubt about the diagnosis, follow D. below.

A. Other etiologies include secondary subarachnoid and intraventricular extension from a primary intracerebral hematoma, vascular malformations, blood disorders, vasculitis, drug abuse, rupture of a "fusiform" atherosclerotic aneurysm, amyloid angiopathy in the elderly, and hemorrhage within a primary or metastatic tumor. Head trauma is the most frequent cause of SAH. Alteration in the level of consciousness, focal neurologic deficit, and CT (Fig. 1) or MRI findings differentiate all these lesions from primary SAH. CT is a better indicator of recent bleeding than MRI. MRI detects small vascular malformations.

B. Primary SAH is manifested by acute onset of severe headache, frequently accompanied by a transient loss of consciousness or weakness of the legs. Stiff neck as a sign of meningeal irritation is not an early and reliable sign, since it is not found early in the ictus. In elderly patients, a stiff neck is most often due to osteoarthritis of the cervical spine. However, if neck stiffness is due to blood accumulation, the neck is maximally stiff in flexion, whereas in cervical osteoarthritis the neck is stiff in flexion as well as in lateral rotation.

C. Early and more reliable meningeal signs of SAH are photophobia and miosis of pupils. Subhyaloid retinal hemorrhages, when present, indicate intracranial bleeding.

D. In any patient with an acute, excruciating, different type of headache; supple neck; and no focal neurologic deficit, look for photophobia, miosis, or subhy-

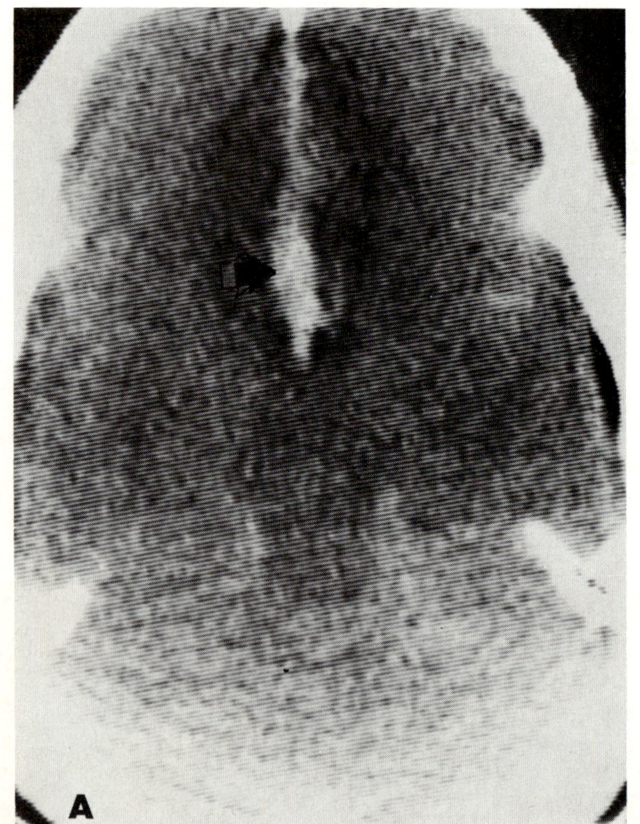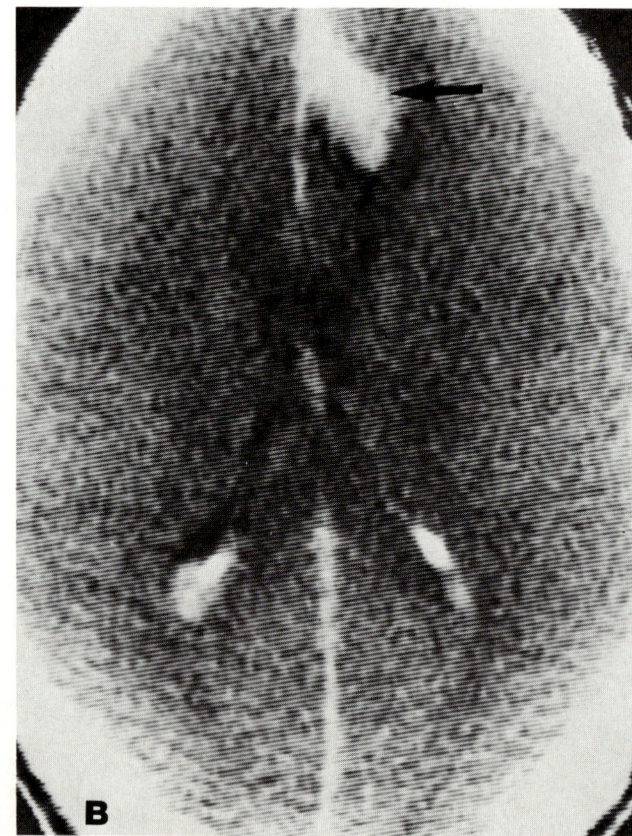

Figure 1 CT scan shows blood in the interhemispheric fissure *(A)* and right frontal lobe *(B)* due to a ruptured anterior cerebral–anterior communicating artery aneurysm.

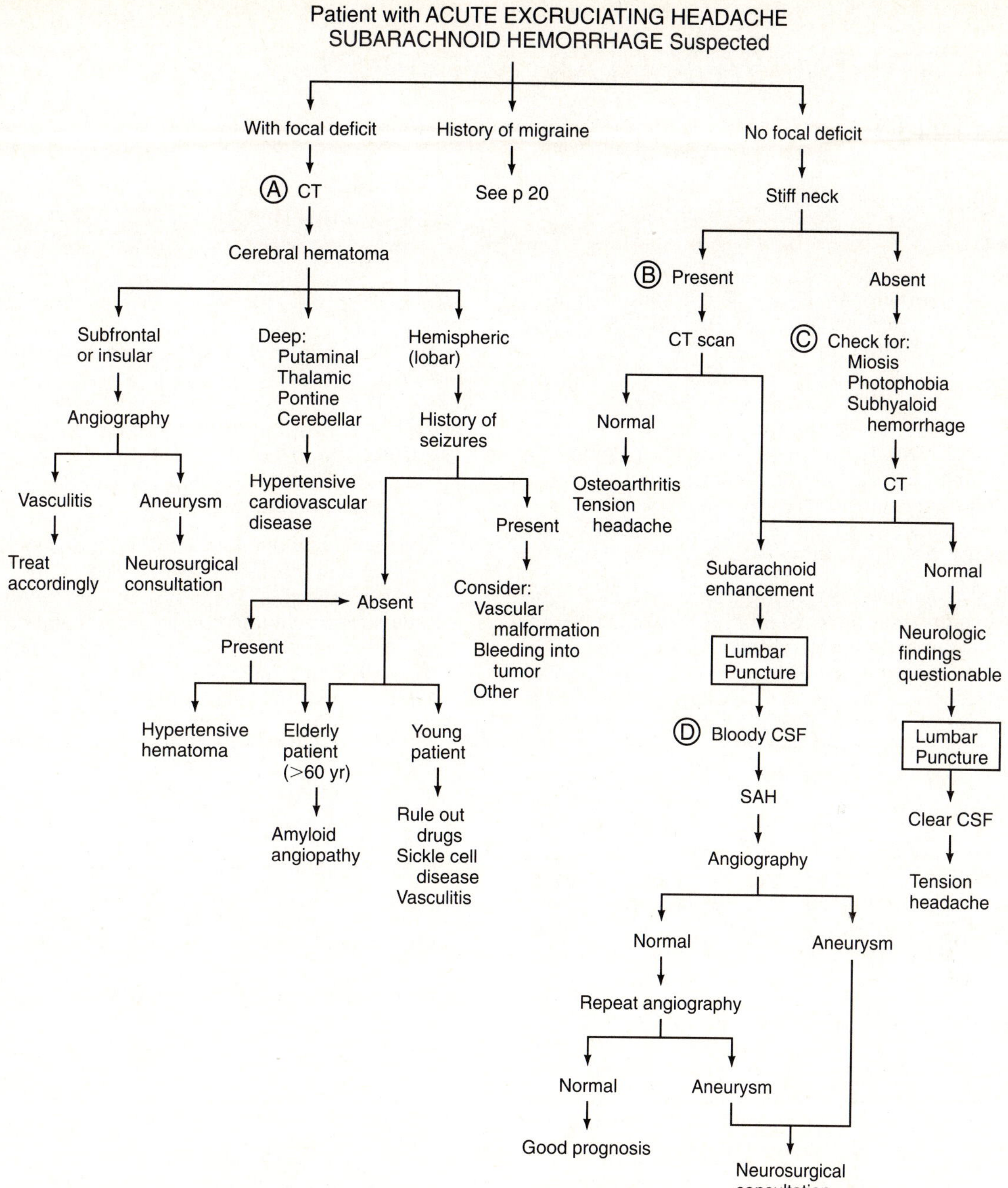

aloid hemorrhage in the eyeground. If any of these signs is present or if there is any doubt of its presence, obtain a CT scan of the head. Subarachnoid enhancement indicates SAH or meningitis. The lumbar puncture (LP) may confirm SAH; a cerebral angiogram is the next step. If there is no subarachnoid enhancement but there is a doubt about the neurologic findings, do an LP. If the LP yields a normal (clear) CSF without red blood cells or xanthochromia, the patient can go home with a prescription for analgesics. If the CSF is bloody, the patient has SAH and must be hospitalized. Cerebral angiography may reveal aneurysm(s) and the patient should be under the care of a neurosurgeon. Regulation of blood pressure (if the patient is hypertensive), sedation, and laxatives are necessary. If no lesions are seen on cerebral angiography, the cause of the bleeding may not be found and the prognosis with medical treatment is usually good. Angiography may not detect the aneurysms for several reasons: technical angiographic factors (appropriate oblique views may be necessary to detect anterior cerebral and anterior communicating artery aneurysms), spasm of vessels with inadequate dye delivery to the cerebral vessels, or spontaneous thrombosis of an aneurysm. Some vascular malformations may undergo spontaneous thrombosis after bleeding and may not be detected by angiography. If no aneurysm is detected on initial study, angiography is repeated.

References

Juul R, Fredriksen TA, Ringkjob R. Prognosis of subarachnoid hemorrhage of unknown etiology. J Neurosurg 1986; 64:359.

Sengupta RP, McAllister VL. Subarachnoid hemorrhage. Berlin: Springer-Verlag, 1986.

INTRACRANIAL SACCULAR ANEURYSM: RUPTURED

Carlos A. Garcia, M.D.

Subarachnoid hemorrhage (SAH) is the most frequent complication of symptomatic aneurysms. Risk factors for the production of SAH include age (the incidence of hemorrhage increases steadily with age), female gender, hypertension, orally administered contraceptives, cigarette smoking, alcohol consumption, and the size of the aneurysm (10 to 15 mm). The most frequent locations of aneurysms that rupture are the internal carotid artery, anterior communicating artery, middle cerebral artery, caput of the basilar artery, and vertebrobasilar trunk. Signs and symptoms of SAH are described on page 142.

A. Rupture of an aneurysm may produce pure subarachnoid hemorrhage (see p 142) or SAH associated with an intracerebral or intraventricular hematoma. The aneurysm ruptures directly into the brain parenchyma and produces a hematoma, which may rupture into the ventricle. It may also produce a subdural hematoma, which occurs when the aneurysm ruptures directly into the subdural space, after the aneurysm has leaked, causing adhesions to form between the arachnoidal membrane and the aneurysmal sac. Finally, aneurysmal rupture may lead to focal late ischemia. This may occur in the arterial territory of the parent vessel and is frequently associated with severe spasm of that vessel. Microemboli from the aneurysmal sac have also been described as a cause of transient ischemia.

B. Signs and symptoms of a ruptured vascular aneurysm vary according to the location of the aneurysm, presence of intracerebral hematoma, spasm, etc. Grading of patients according to their neurologic function (Hunt and Hess) is of help for determining the appropriate management and the prognosis:

Grade 1 Patients are asymptomatic or are alert and oriented and have mild headache, slight neck stiffness, and no motor or sensory deficit.

Grade 2 Patients have moderate to severe headache and major meningeal signs, mild alterations in sensorium, and no neurologic deficit other than cranial nerve palsy.

Grade 3 Patients are drowsy or confused or have a mild focal deficit.

Grade 4 Patients show stupor, moderate to severe hemiparesis, possible early decerebrate rigidity, and vegetative disturbances.

Grade 5 Patients are in a deep coma, with decerebrate rigidity and moribund apperance.

The number of patients who die during the first ictus and the time of death (sudden death) are difficult to assess. Rebleeding occurs in approximately 10% of patients before admission to the hospital and continues as a high-risk event in the first week. During rebleeding an intracerebral hematoma usually occurs and the prognosis becomes dismal.

C. Medical management, aimed at early diagnosis and the prevention of rebleeding, consists of stabilization of the blood pressure, total bed rest, sedation, and laxatives. The timing of surgery, the surgical procedure, and the immediate preoperative and postoperative management vary, depending on the clinical grade. There is also variance among neurosurgeons about how to manage each case. However, early referral and early surgery combined with anti-ischemic treatment with nimodipine or hemodilution significantly improve the outcome.

References

Longstreth WT, Kaepsell TD, Yerby MS, Belle G. Risk factors for subarachnoid hemorrhage. Stroke 1985; 16:377.

Masson RL, Day AL. Aneurysmal intracerebral hemorrhage. Neurosurg Clin North Am 1992; 3:539.

Sundt TM, Whisnant JP. Subarachnoid hemorrhage from intracranial aneurysms. Surgical management and natural history of disease. N Engl J Med 1978; 299:116.

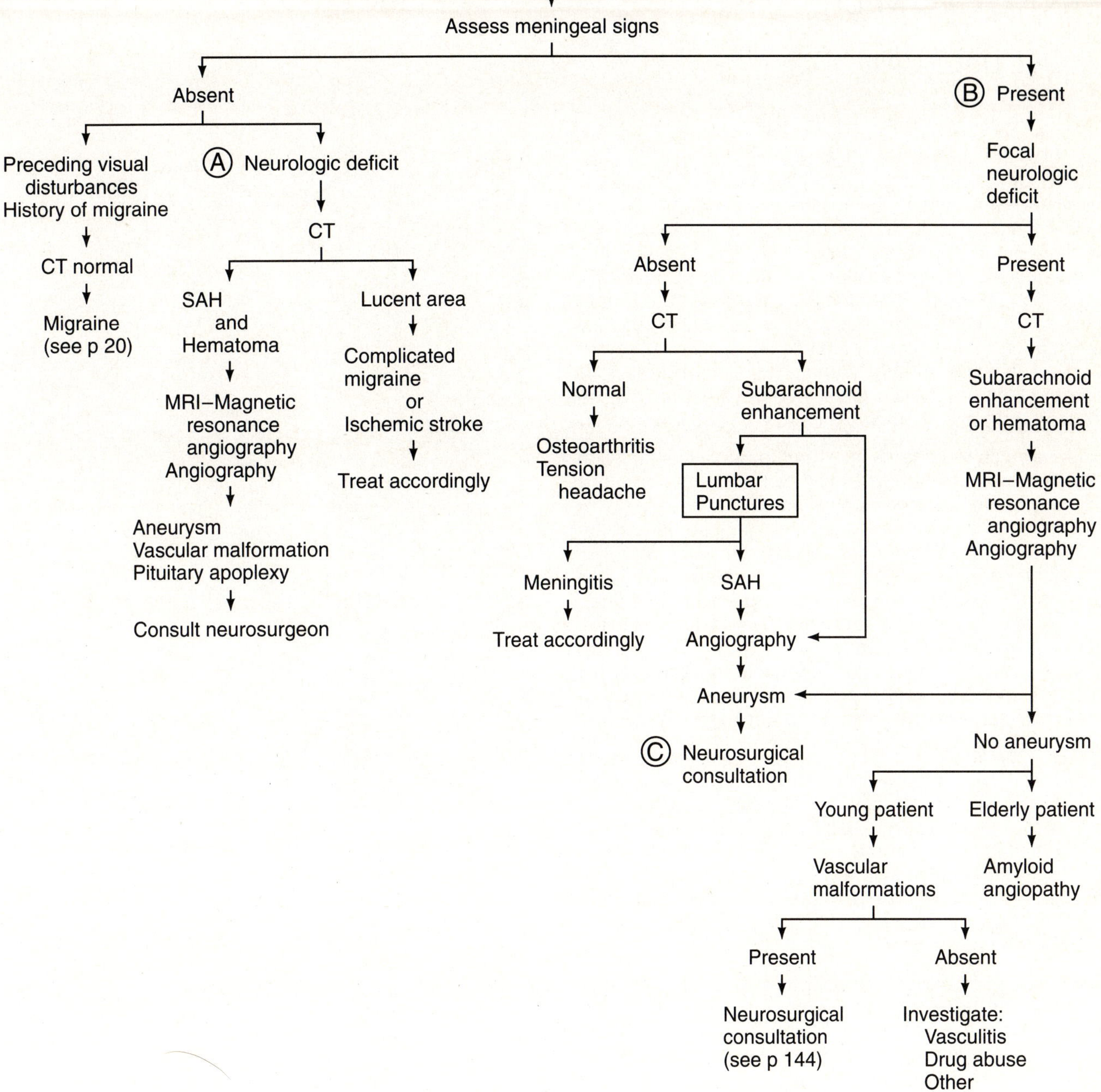

Patient with ACUTE EXCRUCIATING HEADACHE;
RUPTURED INTRACRANIAL SACCULAR ANEURYSM Suspected

Assess meningeal signs

Absent

Ⓑ Present

Preceding visual
disturbances
History of migraine

Ⓐ Neurologic deficit

Focal
neurologic
deficit

CT normal

CT

Migraine
(see p 20)

SAH
and
Hematoma

Lucent area

Absent

Present

Complicated
migraine
or
Ischemic stroke

CT

CT

MRI—Magnetic
resonance
angiography
Angiography

Treat accordingly

Normal

Subarachnoid
enhancement

Subarachnoid
enhancement
or hematoma

Aneurysm
Vascular malformation
Pituitary apoplexy

Osteoarthritis
Tension
headache

Lumbar
Punctures

MRI—Magnetic
resonance
angiography
Angiography

Consult neurosurgeon

Meningitis

SAH

Treat accordingly

Angiography

Aneurysm

Ⓒ Neurosurgical
consultation

No aneurysm

Young patient

Elderly patient

Vascular
malformations

Amyloid
angiopathy

Present

Absent

Neurosurgical
consultation
(see p 144)

Investigate:
Vasculitis
Drug abuse
Other

INTRACRANIAL SACCULAR ANEURYSM: UNRUPTURED

Carlos A. Garcia, M.D.

Saccular aneurysms are dilatations of the wall of large arteries at the base of the brain. The lesions are found at bifurcations, usually in the anterior portion of the circle of Willis. Saccular aneurysms are found in approximately 5% of the general population. They occur in either sex, and symptoms are seen most frequently in 30- to 50-year-olds. They are rarely seen in infancy or childhood. The lesions arise at sites where the muscular layer is absent (congenital defect) and where degeneration of the elastic layer often occurs. The roles of hypertension, hemodynamic factors, and the type of collagen found in these areas are not yet clear. Aneurysms are multiple in 20% of the patients.

A. Saccular aneurysms may be found incidentally at autopsy (often at the middle cerebral artery), may be asymptomatic and found on CT scans, MRI, or cerebral angiography (frequently the carotid and anterior communicating arteries), or may be found in rare cases in which there is a family history of aneurysms. The surgical management of an asymptomatic lesion found on angiography is directed to the prevention of its rupture. The size of the aneurysm seems to be an important risk factor for bleeding; the risk increases as the lesion approaches 10 mm in diameter. Figure 1 depicts an angiogram showing a middle cerebral artery aneurysm.

B. Saccular aneurysms may compress surrounding structures. The oculomotor cranial nerve is the structure most often compressed by aneurysms arising in the junction of the internal carotid artery with the posterior communicating artery. The patient usually complains of acute painful ptosis, and on examination there is a dilated pupil, with abduction and downward rotation of the affected eye.

C. Aneurysms arising in the cavernous sinus portion of the carotid artery may compress the oculomotor, trochlear, and abducent nerves and the ophthalmic branch of the trigeminal nerve. Spontaneous rupture of the lesion produces a cavernous sinus fistula with a pulsating exophthalmous and a bruit in the eye and around the orbit. Carotid artery and anterior communicating aneurysms may compress the optic chiasm or optic nerves. Basilar artery aneurysms may compress the brain stem.

D. A giant aneurysm (>3 cm) may compress brain tissue; produce seizures; block CSF pathways, producing

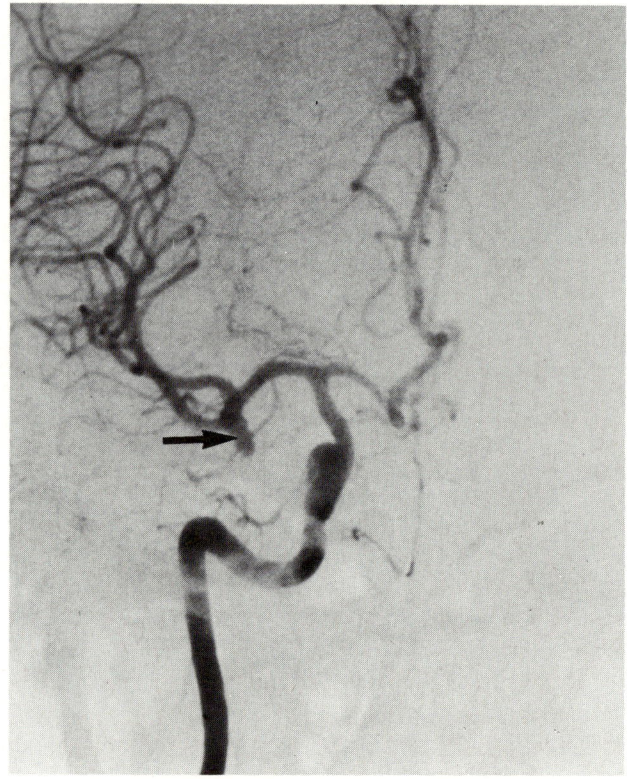

Figure 1 Angiography shows a middle cerebral artery aneurysm.

hydrocephalus; and present as a mass lesion. A CT scan, MRI, and angiography aid in the diagnosis of most of these lesions. Surgery benefits some patients. The mechanism of headache in an "unruptured" aneurysm can be rapid expansion of the aneurysm (an ominous sign) or leakage of the aneurysm without full rupture (an equally ominous sign).

References

Crevel van H, Habema JDF, Braakman R. Decision analysis of the management of incidental intracranial saccular aneurysms. Neurology 1986; 36:1335.

terBerg HWM, Dippel DWJ, Limburq M, et al. Familial intracranial aneurysms: A review. Stroke 1992; 23:1024.

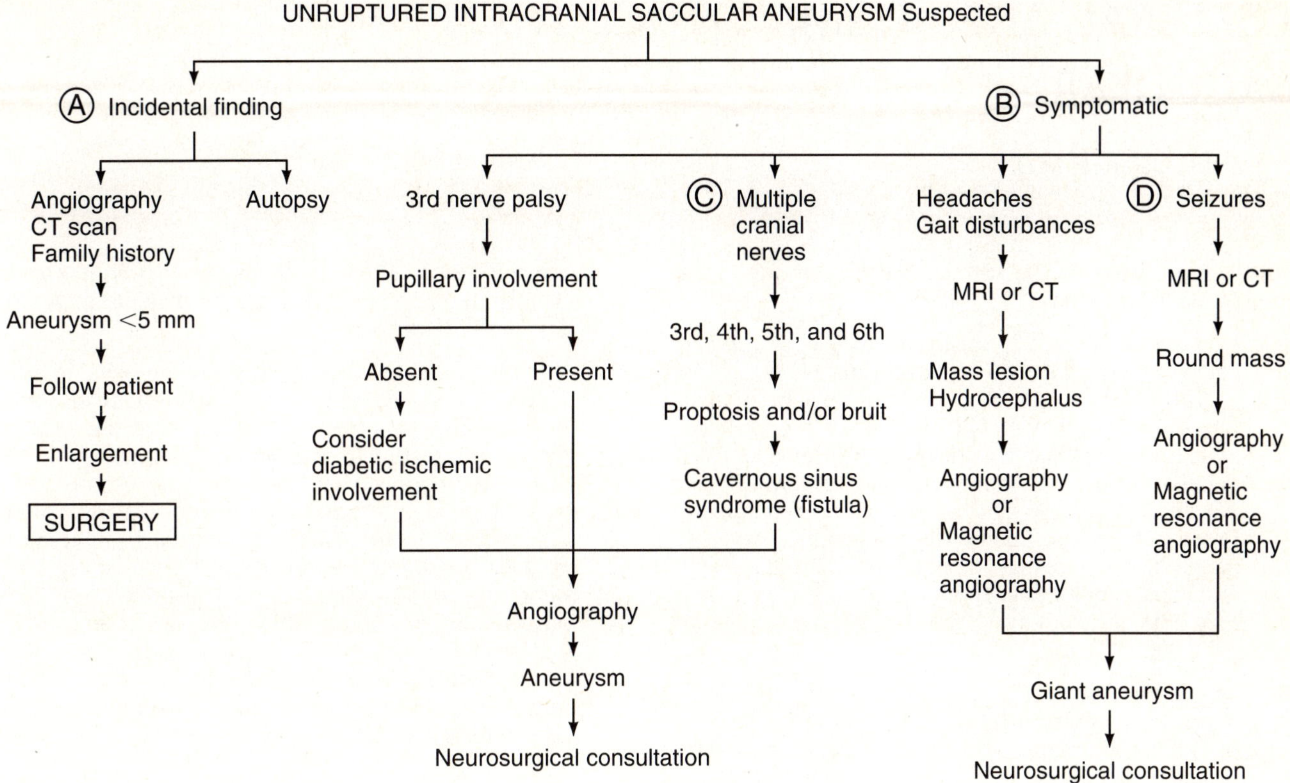

UNRUPTURED INTRACRANIAL SACCULAR ANEURYSM Suspected
A Incidental finding
B Symptomatic
Angiography
CT scan
Family history
Aneurysm <5 mm
Follow patient
Enlargement
SURGERY
Autopsy
3rd nerve palsy
Pupillary involvement
Absent
Present
Consider diabetic ischemic involvement
Angiography
Aneurysm
Neurosurgical consultation
C Multiple cranial nerves
3rd, 4th, 5th, and 6th
Proptosis and/or bruit
Cavernous sinus syndrome (fistula)
Headaches
Gait disturbances
MRI or CT
Mass lesion
Hydrocephalus
Angiography
or
Magnetic resonance angiography
D Seizures
MRI or CT
Round mass
Angiography
or
Magnetic resonance angiography
Giant aneurysm
Neurosurgical consultation

CEREBRAL ANEURYSMS OTHER THAN SACCULAR

Carlos A. Garcia, M.D.

Aneurysms other than the saccular variety are rare in the intracranial circulation.

A. Infectious ("mycotic") aneurysms may be caused by bacteria *(Staphylococcus* or *Streptococcus),* fungi *(Aspergillus),* or parasites *(Acanthamoeba).* These aneurysms are formed by embolic infectious fragments that attack and infiltrate the vessel wall. These types of aneurysms are small, have a spindle (fusiform) shape, are distal in the circulation, and are seen frequently in a branch of the middle cerebral artery. They may be multiple, and may rupture and present as subarachnoid hemorrhage. Other infectious aneurysms may originate from meningitis, osteomyelitis, pharyngitis, etc.

B. Severe head or neck trauma may be associated with minor lacerations of the cerebral arteries. Leaking of blood and formation of a clot around the vessel produce a "pseudoaneurysm" that becomes organized and adherent to the parent vessel.

C. Dissecting aneurysms of the carotid or vertebral arteries may be spontaneous and are usually associated with fibromuscular dysplasia or polycystic kidney disease, but may result from blunt neck or head trauma or neck manipulation. The clinical presentation consists of cerebral ischemic events associated with headache, syncope, and neck pain. Completed cerebral infarction or Horner's syndrome may occur. Bleeding of these lesions is rare. Cerebral angiography is diagnostic and demonstrates elongated, irregular, tapered narrowing of the lumen of the affected artery. The prognosis is good, with spontaneous recovery in most patients. Antiplatelet drugs may be of benefit in some. Anticoagulation and surgery may be helpful in selected cases. There is an increased frequency of saccular intracranial aneurysms in patients with carotid artery dissection.

D. Atherosclerotic fusiform aneurysms are seen in patients with severe generalized atherosclerosis and long-standing hypertension. Damage of the elastic (intima) and medial (muscular) layers by atherosclerosis dilates, uncoils, and elongates the vessel wall, producing "ectasia" and then aneurysmal dilatation with compression of adjacent structures. These lesions are most frequently found in the basilar artery and intracranial part of both internal carotid arteries, and occasionally may bleed. They have also been associated with tic douloureux, atypical facial pain, and facial spasms. Fusiform aneurysms of the carotid arteries have been described after radiation or radical surgery for craniopharyngiomas.

References

Azzarelli B, Moore J, Gilmor R, et al. Multiple fusiform intracranial aneurysms following curative radiation therapy for suprasellar germinoma. Case report. J Neurosurg 1984; 61:1141.

Clare CE, Barrow DL. Infectious intracranial aneurysms. Neurosurg Clin North Am 1992; 3:551.

Ramadan NM, Tietgen GE, Levine SR, Welch KMA. Scintillating scotomata associated with internal carotid artery dissection: Report of three cases. Neurology 1991; 41:1084.

Schievink WI, Mokri B, Piepgras DG. Angiographic frequency of saccular intracranial aneurysms in patients with spontaneous cervical artery dissection. J Neurosurg 1992; 76:62.

Patient with HEADACHE OR PROGRESSIVE NEUROLOGIC DEFICIT

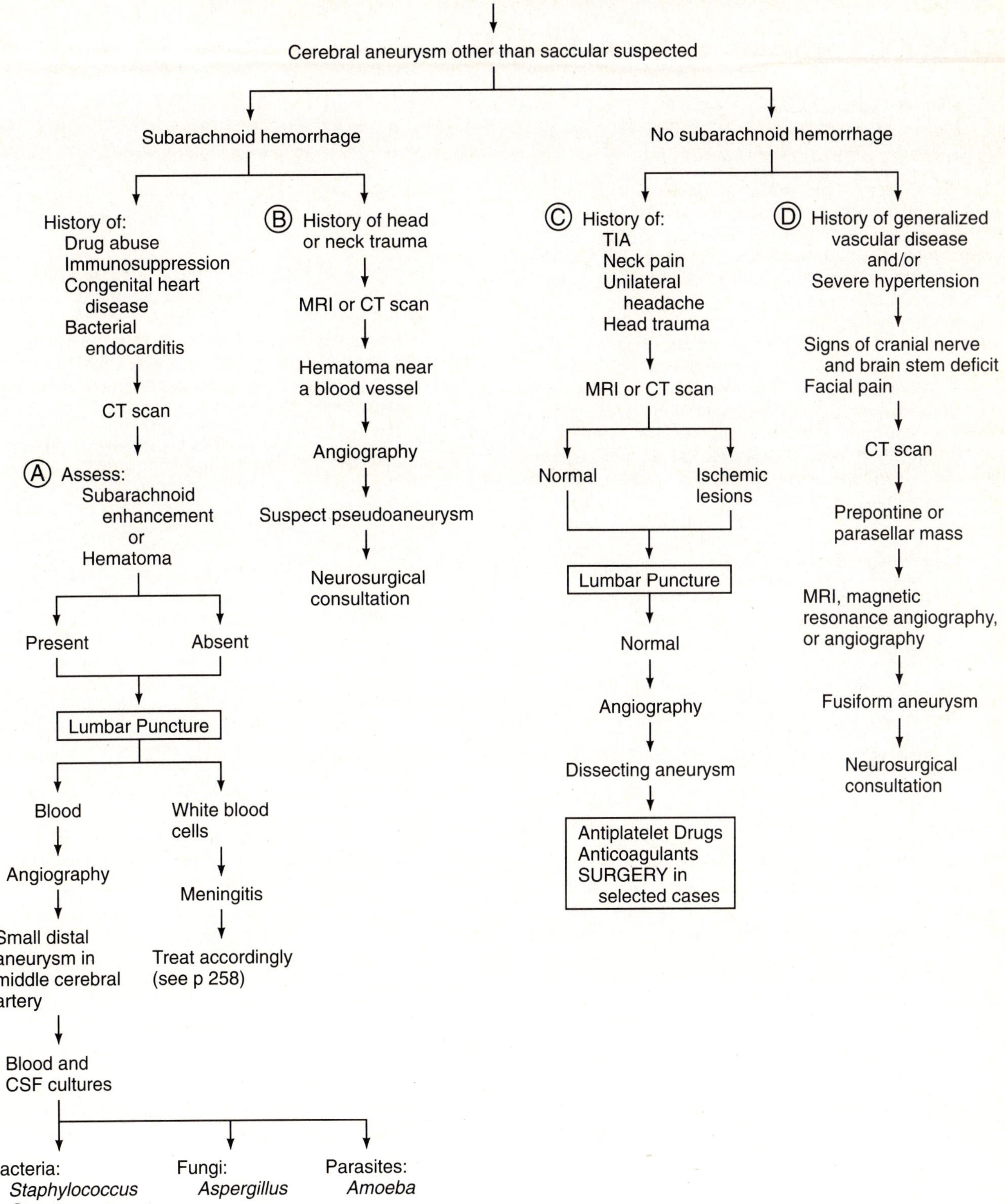

VASCULAR MALFORMATIONS: DIAGNOSIS AND MANAGEMENT

Carlos A. Garcia, M.D.

Vascular malformations (VMs) are developmental anomalies of CNS blood vessels due to lack of involution of embryonic vascular networks. VMs vary in size, site, and components of abnormal vessels. Telangiectases are small and composed of excessive dilated capillaries separated by normal neuronal tissue. Cavernous angiomas are easily identified, may have areas of calcification, and are formed by sinusoidal blood vessels with gliotic intervening neuronal tissue with evidence of previous bleeding. Venous angiomas (venous varices) are formed by anomalous veins separated by normal neuronal tissue, with no evidence of direct arterial input. Arteriovenous malformations (AVMs) are formed by masses of arteries and arterialized veins separated by gliotic neuronal tissue. This is the most clinically significant malformation.

A. VMs may be asymptomatic and be found incidentally at autopsy or during CT, MRI, or angiography.

B. Other VMs are symptomatic and present in childhood as an intracerebral hemorrhage or in early adulthood with focal or generalized seizures. Approximately 50% of VMs present clinically as intracerebral hemorrhages with some subarachnoid extension. Hemorrhage from VMs is not as devastating as subarachnoid hemorrhages of aneurysms; the mortality rate from first bleed is 10% to 15% compared with 30% in aneurysms. Rebleeding in VMs is 6% during the first year and 3% per year thereafter. The morbidity and mortality are related to the location, size, and configuration and the age and neurologic condition of the patient. Whether rupture is precipitated by rigorous activity, whether seizures increase the chance of bleeding, and whether there is a relationship to headaches has not been unequivocally proved. Occipital lobe AVMs may have some association with migraine symptoms.

C. Saccular aneuryms occur at twice the normal frequency in patients with AVM and usually occur in a large feeder vessel. Differentiation of the source of the bleeding is difficult when an AVM and aneurysm are found in the same patient, but imaging studies may help to localize the culprit. Bleeding in AVM occurs with less frequency after middle age; however, younger patients with hemorrhage recover better than adults.

D. The progressive neurologic deficit seen in some large AVMs has been explained as being produced by the "steal phenomenon" (shunting of blood from arteries to low-resistance channels producing ischemia), obstructive hydrocephalus produced by ventricular compression, venous hypertension, or mass effect produced by bleeding and edema.

E. Most lesions are neurosurgical lesions. However, management should be via a team approach with a neurosurgeon, an interventional neuroradiologist, and a radiotherapist. Most surgical procedures should be elective and carefully planned unless there is an intracerebral or subdural hematoma. Drainage of the hematoma may be accomplished with total resection of small superficial lesions. Brain swelling and diffuse or focal hemorrhage in the adjacent normal parenchyma may occur after resection of an AVM. The so-called "perfusion breakthrough" may be prevented by reducing the blood supply of the malformation by stages ("staging") through either surgical resection, occlusion of the feeders, or embolization of the lesion. Embolization through arterial catheters has been done with Silastic spheres and balloons by expert interventional neuroradiologists. Radiosurgery with proton beam therapy, or highly collimated gamma irradiation delivered via Leksell's stereotactic method, is used in specialized centers. Radiosurgery has been used effectively in deep, small (<3-cm) lesions.

References

OJemann RG, Heros RC, Crowell RM. Surgical management of cerebrovascular disease. 2nd ed. Baltimore: Williams & Wilkins, 1988.

Rubinstein L. Tumors of the central nervous system, 2nd series. Washington, DC: Armed Forces Institute of Pathology, 1972.

Wilson CB, Stein B. Intracranial arteriovenous malformations. Baltimore: Williams & Wilkins, 1984.

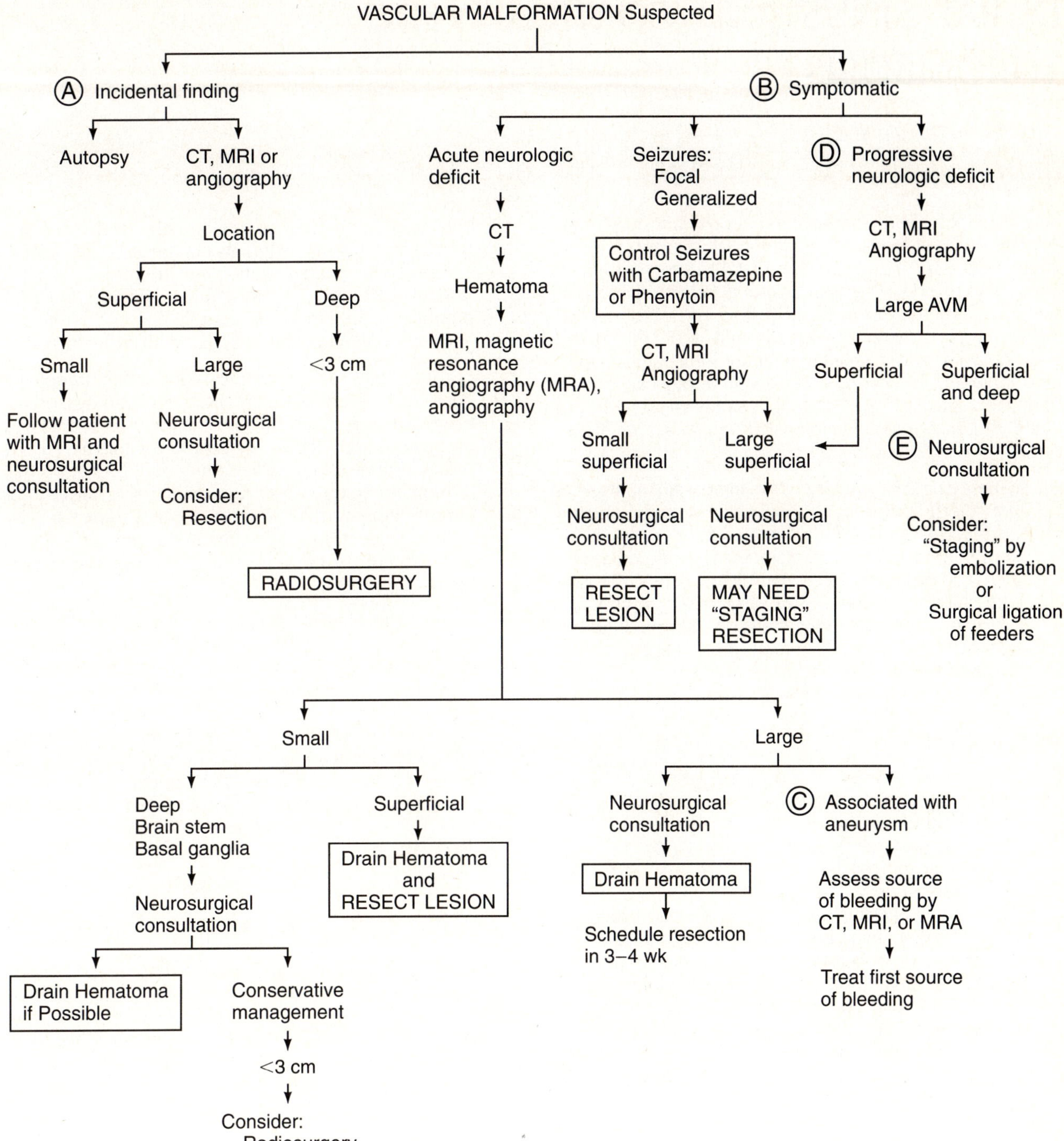

VASCULAR MALFORMATION Suspected

A Incidental finding

Autopsy

CT, MRI or angiography

Location

Superficial

Deep

Small

Large

<3 cm

Follow patient with MRI and neurosurgical consultation

Neurosurgical consultation

Consider: Resection

RADIOSURGERY

B Symptomatic

Acute neurologic deficit

CT

Hematoma

MRI, magnetic resonance angiography (MRA), angiography

Seizures: Focal Generalized

Control Seizures with Carbamazepine or Phenytoin

CT, MRI Angiography

Small superficial

Large superficial

Neurosurgical consultation

Neurosurgical consultation

RESECT LESION

MAY NEED "STAGING" RESECTION

D Progressive neurologic deficit

CT, MRI Angiography

Large AVM

Superficial

Superficial and deep

E Neurosurgical consultation

Consider: "Staging" by embolization or Surgical ligation of feeders

Small

Deep Brain stem Basal ganglia

Superficial

Neurosurgical consultation

Drain Hematoma and RESECT LESION

Drain Hematoma if Possible

Conservative management

<3 cm

Consider: Radiosurgery

Large

Neurosurgical consultation

C Associated with aneurysm

Drain Hematoma

Schedule resection in 3–4 wk

Assess source of bleeding by CT, MRI, or MRA

Treat first source of bleeding

DURAL SINUS AND CORTICAL VEIN THROMBOSIS

Carlos A. Garcia, M.D.

Because of the abundant collateral circulation, dural sinus thrombosis may have a spectrum of clinical findings ranging from asymptomatic to a fatal course. Localized thrombosis of a dural sinus or a cortical vein rarely leads to a cerebral lesion. Complete occlusion of one or several sinuses impairs venous drainage and CSF absorption, producing hemorrhagic infarctions or intracranial hypertension. Dural sinuses and cortical vein thrombosis may be septic or nonseptic. Septic thrombosis may be secondary to meningitis or to infections in nearby structures, mainly air sinuses or middle ear infections.

A. Patients present with signs of increased intracranial pressure (ICP) (headache, nausea, vomiting) and on examination show papilledema, with or without bilateral sixth cranial nerve weakness. They are otherwise alert and show no other neurologic deficit. CT and MRI may show the lesions and small compressed ventricles. A lumbar puncture shows normal fluid but increased pressure. Cerebral angiography shows thrombosis of the lateral sinus(es). "Otitic hydrocephalus" is often associated with chronic middle ear or mastoid infection. This entity is most commonly seen in young patients.

B. If the patient has signs of increased ICP, is comatose, and is having seizures (usually generalized), there may be thrombosis of most if not all dural sinuses. CT or MRI and delayed venous phase angiography help confirm the diagnosis. Prediagnostic risk factors include birth control pills in young females, polycythemia, congestive heart failure, sickle cell disease, malnutrition, dehydration, and head trauma. All these factors may work in isolation or in combination. If the patient is known to have meningitis, the dural sinus is septic. Treatment consists of specific therapy for the underlying factor(s). In some patients, focal findings may consist of hemiparesis or paraparesis. The patient may be alert or comatose. Seizures are frequent. MRI and magnetic resonance angiography (MRA) confirm the diagnosis. Anticoagulants may be used in selected cases. Local administration of fibrinolytic agents (urokinase) is safe, but systemic administration may produce major neurologic complications. Puerperium and later pregnancy are well-known risk factors.

C. Focal findings such as proptosis and ophthalmoplegia may indicate involvement of the cavernous sinus. Bruits around the orbit and in the eye indicate a cavernous sinus fistula. Aneurysm of the cavernous sinus portion of the carotid artery may present in this fashion (spontaneous fistula) without a history of trauma. However, head trauma may produce a cavernous sinus fistula. Treatment consists of balloon embolization of the lesion or ligation of the carotid artery at the neck.

D. Poorly controlled adult diabetes may present with a cavernous sinus syndrome, but there is also contralateral hemiplegia and the patient is comatose. Mucormycosis is a frequent etiologic agent in these cases. The fungi thrombose the carotid artery and produce an extensive and massive cerebral infarction. Immunosuppressed patients receiving chemotherapy for leukemia, lymphoma, or other tumors are at risk of developing a cavernous sinus infection, usually by *Aspergillus*. Fungal infections respond poorly to therapy.

References

Barnwell SL, Higashida RT, Halbach UV, et al. Direct endovascular thrombolitic therapy for dural sinus thrombosis. Neurosurgery 1991; 28:135.

Kalgab RM, Woolf AL. Thrombosis and thrombophlebitis of cerebral veins and dural sinuses. In Vinken, Bruyhn, eds. Handbook of clinical neurology. 1972:422.

DURAL SINUS AND CORTICAL VEIN THROMBOSIS Suspected

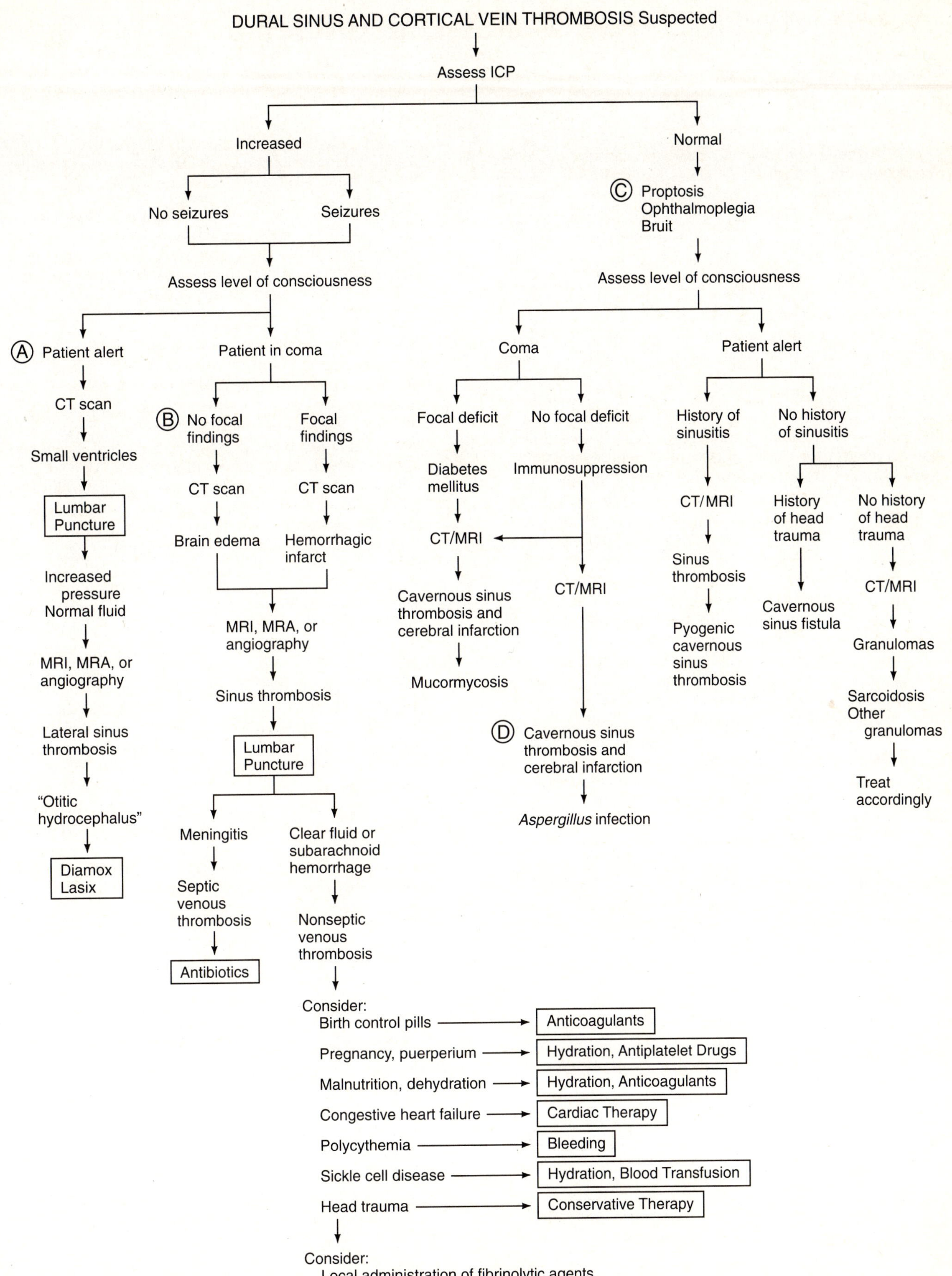

ACUTE HYPERTENSIVE VASCULAR CRISIS

Leon A. Weisberg, M.D.

Acute hypertensive vascular crisis may cause acute encephalopathy precipitated by a sudden dramatic rise in blood pressure (BP). This usually occurs in the presence of end-organ (CNS, myocardial, renal, retinal) damage; rarely are these complications absent. In hypertensive encephalopathy, systolic BP is usually >200 mm Hg and diastolic BP is >130 mm Hg. An acute rise in BP may cause neurologic symptoms within several hours; symptoms of hypertensive encephalopathy reflect cerebral edema and breakdown of cerebrovascular autoregulation. Early symptoms are headache, vomiting, and visual disturbances. Visual symptoms include bilateral blurring or dimming of vision or scintillating scotomata; these are believed due to retinal or optic nerve ischemia. The mental state may be normal in early stages; confusion and seizures develop later. Funduscopy shows hypertensive retinopathy (arterial narrowing, cotton wool exudates, hemorrhages, retinal edema). Focal signs occasionally occur but are usually transient; their persistence suggests ischemia or hemorrhage complicating hypertensive vascular crisis.

A. Hypertensive encephalopathy rarely occurs in previously normotensive individuals. When it does, seek a drug history and perform toxicology tests. Cocaine and other sympathomimetic drugs (amphetamine, phencyclidine, diet pills) may precipitate hypertensive crisis. Consider acute renal insufficiency, eclampsia, pheochromocytoma, aortic dissection, monoamine oxidase (MAO) (antidepressant medication) interaction with tyramine-containing food substances or drugs such as meperidine (Demerol), or abrupt withdrawal of certain antihypertensive medications (e.g., clonidine [Catapres], propranolol [Inderal]).

B. The retinal edema of hypertensive retinopathy is difficult to differentiate from papilledema that is due to primary intracranial disorder causing elevated intracranial pressure. Subhyaloid hemorrhages in the retina suggest sudden BP increase; they are also commonly seen in subarachnoid hemorrhage (SAH). In patients with hypertensive encephalopathy and papilledema, bradycardia and respiratory abnormalities suggest Cushing reflex (due to tonsillar herniation). In this case, arterial hypertension may be secondary to an intracranial lesion, such as a posterior fossa mass (neoplasm, hemorrhage), which is diagnosed by CT/MRI.

C. Focal signs and nuchal rigidity may occur in hypertensive encephalopathy and suggest complicating intracranial hemorrhage. If CT shows no bleeding, lumbar puncture is necessary to exclude SAH.

D. If CT shows intracerebral bleeding, treatment is different from that of uncomplicated hypertensive encephalopathy. Rapidly lower BP and use antiedema drugs; improvement may be less complete because there has been brain injury from the intracerebral bleeding (see p 134).

E. If there are no focal signs or nuchal rigidity, attempt immediate and rapid reduction of BP. Treat these acute hypertensive crisis patients in the intensive care unit; monitor renal and cardiac function to prevent oliguria, heart failure, and myocardial ischemia. The goal of therapy is to lower arterial BP by 25% or to lower diastolic BP to 100 to 110 mm Hg. Use sodium nitroprusside infusion; adjust the rate according to clinical response. If the neurologic condition worsens, this may result from decreased cerebral perfusion due to rapid lowering of BP. If the neurologic status improves as BP rises, adequate cerebral perfusion may require a higher BP than in normotensive patients. Alternative mechanisms for neurologic deterioration that may occur during treatment of hypertensive encephalopathy include CNS depression by drugs, worsening of cerebral edema, and seizure activity. The development of focal signs during treatment suggests cerebral ischemia. If the neurologic condition does not improve with nitroprusside, use antiedema drugs and switch to an alternative antihypertensive drug (labetalol, diazoxide). EEG is necessary to exclude seizure activity. The choice of anticonvulsant medication requires careful consideration. Phenobarbital depresses consciousness; phenytoin and diazepam have potential cardiac toxicity. If acute hypertensive crisis is successfully managed, a full neurologic recovery should result.

References

Calhoun DA, Oparil S. Treatment of hypertensive crisis. N Engl J Med 1990; 323:1177.

Chester EM, Agamanolis DP, Banker BD. Hypertensive encephalopathy: A clinicopathologic study of 20 cases. Neurology 1978; 28:928.

Dinsdale HB. Hypertensive encephalopathy. Neurol Clin North Am 1985; 1:3.

Gifford RW, Westbrook E. Hypertensive encephalopathy: Mechanisms, clinical features and treatment. Prog Cardiovasc Dis 1974; 17:115.

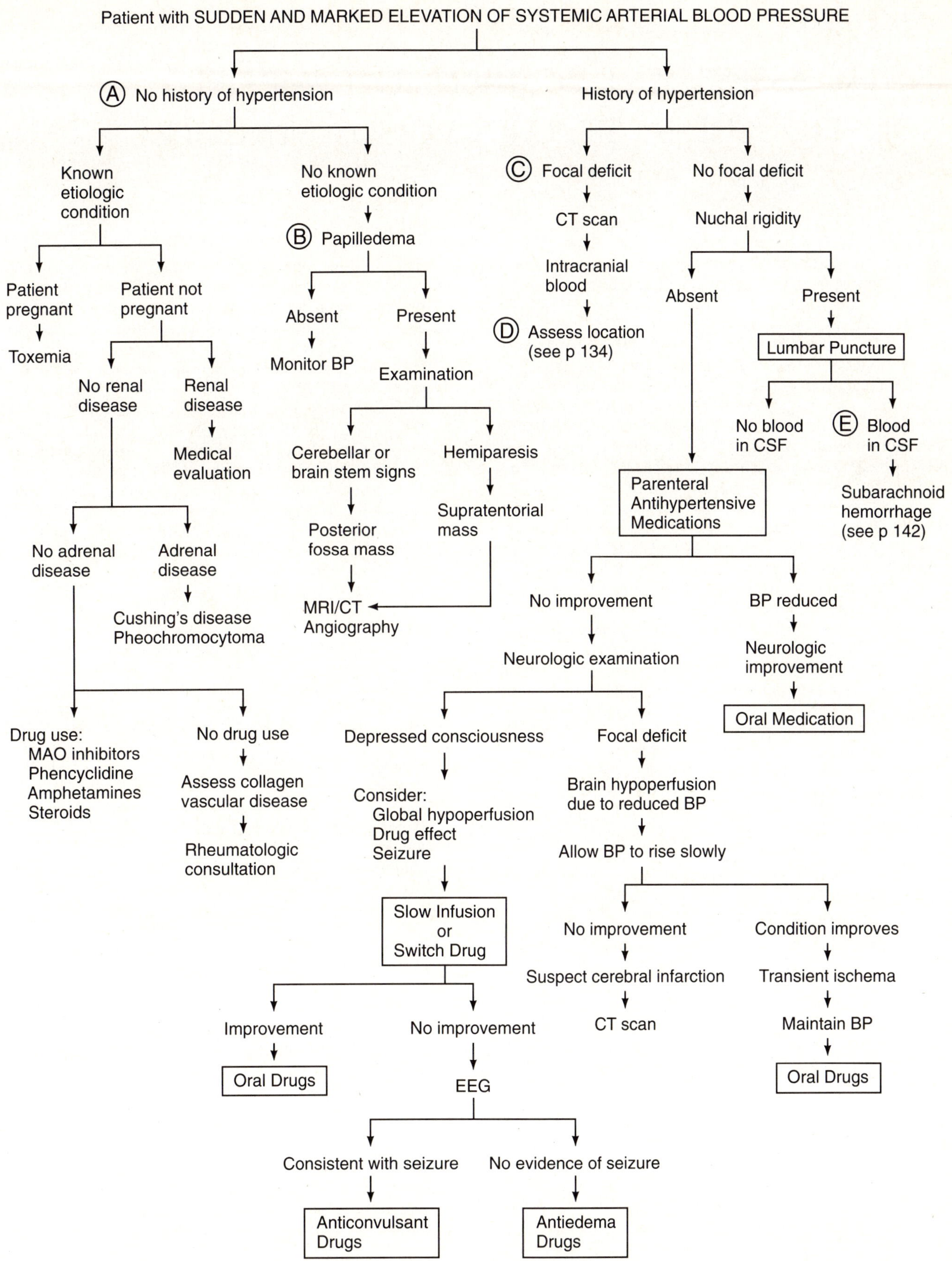

Patient with SUDDEN AND MARKED ELEVATION OF SYSTEMIC ARTERIAL BLOOD PRESSURE
A No history of hypertension
History of hypertension
Known etiologic condition
No known etiologic condition
B Papilledema
C Focal deficit
No focal deficit
Patient pregnant
Patient not pregnant
Toxemia
No renal disease
Renal disease
Medical evaluation
Absent
Present
Monitor BP
Examination
CT scan
Intracranial blood
D Assess location (see p 134)
Nuchal rigidity
Absent
Present
Lumbar Puncture
No blood in CSF
E Blood in CSF
Subarachnoid hemorrhage (see p 142)
No adrenal disease
Adrenal disease
Cushing's disease
Pheochromocytoma
Cerebellar or brain stem signs
Hemiparesis
Posterior fossa mass
Supratentorial mass
MRI/CT Angiography
Parenteral Antihypertensive Medications
No improvement
BP reduced
Neurologic examination
Neurologic improvement
Oral Medication
Drug use:
MAO inhibitors
Phencyclidine
Amphetamines
Steroids
No drug use
Assess collagen vascular disease
Rheumatologic consultation
Depressed consciousness
Focal deficit
Consider:
Global hypoperfusion
Drug effect
Seizure
Brain hypoperfusion due to reduced BP
Allow BP to rise slowly
No improvement
Condition improves
Slow Infusion or Switch Drug
Suspect cerebral infarction
Transient ischema
CT scan
Maintain BP
Oral Drugs
Improvement
No improvement
Oral Drugs
EEG
Consistent with seizure
No evidence of seizure
Anticonvulsant Drugs
Antiedema Drugs

INITIAL ASSESSMENT OF TRANSIENT IMPAIRED CONSCIOUSNESS: SEIZURES VERSUS SYNCOPE

Leon A. Weisberg, M.D.

Seizures are sudden paroxysmal episodes of altered neurologic function followed by complete recovery. They are caused by abnormal electrical excitatory activity. During a seizure, EEG is *always* abnormal; between seizures, EEG may show no abnormalities. Seizure stages are (1) prodrome: interval before seizures when behavior, mood, or attitude changes may occur; (2) aura: initial seizure phase which may be characterized by motor or somatosensory disturbances such as localized muscle twitching or tingling sensation; abnormal visceral sensations involving abdomen or head regions; and affective or behavioral symptoms such as fear, anger, distortions of size or time, hallucinations, or dream-like states; (3) ictus: seizure episode, usually characterized by impaired consciousness and abnormal motor manifestations; (4) postictal stage during which the patient may be confused or show focal signs (Todd's postictal paralysis) but then returns to baseline condition; and (5) interictal stage during which patients show no clinical abnormalities and EEG may show intermittent spikes or slow waves or be normal.

In delineating the type of seizure and differentiating it from other paroxysmal disorders (syncope, narcolepsy, migraine, vertigo), describe the clinical characteristics of each stage. Because patients may have impaired consciousness during clinical episodes and may be confused or amnestic postictally, their description of the seizure may be incomplete and fragmented. Question observers who have witnessed a clinical episode. Seizure is the most likely diagnosis if the patient reports an aura, if rhythmic jerking motor activity is observed, if tongue maceration and incontinence occur, if confusion follows the episode, and if the patient reports postepisode headache and myalgias.

A. Prodromal symptoms (dizziness, weakness, perioral paresthesias, light-headedness, weakness) suggest syncope. Episodes that occur during periods of emotional stress or are associated with postural change are consistent with syncope. Abnormal visceral (including cephalic and abdominal) sensations suggest seizure disorder. Chest pain, palpitations, and shortness of breath suggest cardiac-related syncope or possibly hyperventilation induced by an anxiety state.

B. In major motor or grand mal seizures, patients fall to the ground and develop increased body tone (tonic phase) and may injure themselves; in syncope, patients become limp (hypotonic) and are not usually injured. If a patient falls from a height (ladder, roof), injury may occur in either seizure or syncope. It is extremely important to diagnose accurately an episode of transient loss of consciousness (LOC) with spontaneous recovery (no cardiopulmonary resuscitation or drug intervention required to terminate the episode) as either a primary brain dysfunction (seizure) or an episode of reduced brain activity (syncope), which is usually due to a systemic non-neurologic disorder. Seizures require neurodiagnostic evaluation and usually treatment with antiepileptic medication; syncope represents a systemic (*not* primary brain disturbance) disorder that may be benign (self-limited but sometimes recurrent) or more malignant (life-threatening, especially if there is a cardiac cause). In several studies, syncope of cardiac etiology carries a 18% to 33% mortality rate. Syncope may also be secondary to metabolic dysfunction or drug effect (vasodilators, diuretics, antihypertensives). History and physical examination provide the most useful diagnostic information in 85% of patients with transient LOC of established etiology.

C. Incontinence occurs with seizures or syncope if the bladder is full; it is more common with seizures.

D. After seizures, patients are usually confused for several minutes to hours. Transient focal signs (Todd's postictal paralysis) indicate an underlying lesion. Focal neurologic signs are most unusual after syncope. Myalgias (due to intense muscle contraction) and headache (due to cerebral vasodilation) are common after seizures. Absence of postictal confusion suggests pseudoseizure (hysterical reaction) rather than a true seizure. If pseudoseizure is considered, monitor the patient with videotelemetric EEG. If an episode occurs during monitoring and EEG remains normal, "pseudoseizure" is confirmed.

E. In major motor seizures the tonic phase is followed by rhythmic myoclonic jerks. Random, irregular, non-rhythmic myoclonic jerks may occur in syncopal disorders as a result of cerebral hypoxia. Tonic spasms (decerebration) without rhythmic myoclonic jerks may occur either in tonic seizures or with brain stem ischemia (anoxic seizures). Differentiation of these two disorders requires EEG monitoring.

F. In partial complex seizures, patients appear confused and may act inappropriately; consciousness may not be completely lost and they report being in a twilight zone, aware of things going on around them but unable to respond appropriately. Purposeful goal-directed activity is impossible during seizures.

G. When transient LOC occurs suddenly and without warning and no cardiac abnormalities are identified,

Patient with **EPISODE OF TRANSIENT IMPAIRED CONSCIOUSNESS**

(A) Assess warning symptoms

Absent → (B) Assess motor activity

- Clonic jerks
  - Rhythmic → Assess tongue maceration
    - Present → (C) Assess incontinence
      - Present → (D) Assess postepisode confusion
        - Present → Assess amnesia for episode
          - Present → Assess headache
            - Present → Assess myalgia
              - Present → Diagnosis of seizure clinically confirmed
              - Absent → Seizure still most likely
            - Absent → Consider: Syncope or pseudoseizure
          - Absent → Consider: Syncope or pseudoseizure
        - Absent → Seizure still most likely
      - Absent → Seizure still most likely
    - Absent → Seizure still most likely
  - Arrhythmic → Consider: Convulsive syncope
- No clonic jerks → Assess loss of muscle tone in legs
  - (E) Present → Consider: Syncope, Drop attack, Cataplexy, Pseudoseizure
  - Absent → Consider seizure: Petit mal, Psychomotor (partial complex), Pseudoseizure
    - (F) Observe rhythmic eyelid blinking
      - Absent → Assess semipurposeful motor activity
        - Absent → Consider: Psychomotor seizure, Pseudoseizure → Assess EEG for epileptic findings
          - Absent → Pseudoseizure more likely than psychomotor seizure → Video moitoring
            - Episode not captured → No diagnosis possible
            - Episode captured → Assess EEG
              - No changes → Pseudoseizures (see p 164)
              - Changes → Psychomotor seizures
          - Present → Psychomotor seizure
        - Present → Psychomotor seizure (see p 170)
      - Present → Petit mal (see p 164)

Present → (G) Neurologic → Consider: Seizure, Cerebrovascular episode, Migraine

Generalized → Consider: Syncope

consider subarachnoid hemorrhage (SAH); however, rapid and full recovery is unusual and severe headache is present in SAH patients. Syncope may occur with migraine, but rarely as the initial symptom and rarely without headache. Sudden LOC with spontaneous recovery and no focal neurologic signs is almost never seen with ischemic or hemorrhagic stroke.

References

Day SC, Cook EF, Funkenstein H. Evaluation and outcome of emergency room patients with transient loss of consciousness. Am J Med 1982; 73:15.

Gastaut H. Clinical and electroencephalographic classification of epileptic seizures. Epilepsia 1981; 22:489.

Kapoor WN, Karpf M, Wicand S. Prospective evaluation and follow-up of patients with syncope. N Engl J Med 1983; 309:197.

ANTIEPILEPTIC MEDICATION MANAGEMENT: GENERAL PRINCIPLES

Leon A. Weisberg, M.D.

The goal in selecting the appropriate antiepileptic drug (AED) is to achieve full control of seizures while avoiding drug toxicity. An AED has relative specificities; the drug used should be effective for the particular seizure type. The severity of epilepsy is variable: two individuals may have different responses despite having the same epileptic disorder and being treated with the same medication. Before initiating AED treatment, make sure the diagnosis of epilepsy is well established. A "therapeutic trial" of AED when the diagnosis of epilepsy is "possible" but not established is rarely successful. Be certain that seizure diagnosis is established on the basis of clinical episodes and EEG findings. The patient should understand the goals of therapy, drug administration schedule, and potential side effects (including possible interaction of AED with other drugs). Noncompliance (not taking medication as prescribed) is the most common cause of treatment failure.

A. Treat with one drug (monopharmacy) at a low dosage and slowly increase the dosage. Plasma clearance of AED may be lower early in treatment. After 1 month, induction of liver enzyme systems increases and a higher dosage may be necessary. For primary generalized tonic-clonic seizures, begin with phenobarbital, phenytoin, valproic acid, or carbamazepine; for absence attacks, valproic acid or ethosuximide; for partial seizures, phenytoin or carbamazepine. The frequency of administration is determined by drug half-life. There may be significant variation in individual patient dosages owing to differences in gastrointestinal absorption, protein binding, and metabolism. If seizures are controlled, follow the patient for side effects, neurologic condition, or changed attitude toward medication. If seizures are controlled, it is not essential to check blood levels; however, periodic monitoring for hematologic, hepatic, or metabolic effects is necessary. Avoid using medications that have unpleasant side effects for the individual patient. For example, gum hyperplasia and body hair growth due to phenytoin are poorly tolerated by adolescents. Choose medications that minimally interfere with the patient's life style. Once-daily administration of phenytoin is easier than multiple-dose administration of valproate or carbamazepine.

B. If seizures are controlled but adverse reactions occur, determine whether the reactions are dose dependent. If there are hypersensitivity or toxic (non−dose-dependent) reactions, switch drugs. If the effect is dose related, lower the dosage or use the same dosage but divide the total throughout the day. If seizures recur, switch to an alternative drug or start a second drug while maintaining the first at the tolerated dosage. Polypharmacy (multiple AEDs) increases the need for drug level monitoring, because the potential for metabolic interaction between drugs is greater. Polypharmacy is sometimes necessary if patients have multiple types of seizures. If seizures are not controlled with two drugs, increase the dosage of the second drug or introduce a third drug.

C. If seizures are not controlled satisfactorily despite adequate drug levels, consider pseudoseizures; video monitoring is indicated if this diagnosis is possible. If seizures are accompanied by abnormal electrical discharges, reassess the patient's condition, and include repeat diagnostic studies. If seizures change in pattern or if neurologic signs develop, periodic reassessment is indicated.

D. Rapid seizure control is associated with a good clinical outcome; multiple seizures may damage brain tissue. In patients with frequent episodes of status epilepticus, a neurologic deficit may develop as a consequence of hypoxic-ischemic brain injury. Neurologic deficit does not usually result from multiple recurrent seizures; if it occurs, consider an underlying structural brain lesion.

E. If seizures are not controlled, consider noncompliance. This may be documented by low AED levels and a dramatic increase if the patient is given medication in a controlled environment (inpatient hospitalization). Noncompliance may be managed by a frank discussion with the patient about the importance of taking medication as prescribed. When poor seizure control occurs, consider use of drugs by the patient that may lower the seizure threshold (antihistamines, antidepressants, antipsychotics, aminophylline); this includes prescription and over-the-counter medications. Alcohol and illicit drugs may lower the seizure threshold.

F. If the patient is seizure free for 2 years, consider discontinuing AED (see p 162).

References

Escueta AV, Treiman DM, Walsh GO. The treatable epilepsies. N Engl J Med 1977; 308:1508.

Shinnar S, Vining E, Mellits D, et al. Discontinuing antiepileptic medication in children with epilepsy after two years without seizures. N Engl J Med 1985; 316:976.

So EL, Penry JK. Epilepsy in adults. Ann Neurol 1981; 9:3.

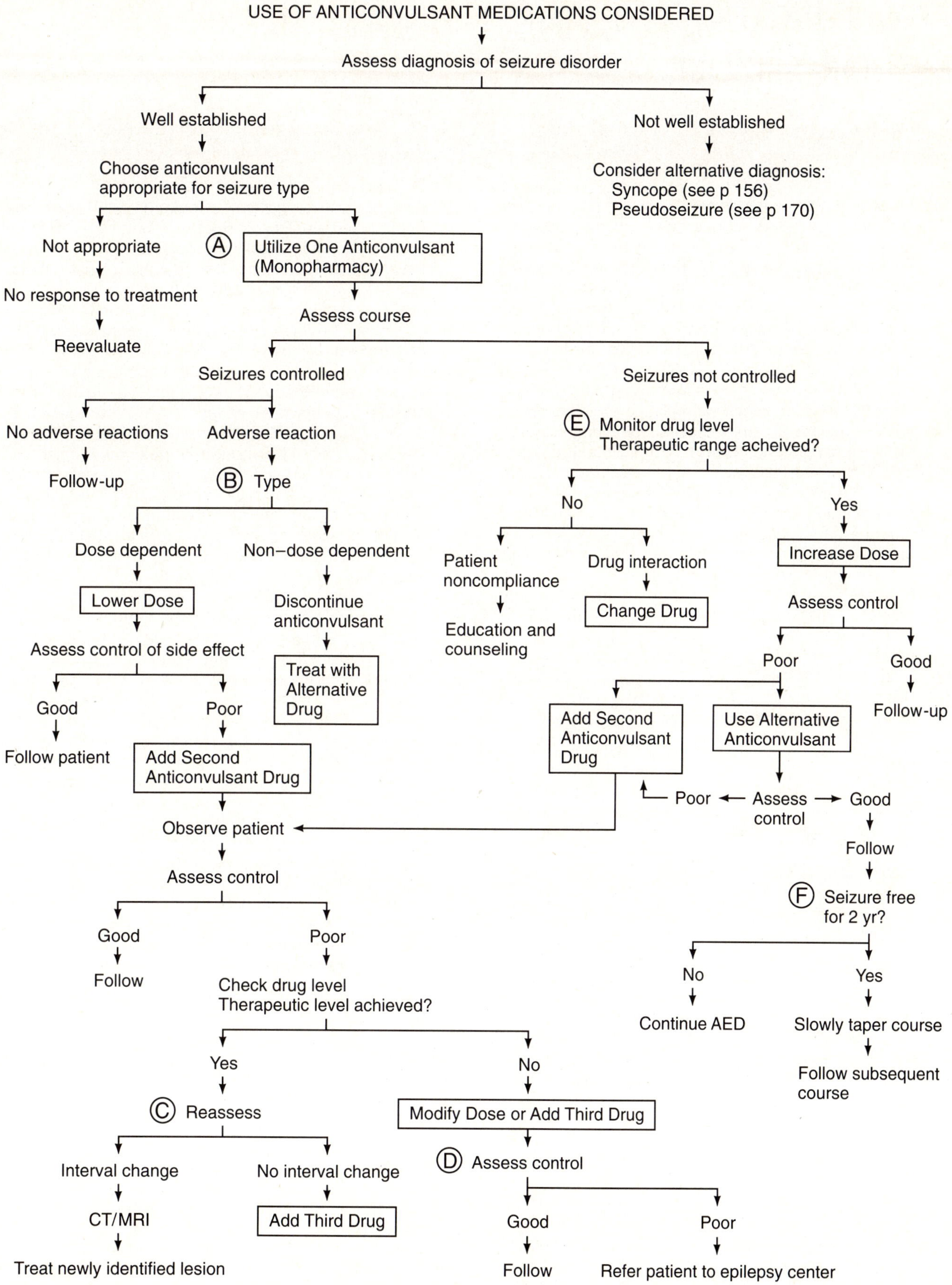

USE OF ANTICONVULSANT MEDICATIONS CONSIDERED

Assess diagnosis of seizure disorder

Well established

Choose anticonvulsant appropriate for seizure type

Not appropriate → No response to treatment → Reevaluate

Ⓐ Utilize One Anticonvulsant (Monopharmacy)

Assess course

Seizures controlled

No adverse reactions → Follow-up

Adverse reaction → Ⓑ Type

Dose dependent → Lower Dose → Assess control of side effect

Good → Follow patient

Poor → Add Second Anticonvulsant Drug

Non–dose dependent → Discontinue anticonvulsant → Treat with Alternative Drug

Observe patient

Assess control

Good → Follow

Poor → Check drug level — Therapeutic level achieved?

Yes → Ⓒ Reassess

Interval change → CT/MRI → Treat newly identified lesion

No interval change → Add Third Drug

No → Modify Dose or Add Third Drug → Ⓓ Assess control

Good → Follow

Poor → Refer patient to epilepsy center

Not well established

Consider alternative diagnosis:
Syncope (see p 156)
Pseudoseizure (see p 170)

Seizures not controlled

Ⓔ Monitor drug level — Therapeutic range acheived?

No:

Patient noncompliance → Education and counseling

Drug interaction → Change Drug

Yes → Increase Dose → Assess control

Poor:

Add Second Anticonvulsant Drug

Use Alternative Anticonvulsant → Assess control

Poor → (to Observe patient)

Good → Follow → Ⓕ Seizure free for 2 yr?

No → Continue AED

Yes → Slowly taper course → Follow subsequent course

Good → Follow-up

ADULT PATIENT WITH FIRST SINGLE MAJOR MOTOR SEIZURE

Leon A. Weisberg, M.D.

A. If a patient is evaluated immediately after a first seizure and has meningeal signs or fever, perform lumbar puncture. Perform CT if there are focal neurologic signs or papilledema. Neurologic signs that persist after seizures (even if transient, e.g., Todd's postictal paralysis) suggest an underlying structural brain lesion, which may be demonstrated by CT or MRI. The lesion may be macroscopic and demonstrated by neuroimaging studies (CT, MRI) or microscopic, in which case neuroimaging studies are usually normal. If a lesion (neoplasm, abscess, cyst) is present, appropriate therapy is indicated; antiepileptic drug (AED) treatment should also be initiated. It is commonly believed that seizures due to a structural brain lesion are most difficult to treat effectively. Negative neuroimaging studies do not rule out an underlying brain lesion, especially glioma or metastasis. In some patients, these may not be visualized on initial CT or MRI. Malignant gliomas may be infiltrating and cause minimal mass effect; thus, they may not be initially detected. MRI may be more sensitive than CT in demonstrating lesions in patients with seizures. If neuroimaging studies are negative in patients with seizures, initiate AED. Indications for periodic reassessment in seizure patients include development of new neurologic signs, uncontrolled seizures despite adequate blood levels of AED, and change in seizure pattern.

B. If the neurologic examination is normal, perform EEG. If EEG shows no abnormality, obtain a careful history for risk factors that may precipitate seizures (sleep deprivation, alcohol, drugs, emotional stress, fever, diet). Order laboratory studies to exclude metabolic factors (abnormality of glucose, sodium, or calcium; liver or renal dysfunction). If no abnormal metabolic factors are identified, obtain a history of drug use, both prescription (antihistamines, anticholinergics, amphetamines, antidepressants, antipsychotics) and illicit (phencyclidine, marijuana, cocaine, amphetamines, Ts and Blues containing Talwin and Pyribenzamine), supplemented by blood and urine toxicology tests. Patients with a single seizure precipitated by a toxic, drug, or metabolic condition who have a normal neurologic examination and normal EEG do not require AED. In patients with drug-induced seizures, EEG may show abnormalities due to drug effect for several days, but this usually normalizes within 1 week. If EEG abnormalities persist, the patient probably has underlying epilepsy triggered by a precipitating factor; treatment with AED is warranted. If the neurologic examination and EEG are normal, the probability of detecting abnormalities with CT and CSF examination is low (if the patient is systemically well and has a negative syphilis serologic test).

C. Five percent of general population will have one unprovoked nonfebrile seizure. The risk of seizure recurrence after the single seizure is not known. Several studies have reported a recurrence risk ranging from 33% to 71%. This depends on multiple factors: age of the patient when the seizure initially occurs, neurologic findings, EEG findings, duration of follow-up, and seizure type. The decision to treat the first seizure is based on (1) belief that there is a high risk of seizure recurrence, (2) fear that the next seizure episode may be status epilepticus, (3) awareness that early treatment reduces the risk of recurrence, (4) the low toxicity of AED, and (5) the potential danger and effect on the patient's life if seizure recurs (need to drive, risk of job loss, patient living alone). Recurrence of seizure usually develops within 36 months. If a patient remains seizure free during this time on medication, discontinuation of AED may be safely attempted. One may decide not to treat because relatively few patients have seizure recurrence, and because AED may interfere with normal neurologic function (alertness, intellectual and cognitive activities) and may cause systemic side effects in >30% of patients requiring discontinuation of AED. The exact incidence of seizure recurrence after a single seizure is unknown; the most recent estimate is 30%. It is believed that 60% to 85% of patients diagnosed as having epilepsy (defined as recurrent and multiple seizures) have suffered multiple seizures before seeking neurologic evaluation. Of patients experiencing a single seizure, seizure recurs within 6 months of the initial seizure. It appears safe to wait until a second seizure before exposing the patient to a 30% risk of adverse effects of AED. The risk of a second seizure interfering with activities of daily living may be estimated by determining when the seizure occurred (awake or sleep state) and whether a prodrome or aura occurred. For example, the risk of a second seizure occurring while the patient is driving appears low, especially if the seizure is preceded by an aura.

References

Elwes RD, Chesterman P. Prognosis after a first untreated tonic-clonic seizure. Lancet 1985; 2:752.

Hauser WA. Should people be treated after a first seizure? Arch Neurol 1986; 43:1287.

Hauser WA, Anderson E, Loewenson BB, et al. Seizure recurrence after a first unprovoked seizure. N Engl J Med 1982; 307:522.

Hopkins A, Garman A, Clarke C. The first seizure in adult life. Lancet 1988; 1:721.

Shinnar S, Berg AT. The risk of seizure recurrence following a first unprovoked seizure. Neurology 1991; 41:965.

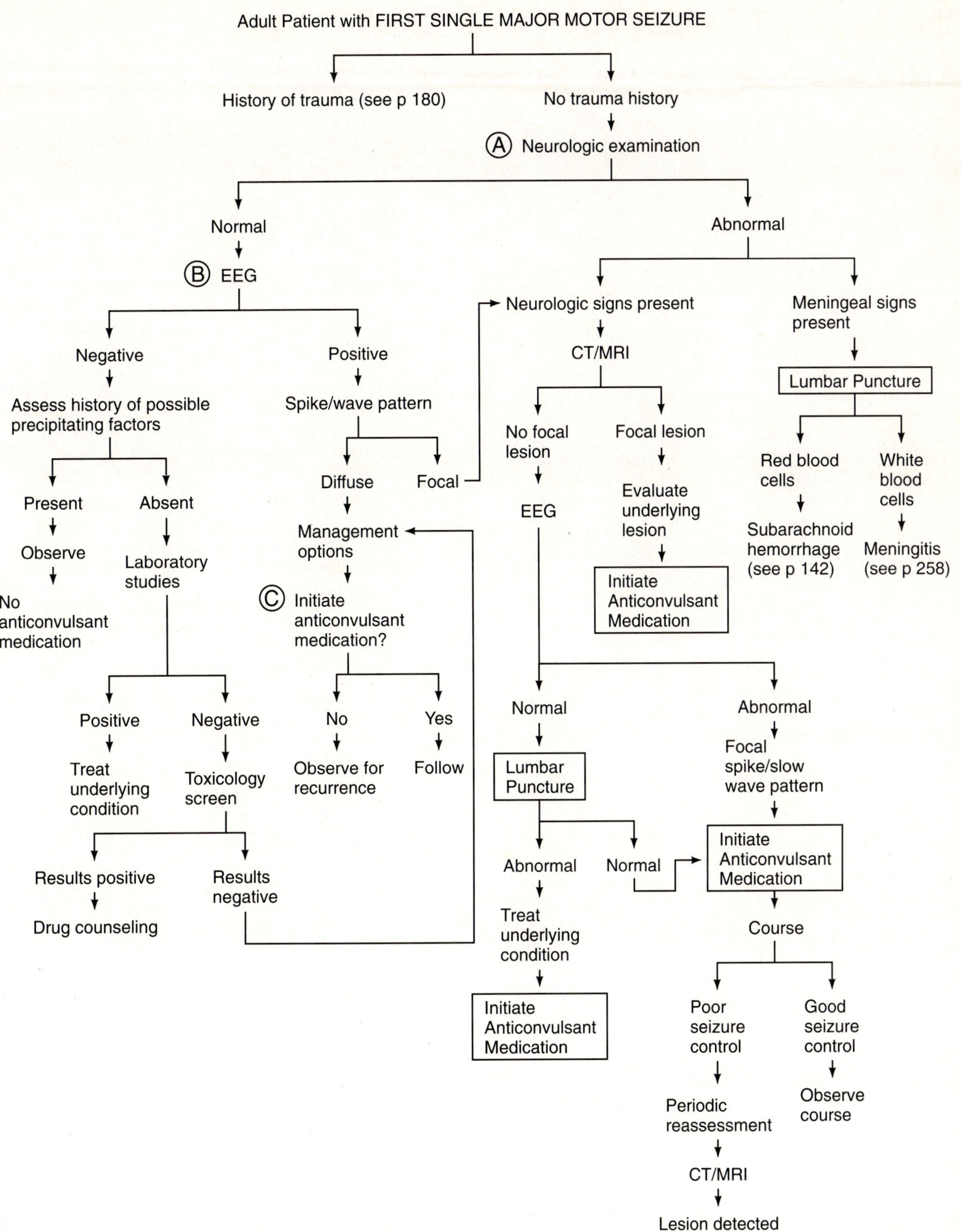

Adult Patient with FIRST SINGLE MAJOR MOTOR SEIZURE
History of trauma (see p 180)
No trauma history
A Neurologic examination
Normal
Abnormal
B EEG
Negative
Positive
Neurologic signs present
Meningeal signs present
Assess history of possible precipitating factors
Spike/wave pattern
CT/MRI
Lumbar Puncture
Present
Absent
Diffuse
Focal
No focal lesion
Focal lesion
Red blood cells
White blood cells
Observe
Laboratory studies
Management options
EEG
Evaluate underlying lesion
Subarachnoid hemorrhage (see p 142)
Meningitis (see p 258)
No anticonvulsant medication
C Initiate anticonvulsant medication?
Initiate Anticonvulsant Medication
Positive
Negative
No
Yes
Treat underlying condition
Toxicology screen
Observe for recurrence
Follow
Normal
Abnormal
Results positive
Results negative
Lumbar Puncture
Focal spike/slow wave pattern
Drug counseling
Abnormal
Normal
Initiate Anticonvulsant Medication
Treat underlying condition
Course
Initiate Anticonvulsant Medication
Poor seizure control
Good seizure control
Periodic reassessment
Observe course
CT/MRI
Lesion detected

DECISION TO DISCONTINUE ANTIEPILEPTIC THERAPY

Leon A. Weisberg, M.D.

Antiepileptic drugs (AEDs) have the potential to cause adverse effects, especially when used for many decades. Chronic side effects include possible teratogenicity for women of child-bearing age, reduced fertility in men, adverse interactions with other drugs, and neuropsychological and behavioral disorders. These effects should provide an incentive for assessing whether AEDs can be discontinued with a low risk of seizure relapse. If AEDs are successfully discontinued, the stigma of "epilepsy" or "nervous illness" is removed, enhancing the patient's esteem and self-confidence. These advantages must be balanced against the risk of seizure relapse, which might adversely influence the patient's job or driving status. It is important to analyze factors that influence the decision to continue or discontinue AEDs in adult epileptic patients.

A. It is believed that the longer patients are seizure free, the lower is the relapse rate if AEDs are discontinued. It is usually believed that patients should be seizure free for at least 2 years before drug withdrawal is attempted. This suggests that this duration of inhibitory activity by AEDs is required to prevent repeated seizures.

B. A normal neurologic examination and normal neuroimaging studies suggest that there is no structural brain injury. It is believed that primary generalized epilepsies are more easily controlled than are partial epilepsies. If there is structural brain injury, the epileptogenic potential is greater than if there is a physiologic or biochemical propensity to develop seizures without an underlying structural abnormality. For example, some patients have seizures only with alcohol consumption, sleep deprivation, or use of certain prescription or illicit drugs. If these precipitating factors are avoided, the patient may remain seizure free without an AED. If the patient refuses to recognize the need for avoidance, it may be necessary to continue the AED. It is believed that the prognosis for successful withdrawal of an AED is better if the cause of seizures is unknown than if there is structural brain disease.

C. EEG is considered useful in predicting seizure relapse. If EEG shows persistent paroxysmal discharges, the chance of seizure relapse is increased; however, there is no correlation with initial EEG findings when seizure diagnosis is initially established. If EEG is normal when the patient takes an AED, but shows paroxysmal discharges after the AED is withdrawn, the chances of seizure relapse are increased.

D. There is no evidence that the duration of withdrawal influences prognosis. AEDs should be gradually tapered, but whether this is done over 8 weeks or 8 months is not a prognostic factor. Never abruptly discontinue the AED, because this may precipitate withdrawal seizures. The presence of neuropsychological and behavioral side effects of an AED makes the need to discontinue it more urgent; however, since these are chronic effects, there is usually no need to taper drugs rapidly.

E. Patients who have fewer seizures and those in whom seizure control is achieved most rapidly are considered better candidates for successful discontinuation of AEDs than those who have more seizures and greater difficulty in achieving seizure-free status. Successful discontinuation is thought to be more likely in patients who achieved control with a single AED than in those treated with polypharmacy.

F. The seizure relapse rate in adult epileptic patients has varied in several studies but is generally accepted to be 25% to 33%. This probably depends on the individual patient, seizure type, and seizure etiology. For example, most absence attacks stop spontaneously, but some patients may develop major motor seizures. If partial seizures are controlled completely for 2 years, the relapse rate is lower than for generalized seizures. Partial seizures without secondary generalization have a better prognosis than those with generalization. It is important in evaluating clinical studies of AED discontinuation to use clinical data derived *only* from adult patient studies if considering this decision for adult patients.

References

Callaghan N, Garrett A, Goggin T. Withdrawal of anticonvulsant drugs in patients free of seizures for two years. N Engl J Med 1988; 318:942.

Pedley T. Discontinuing antiepileptic drugs. N Engl J Med 1988; 318:982.

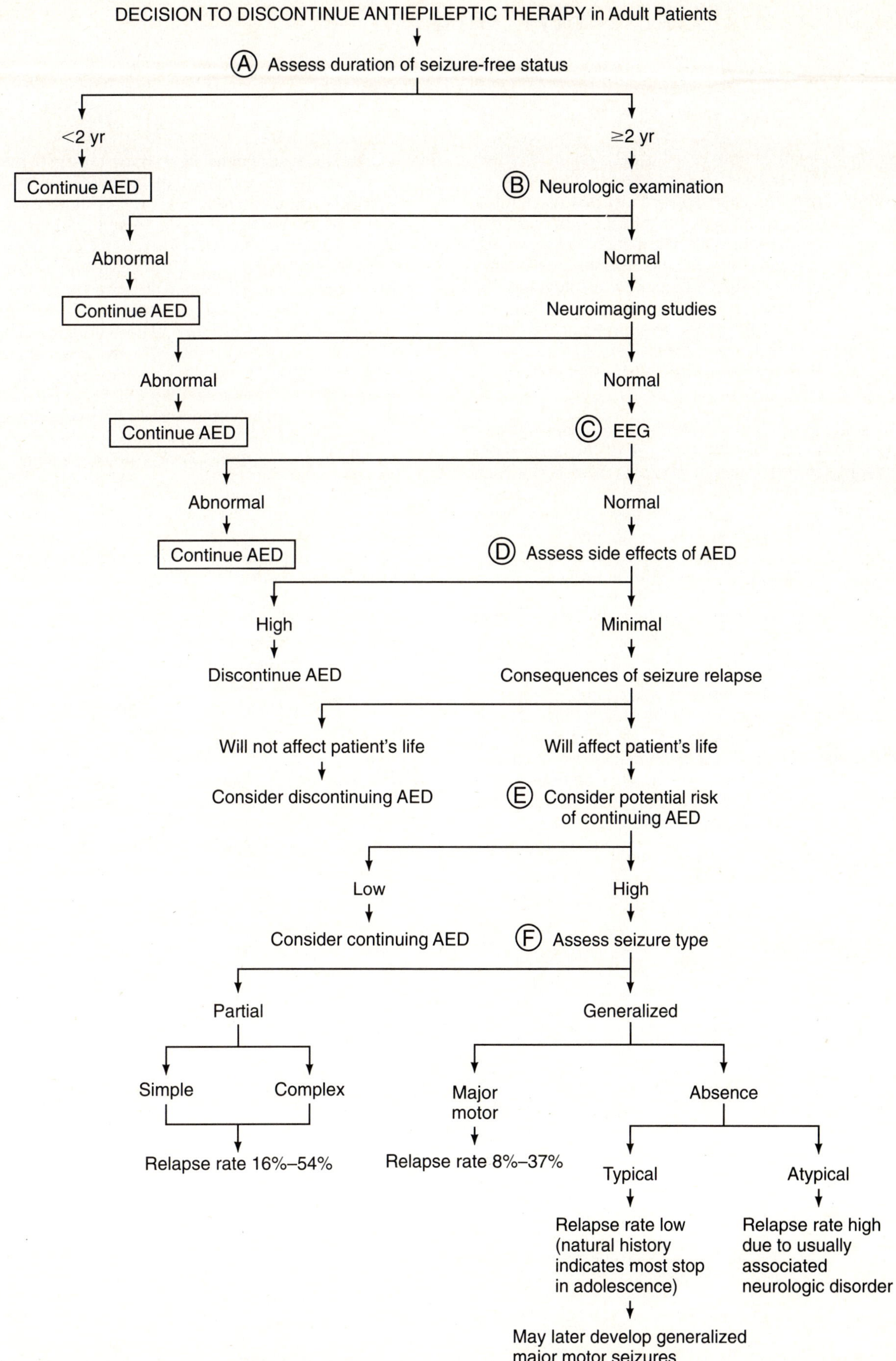

DECISION TO DISCONTINUE ANTIEPILEPTIC THERAPY in Adult Patients
A Assess duration of seizure-free status
<2 yr
≥2 yr
Continue AED
B Neurologic examination
Abnormal
Normal
Continue AED
Neuroimaging studies
Abnormal
Normal
Continue AED
C EEG
Abnormal
Normal
Continue AED
D Assess side effects of AED
High
Minimal
Discontinue AED
Consequences of seizure relapse
Will not affect patient's life
Will affect patient's life
Consider discontinuing AED
E Consider potential risk
of continuing AED
Low
High
Consider continuing AED
F Assess seizure type
Partial
Generalized
Simple
Complex
Major
motor
Absence
Relapse rate 16%–54%
Relapse rate 8%–37%
Typical
Atypical
Relapse rate low
(natural history
indicates most stop
in adolescence)
Relapse rate high
due to usually
associated
neurologic disorder
May later develop generalized
major motor seizures

ABSENCE SEIZURE (PETIT MAL)

Leon A. Weisberg, M.D.

Absence (petit mal) attacks usually develop in children between 5 and 10 years of age and are characterized by sudden brief periods of unresponsiveness that usually last <1 minute. They occur without warning or postictal confusion. After the episode, the patient resumes the activities performed before the attack. Absence attacks result from inherited diffuse (nonfocal) epileptogenic disturbances and therefore are not caused by focal structural brain lesions. CT or MRI does not show structural brain lesions in petit mal seizure patients. Because there is no structural brain lesion, these seizures may stop completely and spontaneously.

A. The initial absence attack almost always occurs before age 10 years. When "staring spells" begin in older patients, consider partial complex seizures, which show the following features not usually seen in absence seizures: (1) aura, (2) longer episode duration (several minutes or more), (3) incontinence, (4) post-ictal confusion, (5) automatic motor behavior, and (6) secondary generalization to major motor attacks.

B. In absence attacks, onset is sudden, without warning or aura; in partial complex seizures, there is an aura.

C. In most absence attacks, there are no abnormal movements or alterations in body tone. There may rarely be atonic features (head drops, trunk slumps forward, generalized weakness). There is not sufficient loss of body tone to cause drop attacks. There often is rhythmic eyelid blinking or mouth twitching in absence seizures. Automatic activity with lip smacking, chewing movements, or nonpurposeful finger movements may be seen in absence attacks; these are common in partial complex seizures.

D. During absence attacks, EEG shows a 3-cps symmetric spike and wave pattern (Fig. 1). Between episodes (interictally), there may be similar short spike-and-wave bursts without clinical manifestations. In patients with characteristic clinical and EEG manifestations of absence attacks, CT and MRI are not usually necessary. In rare patients with absence attacks, EEG shows a slow (<2.5-cps) spike and wave pattern (Lennox-Gastaut syndrome). These patients may also have minor motor seizures with drop attacks in addition to staring spells (absence seizures). They usually have an abnormal interictal EEG, developmental delay, and mental retardation. CT frequently shows structural brain abnormality, including brain atrophy; the clinical prognosis is poor in these patients.

E. Absence attacks often impair mental alertness. These patients may be mistakenly accused of "daydreaming" or being inattentive children with behavior problems. Because absence seizures may occur often enough to interfere with concentration, they may result in poor school performance. The clinician may provoke an absence attack by inducing the patient to hyperventilate; continue this for as long as 3 minutes before concluding that there has been a negative result. The diagnosis of absence attacks is confirmed by EEG; this shows a 3-cps spike and wave pattern. Initiate treatment with ethosuximide (Zarontin) or valproic acid (Depakote).

F. Absence attacks usually cease spontaneously in adolescence. Fifty percent of patients develop tonic-clonic major motor seizures. It cannot be predicted which patients are at risk for developing major motor seizures. Girls have the highest risk of a seizure

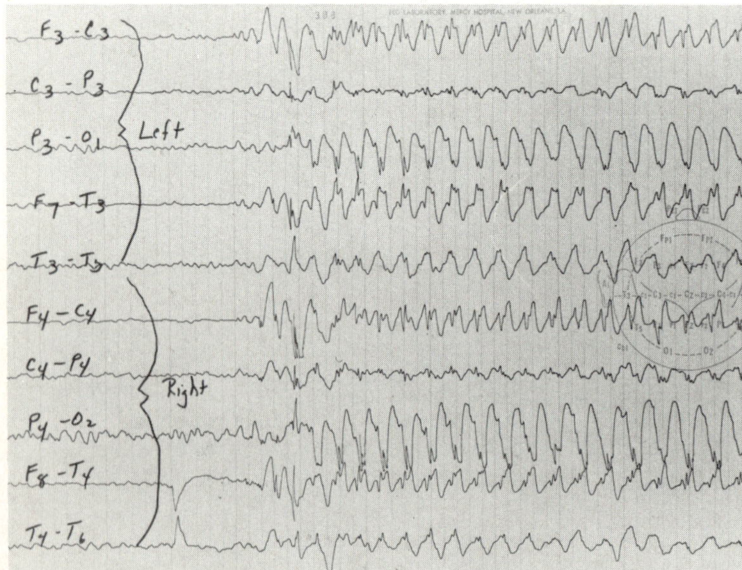

Figure 1 EEG of an older patient who has continued to have absence seizures. EEG shows a spike and slow wave pattern similar to the classic 3-per-second bursts seen in children.

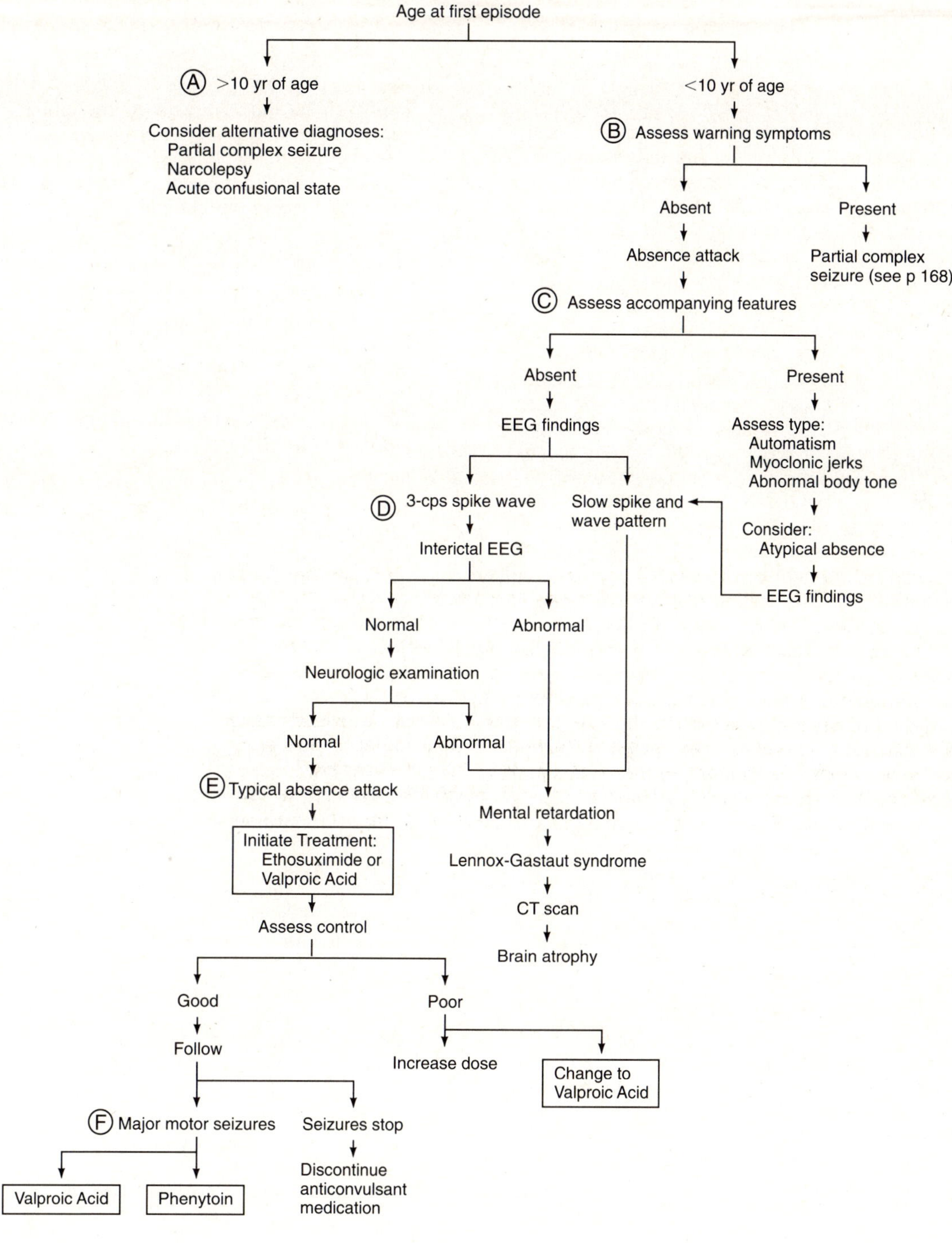

occurring at menarche, whereas boys are at equal risk throughout adolescence. It may be better to treat absence attacks with valproic acid than with ethosuximide; the former may suppress development of tonic-clonic seizures and control absence attacks. Phenytoin and phenobarbital are contraindicated in absence seizures.

References

Hertott P. Clinical, EEG and social prognosis in petit mal epilepsy. Epilepsia 1963; 4:298.

Levy SR. Epileptic syndromes and seizure types in children. Semin Neurol 1990; 10:380.

Penry JK, Porter RJ, Dreifuss FE. Simultaneous recording of absence seizures with video tape and EEG. Brain 1975; 98:427.

SIMPLE PARTIAL (FOCAL) SEIZURE

Leon A. Weisberg, M.D.

Simple partial (focal) seizures (SPS) are caused by a discrete lesion in or near primary cerebrocortical regions. This may cause motor, somatosensory, or special sensory symptoms (including visual, auditory, or vertiginous types), autonomic symptoms, psychic symptoms, or symptoms of disturbed higher cortical function. Toxic or metabolic disorders do *not* usually cause partial seizures. In adults, SPS are symptomatic of unilateral localized epileptogenic lesions; these may be macro- or microscopic. Some lesions (neoplasm, angioma, cyst, abscess) may be detected by CT or MRI in 30% of patients; others including hamartomas, post-traumatic brain lesions, and cortical heterotopias, are detected only by pathologic examination (surgical excision, autopsy). These structural brain lesions may be static (not increasing in size) or progressive (increasing in size). The most common pathologic lesion in patients with partial seizures is mesial temporal lobe sclerosis; this occurs in patients with complex partial seizures.

Patients with partial seizures initially develop an aura. This is the initial ictal event and may be associated with EEG abnormalities; however, these often may not be detected with scalp-recorded EEG and may require depth electrodes. Partial seizures may be classified into three types: (1) SPS characterized by sensory, motor, or autonomic symptoms without impairment of consciousness; (2) complex partial seizures manifested by impaired consciousness; and (3) partial seizures progressing to secondary generalized tonic-clonic seizures. SPS may originate in any discrete cortical region; complex partial seizures originate in the temporal lobe in 80% of patients. Complex partial seizures should not be referred to as temporal lobe seizures because they may originate in an extratemporal region, most commonly frontal lobes. Partial epilepsies are more refractory to medical therapy than primary generalized epilepsies, and certain patients with partial epilepsy may require surgical treatment.

A. In SPS, the differential diagnosis includes migraine and TIA. In migraine, neurologic symptoms spread more slowly than with seizures. There is a unilateral headache, and a focal slow wave EEG focus without spikes may be seen. In TIA, neurologic symptoms develop rapidly without spread so that they are maximal at onset, headache is not usually prominent, and EEG is usually normal. In SPS, clinical manifestations are more likely to be "positive" phenomena, including sensory (tingling sensation, paresthesias), motor (myoclonic jerks, shaking), and visual (flashing lights), rather than "negative" phenomena, including sensory (numbness), motor (weakness), and visual (blindness) phenomena as seen in vascular disturbances, including migraine. Seizures are stereotyped, recurrent, and unpredictable events.

B. In patients with suspected SPS, initial management should confirm the diagnosis of seizure and classify the seizure type. There is a surprisingly low incidence of ictal scalp-recorded EEG abnormalities in patients with SPS. This indicates that ictal EEG may not be entirely reliable in differentiating SPS from nonepileptic disturbances. This is contrasted with complex partial seizures in which ictal surface EEG abnormalities occur in 90%.

C. In SPS patients, antiepileptic drugs (AEDs) of choice are carbamazepine and phenytoin. Because these seizures are caused by structural brain abnormalities, control may require a higher-dose AED than in patients with generalized epilepsy. Use monotherapy, and if one drug is unsuccessful, switch to another to avoid polypharmacy. Use of a second drug is associated with improved seizure control in *few* patients, and development of drug toxicity in *many*. Less effective AEDs for partial seizures include valproate, phenobarbital, and primidone; clonazepam and clorazepate are rarely used.

D. In patients with medically refractory (intractable) partial seizures, surgical ablative procedures such as resection of the focal epileptogenic cortex may be performed, but only after maximal medical management has been attempted. This is appropriate only if seizures originate from a cortical region that can be resected without causing neurologic dysfunction or worsening pre-existing neurologic impairment. Treat SPS aggressively, because the longer an intractable seizure disorder exists, the greater is the degree of epileptogenicity established and the less the chance of success with surgery.

References

Cascino GD. Intractable partial epilepsy: Evaluation and treatment. Mayo Clin Proc 1990; 65:1578.

Devinsky D, Kelley K, Porter RJ. Clinical and EEG features of simple partial seizures. Neurology 1988; 38:1347.

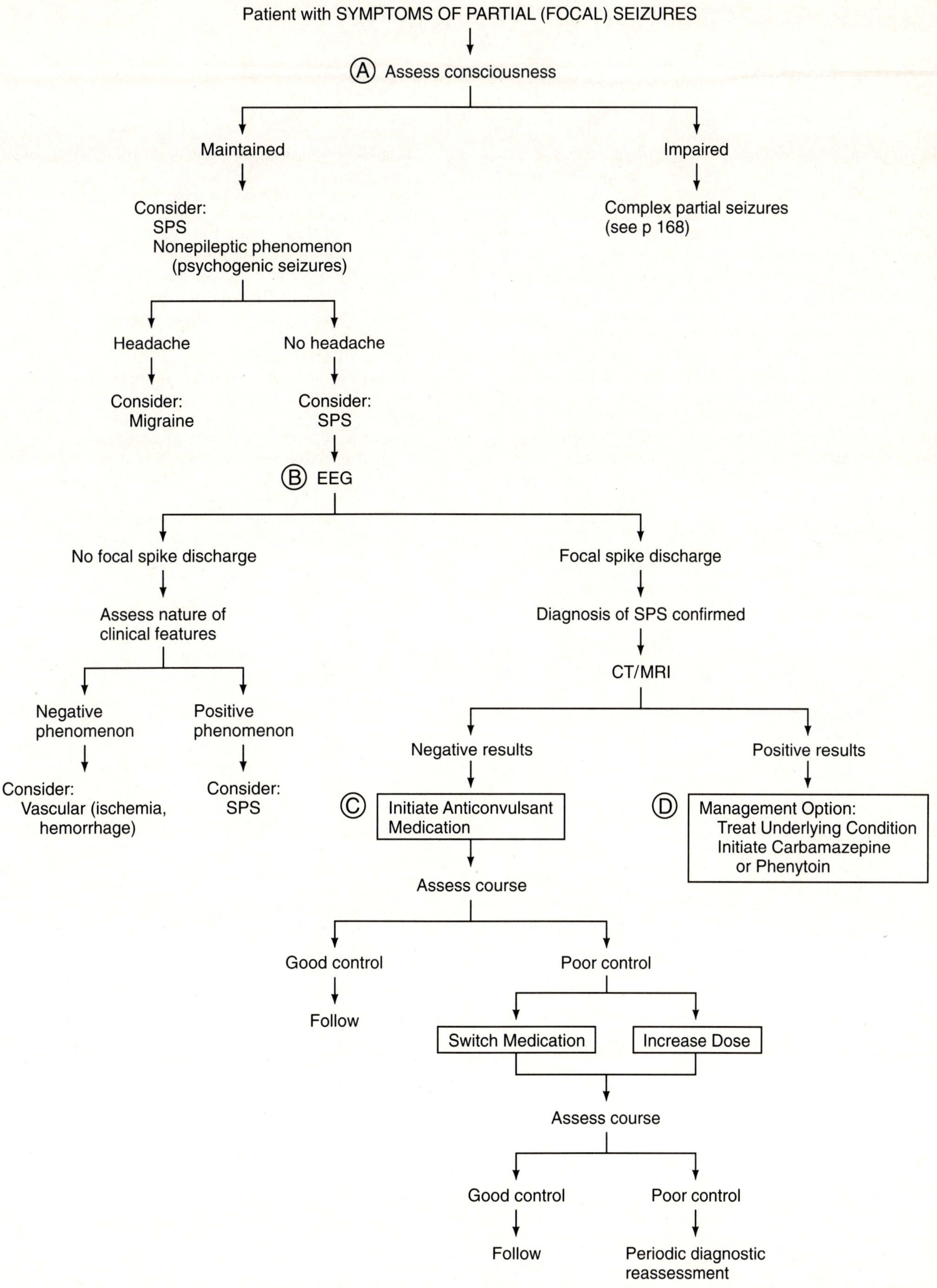

Patient with SYMPTOMS OF PARTIAL (FOCAL) SEIZURES
A Assess consciousness
Maintained
Impaired
Consider:
SPS
Nonepileptic phenomenon
(psychogenic seizures)
Complex partial seizures
(see p 168)
Headache
No headache
Consider:
Migraine
Consider:
SPS
B EEG
No focal spike discharge
Focal spike discharge
Assess nature of
clinical features
Diagnosis of SPS confirmed
CT/MRI
Negative
phenomenon
Positive
phenomenon
Negative results
Positive results
Consider:
Vascular (ischemia,
hemorrhage)
Consider:
SPS
C Initiate Anticonvulsant
Medication
D Management Option:
Treat Underlying Condition
Initiate Carbamazepine
or Phenytoin
Assess course
Good control
Poor control
Follow
Switch Medication
Increase Dose
Assess course
Good control
Poor control
Follow
Periodic diagnostic
reassessment

COMPLEX PARTIAL (FOCAL) SEIZURE

Leon A. Weisberg, M.D.

In complex partial seizures (CPS), consciousness or responsiveness is impaired at some time during the seizure episode. It is possible to begin with a simple partial seizure and evolve to a CPS. The aura of CPS may include hallucinations (olfactory, auditory, visual), distortions of space or size (micropsia, macropsia), or time (déjà vu, déjà jamais). Affective or behavioral experiences may be part of the aura. During CPS, patients may perform automatic motor behavior consisting of semipurposeful movements. After these episodes, patients appear dazed or confused; they may be amnestic for the entire seizure. During simple or complex partial seizures, EEG usually shows focal spike discharges (Fig. 1); EEG may be normal between episodes. Focal spikes may be intermittent if the epileptic focus is small or at some distance (deep) from the cerebral cortex surface. Most CPS originate in temporal lobes, but some originate in extratemporal sites, most commonly frontal lobes.

A. CPS may cause diagnostic problems. There may be varied and behaviorally complex ictal manifestations. It is very important to establish the diagnosis of CPS, because other nonepileptic conditions simulating CPS do not respond to antiepileptic drugs (AEDs). In patients with intermittent confusional episodes and prominent headache, consider migraine. If the patient appears confused and if memory impairment is prominent, consider transient global amnesia (TGA). TGA may last several hours and resolve completely. This condition results from vascular ischemia of the posterior cerebral arteries involving the mesial temporal cortex. TGA may be an isolated event; rarely, it is the harbinger of a completed stroke.

B. If patients exhibit violent behavior for which they are amnestic, consider episodic dyscontrol syndrome. In this condition, violent behavior is random and not premeditated; EEG does not show temporal spikes. If there is a gradual build-up of bizarre or unusual behavior (with or without hallucinations) that lasts for a prolonged time, consider psychosis. In psychotic states, EEG is usually normal. Psychoses may be drug precipitated. In patients with reduced responsiveness and episodes of abnormal behavior, consider narcolepsy and other REM-behavioral sleep disorders. In narcolepsy, it is usually possible to awaken patients during attacks, and automatisms are not usually present; sleep studies may be necessary. Psychiatric "fugue states" may simulate CPS; however, EEG is normal, and the response to an amobarbital (Amytal) interview may confirm this psychiatric diagnosis. In some cases, EEG-video monitoring that captures a clinical "spell" is necessary to establish the mechanism of the behavioral disorder.

C. Ictal EEG is almost always abnormal during CPS, but it may be necessary to use sphenoidal or nasopharyngeal electrodes to demonstrate medial temporal spikes. The absence of change in EEG pattern during ictal and postictal periods makes a diagnosis of CPS highly unlikely.

D. Treatment for CPS includes carbamazepine (Tegretol), three or four times daily. It is necessary to monitor liver function and hematologic status regularly. Phenytoin, phenobarbital, and primidone are also effective in CPS patients. CPS may sometimes be medically refractory. Be certain that the patient is compliant with the prescribed AED before concluding that the seizure disorder is medically refractory. It may be necessary to increase AED dosage to high levels that may exceed the expected therapeutic range. High blood AED levels alone are not an indication to reduce dosage unless the patient also shows clinical toxic drug effects. If carbamazepine is ineffective or cannot be tolerated owing to toxic effects, switch to phenytoin. Avoid polypharmacy, which often causes toxicity and adds little to seizure control. If seizures are not controlled within 24 months, consider referral to a comprehensive epilepsy management program for possible temporal lobe surgery. Only patients with a *unilateral* temporal lobe focus are surgical candidates.

References

Currie S, Heathfield KWG, Henson RA. Clinical course and prognosis of temporal lobe epilepsy. Brain 1971; 94:173.

Ouesney LF. Clinical and EEG features of complex partial seizures of temporal lobe origin. Epilepsia 1986; 27(Suppl 2):S27.

Theodore WH, Porter RR, Penry JK. Complex partial seizures: Clinical characteristics and differential diagnosis. Neurology 1983; 33:1115.

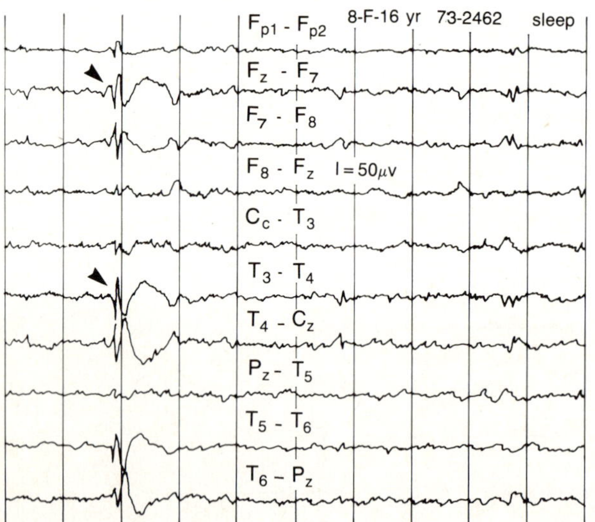

Figure 1 EEG of a patient with temporal lobe epilepsy (partial complex seizures). Spike focus is present in the anterior temporal lobe on the left, F7 *(top arrow)*, and in the midtemporal area on the right, T4 *(lower arrow)*.

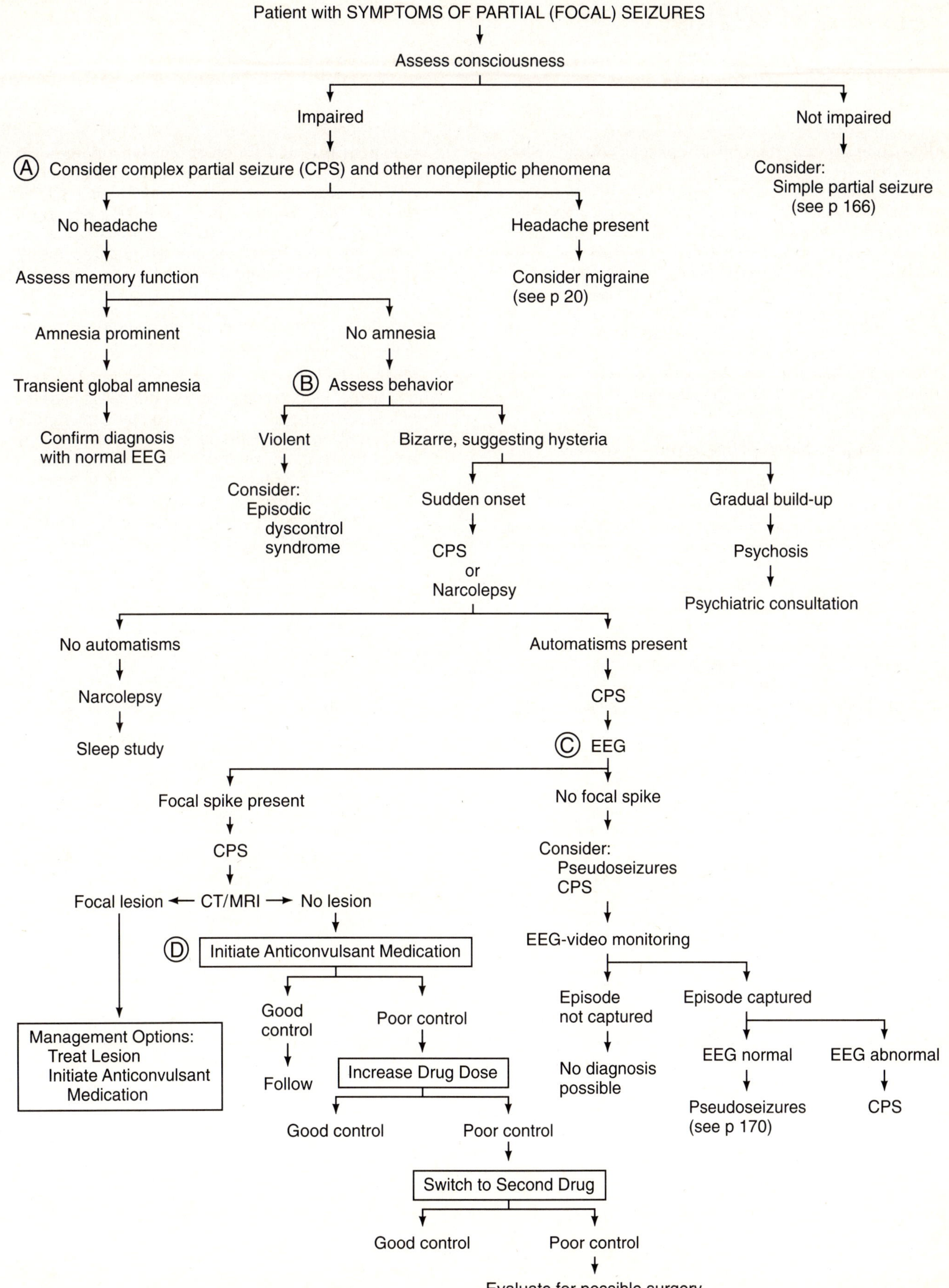

Patient with SYMPTOMS OF PARTIAL (FOCAL) SEIZURES
Assess consciousness
Impaired
Not impaired
A Consider complex partial seizure (CPS) and other nonepileptic phenomena
Consider:
Simple partial seizure
(see p 166)
No headache
Headache present
Assess memory function
Consider migraine
(see p 20)
Amnesia prominent
No amnesia
Transient global amnesia
B Assess behavior
Confirm diagnosis
with normal EEG
Violent
Bizarre, suggesting hysteria
Consider:
Episodic
dyscontrol
syndrome
Sudden onset
Gradual build-up
CPS
or
Narcolepsy
Psychosis
Psychiatric consultation
No automatisms
Automatisms present
Narcolepsy
CPS
Sleep study
C EEG
Focal spike present
No focal spike
CPS
Consider:
Pseudoseizures
CPS
Focal lesion ← CT/MRI → No lesion
EEG-video monitoring
D Initiate Anticonvulsant Medication
Episode
not captured
Episode captured
Good
control
Poor control
No diagnosis
possible
EEG normal
EEG abnormal
Management Options:
Treat Lesion
Initiate Anticonvulsant
Medication
Follow
Increase Drug Dose
Pseudoseizures
(see p 170)
CPS
Good control
Poor control
Switch to Second Drug
Good control
Poor control
Evaluate for possible surgery

PSEUDOSEIZURE

Richard L. Strub, M.D.

All seizures are not true organic epileptic seizures; some are purely psychogenic, hysteric pseudoseizures. Some basic facts and a systematic approach to evaluation can usually distinguish the organic from the pseudoseizure. Many patients who have pseudoseizures have true epilepsy as well; thus, the mere identification of a single pseudoseizure does not justify stopping medication and labeling the patient hysteric. The following are some useful background facts. Most pseudoseizures occur in females 15 to 35 years of age; at least half the patients have significant psychiatric problems (depression or hysteria); in most cases, emotional stress triggers the seizure; they rarely occur at night; they usually occur when there is someone with the patient who will respond with sympathy.

A. If there is no history of true seizures in childhood or no positive EEG findings, be suspicious.

B. Actual observation or an accurate report of the seizure is the most important factor in the diagnosis. Pseudoseizures do not look real to the practiced eye. The true generalized tonic-clonic seizure is limited in its expression; it starts with a cry and then a fall, with tonic movements followed by clonic (rhythmic symmetric jerking) movements. There is then often a loss of bowel and bladder control, tongue biting, and a period of postictal confusion that is not remembered by the patient. The pseudoseizure is bizarre, often characterized by purposeful movements, and involves random flailing and thrashing movements with the head thrown side to side, and aimless kicking. Patients often remember the seizure and tell of people talking to them during the episode. Sometimes they stop if told to. No tongue biting, incontinence, or postictal confusion is seen. Partial seizures are equally atypical; the eyes may rove rather than exhibit a forced lateral gaze.

C. In pseudoseizure, the findings on neurologic examination are normal in the postictal period.

D. The interictal EEG is normal in a pure pseudoseizure, but a single interictal EEG cannot confirm the diagnosis. It is best to obtain an EEG during the seizure; this is frequently possible in pseudoseizures because many such patients are suggestible and obligingly have a seizure in the EEG laboratory. During the pseudoseizure there is no epileptic activity on the EEG (this is often difficult to assess because of movement artifact), and the postictal EEG is normal instead of slow.

References

Desai BT, Porter RJ, Penry K. Psychogenic seizures: A study of 42 attacks in six patients, with intensive monitoring. Arch Neurol 1982; 39:202.

Gates JR, Ramani V, Whalen S, Loewenson R. Ictal characteristics of pseudoseizure. Arch Neurol 1985; 42:1183.

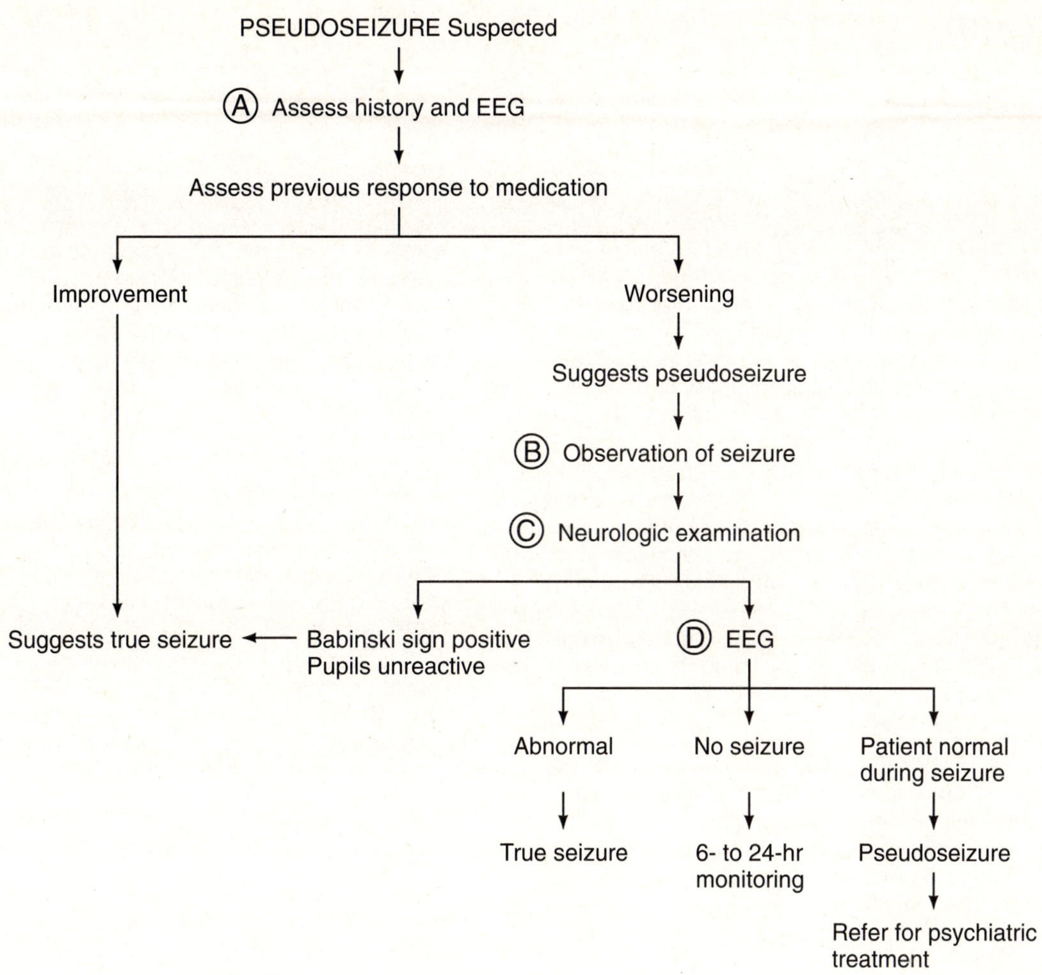

PSEUDOSEIZURE Suspected
A Assess history and EEG
Assess previous response to medication
Improvement
Worsening
Suggests pseudoseizure
B Observation of seizure
C Neurologic examination
Suggests true seizure
Babinski sign positive
Pupils unreactive
D EEG
Abnormal
No seizure
Patient normal
during seizure
True seizure
6- to 24-hr
monitoring
Pseudoseizure
Refer for psychiatric
treatment

SYNCOPE

Richard L. Strub, M.D.*
Freddy Abi-Samra, M.D.

The syncopal or fainting spell is caused by a sudden drop in blood flow to the brain. The most common etiologies are cardiogenic (arrhythmia, acute myocardial infarct, or low cardiac output) or hypotensive (vasodepressive). Clinically, syncope is a sudden transient loss of consciousness without neurologic findings. Patients often feel faint or light-headed a few seconds before the attack, but then become unconscious and fall. Usually they lie still for a few seconds and then quickly regain consciousness. If the blood supply to the brain is prolonged or extensive, patients may exhibit twitching or mild generalized convulsive movements after they have fallen. There may also be a short period of confusion after simple syncope, although this is unusual. If the history of the event suggests a seizure, a neurologic evaluation is necessary. However, most syncopal events are cardiovascular and should be evaluated by a cardiologist. Many cases can be explained after careful evaluation, but some remain idiopathic.

A. The history is very important in evaluating patients with a loss of consciousness. Patients' accounts of the attack plus the reports of observers are of utmost importance. The history of the situation provoking the "spell," if there is one; the history of medication use; the age of the patient; and any history of previous heart disease are all important in guiding the decision-making process.

B. Cerebrovascular disease is rarely a cause of a transient loss of consciousness. If it is, it stems from a combination of severely stenotic major vessels (carotids or basilar arteries) in conjunction with a decrease in blood supply, as can occur with rapid rising, or bradycardia. On equally rare occasions in which patients have severely impaired focal cerebral perfusion secondary to intracranial vascular stenosis, those with simple syncope may have accompanying transient neurologic symptoms. One clinical situation that must be differentiated from syncope is the classic 'drop attack' in which the patient suddenly loses all strength in the legs and falls to the floor but does not lose consciousness. The mechanism of drop attacks is far from clear but is likely to be secondary to ischemia in the ventral pons.

C. Several classic situations provoke syncopal attacks in some people; high emotion, fright, hot sun, and venipuncture are the most common. In these cases, blood vessel tone decreases and blood pressure drops; the pulse rate remains unchanged or may decrease. Vasovagal syncope is the most common term used to describe the mechanism of these attacks, which often occur in young people. This term implies that vagus-induced bradycardia is the initiating mechanism. In fact, it appears that bradycardia (if and when it occurs) is only a late phenomenon. The pathophysiology is somewhat complex and appears to involve an initial sympathetic overstimulation followed by left ventricular C-fiber stimulation and efferent vagal outflow resulting primarily in vasodilation and hypotension. A better term is vasodepressor syncope.

D. Miscellaneous forms of situational syncope include tussive, deglutition, and micturition syncope. These are uncommon and have a complex pathophysiology. A somewhat more common cause is carotid sinus syncope, which is usually brought on by an activity that massages the carotid sinus (e.g., shaving or holding the telephone receiver with one's chin). Full evaluation for other causes should probably be undertaken before making this diagnosis. The cardiogenic and mixed types of carotid sinus syncope are adequately prevented by single- and dual-chamber pacing, respectively. There is currently no known effective prophylaxis for the purely or predominantly vasodepressive type of this disorder.

E. Vasodepressive syncope can be induced by other nonclassic situational triggers such as venous pooling (orthostasis) or hypovolemia (anemia, diuretics). These are often unheralded (without premonitory symptoms) and must be differentiated from arrhythmic causes of syncope. Tilt testing is very useful in these settings.

F. Cardiogenic syncope is a potentially very malignant symptom carrying a 25% 1-year mortality rate. Although obvious structural lesions such as mitral or aortic stenosis, pulmonary embolization, and cardiac tamponade may be causative, most events are secondary to malignant brady- or tachydysrhythmias. Older patients and patients with low left ventricular ejection fractions with recent-onset syncope need full cardiac evaluation (often including electrophysiologic testing).

G. Idiopathic orthostatic hypotension is a major problem in the elderly. In the Shy-Drager syndrome, there is degeneration in the sympathetic neurons of the spinal cord and clinically severe orthostatic hypotension. In some patients, parkinsonism, dementia, and other neurologic illness are seen (multisystem atrophy). In patients with peripheral neuropathy from diabetes or other causes, an autonomic neuropathy can also develop with secondary orthostatic syncope.

References

Abi-Samra F, Sweeney P, Maloney JD. Syncope: A pathophysiological approach. In Furlan A, Conomy JD, eds. The heart and stroke. New York: Springer-Verlag, 1987:249.

Kapoor WN, Karpf M, Wieand S, et al. A prospective evaluation and follow-up of patients with syncope. N Engl J Med 1983; 309:197.

Noble RJ. The patient with syncope. JAMA 1977; 237:1372.

Silverstein MD, et al. Patients with syncope admitted to medical intensive care units. JAMA 1982; 248:1185.

*Staff Electrophysiologist, Department of Cardiology, Ochsner Clinic, New Orleans, Louisiana.

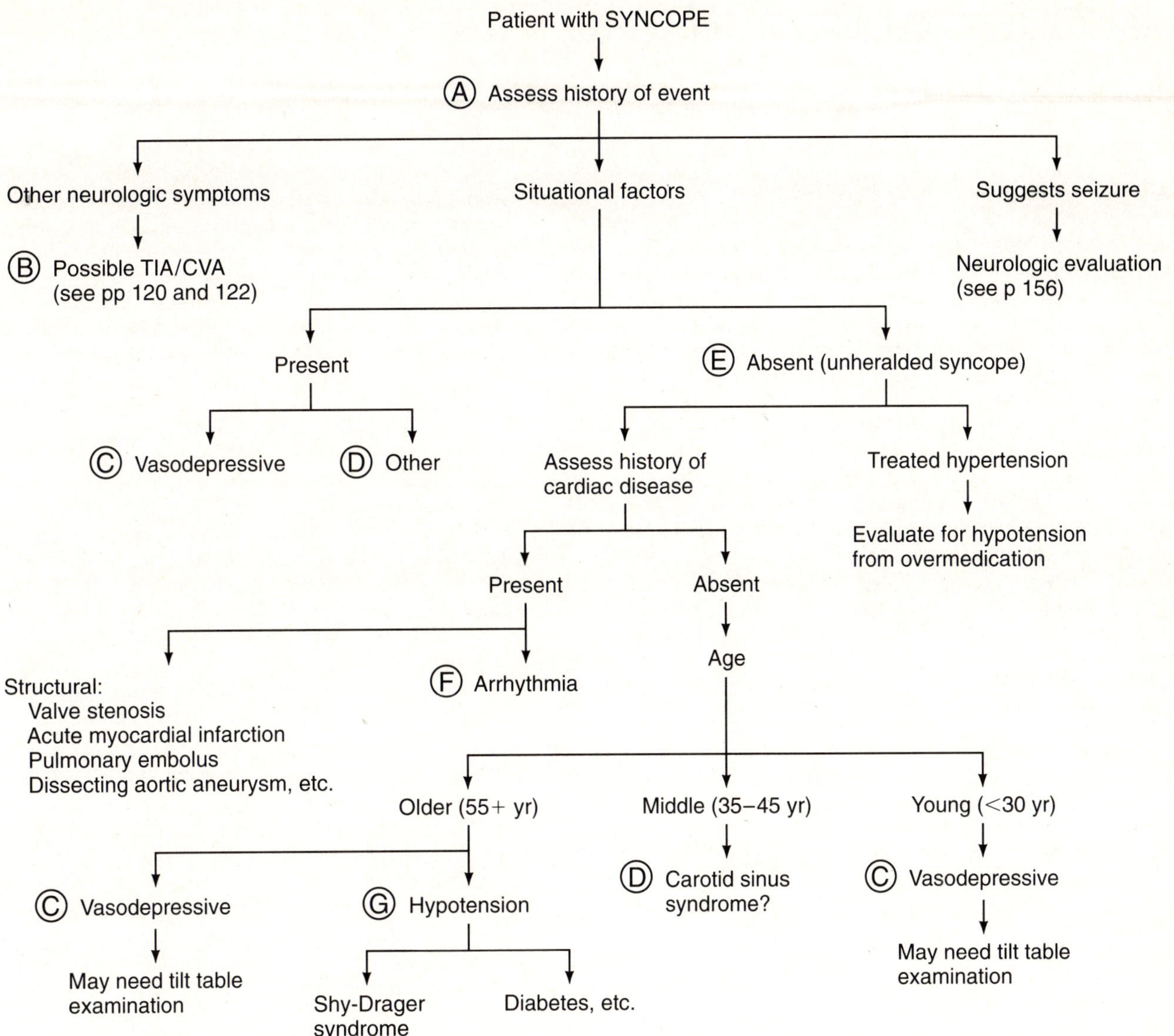

Patient with SYNCOPE
A Assess history of event
Other neurologic symptoms
Situational factors
Suggests seizure
B Possible TIA/CVA
(see pp 120 and 122)
Neurologic evaluation
(see p 156)
Present
E Absent (unheralded syncope)
C Vasodepressive
D Other
Assess history of
cardiac disease
Treated hypertension
Evaluate for hypotension
from overmedication
Structural:
Valve stenosis
Acute myocardial infarction
Pulmonary embolus
Dissecting aortic aneurysm, etc.
Present
Absent
F Arrhythmia
Age
Older (55+ yr)
Middle (35−45 yr)
Young (<30 yr)
C Vasodepressive
G Hypotension
D Carotid sinus
syndrome?
C Vasodepressive
May need tilt table
examination
Shy-Drager
syndrome
Diabetes, etc.
May need tilt table
examination

ALCOHOL-RELATED SEIZURE

Leon A. Weisberg, M.D.

Alcohol withdrawal seizures occur within 48 hours after alcohol intake is reduced, most commonly 12 to 24 hours after a heavy alcoholic binge. Seizures are usually generalized. In 40% of cases, there is a single seizure; in 60%, there are multiple seizures. Rarely, status epilepticus develops as a manifestation of alcohol withdrawal seizures. Focal seizures are uncommon; when present, they indicate a possible underlying structural brain lesion, which must be excluded by neurodiagnostic studies. In 90% of patients with alcohol withdrawal seizures, interictal EEG is normal within 1 week. In 50% of such patients, there is a photomyoclonic response, involving myoclonic twitching of the eye, face, or extremities in response to photic stimulation. This rapidly disappears within 1 week after alcohol consumption stops. In addition to being a direct effect of alcohol withdrawal, seizures in alcoholics are also caused by metabolic disturbances (electrolyte imbalance, hypoglycemia, hepatic failure), neurologic conditions (meningitis, cerebral contusions, subdural hematoma), and alcohol-precipitated seizures in patients with preexisting epilepsy.

A. Alcoholic patients may stop drinking because they run out of money to purchase alcohol or because they develop intercurrent medical complications (gastritis, meningitis, pneumonia, pancreatitis, hepatitis). Alcohol-induced hypoglycemia is an important cause of seizures; IV glucose should be supplemented with thiamine. This avoids precipitation of Wernicke's encephalopathy. This disorder may develop because alcoholics are thiamine deficient and rapid glucose infusion utilizes already depleted brain thiamine sources of these alcoholic patients.

B. In patients with suspected alcoholic withdrawal seizures, the following are indications for neurodiagnostic studies: (1) focal seizures, (2) focal neurologic signs, and (3) focal EEG abnormality. In most patients with typical alcohol withdrawal seizures, CT and lumbar puncture are not cost effective; however, they probably should be performed after the *initial* alcohol withdrawal seizure even if the seizures are generalized and have no focal clinical or EEG features. Alcohol may cause coagulation or hematologic disturbances with impaired hemostasis; this may result in intracranial hemorrhage.

C. Treatment of alcohol withdrawal seizures with phenytoin has been advocated, but Librium (chlordiazepoxide) has also been used to treat withdrawal seizures as well as other symptoms of major withdrawal syndrome. Librium is a weak anticonvulsant in most other circumstances and is rarely used as an antiepileptic drug (AED) in other seizure patients. If phenytoin is used, quickly load the patient to achieve rapid adequate blood level, because the greatest risk of seizure recurrence is within 3 days of cessation of drinking. If treatment with phenytoin is initiated, use a loading dose (1 g on the first day, 600 mg on the second day, 400 mg on subsequent days) to achieve the adequate blood levels rapidly. If treatment is initiated with a daily maintenance dose of 300 to 400 mg, adequate blood levels are not achieved for 5 to 10 days, when the greatest risk of seizure recurrence has already passed. Despite common use of phenytoin, there is no convincing evidence to support its effectiveness for alcohol withdrawal seizures. Paraldehyde may control both seizures and withdrawal symptoms. Diazepam may stop seizure activity, but its short half-life limits its prophylactic anticonvulsant capability. Susceptibility to seizures due to alcohol effect usually lasts 24 to 48 hours. Treatment with AEDs for alcoholic patients on a chronic basis is not beneficial. When alcoholics go on a drinking binge, they usually stop taking AEDs. Alcohol intake and rapid discontinuation of anticonvulsant medication are two reasons that seizures occur in the withdrawal phase.

D. Seizures that occur when patients are not drinking cannot be attributed to alcohol withdrawal. A seizure that occurs more than 1 week after cessation of alcohol should *not* be considered a result of alcohol withdrawal. One or two drinks do not usually precipitate seizures in normal patients but may exacerbate seizures in epileptics. Some patients are predisposed to seizures after one or two drinks. These should avoid alcohol, and an AED is unnecessary in this clinical setting. In rare instances, nonalcoholic, nonepileptic patients experience seizures after moderate or large consumption of alcohol. It is possible that these patients have a predisposition to epilepsy; an AED is probably not required if these patients remain abstinent. These individuals are advised to avoid alcohol consumption, because alcohol lowers the seizure threshold. Epileptic alcoholic patients should be treated with AEDs and told to avoid alcohol; 85% of epileptic patients have seizures after taking five or six alcoholic beverages. Alcohol should be consumed by epileptic patients only in moderation.

References

Alldredge BK, Lowenstein DH, Simon RP. Placebo controlled trial of intravenous phenytoin for short-term treatment of alcohol withdrawal seizures. Am J Med 1989; 87:645.

Feussner JR, Linfors EW, Blessing CL. CT in alcohol withdrawal seizures. Ann Intern Med 1981; 94:519.

Mattson RH. Effect of alcohol intake on nonalcoholic subjects. Neurology 1975; 25:351.

Thompson WL. Management of alcohol withdrawal syndromes. Arch Intern Med 1975; 138:278.

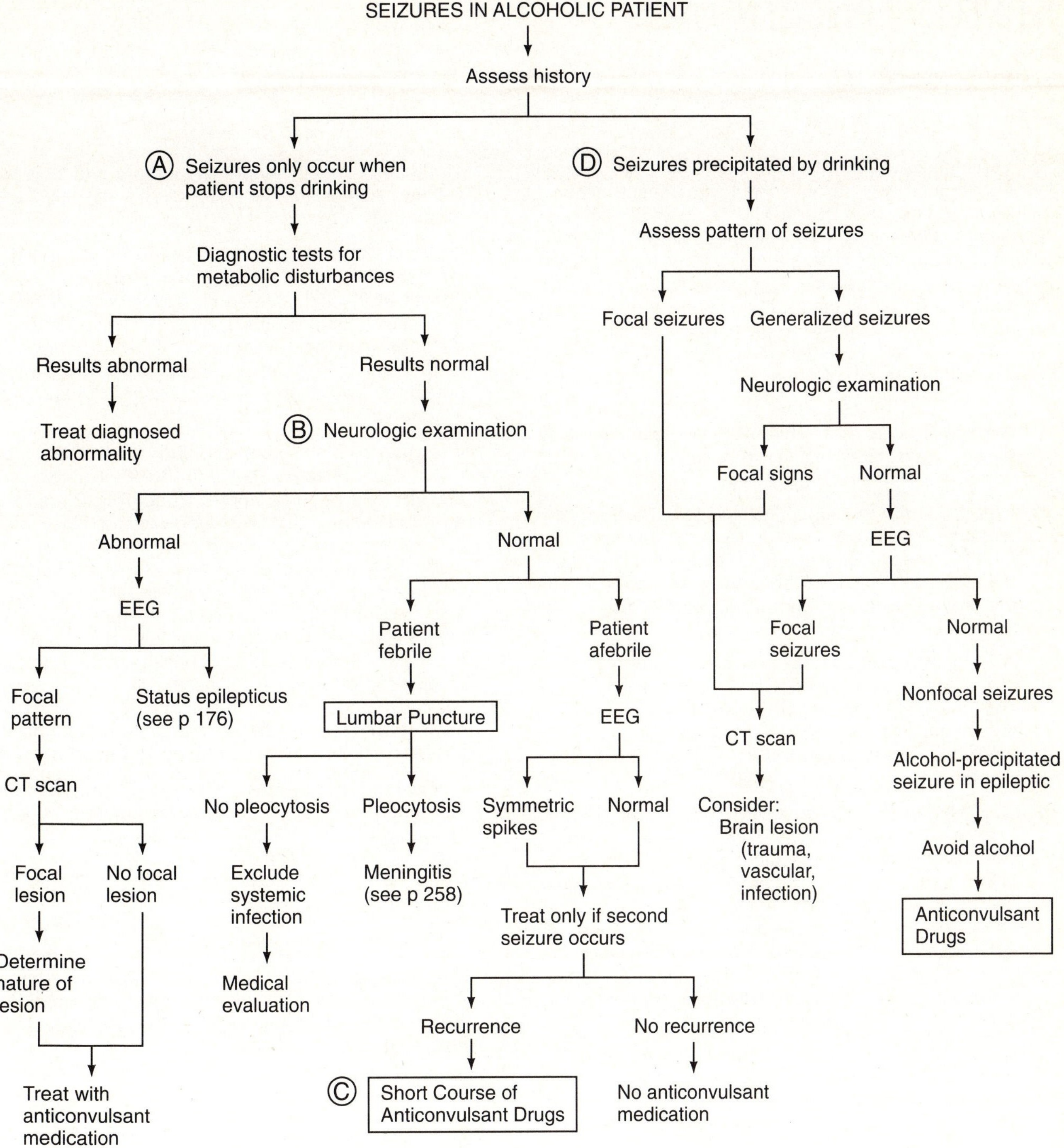

SEIZURES IN ALCOHOLIC PATIENT
Assess history
A Seizures only occur when patient stops drinking
D Seizures precipitated by drinking
Diagnostic tests for metabolic disturbances
Assess pattern of seizures
Results abnormal
Results normal
Focal seizures
Generalized seizures
Treat diagnosed abnormality
B Neurologic examination
Neurologic examination
Abnormal
Normal
Focal signs
Normal
EEG
EEG
Focal pattern
Status epilepticus (see p 176)
Patient febrile
Patient afebrile
Focal seizures
Normal
CT scan
Lumbar Puncture
EEG
CT scan
Nonfocal seizures
Focal lesion
No focal lesion
No pleocytosis
Pleocytosis
Symmetric spikes
Normal
Consider: Brain lesion (trauma, vascular, infection)
Alcohol-precipitated seizure in epileptic
Determine nature of lesion
Exclude systemic infection
Meningitis (see p 258)
Treat only if second seizure occurs
Avoid alcohol
Medical evaluation
Recurrence
No recurrence
Anticonvulsant Drugs
Treat with anticonvulsant medication
C Short Course of Anticonvulsant Drugs
No anticonvulsant medication

STATUS EPILEPTICUS

Carlos A. Garcia, M.D.

Status epilepticus is a condition in which there is continuous seizure activity with or without impairment of consciousness lasting >30 minutes. It is one of the few neurologic emergencies and should be controlled within 60 minutes to avoid irreversible brain damage. Prolonged convulsions can also produce myoglobinuria due to muscle fiber necrosis. Probably the most common cause of status epilepticus is the stopping of medication in known epileptics. Epileptics may stop their medication voluntarily or because of intercurrent infections.

A. The convulsive state, either generalized or partial, is easy to diagnose. Nonconvulsive status epilepticus is a diagnostic challenge and may present as a confusional state to be confirmed only by EEG.

B. In nonconvulsive status epilepticus, EEG monitoring is required. In an absence status case, give IV diazepam (DZP) at a rate of 2 mg/min until control is achieved or until 10 mg is given. Add oral doses of ethosuximide or valproic acid, or both if necessary, to obtain therapeutic blood levels.

C. As soon as the diagnosis of convulsive status is made, assess cardiorespiratory function, administer oxygen, and intubate the patient if necessary. Insert an indwelling IV catheter. The timing of treatment is important; 0 time is the time at seizure onset (see time values on the decision tree).

D. Draw blood for a complete blood count (CBC), calcium, electrolytes, and glucose (SM_7) levels, anticonvulsant levels, if the patient is a known epileptic under treatment, and toxicology screening for drugs and alcohol levels. Order blood cultures. Perform a Dextrostix test; if hypoglycemia is found, infuse a bolus of 50 ml 50% glucose. Start a normal saline IV drip containing vitamin B complex and 100 mg of thiamine. If you suspect that the patient is an alcoholic, add magnesium sulfate, 2 ml IM.

E. If a metabolic abnormality is found (hyperosmolarity, nonketotic coma, electrolyte disturbance), correct the metabolic problem. There is no need for anticonvulsants in the acute phase or in the future because there is no response to anticonvulsants.

F. Begin a slow IV push (IVP) of phenytoin (PHT) at a rate of 50 mg/min to a total of 18 mg/kg, approximately 1,000 mg. Carefully monitor vital signs; if there is any change, slow or stop the infusion. This may take 20 to 40 minutes.

G. If seizures stop, evaluate the neurologic status. Look for localizing signs, a dilated pupil, and hemiplegia. Obtain a CT scan; if a lesion is found, try to identify it (e.g., acute trauma, neoplasm). If a mass lesion is identified, call the neurosurgeon. If the scan shows no mass lesion and no mass effect, perform a lumbar puncture; if meningitis or encephalitis is found, treat accordingly.

H. If seizures continue while PHT (IVP) is used, there are two options: **Plan 1:** Start a DZP IVP at a rate of 2 mg/min until seizures stop or a total of 20 mg/kg is given. Remember that DZP depresses respiration, and at this time reconsider intubation. Also remember that DZP's anticonvulsant effect is very short acting; thus, continue using other anticonvulsants simultaneously. If seizures stop, follow the recommendations at G in the decision tree. **Plan 2:** Start lorazepam (LZP), 4 to 8 mg IV. Remember that LZP depresses respiration, but its duration of action is longer than DZP. If seizures continue, start a phenobarbital IVP at a rate of 100 mg/min until seizures stop or a total dose of 20 mg/kg has been infused. Monitor respiratory function.

I. At this stage, you are most likely 50 to 60 minutes from the start of treatment. If seizures continue, consider a mannitol IVP and call the anesthesiologist.

J. General anesthesia should be used with halothane and a neuromuscular blockade. Continue with baseline anticonvulsants and consider hyperventilation to reduce intracranial hypertension.

K. If seizures are not controlled, use general anesthesia. It may be necessary to communicate with a regional epilepsy center for further advice. The prognosis at this point is dismal.

References

Dalgado-Escueta AV, Westerlain C, Treiman DM, Porter RJ. Management of status epilepticus. N Engl J Med 1982; 306:1337.
Med Lett 1986; 28:91.

TABLE 1 Drugs for Treatment of Status Epilepticus

	Phenytoin	Diazepam	Lorazepam	Phenobarbital
Dose	15-20 mg/kg	0.3-0.5 mg/kg	0.05-0.2 mg/kg	10-20 mg/kg
Ease of IV administration	+	++ to ++	++ to +++	++++
Entry into brain	Rapid	Very rapid	Rapid	
Duration of action	Long	Very short	1/2 life = 15 hrs	Very long
Maintenance use	Yes	No	No	Yes
Adverse reaction	Arrhythmia	Respiratory arrest	Respiratory arrest	Sedation

HEAD TRAUMA

CLOSED HEAD INJURY

Richard L. Strub, M.D.

Closed head injury is a common occurrence in our society and a problem for all physicians. With the increase in lawsuits in head injury cases (particularly in the United States), physicians are forced to take a defensive posture and order more skull x-ray films and brain scans and to admit more patients to the hospital than indicated on a strictly clinical basis.

A. The definition of concussion varies, but the term implies that the blow to the head has caused some disturbance in neurologic function: usually loss of consciousness, memory loss, confusional behavior, or other neurologic abnormalities. Inspect for spinal fluid leakage (nose or ear) or bruises over the mastoid area (Battle sign, usually a delayed sign). These are signs of basal or subfrontal skull fracture.

B. The important features to watch for in the examination are the level of alertness, orientation, and focal neurologic signs. A decreased level of alertness is often the first sign of an intracranial blood clot and must be assessed frequently.

C. Any patient with focal neurologic findings or a decreased level of consciousness after being brought to the hospital and examined should undergo some type of brain scanning. Scanning in a patient with a skull fracture but no abnormalities on neurologic examination is controversial.

D. Epidural clots are extremely dangerous and must be promptly evacuated. Subdural clots are often less urgent, but a neurosurgeon should make the decision when to operate. In some cases of epidural clot, patients have a lucid interval after the initial concussion before they again experience a decrease in level of consciousness as the clot forms.

E. Small-to-medium clots usually resorb with less residual brain damage than if surgically removed. In patients who are improving, it is best to observe rather than operate. If the level of consciousness is low or deteriorating, surgery may be indicated. Each case should be managed on an individual basis and neurosurgeons should follow patients closely and re-evaluate frequently.

References

Becker DP, Miller JD, Young HF, et al. Diagnosis and treatment of head injury in adults. In Youmans JR, ed. Neurological surgery. 2nd ed. Philadelphia: WB Saunders, 1982:1938.

Jennett B, Teasdale G. Management of head injuries. Philadelphia: FA Davis, 1981.

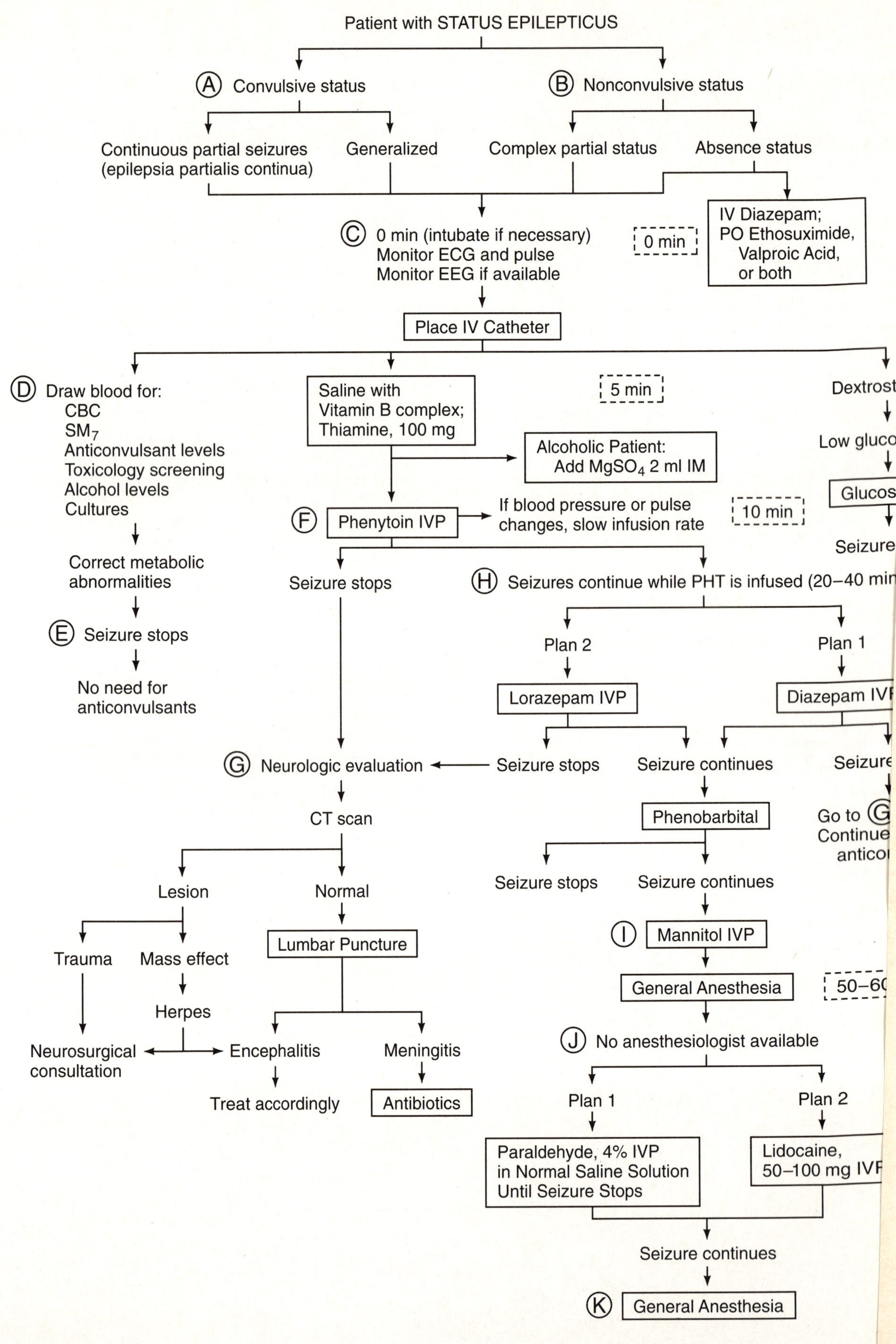

Patient with STATUS EPILEPTICUS
A Convulsive status
B Nonconvulsive status
Continuous partial seizures (epilepsia partialis continua)
Generalized
Complex partial status
Absence status
C 0 min (intubate if necessary) Monitor ECG and pulse Monitor EEG if available
0 min
IV Diazepam; PO Ethosuximide, Valproic Acid, or both
Place IV Catheter
D Draw blood for:
CBC
SM7
Anticonvulsant levels
Toxicology screening
Alcohol levels
Cultures
Saline with Vitamin B complex; Thiamine, 100 mg
5 min
Dextrosti
Low glucos
Alcoholic Patient: Add MgSO4 2 ml IM
Glucose
Correct metabolic abnormalities
F Phenytoin IVP
If blood pressure or pulse changes, slow infusion rate
10 min
Seizure
E Seizure stops
Seizure stops
H Seizures continue while PHT is infused (20–40 min
No need for anticonvulsants
Plan 2
Plan 1
Lorazepam IVP
Diazepam IVP
G Neurologic evaluation
Seizure stops
Seizure continues
Seizure
CT scan
Phenobarbital
Go to G
Continue
anticol
Lesion
Normal
Seizure stops
Seizure continues
Trauma
Mass effect
Lumbar Puncture
I Mannitol IVP
Herpes
General Anesthesia
50–60
Neurosurgical consultation
Encephalitis
Meningitis
J No anesthesiologist available
Treat accordingly
Antibiotics
Plan 1
Plan 2
Paraldehyde, 4% IVP in Normal Saline Solution Until Seizure Stops
Lidocaine, 50–100 mg IVP
Seizure continues
K General Anesthesia

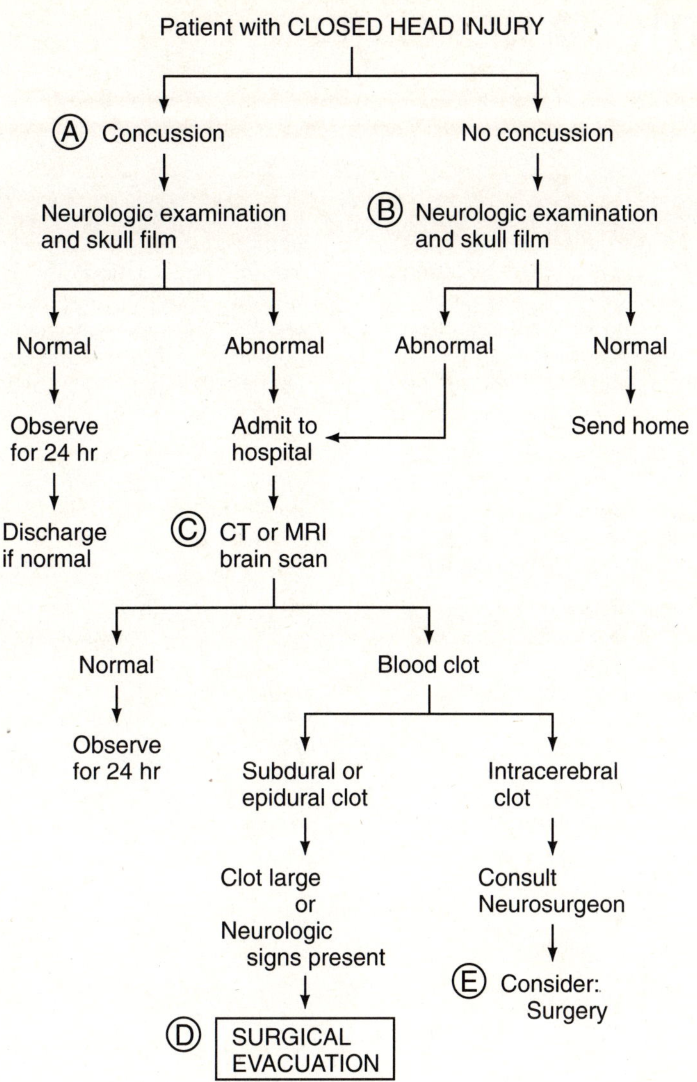

Patient with CLOSED HEAD INJURY
A Concussion
No concussion
Neurologic examination and skull film
B Neurologic examination and skull film
Normal
Abnormal
Abnormal
Normal
Observe for 24 hr
Admit to hospital
Send home
Discharge if normal
C CT or MRI brain scan
Normal
Blood clot
Observe for 24 hr
Subdural or epidural clot
Intracerebral clot
Clot large or Neurologic signs present
Consult Neurosurgeon
D SURGICAL EVACUATION
E Consider: Surgery

POST-TRAUMATIC SYNDROME

Richard L. Strub, M.D.

After a closed head injury, some patients develop lingering symptoms, most commonly headache, dizziness, fatigue, and difficulty concentrating. These symptoms are often exacerbated by stress and physical exertion and can be annoying at best, but at worst may prevent patients from returning to their regular routine. Psychological and legal factors play a part in many cases, but the symptoms are often organic.

A. Although post-traumatic headache and dizziness can start after the patient is home, this suggests that a new problem may have arisen (e.g., subdural hematoma, hydrocephalus). It is probably wise to obtain a CT brain scan even if examination findings are normal.

B. Post-traumatic symptoms are often exacerbated by such normal circumstances as having an alcoholic drink, sneezing, exercising, or being under psychological stress. At times the only treatment necessary is a temporary change in life and work style until symptoms clear.

C. With chronic headaches (lasting many months) it is wise to explore psychological difficulties. At times these cause the headaches; in other cases the continued headaches produce emotional problems. Regardless of the situation, the problem at this point has become much more complex. Be careful not to escalate the doses of analgesics; it is all too easy to continue to increase the strength of medication until the patient is dependent on large doses of narcotic and psychotropic drugs.

D. Tricyclic antidepressants such as amitriptyline, doxepin, and nortriptyline can be very useful in treating these chronic headaches.

References

Becker DP, Miller JD, Young HF, et al. Diagnosis and treatment of head injury in adults. In Youmans JR, ed. Neurological surgery. 2nd ed. Philadelphia: WB Saunders, 1982:1938.

Jennett B, Teasdale G. Management of head injuries. Philadelphia: FA Davis, 1981.

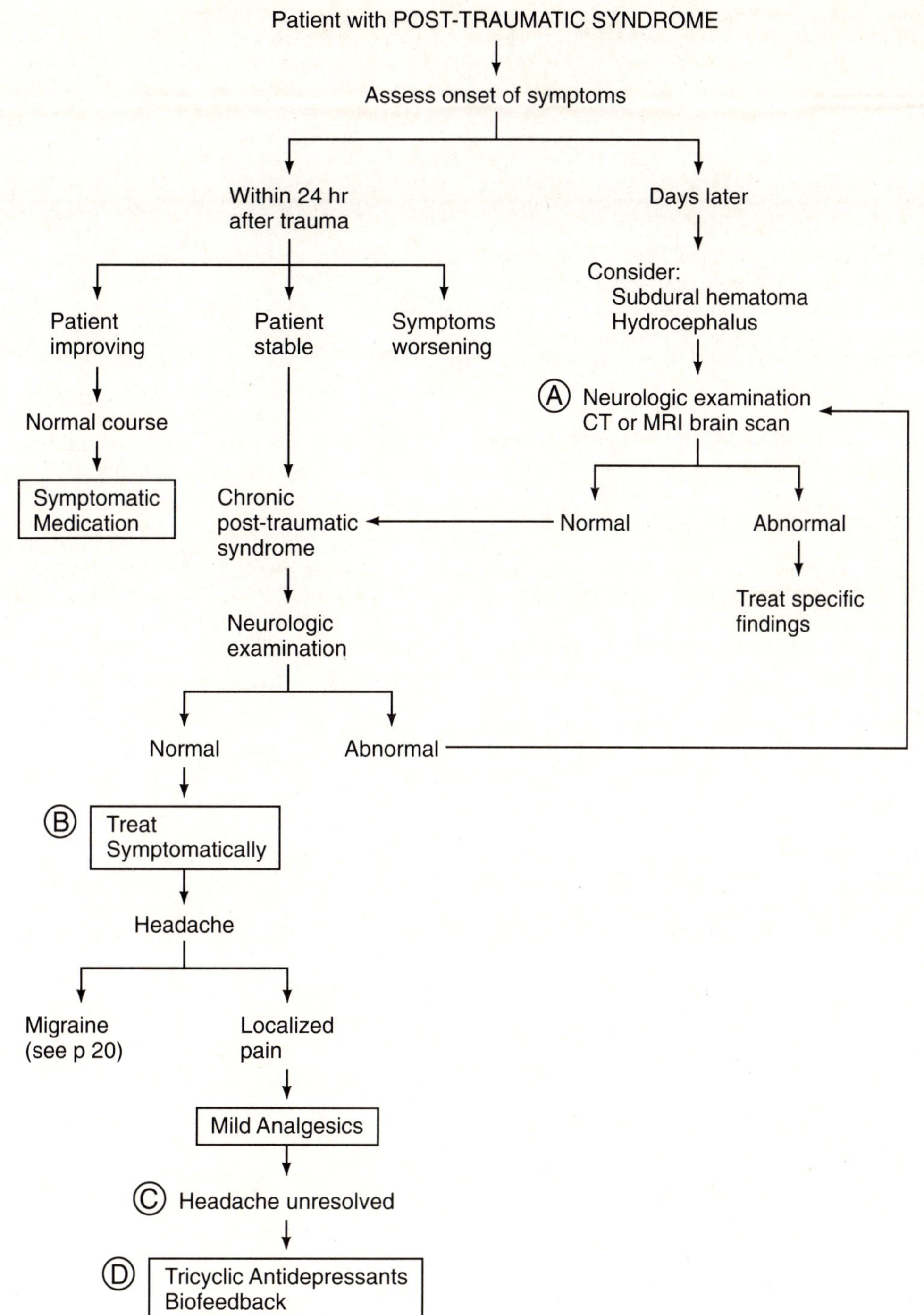

Patient with POST-TRAUMATIC SYNDROME
Assess onset of symptoms
Within 24 hr after trauma
Days later
Patient improving
Patient stable
Symptoms worsening
Consider:
Subdural hematoma
Hydrocephalus
Normal course
A Neurologic examination CT or MRI brain scan
Symptomatic Medication
Chronic post-traumatic syndrome
Normal
Abnormal
Treat specific findings
Neurologic examination
Normal
Abnormal
B Treat Symptomatically
Headache
Migraine (see p 20)
Localized pain
Mild Analgesics
C Headache unresolved
D Tricyclic Antidepressants Biofeedback

POST-TRAUMATIC MENTAL SYMPTOMS

Richard L. Strub, M.D.

Brain trauma frequently causes some behavioral change, which fortunately is usually transient and mild. Mild confusion and amnesia are often seen in the minutes or hours after a blow to the head. It is when mental symptoms persist or develop late that the physician must be concerned. It is important to appreciate the changes, for they are often the limiting factor in complete social reintegration.

A. Mild trauma refers to a short period (minutes) of loss of consciousness and amnesia of a few hours at most. Post-traumatic amnesia constitutes the total of retrograde (before trauma) and anterograde (after trauma) amnesia.

B. Late-onset worsening or reappearance of symptoms should alert the physician to a physiologic change. This may be due to medications, but do not overlook a structural lesion.

C. Some patients become obsessed with their accident and have nightmares and recurring fears about it. This post-traumatic stress disorder often requires psychiatric help.

D. Mild head trauma should not produce significant behavioral change on a pathologic basis. In elderly patients it may at times, but some of these cases may be early unrecognized dementia. Serial observations are necessary.

E. A moderate-to-severe head injury results in at least 24 hours of amnesia but may last for >1 week. Loss of consciousness may last for hours.

F. Confusion resulting from the blow may last a few hours, but when symptoms do not clear in a few days, some type of brain damage is probable.

G. The most common changes resulting from higher grades of head injury are the onset of frontal lobe behavior and personality change (usually apathy), recent memory loss, difficulty in concentrating, and general nonspecific loss of intellectual acuity.

H. If the problem is significant and long-term rehabilitation necessary, or if patients have trouble reintegrating into a normal routine, it is important to obtain a full neuropsychological profile of their intellectual and emotional problems.

I. The prognosis is difficult to render in the first few months, particularly in younger patients (ages 10 to 30 years). Much spontaneous recovery occurs in the first year and can continue for 3 to 5 years.

References

Brooks N, ed. Closed head injury. New York: Oxford University Press, 1984.

Levin HS, Benton AL, Grossman RG. Neurobehavioral consequences of closed head injury. New York: Oxford University Press, 1982.

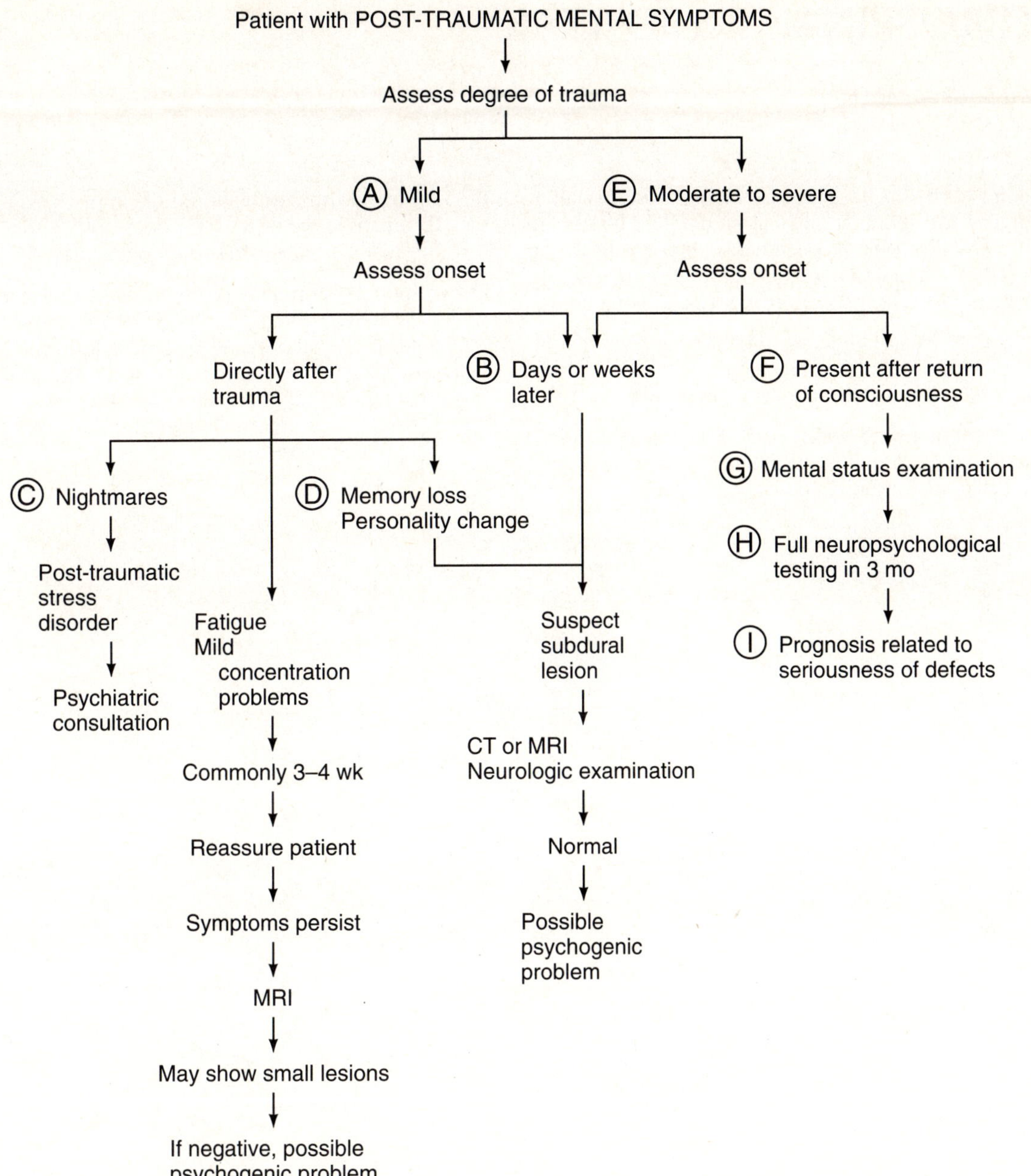

Patient with POST-TRAUMATIC MENTAL SYMPTOMS
Assess degree of trauma
A Mild
E Moderate to severe
Assess onset
Assess onset
Directly after trauma
B Days or weeks later
F Present after return of consciousness
C Nightmares
D Memory loss Personality change
G Mental status examination
Post-traumatic stress disorder
Psychiatric consultation
Fatigue Mild concentration problems
Commonly 3–4 wk
Reassure patient
Symptoms persist
MRI
May show small lesions
If negative, possible psychogenic problem
Suspect subdural lesion
CT or MRI Neurologic examination
Normal
Possible psychogenic problem
H Full neuropsychological testing in 3 mo
I Prognosis related to seriousness of defects

CEREBROSPINAL FLUID LEAK

Richard L. Strub, M.D.

Fluid leaking from the nose occurs in head trauma after cranial surgery and spontaneously. A spinal fluid leak is an important medical problem, because such patients are at risk for the development of bacterial meningitis. In general, spinal fluid leaks are best managed by a neurosurgeon.

A. If a patient has sustained significant head trauma and clear or bloody fluid is leaking from the nose, it can usually be safely assumed to be spinal fluid.

B. In spontaneous fluid leaks, establishing and locating the leak are more of a diagnostic challenge. At times, the clear fluid is mucus and not CSF.

C. An otolaryngologist should place pledgets under each turbinate in the nose. If CT does not identify the site of the leak, the CSF soaked pledgets may.

D. Although meningitis is a definite risk with a CSF leak, it is controversial whether prophylactic doses of antibiotics can prevent it. Some studies show that such prophylactic therapy does not help and that the meningitis that does develop in treated patients is caused by a more malignant and more resistant "hospital" bacterium.

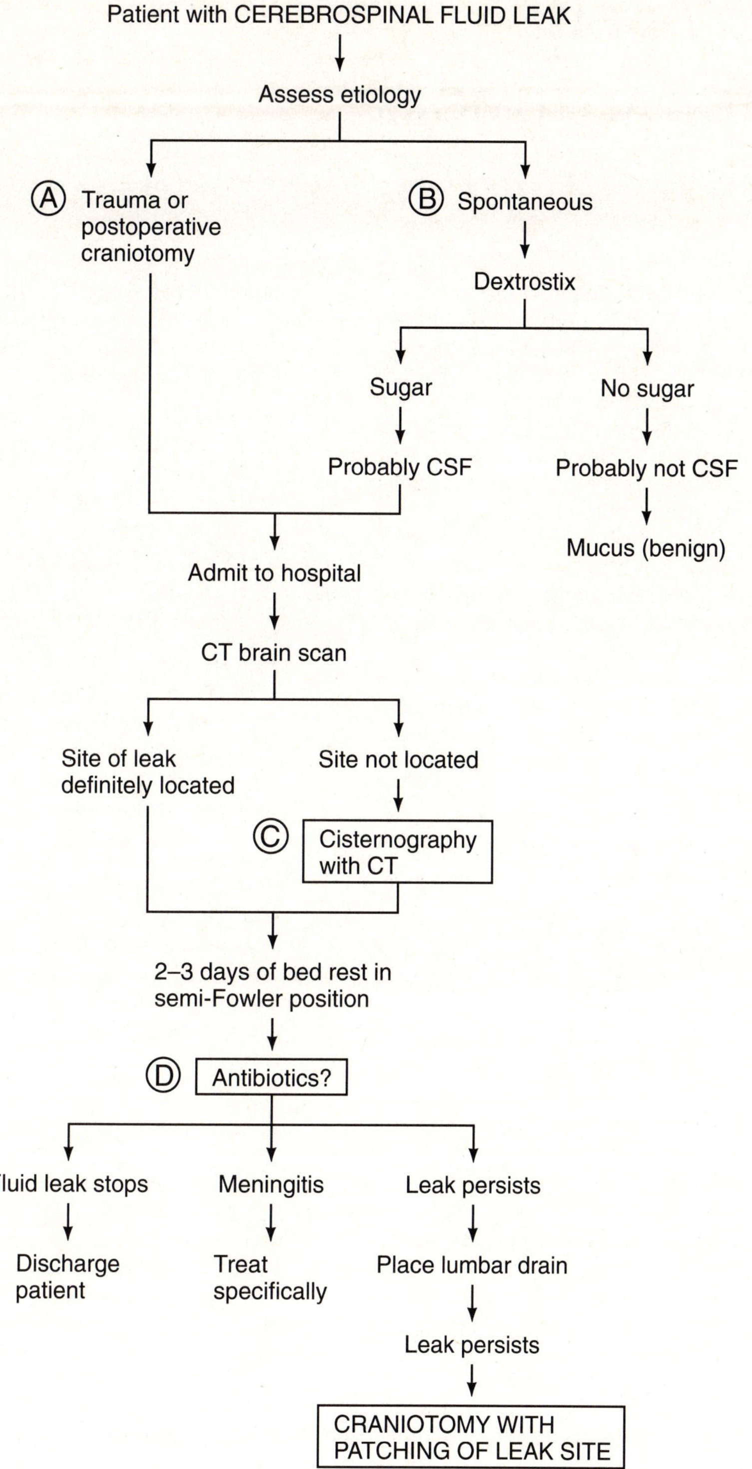

Patient with CEREBROSPINAL FLUID LEAK
Assess etiology
A Trauma or postoperative craniotomy
B Spontaneous
Dextrostix
Sugar
No sugar
Probably CSF
Probably not CSF
Mucus (benign)
Admit to hospital
CT brain scan
Site of leak definitely located
Site not located
C Cisternography with CT
2–3 days of bed rest in semi-Fowler position
D Antibiotics?
Fluid leak stops
Meningitis
Leak persists
Discharge patient
Treat specifically
Place lumbar drain
Leak persists
CRANIOTOMY WITH PATCHING OF LEAK SITE

NEOPLASTIC DISEASE

SUPRATENTORIAL TUMORS

Carlos A. Garcia, M.D.

Most tumors (70%) in adults are supratentorial. These include primary tumors, of which gliomas and meningiomas are the most common, and secondary or metastatic tumors from systemic cancer. The risk of developing a symptomatic primary tumor increases with age; there is a peak at 60 years of age. The age-adjusted incidence shows that primary tumors are more frequent in men than in women. However, meningiomas and pituitary tumors occur more frequently in young adult females, whereas gliomas and nerve sheath tumors occur more often in males over the age of 40.

The clinical features of a brain tumor depend on the location of the tumor, its histologic type and differentiation, its growth rate, the degree of infiltration and invasion of normal neural parenchyma, and the mass effect and increased intracranial pressure (ICP). Small tumors (meningiomas) may be found incidentally on neuroradiologic studies or autopsy and may cause no symptoms. Others may cause seizures without a focal neurologic deficit, and CT or MRI may show no change in size. On the other hand, a strokelike presentation may be seen in tumors that grow rapidly enough to outstrip the blood supply of the neoplasm and bleed (metastatic, glioblastomas). The most common presentation is a progressive deterioration of mental, sensorimotor, or visual function. There may be irritative effects, which present as a seizure disorder of a localized or generalized nature, or the tumor may produce generalized effects owing to space occupation, edema, or obstruction of CSF flow, causing increased ICP. The type of tumor (slow or fast-growing) and the location (superficial, deep, infiltrative) are the main factors in the clinical presentation. Secondary (metastatic) tumors are an important group described separately (see p 196).

A. Glioblastoma multiforme is the most common primary tumor in adult patients, particularly affecting males over 40 years of age. This highly malignant, rapidly growing tumor has a predilection for the frontotemporal lobes, is highly infiltrative, and tends to spread to the opposite hemisphere, infiltrating across the corpus callosum (butterfly glioma). When these tumors are frontally located, they may cause progressive dementia and gait disturbance. If they are in the temporoparietal region, hemiparesis and language disturbance may occur. Seizures may be the first manifestation or may occur during the course of the disease. Peritumor hemorrhage may cause an exacerbation of the symptoms or may be the first manifestation of the tumor. CT or MRI demonstrates a solitary hemispheric lesion with contrast enhancement and surrounding cerebral edema, but the imaging appearance does not make it possible to confirm the histologic diagnosis without biopsy. Cerebral edema surrounding the glioma re-sponds to steroids. The prognosis is dismal regardless of the form of treatment because of the rapid growth and tissue infiltration; 90% of patients die within 2 years after diagnosis.

B. Meningiomas are the third most common CNS tumor in adults, after metastatic disease and glioblastoma multiforme. The tumor is frequent in young adult females; it is a slow-growing, histologically benign tumor that originates in the arachnoidal cells of the meninges and attaches to the dura mater. It is nodular, well circumscribed, and sharply demarcated. It frequently is associated with changes in the overlying bone (hyperostosis) and compresses, indents, and distorts the brain tissue (extra-axial, extraparenchymal). The tumor is most often found in the parasagittal and lateral cerebral hemispheric convexity regions but may also arise in the subfrontal area, sphenoid ridge, tuberculum sellae, tentorium, and foramen magnum or within the ventricular system. The tumor grows slowly and may reach a great size before producing symptoms. Focal or generalized seizures, dementia, and progressive ocular and motor deficits may be the clinical presentation. Imaging studies demonstrate a sharply marginated, homogeneous lesion. A resection biopsy (when possible) may confirm the diagnosis. Steroid-responsive vasogenic edema may be seen around the tumor. Bleeding and calcifications are rare.

C. Gliomas other than glioblastoma multiforme may occur in the cerebral hemispheres. Most are slow-growing astrocytomas. These tumors are infiltrative and slow growing and may arise in any area of the cerebral hemispheres. Gemistocytic astrocytomas (arising from "plump" astrocytes) are of importance because of their tendency to become malignant and their predilection for the temporal lobe. Cystic or solid astrocytomas may originate anywhere. Tomography may fail to reveal these isodense lesions. MRI may demonstrate this lesion earlier. Surgical resection in accessible areas is recommended. Oligodendrogliomas are seen in young adults of either sex, predominantly in the frontal lobes, and frequently show calcifications. Longer survivals are seen in patients with highly calcified lesions (calcium seen on simple skull x-ray views) and when the tumor is localized and most of the lesion is resected. There has been a dramatic rise in the incidence of primary CNS lymphomas, both in therapeutically immunosuppressed patients (transplants, etc.) and in AIDS patients. These tumors may be multicentric, are seen in the periventricular corpus callosum areas, and show a partial response to radiotherapy and chemotherapy.

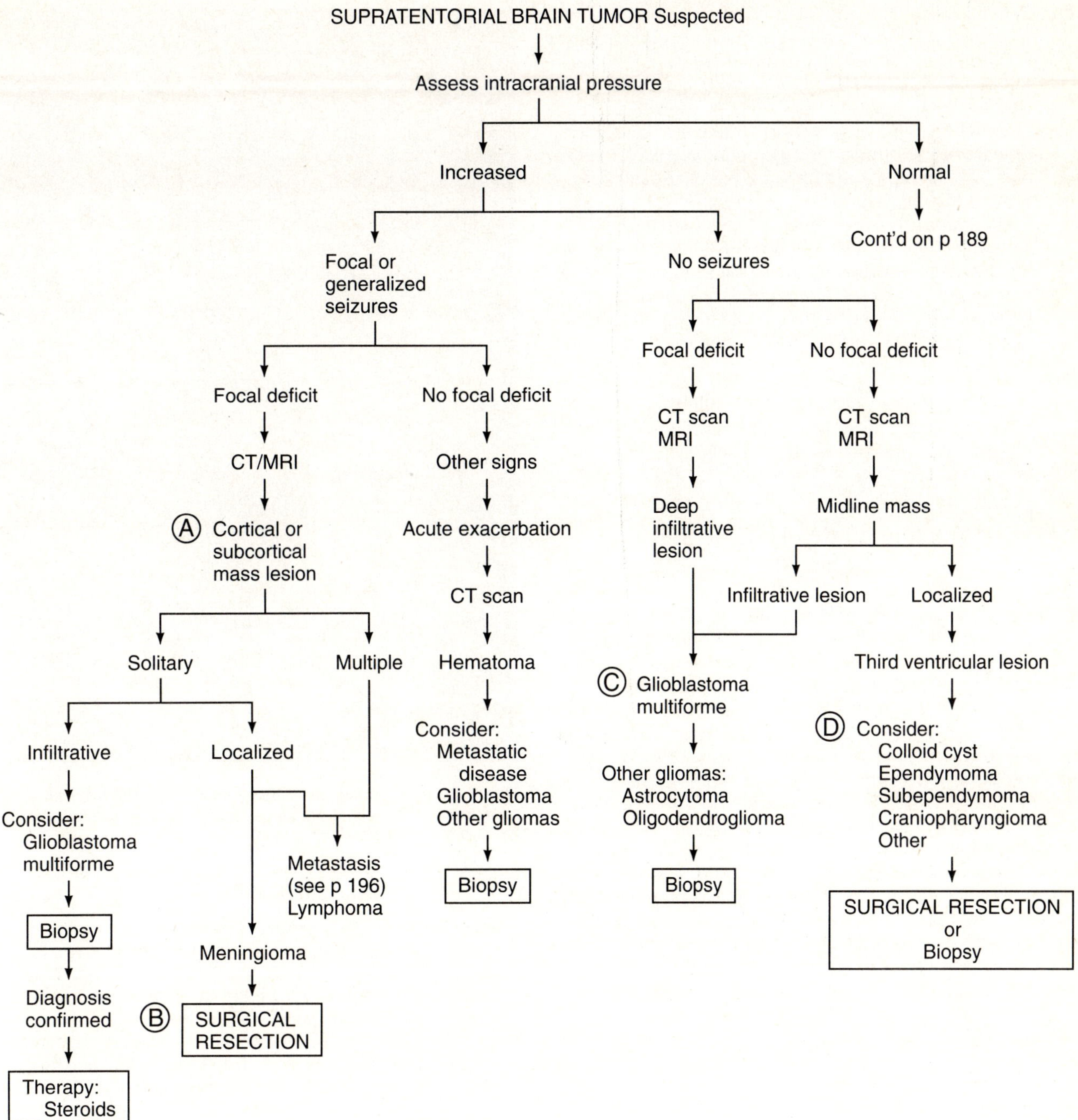

SUPRATENTORIAL BRAIN TUMOR Suspected
Assess intracranial pressure
Increased
Normal
Cont'd on p 189
Focal or generalized seizures
No seizures
Focal deficit
No focal deficit
Focal deficit
No focal deficit
CT/MRI
Other signs
CT scan MRI
CT scan MRI
A Cortical or subcortical mass lesion
Acute exacerbation
Deep infiltrative lesion
Midline mass
CT scan
Infiltrative lesion
Localized
Solitary
Multiple
Hematoma
Third ventricular lesion
Infiltrative
Localized
Consider:
Metastatic disease
Glioblastoma
Other gliomas
C Glioblastoma multiforme
D Consider:
Colloid cyst
Ependymoma
Subependymoma
Craniopharyngioma
Other
Consider:
Glioblastoma multiforme
Metastasis (see p 196)
Lymphoma
Other gliomas:
Astrocytoma
Oligodendroglioma
Biopsy
Biopsy
Biopsy
Diagnosis confirmed
Meningioma
B SURGICAL RESECTION
SURGICAL RESECTION
or
Biopsy
Therapy:
Steroids

D. Patients may present with signs of nonlocalized increased ICP. This is most common in young adults. CT shows a third ventricular (midline) lesion producing hydrocephalus. The differential diagnosis of anterior third ventricular tumors includes colloid cyst and craniopharyngioma, posterior third ventricular tumor, pinealoma, teratoma, and germinoma. Ocular findings such as upward gaze paralysis (Parinaud's syndrome) may be seen with a posterior third ventricular tumor that compresses the quadrigeminal areas. Neurosurgical treatment should be directed toward relieving the hydrocephalus, or the lesion should be excised when possible. Herniation secondary to displacement of brain tissue from one compartment to another is the result of a mass effect with increased intracranial pressure (Fig. 1).

E. Pituitary tumors, the fourth most common tumor in adults, are usually seen in young females. These tumors and parasellar tumors are described on page 192.

MANAGEMENT OF PATIENTS WITH BRAIN TUMORS

Differentiation between primary and secondary tumors is important and is easier when multiple lesions are found. However, remember that primary lymphomas and rare cases of gliomas and meningiomas may be multicentric. In most metastatic lesions the primary source can be identified, but in some cases a brain biopsy may be necessary to arrive at the correct diagnosis. With primary tumors the aim of neurosurgery is to make a definite histologic diagnosis and to cure by excision when possible. In some cases the curative surgical resection is not possible, even in some benign tumors. In these, adjuvant therapy may palliate symptoms of increased ICP (edema-responsive steroids). Chemotherapy and radiation therapy have prolonged the survival time in some malignant gliomas. Cooperative study group trials are being done at the present time to learn more about the behavior of the tumor and the response to different therapies.

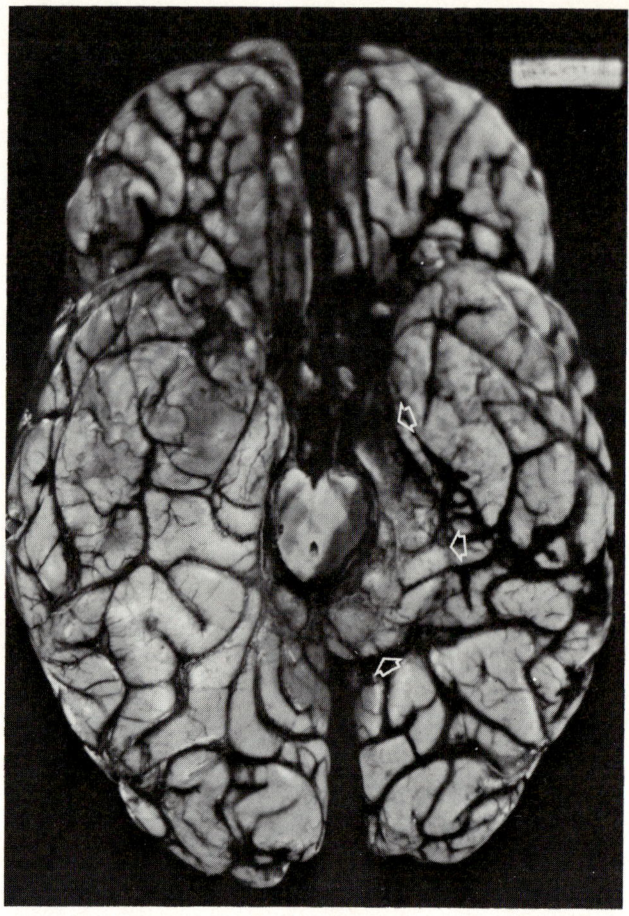

Figure 1 Base of the brain after removal of the brain stem and cerebellum, showing a left hippocampal herniation *(arrows)* secondary to a left hemispheric neoplasm.

References

DeAngelis LM. Primary central nervous system lymphoma: A new clinical challenge. Neurology 1991; 41:619.

Mork SJ, Lindegaard KF, Halvorsen TB, et al. Oligodendrogliomas: Incidence and biological behavior in a defined population. J Neurosurg 1985; 63:881.

Russell DS, Rubinstein LJ. Pathology of tumours of the nervous system. 5th ed. Baltimore: Williams & Wilkins, 1989.

Walker AE, Robins M, Weinfeld FD. Epidemiology of brain tumors: The national survey of intracranial neoplasms. Neurology 1985; 35:219.

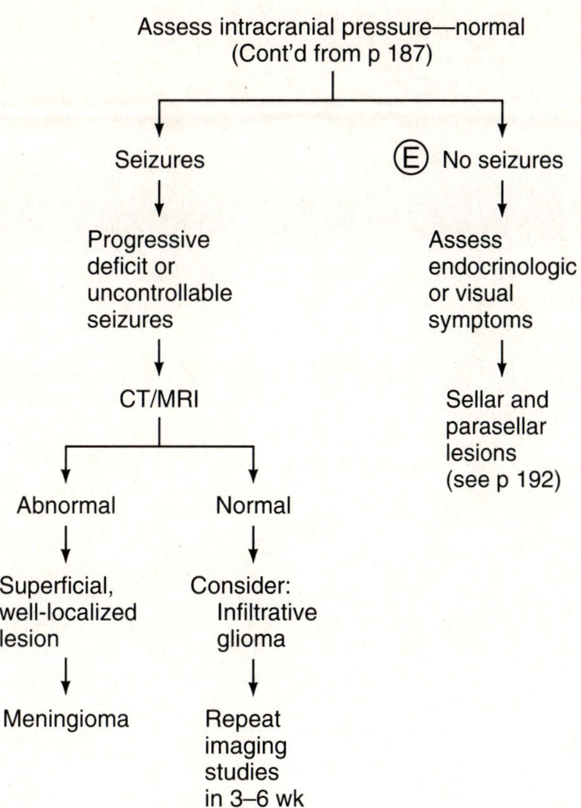

Assess intracranial pressure—normal
(Cont'd from p 187)

Seizures

E No seizures

Progressive
deficit or
uncontrollable
seizures

Assess
endocrinologic
or visual
symptoms

CT/MRI

Sellar and
parasellar
lesions
(see p 192)

Abnormal

Normal

Superficial,
well-localized
lesion

Consider:
Infiltrative
glioma

Meningioma

Repeat
imaging
studies
in 3–6 wk

INFRATENTORIAL TUMORS

Carlos A. Garcia, M.D.

Only 30% of tumors in adults are infratentorial, a figure that contrasts with the 70% incidence of infratentorial tumors in children. Most infratentorial tumors in adults are benign in histologic appearance and behavior, but some are difficult to resect completely because of their location. The tumor produces signs of increased intracranial pressure (ICP) (headache, nausea, vomiting, diplopia) and cerebellar (ataxias) or brain stem signs (corticospinal tract signs, multiple cranial nerve disorders, crossed sensorimotor deficit). The two most common tumors are schwannoma and cerebellar hemangioblastoma, in that order. Metastatic lesions are also common. Less common tumors include meningiomas, chordomas, and epidermoid cysts.

A. Schwannoma of the eighth cranial nerve is also known as acoustic neuroma, acoustic neurinoma, and cerebellopontine (CP) angle tumor. The tumor is benign and slow growing and originates from the Schwann cell or fibroblast of the nerve sheath. It arises most frequently from the vestibular branch of the acoustic (eighth) cranial nerve (acoustic neuroma) and presents with hearing loss, especially for speech discrimination. As the tumor grows, it compresses the adjacent structures, such as the seventh facial nerve (infranuclear facial weakness), fifth nerve (facial numbness), and brain stem (long tract signs). The tumor occupies the CP angle area. Neuroradiologic techniques, including CT and MRI, can detect small lesions before any signs of compression of the brain stem. Schwannoma may also arise from the fifth and seventh cranial nerves, in that order of frequency. When schwannoma is bilateral, suspect von Recklinghausen's disease. Treatment consists of resection of the lesion. Meningioma and chordoma may occupy the CP angle and compress the brain stem.

B. Cerebellar hemangioblastoma is a benign, slow-growing tumor composed of a mixture of endothelial cells and stromal (clear) cells of obscure origin. The tumor frequently involves one cerebellar hemisphere but may arise in the midline (Fig. 1). It is often cystic and contains a mural nodule (Lindau's disease). The lesion either compresses or occupies the fourth ventricle, producing hydrocephalus. Lateralized or midline cerebellar symptoms are seen, depending on the site of the lesion. Signs of increased ICP may precede or follow the cerebellar deficit. Erythropoietin or one of its precursors produced by the tumor has been implicated as the cause of the polycythemia that is frequently associated with the lesion. In 20% of cases, the tumor is familial and is associated with spinal cord tumors, retinal angiomas (von Hippel's disease), pancreatic and hepatic cysts, and renal tumors (von Hippel-Lindau disease). Treatment consists of resection of the lesion(s).

Ependymoma arises from the floor of the fourth ventricle from ependymal cells and tends to occupy the fourth ventricle. The tumor grows slowly and produces late signs and symptoms, mainly an increase in ICP. Recurrences after partial resection are frequent. Other posterior fossa tumors or tumor-like lesions are rare (e.g., the epidermoid tumor found in

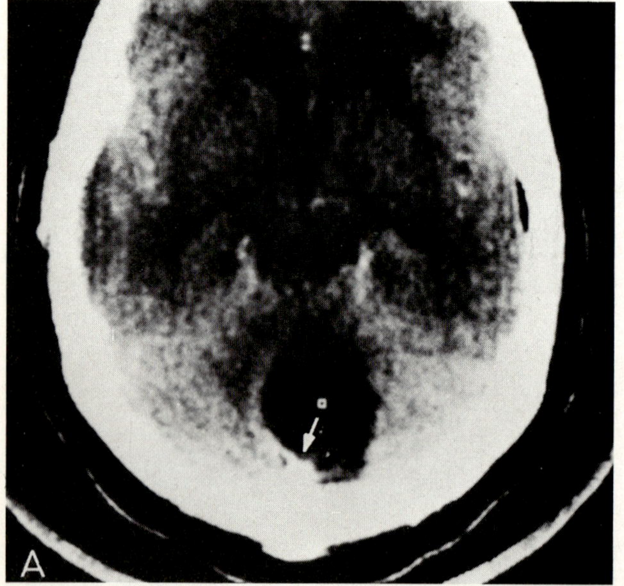
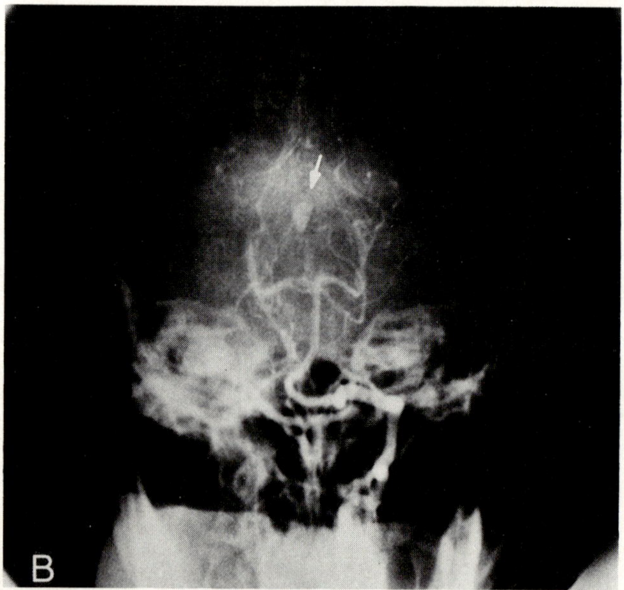

Figure 1 *A,* Brain CT scan showing a midline cerebellar cyst. Arrow shows an enhancing mural nodule in a cerebellar hemangioblastoma. *B,* Vertebral angiogram showing a vascularized nodule *(arrow)* corresponding to a mural nodule seen on CT in a cerebellar hemangioblastoma.

Patient with DECREASED HEARING, HEADACHE or ATAXIA,
↓
Infratentorial tumor suspected
↓
Assess intracranial pressure

Normal

(A) Hearing loss (speech discrimination)

- Corticospinal tract deficit
  - Absent
    - MRI
    - Eighth nerve lesion
    - **SURGERY**
    - Nerve sheath tumor of eighth nerve
  - Present
    - Facial weakness and numbness
    - MRI
    - CP mass
    - Nerve sheath tumor: eighth, seventh, or fifth

No hearing loss

- Corticospinal tract intact
  - Multiple cranial nerves
    - Unilateral
      - MRI
      - CP angle prepontine mass
      - Consider: Nerve sheath tumor / Meningioma / Chordoma / Other
      - **SURGERY / Biopsy**
    - Bilateral
      - MRI
      - Brain stem lesion: Glioma / Metastatic / Other
- No corticospinal tract deficit

Increased

(B) Cerebellar deficit

- Polycythemia
  - MRI / CT scan
  - Cerebellar lesion
    - Cystic
    - Solid
  - Family history
    - Present
      - Retinal (von Hippel's) angioma
      - Other lesions (kidney, spine)
      - **SURGERY**
      - Cerebellar hemangioblastoma (von Hippel-Lindau disease)
    - Absent
      - No other lesions
      - **SURGERY**
      - Cerebellar hemangioblastoma (Lindau's disease)
- No polycythemia
  - MRI / CT scan
  - Solid cerebellar mass
  - Chest CT or MRI
    - Lung lesion
      - Metastatic lesion
    - Normal
      - Consider: Glioma / Other

No cerebellar deficit

- No corticospinal tract deficit
  - MRI or CT
    - Supratentorial lesion (see p 186)
    - Fourth ventricular lesion
      - Epidermoid cyst / Subependymoma
- Corticospinal tract deficit
  - Cranial nerves
  - MRI / CT scan
  - Mass lesion in brain stem or fourth ventricle
  - **SURGICAL EXPLORATION**
  - Consider: Brain stem glioma / Ependymoma / Metastatic disease / Other

the fourth ventricle or parapontine area). Signs of increased ICP and brain stem compression may be seen with or without cerebellar ataxia. CT and MRI differentiate this lesion (low density) from other tumors.

References

Walker AE, Robins M, Weinfeld FD. Epidemiology of brain tumors: The national survey of intracranial neoplasms. Neurology 1985; 35:219.

Whittaker CK, Leutze CM. Vestibular schwannomas. J Neurosurg 1992; 76:897.

SELLAR AND PARASELLAR TUMORS

Carlos A. Garcia, M.D.

Intrasellar tumors originate from tissue within the sella turcica. Parasellar tumors originate from tissue contiguous to or directly above the sella. Extension upward into the suprasellar area may occur with intrasellar tumors. Patients may present with several disorders: endocrinologic dysfunction (hypersecretion or reduced pituitary function), visual disturbances (see pp 132 and 144), and symptoms of intracranial hypertension. An enlarged sella found by imaging studies may be discovered incidentally. Carry out endocrinologic studies, a visual field examination, and MRI with contrast enhancement of the sellar region. Angiography or magnetic resonance angiography (MRA) is used to define the relation of the tumor to blood vessels and to exclude vascular lesions (aneurysms).

Most intrasellar tumors arise from the glandular portion of the pituitary (pituitary adenoma) (Fig. 1). New techniques have made it possible to measure blood hormone levels (radioimmunoassay), to demonstrate a small lesion with MRI and to show hormonal granules in tumors by immunocytochemical (immunoperoxidase) stains. Successful removal of small lesions by the transsphenoidal approach has changed the classification and clinical outcome of patients with these lesions. Microadenomas (<10 mm in size) can be diagnosed and removed with low risk. Pituitary adenomas are classified according to cytoplasmic granules stained by immunocytochemistry. These include prolactin cell adenoma (prolactinoma), growth hormone cell adenoma (and a mixed variety of both), corticotropic cell adenoma, gonadotropic cell adenoma, undifferentiated cell adenoma, and acidophilic stem cell adenoma. Prolactinoma (41%) and growth hormone— (19.5%) and adrenocorticotropic hormone (ACTH)–producing (16.7%) adenomas are the most common and most important tumors. Nonsecreting adenoma (oncocytoma) rarely occurs.

A. Prolactinoma presents with galactorrhea, amenorrhea, and infertility in women; in men it may cause impotence. The serum prolactin level is usually elevated. Microadenoma is diagnosed with MRI (normal-sized sella, and the lesion seen within a normal or slightly enlarged pituitary gland). Transsphenoidal resection of the tumor may be achieved. Prolactinoma may grow to erode and enlarge the sella (macroadenomas). When it becomes large enough, it compresses the optic chiasm, producing visual field defects (bitemporal superior quadrantanopia or hemianopia). As the tumor enlarges, symptoms of reduced pituitary function (panhypopituitarism) may appear. The acute onset of blindness or subarachnoid hemorrhage in a patient known to have a pituitary tumor should alert the clinician to the possibility of bleeding within the tumor (pituitary apoplexy). These tumors may extend laterally and produce diplopia (due to ocular muscle weakness) or may grow down into the sphenoidal sinus to cause cerebrospinal rhinorrhea. The tumor may be resected transsphenoidally or by craniectomy. Bromocriptine may be used to reduce tumor size.

B. The growth hormone—secreting tumor presents with symptoms and signs of acromegaly in adults (enlargement of hands, feet, jaws, and frontal bones) and gigantism in young patients. The tumor may be circumscribed (microadenoma); other tumors enlarge the gland and sella. Endocrinologic studies show an elevated serum growth hormone level. Surgery is required. A patient with a cushingoid appearance ("moon face," hirsutism, hypertension, osteoporosis, "buffalo hump," and diabetes) may harbor an ACTH-secreting adenoma. Endocrinologic studies may confirm hypercortisolism. Most of these lesions are microadenomas; other causes of Cushing's syndrome include drug-induced and primary adrenal disease that can be differentiated by the classic dexamethasone suppression test. At the highest dose of ACTH, those with Cushing's disease suppress cortisol while those with ectopic ACTH-producing lesions and adrenal causes do not. Inferior petrosal venous sampling will help the surgeon to perform hemipituitarectomy. Other tumors include tuberculum sellae meningiomas, choristomas, and metastatic lesions. Tumor-like lesions, such as dermoid and epidermoid cysts, may originate in this area. MRI or MRA may reveal an aneurysm of the carotid artery.

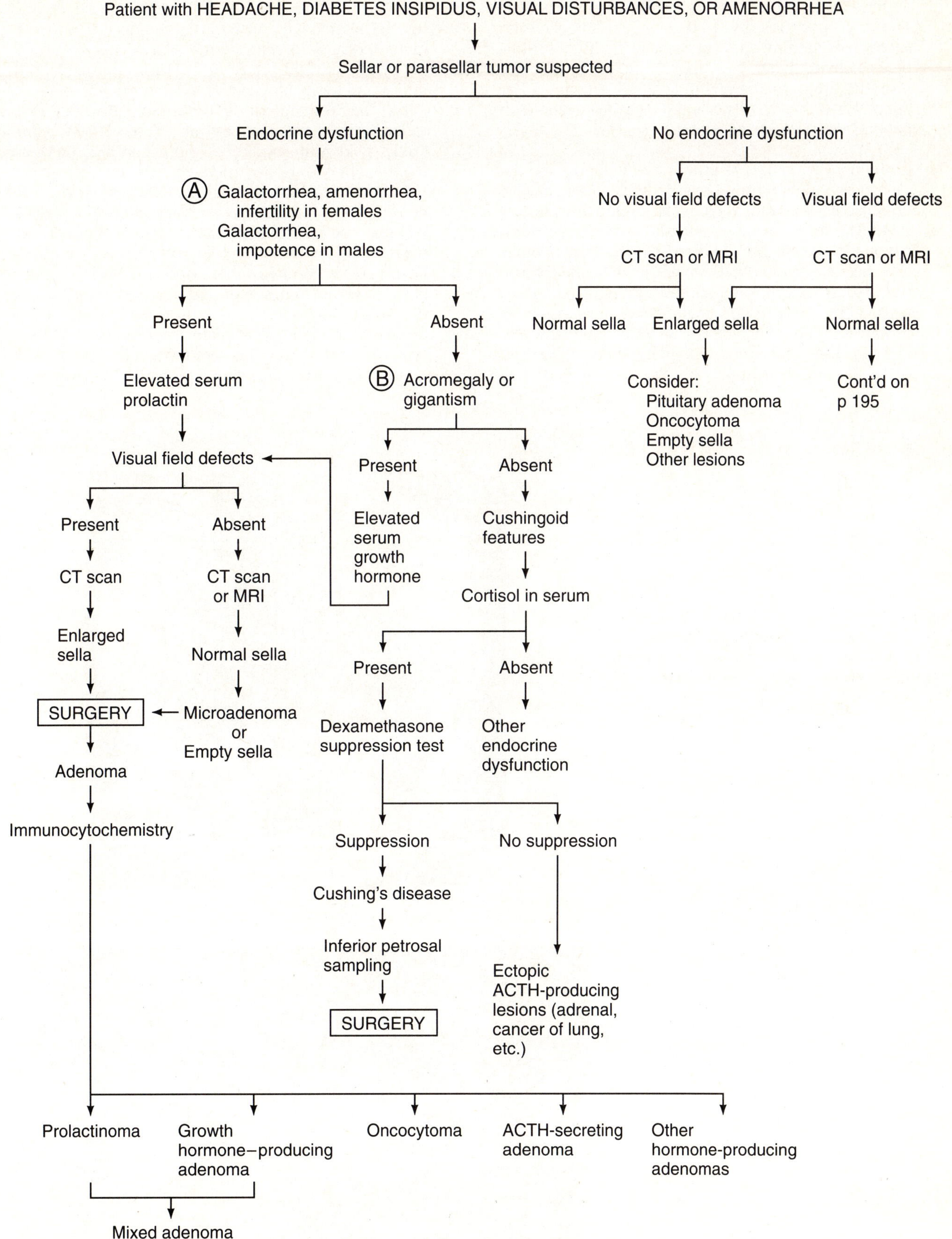

Patient with HEADACHE, DIABETES INSIPIDUS, VISUAL DISTURBANCES, OR AMENORRHEA
Sellar or parasellar tumor suspected
Endocrine dysfunction
No endocrine dysfunction
A Galactorrhea, amenorrhea, infertility in females Galactorrhea, impotence in males
No visual field defects
Visual field defects
CT scan or MRI
CT scan or MRI
Present
Absent
Normal sella
Enlarged sella
Normal sella
Elevated serum prolactin
B Acromegaly or gigantism
Consider:
Pituitary adenoma
Oncocytoma
Empty sella
Other lesions
Cont'd on p 195
Visual field defects
Present
Absent
Present
Absent
Elevated serum growth hormone
Cushingoid features
CT scan
CT scan or MRI
Cortisol in serum
Enlarged sella
Normal sella
Present
Absent
SURGERY
Microadenoma or Empty sella
Dexamethasone suppression test
Other endocrine dysfunction
Adenoma
Immunocytochemistry
Suppression
No suppression
Cushing's disease
Inferior petrosal sampling
Ectopic ACTH-producing lesions (adrenal, cancer of lung, etc.)
SURGERY
Prolactinoma
Growth hormone–producing adenoma
Oncocytoma
ACTH-secreting adenoma
Other hormone-producing adenomas
Mixed adenoma

C. Suprasellar extension occurs less frequently because of early diagnosis by MRI or CT. Patients with suprasellar lesions may present with visual disturbances, hypothalamic symptoms including diabetes insipidus, and increased intracranial pressure. The approach to these patients is similar to that taken with patients with intrasellar lesions.

D. Craniopharyngiomas are usually cystic tumors and are seen predominantly in young patients. These tumors originate from epithelial remnants around the pituitary stalk. The tumor is cystic and shows laminar calcification, especially in children. Craniopharyngiomas may become symptomatic in adults and may not be calcified. The tumor is radioresistant and difficult to resect completely. A chiasmatic tumor may arise from astrocytes within the chiasm or optic nerves (optic glioma). This tumor is seen predominantly in children or young adults. It may be a manifestation of von Recklinghausen's disease. Controversy exists regarding the alternatives of therapy, surgery, or no treatment (because certain tumors have a low growth potential). Carotid artery or anterior communicating artery aneurysm may compress the chiasm or optic nerves laterally, superiorly, or inferiorly. Most of these lesions are giant saccular aneurysms (>2.5 cm). Epidermoid (only epithelial elements) and dermoid (epithelium with glands and hair) cysts may present as intrasellar or suprasellar lesions. Because of the low density, these lesions are easy to detect on CT or MRI. Lipomas are rare tumors but may occur around the hypothalamus; they are diagnosed by CT or MRI. Posterior third ventricular tumors arise from the pineal gland in young males. Germinomas and teratomas are the most common lesions. These lesions may compress the quadrigeminal plate to produce Parinaud's syndrome (paralysis of upward gaze). Germinomas are radiosensitive. Germinomas and teratomas may grow

Figure 1 *A,* Coronal CT scan showing an intrasellar neoplasm (pituitary adenoma) with suprasellar extension. *B,* Sagittal section of a brain showing a pituitary adenoma *(arrows)* with hemorrhage (pituitary apoplexy).

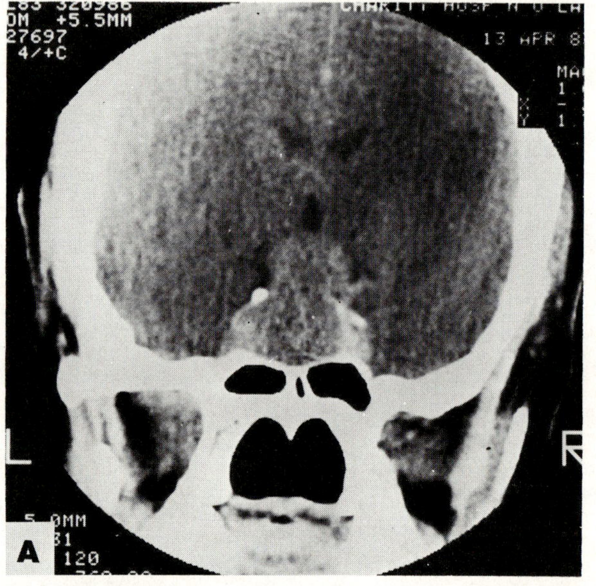

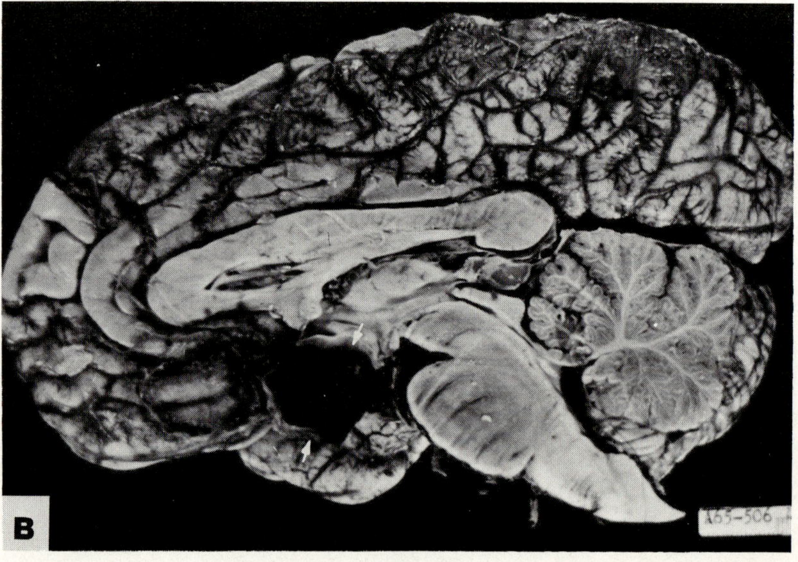

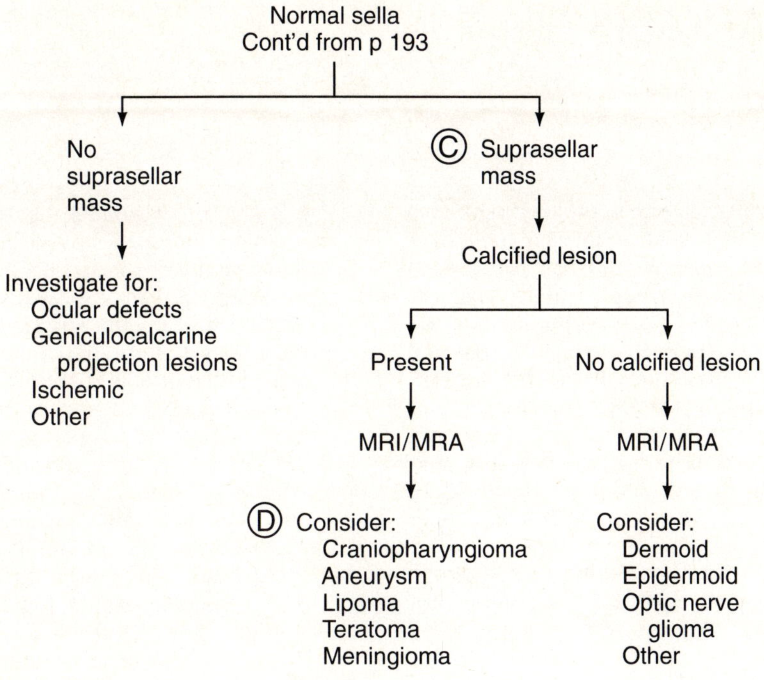

in the suprasellar area (ectopic pinealomas). Teratomas are radioresistant and difficult to resect (calcification is frequent). Granulomas (tuberculous, sarcoid) may occur in the parasellar area. If the sella is enlarged, with or without evidence of erosion, and there are no visual or endocrine symptoms, consider the empty-sella syndrome. It is important to differentiate this from an intrasellar tumor by MRI.

References

Boggan JE, Tyurell JB, Wilson CB. Transsphenoidal microsurgical management of Cushing's disease. J Neurosurg 1983; 59:195.

Ciric I. Pituitary tumors. Neurol Clin North Am 1985; 3:751.

Cutler GB. In: A review of endocrinology: Diagnosis and treatment. NIH Syllabus 1987; 449.

Vic NA, Bigner DD. Neuro-oncology. Neurol Clin North Am 1985; 3:4.

Wilson CB. A decade of pituitary microsurgery. J Neurosurg 1984; 61:814.

BRAIN METASTASIS

Carlos A. Garcia, M.D.

Brain metastases (Fig. 1) are common neurologic problems that seem to be increasing in frequency owing to the longer survival of patients with systemic cancer. Most such metastases are due to hematogenous spread and are multiple; the distribution in the CNS is proportional to the blood supply to the brain: 81% are cerebral, 16% are cerebellar, and only 3% are found in the brain stem. Vasogenic edema surrounding untreated metastases is a constant feature. The edema is often severe and may cause cerebral herniations, but it responds dramatically and rapidly to corticosteroid therapy. Multiple lesions are common and are likely to be associated with lung cancer and melanomas. Solitary metastases are most often seen in cancer of the colon, breast, and kidney. Neurologic symptoms may be the first clinical manifestations of systemic cancer, easily diagnosed with a chest x-ray examination. CT and MRI detect most metastatic lesions and may differentiate metastases from other intracranial lesions (e.g., abscesses, ischemic lesions). Both tests demonstrate solitary or multiple lesions, the size and site of the lesions, and the surrounding cerebral edema and resultant mass effect.

A. The clinical presentation of brain metastasis varies according to the location of the lesion. The onset of symptoms may be insidious, with headache, mental changes, seizures, weakness, and unsteadiness. However, there may also be a sudden onset of deficit with subsequent stabilization and later progressive deterio-ration. The headache is frequently worse in the morning and suggestive of intracranial hypertension. Papilledema occurs in only 25% of patients with brain metastases. CT may show one or multiple intracranial lesions. In a patient suspected of having intracranial metastasis, perform noncontrast and postcontrast studies. Most metastases appear as hypodense or hyperdense lesions on a noncontrast scan. However, 15% may be isodense (not capable of being detected). Because of the impaired blood-brain barrier, a postcontrast scan utilizing iodinated contrast material is necessary for contrast enhancement of these metastatic lesions. The finding of multiple lesions is highly suggestive of metastasis. If the primary site is known, treat the patient as in D. If the patient is known to have systemic cancer but the CT scan is normal, order a delayed CT scan with increased contrast material (double dose), or MRI.

B. If CT or MRI shows evidence of metastatic disease in a patient with no history of systemic cancer, the primary tumor (source) must be sought. Examine the skin for melanoma, palpate the breasts for masses, and obtain chest x-ray views, as well as CT or MRI of the chest, sputum cytologic examination, and an IV pyelogram. Investigate for occult blood in the stool and order biochemical marker examinations. If the primary source is discovered, treat accordingly. If all the tests are negative, brain biopsy of an accessible lesion may be required, especially if the lesion is solitary.

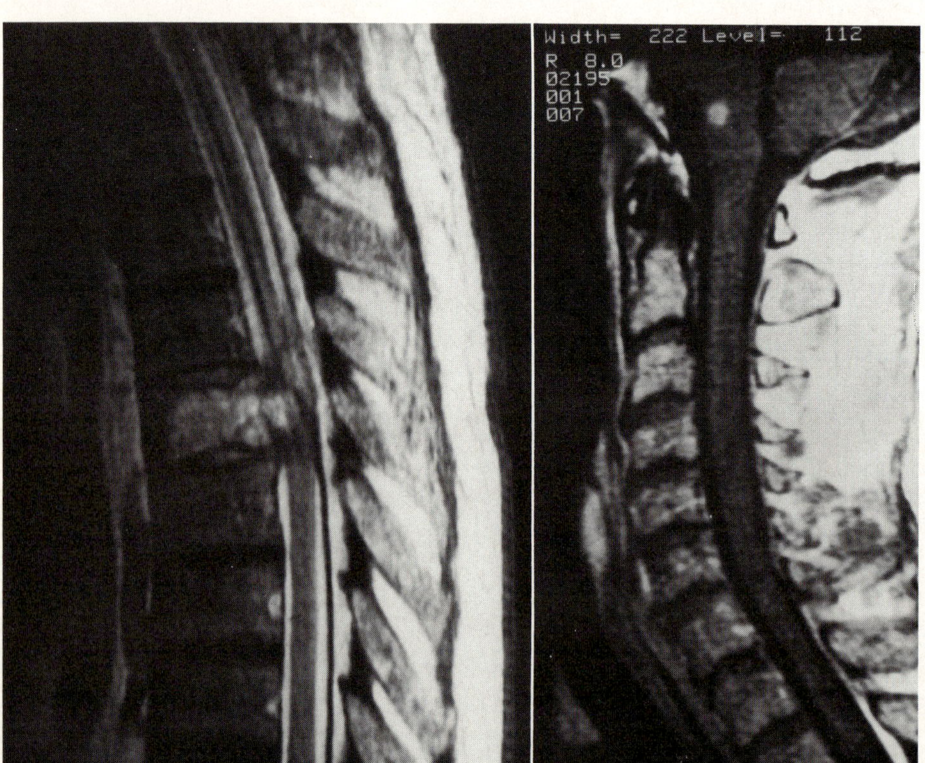

Figure 1 *A*, MRI of the thoracic spine shows a vertebral body lesion causing spinal cord compression. *B*, With the cervical spine MRI, a round, hyperintense medullary brain lesion is also seen. This patient had multiple spinal and brain metastases from adenocarcinoma of the lung.

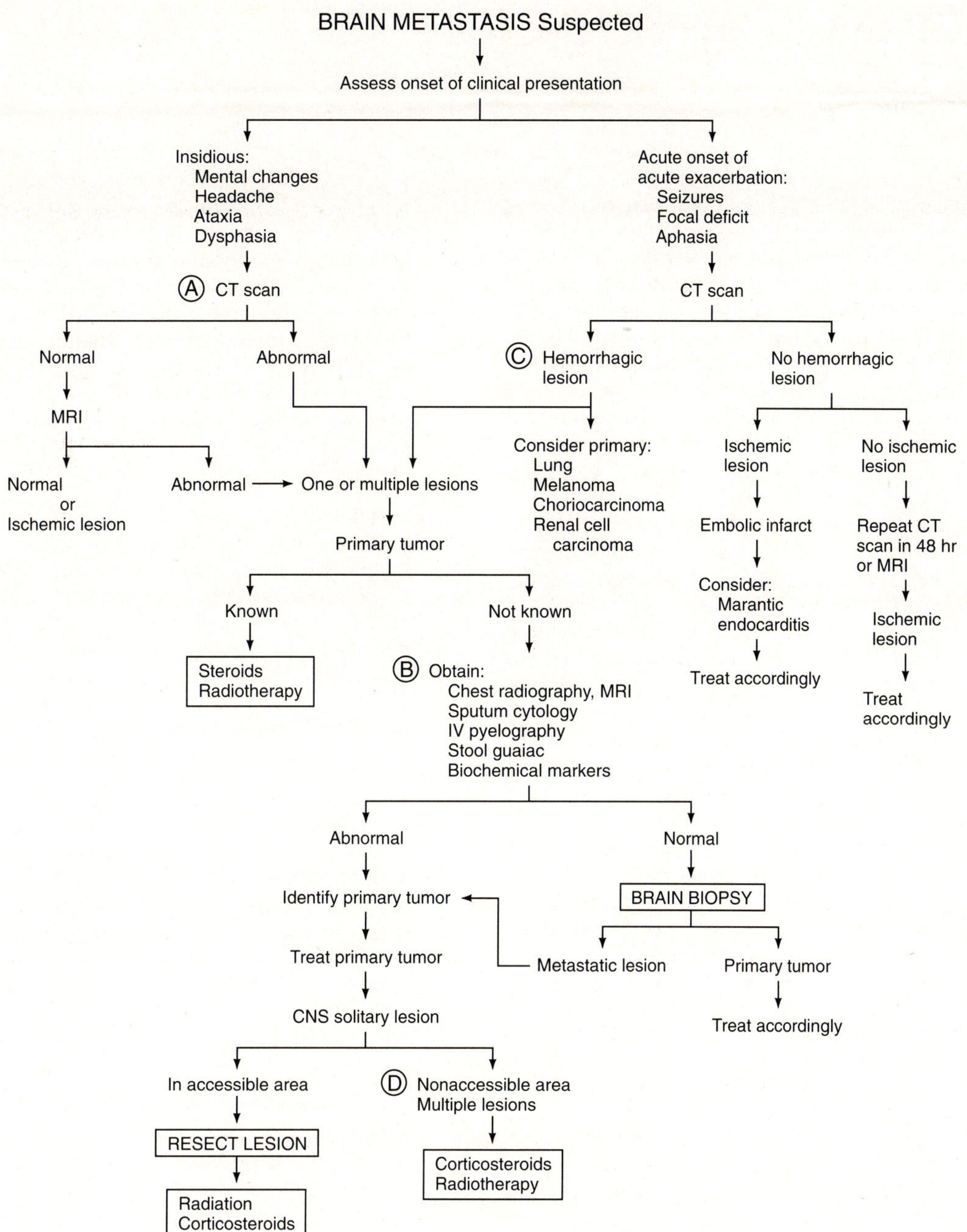

C. There may be an acute onset of neurologic deficit (strokelike presentation) as the first manifestation of a metastasis. An acute exacerbation of neurologic symptoms may also occur in a patient known to have cancer. The sudden onset may be due to either spontaneous bleeding within a metastasis or tumor embolism. CT can confirm the presence of peritumoral bleeding and differentiate it from other lesions. Bleeding is a common occurrence in metastatic melanoma, choriocarcinoma, and renal cell carcinoma, but it may occur in any metastasis. In a patient with systemic cancer in whom there is a sudden onset of neurologic deficit but in whom the CT scan is normal, obtain an MRI. There may be an ischemic rather than a metastatic lesion. Embolic strokes in patients with cancer may originate from nonmarantic bacterial endocarditis. Patients with cancer also may have hypercoagulability that leads to thrombosis.

D. Therapy for metastasis varies according to the extent of the systemic disease, the neurologic status of the patient, and the number and sites of the lesions. Use steroids in all patients to reduce cerebral edema. If a solitary lesion is found and is accessible to surgery, the lesion should be removed and postoperative whole brain radiation therapy carried out. If multiple lesions are found, whole brain irradiation is indicated. Chemotherapy is useful in a few patients.

References

Patchell RA. Brain metastasis. In: Johnson R, ed. Current therapy in neurologic disease. 3rd ed. Philadelphia: BC Decker, 1990:228.

Patchell RA, Posner JB. Neurologic complications of systemic cancer in neurology. Clin Neuro-Oncol 1985; 3:729.

INTRACRANIAL HYPERTENSION

Leon A. Weisberg, M.D.

The intracranial vault contains three compartments: blood vessels (arteries, veins), CSF spaces (ventricles, basal cisterns, sulcal spaces), and brain parenchyma. If there is an increase in size and volume of one or more compartments without a compensatory decrease in another, intracranial hypertension (IH) may result. For example, IH may be due to ventricular obstruction (e.g., obstructive hydrocephalus). IH may result from swelling of brain tissue as may occur in cerebral edema, which may develop with or without an accompanying intracranial mass lesion. IH may result from multiple mechanisms and have many causes. The initial symptom may be headache, which may be in any region, last several hours, be intermittent, fluctuate in intensity, awaken the patient from sleep, or cause nausea and vomiting and visual disturbances (diplopia, visual blurring). The episodic nature of headache may reflect the development of plateau waves of increased intracranial pressure and intermittent and recurring periods of marked IH. These may occur every few hours and each episode may last 20 to 40 minutes. Headache and vomiting may occur during plateau waves and disappear after a fall in CSF pressure. A decrease in the interval between periods of symptoms of IH is an ominous sign that may indicate neurologic deterioration and the development of herniation (transtentorial or tonsillar) syndromes. These syndromes may be due to an expanding intracranial mass lesion that causes distortion and shift of normal brain structures. As a supratentorial mass expands, it compresses and shifts lateral and third ventricles to the opposite side; later, this expanding mass displaces brain structures from one compartment to the other (herniation). In transtentorial herniation, the medial temporal lobe extends through the tentorium to compress the midbrain. Signs of transtentorial herniation are an ipsilateral light-fixed dilated pupil and contralateral hemiparesis. Herniation of cerebellar tonsils downward through the foramen magnum may develop with supratentorial or infratentorial lesions. Signs of tonsillar herniation include elevation of blood pressure, slowing of heart rate, and respiratory depression. These signs are due to medullary compression.

A. If IH develops rapidly, funduscopic examination may not show papilledema. If a patient with IH has meningeal signs (nuchal rigidity, Kernig or Brudzinski sign), lumbar puncture (LP) may be cautiously performed if consciousness is normal and there are no focal signs. Meningitis and subarachnoid hemorrhage (SAH) in the patient with suspected IH may be definitively diagnosed only by CSF examination; very high CSF pressures are frequently recorded in these conditions. In 85% of patients with SAH examined within 48 hours, CT shows intracranial bleeding. CT findings are negative in 15% of cases, and CT is less sensitive as the time after the initial SAH lengthens. In patients with CSF findings consistent with meningitis and funduscopic evidence of papilledema, consider a complicating pathologic process (brain abscess, subdural empyema, venous sinus thrombosis).

B. In patients with initial onset of severe headache (sometimes with visual disturbance, nausea, and vomiting) but without papilledema, nuchal rigidity, or focal signs, consider migraine and SAH. A positive family history and a history of visual disturbance followed by unilateral headache are highly suggestive of migraine. If there are any atypical features in a patient with initial severe headache, LP and CT/MRI may be necessary. In migraine, findings from these studies are normal; in SAH, LP shows bloody or xanthochromic CSF.

C. If papilledema is present with focal signs or impaired consciousness, consider a mass lesion or obstructive hydrocephalus. Depending on the clinical findings, the lesion may be supratentorial or infratentorial and may be midline or lateralized. Gait disturbance and impaired consciousness may result from hydrocephalus alone. The diagnosis of hydrocephalus is established by CT/MRI. Unilateral or bilateral abducens paresis in a patient with papilledema may result from stretching of abducens nerve fibers secondary to IH.

D. Papilledema with gait ataxia, limb ataxia, and incoordination suggests an infratentorial lesion, midline or lateralized. Midline infratentorial tumors (medulloblastoma, ependymoma) may also cause IH without lateralizing signs. Papilledema with hemiparesis, altered consciousness, and seizures indicates a lateralized supratentorial mass. Evidence of IH in the patient with a chiasmal visual field defect is consistent with a midline tumor (craniopharyngioma, juxtasellar tumor such as meningioma, pinealoma).

E. In patients with papilledema but no focal signs, normal blood pressure excludes hypertensive encephalopathy (see p 154). If CT/MRI shows no ventricular abnormalities, perform LP to differentiate pseudotumor cerebri from meningitis or SAH. If hydrocephalus is present, evaluate CT carefully for an intraventricular mass; this may be small and difficult to visualize by CT/MRI. If no mass is seen, consider aqueductal stenosis. It may be difficult to define the cause of ventricular obstruction in aqueductal stenosis even with CT/MRI.

References

Cervos-Novano J, Ferszt R, eds. Brain edema; pathology, diagnosis and therapy. Adv Neurol 1980; 28:1.

Fishman RA. Brain edema. N Engl J Med 1975; 14:706.

Plum F, Posner J. Diagnosis of stupor and coma. Philadelphia: FA Davis, 1986:30.

Weisberg LA. Intracranial neoplasms. Neurol Clin 1984; 2:695.

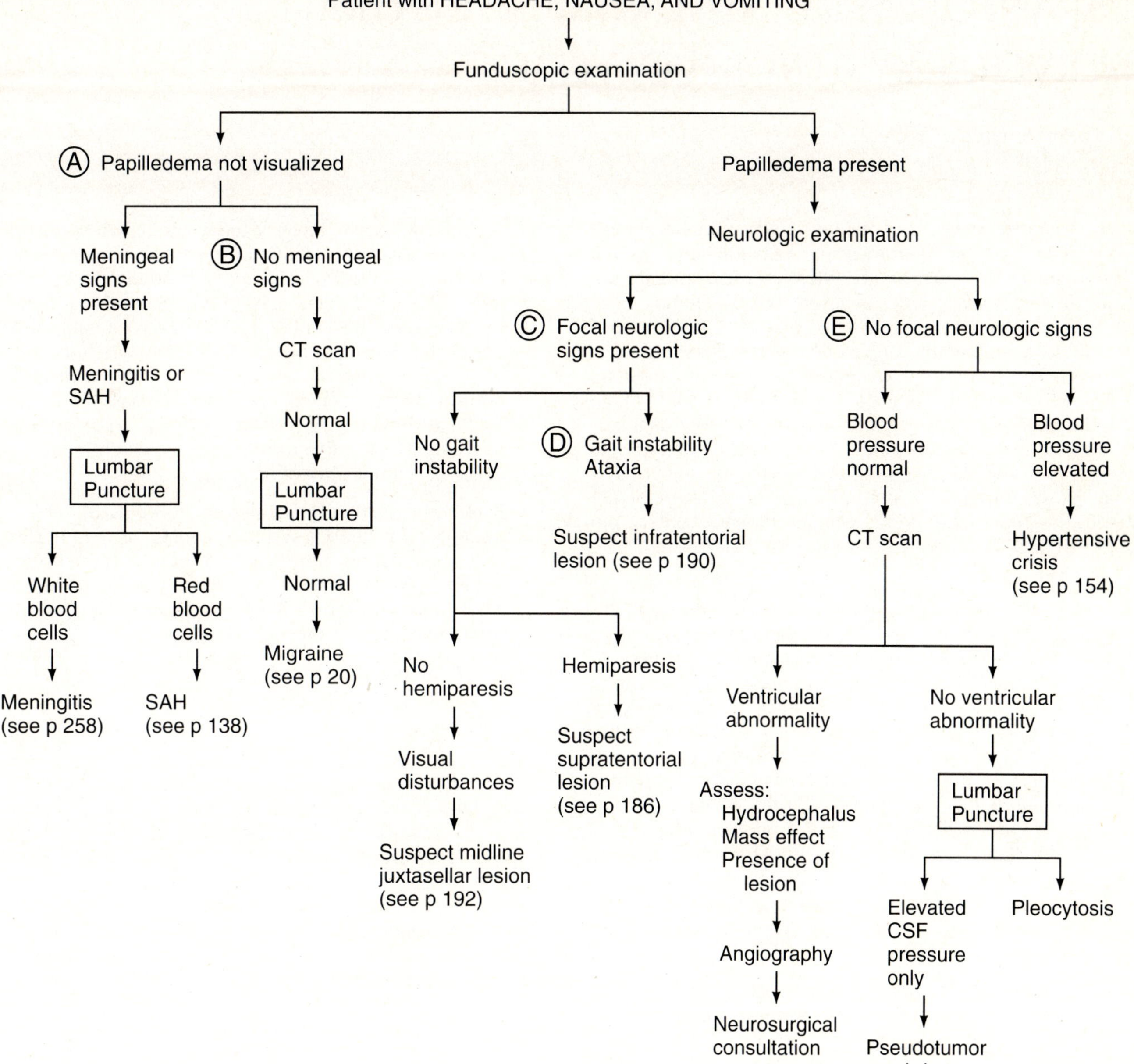

Patient with HEADACHE, NAUSEA, AND VOMITING
Funduscopic examination
A Papilledema not visualized
Papilledema present
Neurologic examination
Meningeal signs present
B No meningeal signs
Meningitis or SAH
CT scan
Normal
Lumbar Puncture
Lumbar Puncture
White blood cells
Red blood cells
Normal
Meningitis (see p 258)
SAH (see p 138)
Migraine (see p 20)
C Focal neurologic signs present
E No focal neurologic signs
No gait instability
D Gait instability Ataxia
Blood pressure normal
Blood pressure elevated
Suspect infratentorial lesion (see p 190)
CT scan
Hypertensive crisis (see p 154)
No hemiparesis
Hemiparesis
Ventricular abnormality
No ventricular abnormality
Visual disturbances
Suspect supratentorial lesion (see p 186)
Assess: Hydrocephalus Mass effect Presence of lesion
Lumbar Puncture
Suspect midline juxtasellar lesion (see p 192)
Angiography
Elevated CSF pressure only
Pleocytosis
Neurosurgical consultation
Pseudotumor cerebri

PARANEOPLASTIC SYNDROMES: CENTRAL NERVOUS SYSTEM INVOLVEMENT

Carlos A. Garcia, M.D.

Paraneoplastic syndromes include CNS, peripheral nervous system (PNS), neuromuscular junction, and muscle abnormalities in patients with systemic cancer that are not due to direct metastatic invasion by the tumor. The abnormalities cannot be explained by the effects of radiotherapy, chemotherapy, or secondary infections in cancer patients. The syndrome is of undetermined etiology, but an immune mechanism has been demonstrated in some of the conditions (myasthenic syndrome and cerebellar degeneration). In approximately half of the patients the neurologic symptoms precede the finding of systemic cancer. The effects may produce symptoms in different areas of the neuromuscular system independent of each other, but more frequently combinations of more than one area are involved.

A. If a patient known to have systemic cancer shows CNS symptoms, there most likely is metastatic disease that can be demonstrated with neuroradiologic studies. If the initial CT scan shows no metastasis, obtain a "double dose" contrast CT scan or carry out MRI. If findings are negative, perform a lumbar puncture for CSF cytologic study. If cytologic examination reveals tumor cells, the most likely diagnosis is carcinomatous leptomeningitis. Remember that this is often secondary to adenocarcinomas (breast, gastrointestinal system); treat accordingly. If the cytologic study is negative for neoplastic cells, the CSF may be normal or may show lymphocytic pleocytosis with a normal glucose level and negative cultures. In such a case, remote effects of cancer in the CNS are most likely.

B. If a patient with known systemic cancer and negative neuroradiologic studies for metastatic disease presents with anxiety, memory loss, and intellectual impairment, you are most likely dealing with the remote effects of cancer. The patient may have seizures and hallucinations, and some individuals may have spinal cord symptoms of encephalomyelitis. The dementia is usually secondary to bilateral atrophic medial temporal lobe lesions.

C. A patient known to have systemic cancer who presents with an insidious onset of a progressive pancerebellar syndrome, including nystagmus, head titubation, dysarthric speech, truncal ataxia, and incoordination and dysmetria of the upper extremities, probably has cerebellar degeneration due to the remote effects of a tumor. Dementia is a frequent associated finding. Some patients develop opsoclonus (erratic, involuntary eye movements that worsen with voluntary eye movements and fixation of sight), which indicates brain stem involvement.

D. Symptoms of spinal cord dysfunction may be seen in patients with known systemic cancer. If neuroradiologic studies do not reveal a tumor mass in the vertebra, epidural space, or cord (negative findings on MRI), there is most likely myelopathy due to the remote effects of cancer.

E. Optic neuropathy (either unilateral but most often bilateral) is an extremely rare remote effect of systemic cancer.

When the patient presents with any of the syndromes described above but is not known to have systemic cancer, try to find a primary tumor. Perform chest x-ray examination, CT or MRI of the chest, and sputum cytologic examination, followed by IV pyelography, CT or MRI of the abdomen, a bone scan, and a bone marrow examination. If all the tests are negative, repeat selected tests in 3 and 6 months according to systemic symptoms or signs. Determination of paraneoplastic autoantibodies in blood and CSF can help in the diagnosis.

References

Furmeau HF, Reich L, Posner JB. Autoantibody synthesis in the central nervous system of patients with paraneoplastic syndromes. Neurology 1990; 40:1085.

Patchell RA, Posner JB. Neurologic complications of systemic cancer. Neurol Clin North Am 1985; 3:729.

PARANEOPLASTIC SYNDROMES:
CENTRAL NERVOUS SYSTEM INVOLVEMENT Suspected

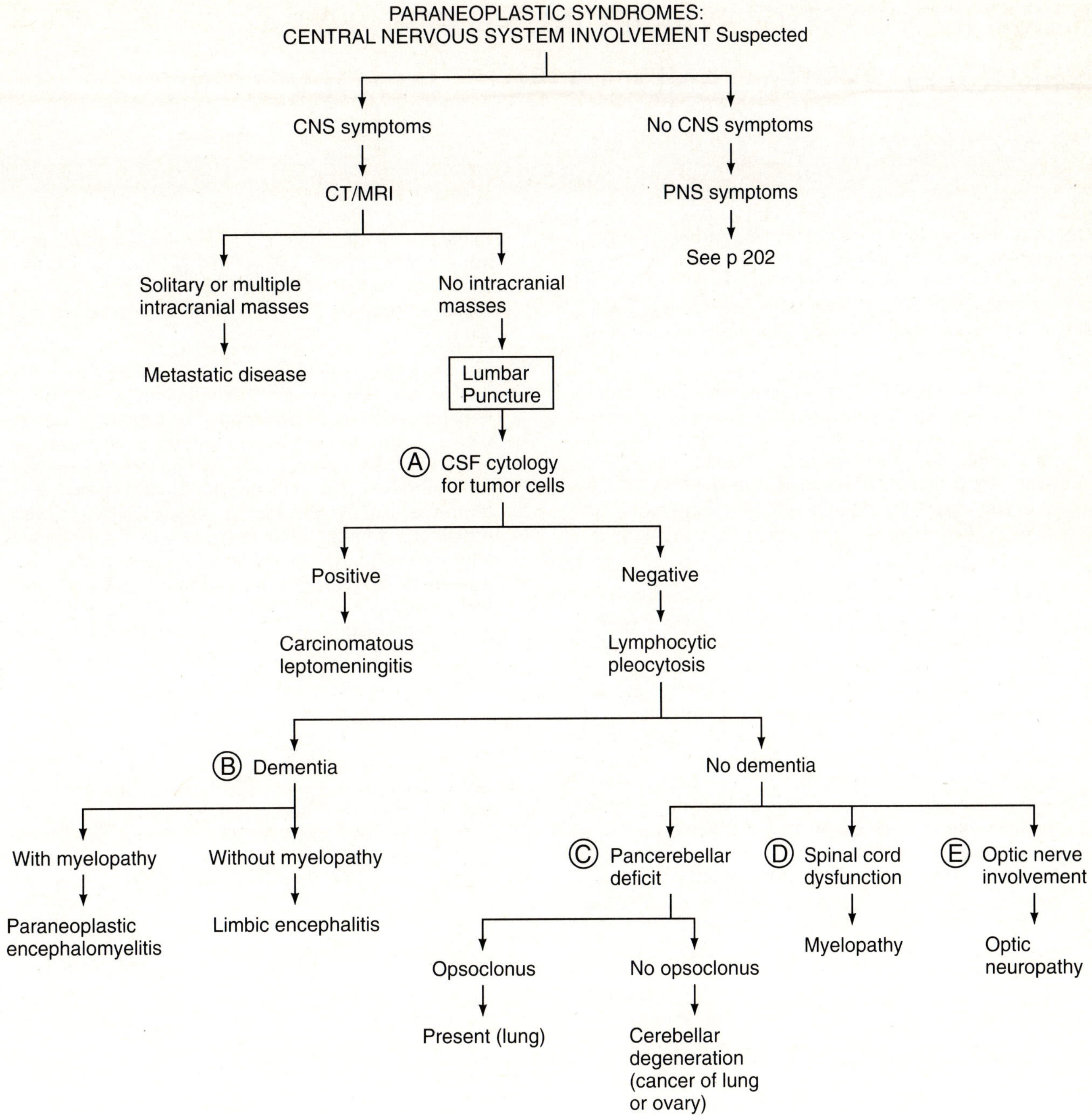

PARANEOPLASTIC SYNDROMES: PERIPHERAL NERVOUS SYSTEM AND MUSCLE INVOLVEMENT

Carlos A. Garcia, M.D.

The peripheral nervous system, muscles, and neuromuscular junctions are more frequently affected than the CNS in paraneoplastic syndromes. When peripheral nerves and plexuses are involved in patients with systemic tumors, the differentiation between direct invasion and paraneoplastic syndromes is difficult.

A. When the diagnosis of dermatomyositis is made in a male >50 years of age, consider an association with a small cell carcinoma of the lung or another tumor. The dermatomyositis does not differ clinically or histologically from that not associated with tumors and may precede discovery of the tumor by several months or years.

B. The peripheral nerves may be affected when there is systemic cancer. Guillain-Barré syndrome most frequently occurs in young patients and rarely is associated with cancer; however, occasional cases have been associated with lymphomas. Most often, a subacute sensory neuronopathy (inflammatory destruction of the dorsal root ganglia) of insidious onset may be associated with systemic cancer. The neuronopathies are manifested by dysesthesias or hypesthesias along with severe appendicular and truncal ataxia dependent on visual cues. Also, painful, predominantly sensory neuropathy may be associated with carcinoma, lymphoma, or osteolytic myeloma. In some patients, autonomic dysfunction may be the first manifestation of a neuropathy, or the symptoms may appear in a patient known to have polyneuropathy associated with systemic cancer. Painless motor neuropathies may be associated with osteosclerotic myeloma.

C. The association of myasthenia gravis with thymoma is well known. The disease predominantly affects young females and is characterized by fatigability, a decremental response of muscle contraction to repetitive nerve stimulation, and anti-acetylcholine (ACh) receptor antibodies. The patient with Eaton-Lambert syndrome is usually an older male who presents with proximal extremity weakness that seems to improve after some activity. There is areflexia, which improves after exercise; there are no antibodies in the serum, and repetitive nerve stimulation shows increments in muscle contraction. Eaton-Lambert syndrome is associated predominantly with small cell tumors of the lung.

References

Antel JP, Moundjiam R. Paraneoplastic syndrome: A role for the immune system. J Neurol 1989; 236:1.

Asbury AK. Sensory neuronopathy. Semin Neurol 1987; 7:58.

Patchell RA, Posner JB. Neurologic complications of systemic cancer. Neurol Clin North Am 1985; 3:729.

PARANEOPLASTIC SYNDROMES:
PERIPHERAL NERVOUS SYSTEM AND MUSCLE INVOLVEMENT Suspected

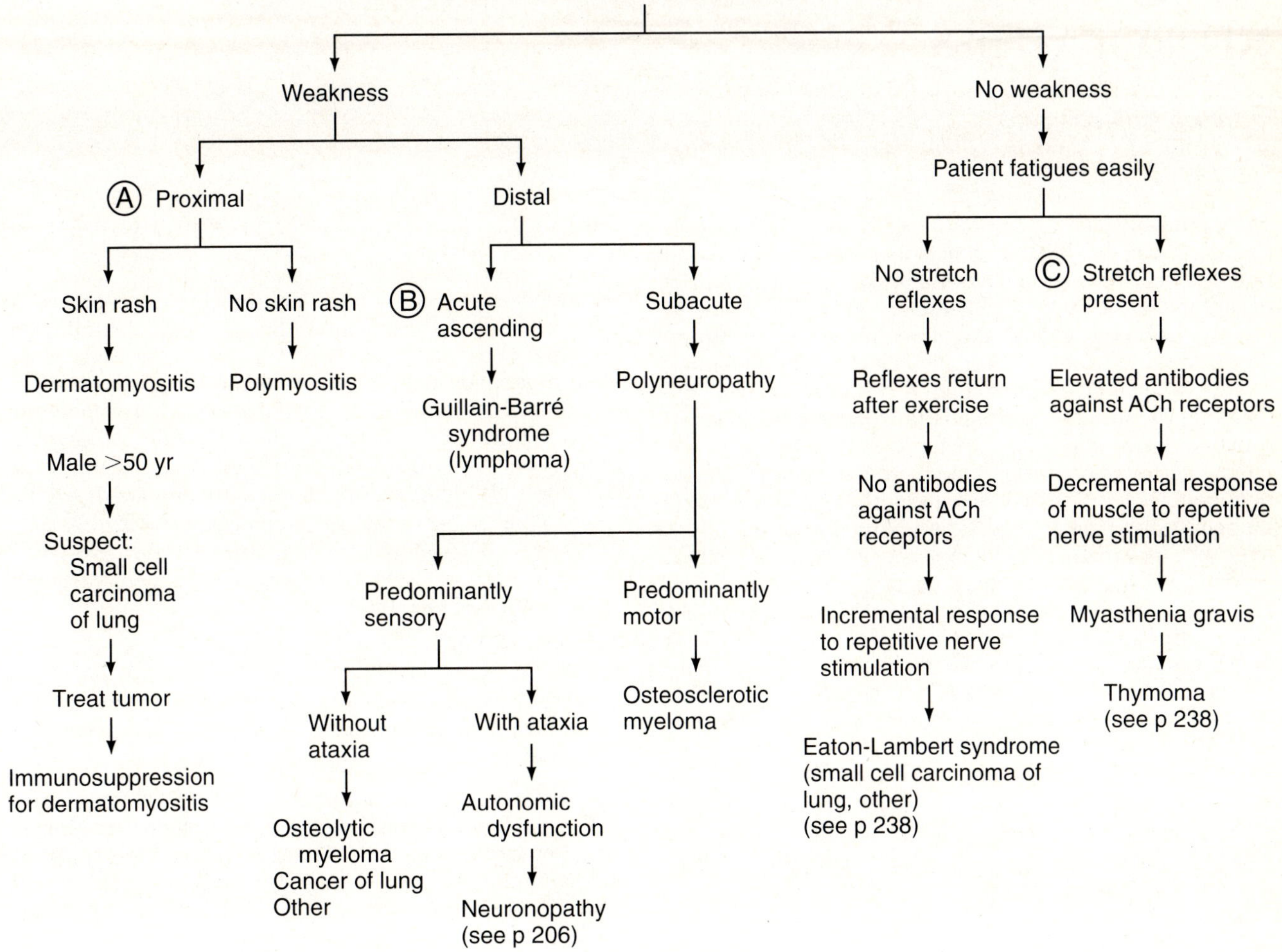

PERIPHERAL NERVOUS DISORDERS

NEUROPATHIES

Carlos A. Garcia, M.D.

The peripheral nerves can be affected by a multitude of disease processes, but the clinical features are limited and nonspecific. The neuropathies usually present with sensory disturbances, including paresthesias or motor disturbances, such as weakness. Examination often reveals both components. Motor disturbances usually begin distally, predominantly in the lower extremities, ascend proximally, and then may involve the hands and trunk. Symmetric polyneuropathies invariably begin in the feet and rarely in the hands. If symptoms begin in the hands, consider localized neuropathies (e.g., carpal tunnel syndrome, cervical radiculopathy) or a spinal cord lesion. Autonomic symptoms may be the main presentation in the dysautonomias (Riley-Day syndrome) or may be part of a more severe polyneuropathy (diabetes). The autonomic symptoms include orthostatic hypotension; heat intolerance associated with excessive sweating or localized anhidrosis; urinary bladder dysfunction manifested by difficulty in voiding or dribbling after urination; sexual impotence or retrograde ejaculation; decreased tearing or pupillary abnormalities; and painless, usually nocturnal diarrhea.

The clinical features of the most common neuropathies include weakness (usually distal), subacute atrophy of affected muscles, areflexia, and sensory deficit in a stocking and glove (polyneuropathies) or neuronal (mononeuropathy) distribution. The diagnosis may be confirmed and better defined by electrophysiologic studies, including nerve conduction velocity and latency studies. Nerve biopsy, when indicated, should be performed by an expert and the specimen processed in a laboratory with experience in the field.

The causes of cranial polyneuropathies include diabetes, sarcoidosis, granulomatosis, and neoplastic meningitis. Diagnostic studies include a blood cell count, chest radiography, blood sugar level, CT or MRI of the head, and lumbar puncture for spinal fluid cytologic study.

A. Once the diagnosis of neuropathy is suspected or established, the examiner should answer the following questions. Is it an isolated lesion of one nerve (mononeuropathy)? Are multiple isolated nerves affected (multiple mononeuropathy, "mononeuritis multiplex")? Or is there symmetric bilateral involvement of nerves (polyneuropathy)? If so, are the spinal roots also involved (polyradiculoneuropathy)? Are the cranial nerves affected (cranial neuropathy) or is an entire plexus affected (plexopathy)? Are the axons affected (axonopathy) or the myelin (demyelinating neuropathy), or both?

B. The evolution of the disease process is also important, since acute lesions are usually compressive, traumatic, or vascular in origin. The subacute form may be infectious; the chronic form is usually genetically determined or of undetermined cause.

C. Answers to all these questions should provide a better idea of the disease process and potential etiologies. Remember that the two most common nonentrapment neuropathies are caused by diabetes mellitus and alcoholism. In at least 25% of patients with polyneuropathy, the cause is never found.

Reference

Thomas PK. Clinical features and differential diagnosis. In: Dyck PJ, Thomas PK, Lambert EH, Bunge R, eds. Peripheral neuropathy. 2nd ed. Philadelphia: WB Saunders, 1984:1169.

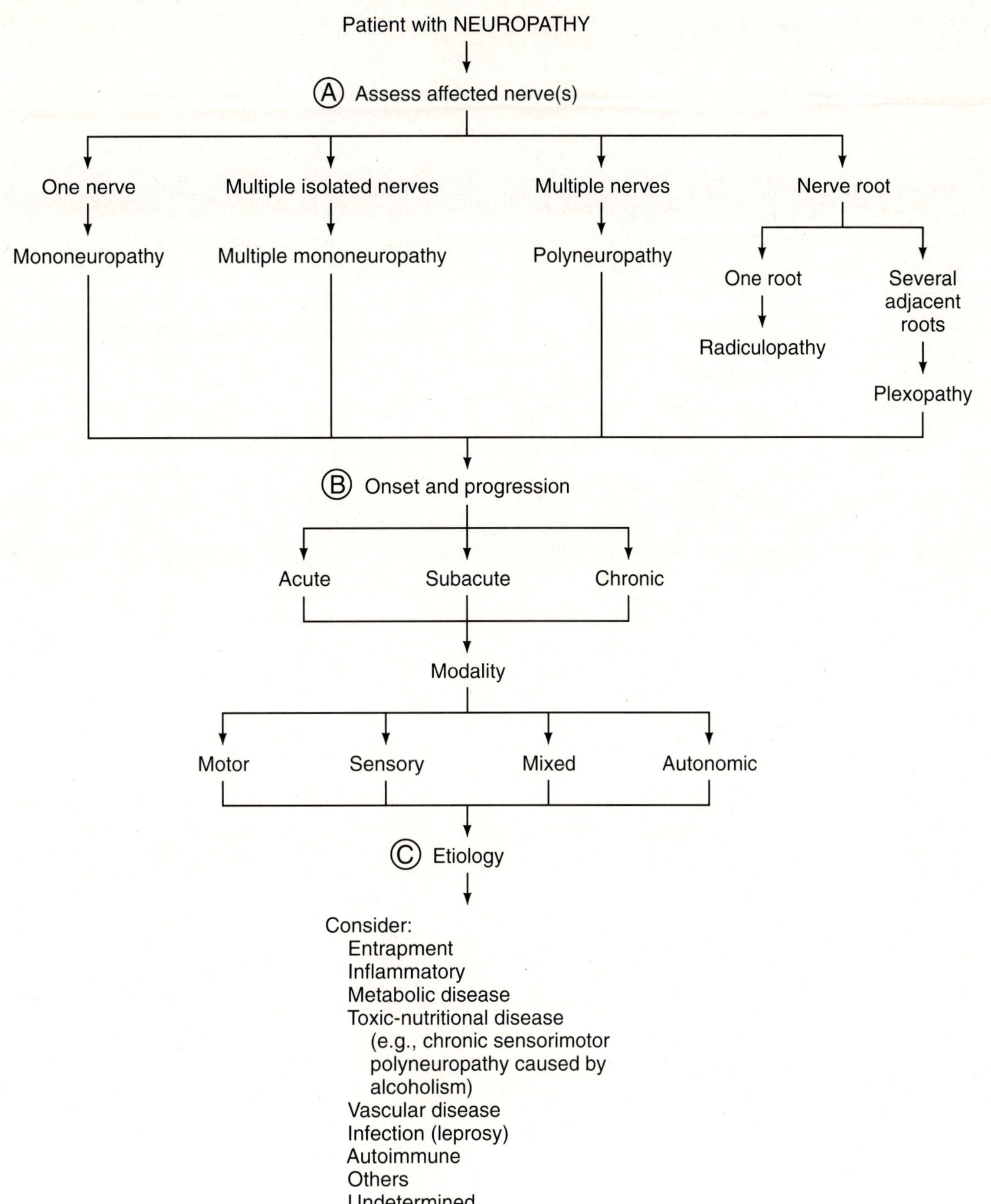

Patient with NEUROPATHY
A Assess affected nerve(s)
One nerve
Multiple isolated nerves
Multiple nerves
Nerve root
Mononeuropathy
Multiple mononeuropathy
Polyneuropathy
One root
Several adjacent roots
Radiculopathy
Plexopathy
B Onset and progression
Acute
Subacute
Chronic
Modality
Motor
Sensory
Mixed
Autonomic
C Etiology
Consider:
Entrapment
Inflammatory
Metabolic disease
Toxic-nutritional disease
(e.g., chronic sensorimotor
polyneuropathy caused by
alcoholism)
Vascular disease
Infection (leprosy)
Autoimmune
Others
Undetermined

POLYNEUROPATHIES

Carlos A. Garcia, M.D.

Most polyneuropathies are mixed (sensorimotor) and are distal and symmetric. However, polyneuropathies may have predominant sensory or motor components. Only a few representative varieties are described below. Diabetes may produce any type of neuropathy and is described separately.

A. Diabetic neuropathy is the most common of all neuropathies. The most frequent form is symmetric sensory polyneuropathy, which may present suddenly or insidiously with a sensation of burning feet, mainly during the night. Sensory examination shows decreased sensation to touch, pricking pain, and vibratory stimuli. In some cases the sensory loss is severe and involves all sensory modalities, producing a sensory ataxia that may be associated with painless arthropathy and absence of the pupillary light reflex, resembling tabes dorsalis ("diabetic pseudotabes"). Motor symptoms eventually accompany the sensory polyneuropathy and are manifested as distal motor weakness (motor polyneuropathy). Symptoms of autonomic dysfunction are not unusual and may include pupillary and lacrimal gland dysfunction, postural hypotension, distal anhidrosis, nocturnal painless diarrhea, and urinary bladder dysfunction. Diabetic patients may also present with isolated cranial neuropathies due to ischemia of the cranial nerves. The most common cranial neuropathy is that of the third nerve, followed by that of the sixth nerve. The same ischemic mechanism, vascular occlusion of the nerve vessels, is seen in femoral neuropathy (diabetic amyotrophy), which presents with painful weakness of the quadriceps muscle, early atrophy, and absence of the patellar reflex.

B. Leprosy is an infectious, predominantly sensory polyneuropathy caused by *Mycobacterium leprae*. The neuropathy is often associated with skin lesions, is predominantly sensory, and is seen in cool areas of the skin. The patient often presents with painless injuries. Nerve enlargement is a predominant feature of the disease.

C. Vitamin B_{12} deficiency is usually associated with a myelopathy, and the symptoms and signs may be obscured by the posterior column lesion. Some of the hereditary neuropathies are mainly sensory and extremely rare and usually present as painless injuries or mutilations. Thallium produces a marked dysesthesia and is associated with a striking loss of hair. Arsenic produces predominantly sensory symptoms, usually affecting the lower extremities.

D. In a patient with subacute polyneuropathy that is predominantly motor who has nerve conduction blocks on the nerve conduction velocity test, consider chronic inflammatory demyelinating polyneuropathy (CIDP). The CSF frequently shows elevated CSF protein. CIDP responds to treatment with plasmapheresis, IV immunoglobulin G (IV IgG), or immunosuppressive therapy.

E. Predominantly motor polyneuropathies include the Guillain-Barré syndrome (GBS, see p 208) and, less frequently, porphyria, lead intoxication (wrist drop), and diphtheria. Porphyric neuropathy is a rare neurologic manifestation of the hereditary hepatic porphyrias. The disease is rare and familial and usually begins with motor symptoms involving the upper extremities, mainly weakness of the wrist and finger flexors. Sensory symptoms may be present, and sympathetic overactivity (hypertension, tachycardia) may appear during the disease course. The symptoms of neuropathy are usually preceded by abdominal pain and by restlessness, insomnia, and hallucinations, all suggestive of a psychiatric disturbance. The diagnosis of porphyria is confirmed by the finding of porphobilinogen in the urine and porphyrins in the stools early in the attack. The crisis may be precipitated by ingestion of alcohol or the use of barbiturates.

F. Hereditary motor and sensory neuropathy (HMSN type 1), also known as Charcot-Marie-Tooth (CMT-1), is an autosomal dominantly inherited disease that affects the peroneal nerve, producing foot drop, with a characteristic steppage (equine) gait and the appearance of "stork legs." Atrophy of the hands ("clawed") is a late event. The disease is self-limited.

G. Uremic polyneuropathy, a mixed variety, has an insidious onset, usually correlating with renal failure and improving with dialysis. The patient usually demonstrates weakness and atrophy and decreased sensation in a stocking distribution. Multiple myeloma and other dysproteinemias produce a mixed sensorimotor neuropathy. Symptoms of autonomic dysfunction may be seen as part of a more diffuse disease, as in diabetes mellitus and alcoholism. Autonomic dysfunction may be prominent in amyloid neuropathy and in primary dysautonomias; these are rare diseases.

References

Dyck PJ, Thomas PK, Asbury AK, et al. Diabetic neuropathy. Philadelphia: WB Saunders, 1987.

Thomas PK. Clinical features and differential diagnosis. In: Dyck PJ, Thomas PK, Lambert EH, Bunge R, eds. Peripheral neuropathy. 2nd ed. Philadelphia: WB Saunders, 1984:1169.

VanDoor PA, Brand A, Strengers PFW, et al. High-dose intravenous immunoglobulin treatment in chronic inflammatory demyelinating polyneuropathy: A double-blind, placebo-controlled, crossover study. Neurology 1990; 40:209.

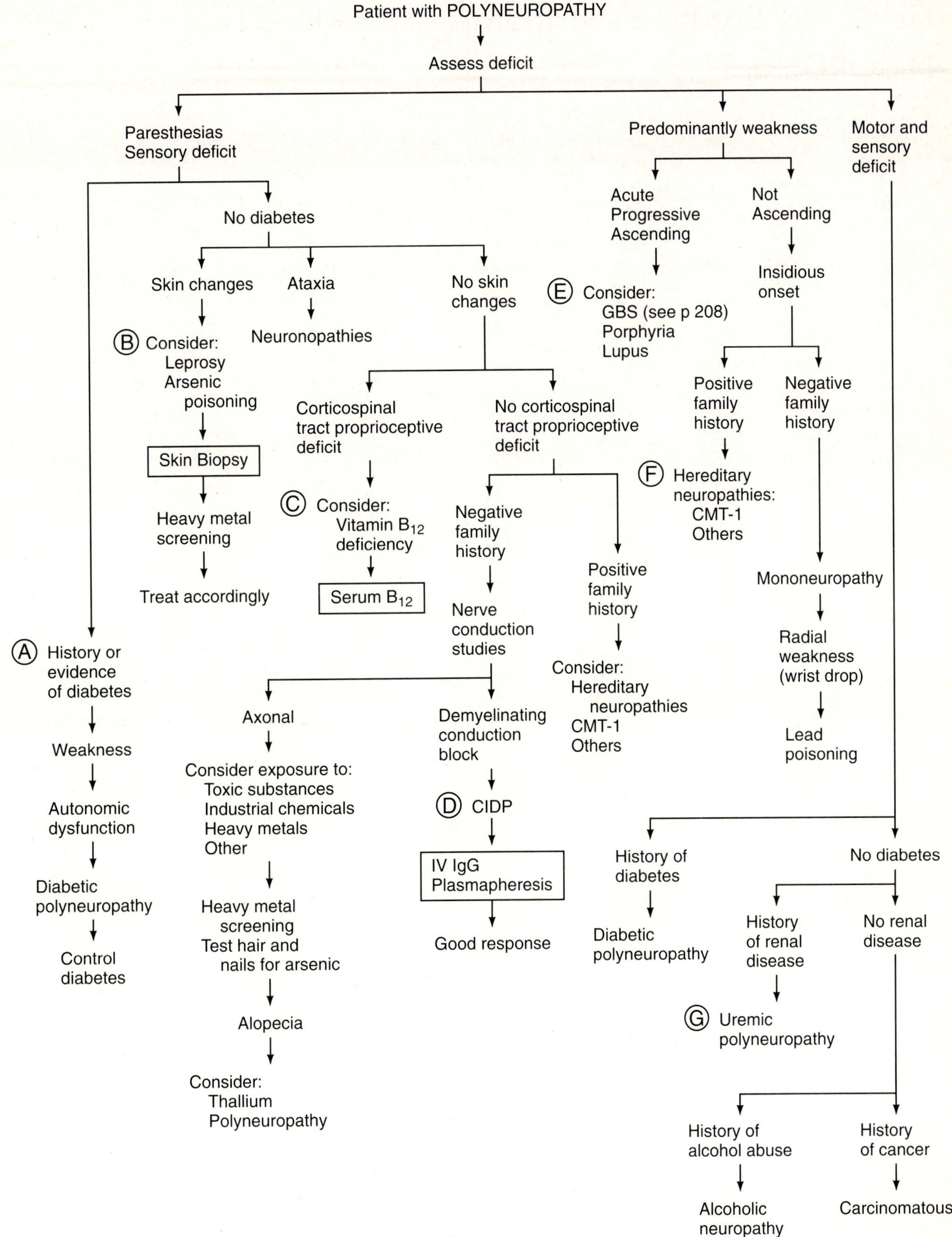

Patient with POLYNEUROPATHY
Assess deficit

Paresthesias
Sensory deficit

Predominantly weakness

Motor and
sensory
deficit

No diabetes

Acute
Progressive
Ascending

Not
Ascending

Skin changes

Ataxia

No skin
changes

E Consider:
GBS (see p 208)
Porphyria
Lupus

Insidious
onset

B Consider:
Leprosy
Arsenic
poisoning

Neuronopathies

Positive
family
history

Negative
family
history

Skin Biopsy

Corticospinal
tract proprioceptive
deficit

No corticospinal
tract proprioceptive
deficit

F Hereditary
neuropathies:
CMT-1
Others

Heavy metal
screening

C Consider:
Vitamin B$_{12}$
deficiency

Negative
family
history

Positive
family
history

Mononeuropathy

Treat accordingly

Serum B$_{12}$

Nerve
conduction
studies

Consider:
Hereditary
neuropathies
CMT-1
Others

Radial
weakness
(wrist drop)

A History or
evidence
of diabetes

Lead
poisoning

Weakness

Axonal

Demyelinating
conduction
block

Autonomic
dysfunction

Consider exposure to:
Toxic substances
Industrial chemicals
Heavy metals
Other

D CIDP

Diabetic
polyneuropathy

IV IgG
Plasmapheresis

History of
diabetes

No diabetes

Control
diabetes

Heavy metal
screening
Test hair and
nails for arsenic

Good response

Diabetic
polyneuropathy

History
of renal
disease

No renal
disease

Alopecia

G Uremic
polyneuropathy

Consider:
Thallium
Polyneuropathy

History of
alcohol abuse

History
of cancer

Alcoholic
neuropathy

Carcinomatous

GUILLAIN-BARRÉ SYNDROME AND RELATED DISORDERS

Carlos A. Garcia, M.D.

Guillain-Barré syndrome (GBS) is a demyelinating polyneuropathy of acute onset and rapid progression that manifests as weakness, which may be ascending when it begins in the legs or descending when it begins in the arms. Although it is primarily a motor neuropathy, paresthesias are often experienced early in the disease, and rare patients have sensory loss. The disease is most likely immunologically mediated and frequently preceded by viral infections, surgery, *Mycoplasma* infections, and vaccinations. Preexisting illnesses include lymphomas, systemic lupus erythematosus (SLE), and Hodgkin's disease.

A. GBS is a frequent cause of acute progressive (usually ascending) paralysis. In some cases the onset of the weakness is proximal and descending (radiculopathy), but it may start in the cranial nerves with bilateral seventh nerve palsy (facial diplegia). Bulbar muscles may be affected early. Papilledema has been found in association with a high CSF protein level. In <5% of cases the disease begins with involvement of the extraocular muscles. Dissemination of the weakness is usually the rule.

B. Clinical features strongly supportive of the diagnosis of GBS include relative symmetry and rapid progression of the weakness, mild sensory symptoms, autonomic dysfunction, and recovery before the fourth week after onset. Monitor respiratory function early in the course of the disease; ideally the patient should be placed in an intensive care unit so that rapid intubation can be carried out when needed. Consider prophylactic tracheostomy if is necessary. Variable symptoms in GBS include fever, severe sensory loss with pain, progression beyond 4 weeks, sphincter dysfunction, and CNS involvement. Spinal fluid albumino-cytologic dissociation with a high protein level and a low blood cell count is usually seen after the first week. Treatment consists of general medical care. Plasmapheresis seems to speed recovery in most patients. IV immunoglobulin (IV IgG) is at least as effective or may be superior to plasma exchange. Physical therapy and respiratory therapy should begin at the bedside. Relapses are rare but occasionally occur after 2 or 3 weeks.

C. In all cases of acute ascending paralysis seen in children and young adults, examine the head and neck for a tick. This is especially suggested when the spinal fluid protein level remains within normal limits. Tick paralysis is rare but should always be kept in mind. Removal of the tick improves the weakness within 7 days.

D. When some atypical features (e.g., decreased sensation) are found, inquire about abdominal pain and personality changes. Order determinations of porphobilinogen and delta-aminolevulinic acid in the urine; all these tests when positive indicate acute intermittent porphyria.

E. Predominant bulbar involvement after a laryngeal infection is highly suggestive of postdiphtheritic polyneuropathy. Other causes of ascending paralysis include SLE and recent exposure to commercial solvents such as *n*-hexane. When wrist drop is a dominant feature, investigate for heavy metal or lead exposure and obtain lead levels.

F. A rare syndrome described by Miller-Fisher consists of the rapid onset of ophthalmoplegia, ataxia, and areflexia with an elevated spinal fluid protein level. The syndrome is usually benign, with fairly complete recovery within weeks to months.

References

Asbury AK. Diagnostic considerations in Guillain-Barré syndrome. Ann Neurol 1981; 9(Suppl):1.

VanDerMeché FGA, Schmitz PIM, Dutch Guillain-Barré Study Group. A randomized trial comparing intravenous immune globulin and plasma exchange in Guillain-Barré syndrome. N Engl J Med 1992; 326:1123.

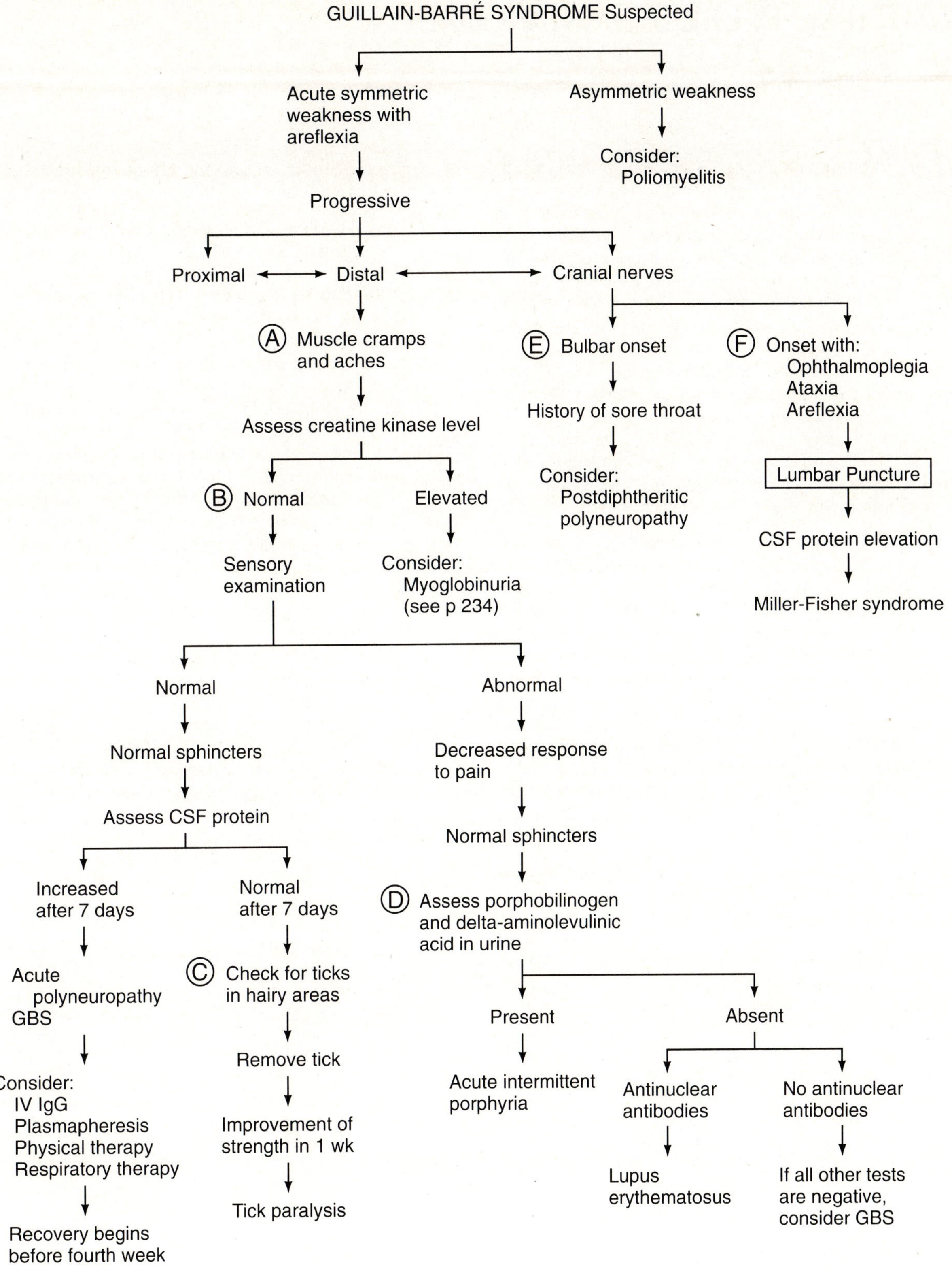

GUILLAIN-BARRÉ SYNDROME Suspected
Acute symmetric weakness with areflexia
Asymmetric weakness
Consider: Poliomyelitis
Progressive
Proximal
Distal
Cranial nerves
A Muscle cramps and aches
E Bulbar onset
F Onset with: Ophthalmoplegia Ataxia Areflexia
Assess creatine kinase level
History of sore throat
Lumbar Puncture
B Normal
Elevated
Consider: Postdiphtheritic polyneuropathy
CSF protein elevation
Sensory examination
Consider: Myoglobinuria (see p 234)
Miller-Fisher syndrome
Normal
Abnormal
Normal sphincters
Decreased response to pain
Assess CSF protein
Normal sphincters
Increased after 7 days
Normal after 7 days
D Assess porphobilinogen and delta-aminolevulinic acid in urine
Acute polyneuropathy GBS
C Check for ticks in hairy areas
Present
Absent
Consider: IV IgG Plasmapheresis Physical therapy Respiratory therapy
Remove tick
Acute intermittent porphyria
Antinuclear antibodies
No antinuclear antibodies
Improvement of strength in 1 wk
Lupus erythematosus
If all other tests are negative, consider GBS
Recovery begins before fourth week
Tick paralysis

BRACHIAL PLEXUS SYNDROME

Carlos A. Garcia, M.D.

In dealing with brachial plexus lesions, be familiar with the anatomy of the structures, the innervation of the muscles of the shoulder and upper extremity, and the sensory mapping. The clinical findings and electromyographic (EMG) changes can aid in localizing the lesion precisely. The superficial location of the plexus and its relation to the shoulder readily expose the structure to multiple and varied traumatic injuries. Most traumatic injuries are self-evident and should be treated in the acute phase by a surgical or orthopedic service. The development of magnification techniques for use during neurosurgical intervention, intra-operative nerve stimulation and recording procedures, and improvement in nerve grafting techniques have improved the management and results in patients with these lesions and made surgical repair more feasible. We deal here only with nonsurgical brachial plexus disorders.

A. Radiation plexopathy usually starts as a painless, slowly progressive weakness of one (unilateral) upper extremity. The lesion usually starts with involvement of the upper plexus (75%) and manifests as weakness of the deltoid, supraspinous, and infraspinous muscles. The disease may progress to involve the entire plexus. Such patients have a history of radiation therapy, usually for breast or lung cancer. There may be induration and scar formation in the supraclavicular fossa. MRI of the upper chest and cervical spine confirms the presence of a brachial plexus lesion. Surgery may be necessary to remove adhesions and fibrosis compressing the brachial plexus and decrease symptoms.

B. Neoplastic brachial plexopathy usually begins as an acute, excruciatingly painful syndrome affecting the arm and hand. The lesion is unilateral and most frequently is caused by carcinoma of the upper lobe of the lung (Pancoast's tumor) or carcinoma of the breast. The pain is usually constant and may be increased by arm movements, but there is no posturing to prevent pain. The lesion affects the lower plexus, producing weakness and atrophy of the hand and arm muscles and a sensory deficit in the ulnar distribution. The disease progresses to involve the entire plexus. Horner's syndrome (ptosis, miosis, and anhydrosis of the face) may be present. CT or MRI of the shoulder and axillary area may reveal the nature of the lesion.

C. Brachial plexus neuropathy (neuralgic amyotrophy), also known as brachial plexitis, is a disease of undetermined etiology. In some cases it is associated with serum inoculations or the use of tetanus toxoid, or may be seen after an infectious illness such as diphtheria, typhus, or chickenpox. The disease has an acute onset with severe excruciating pain in the shoulder, back, neck, and arm. The patient usually guards against pain by immobilizing the upper extremity in a flexion position of the elbow, adduction of the shoulder, and abduction and external rotation of the arm. Movements of the affected extremity increase or trigger the onset of pain. The pain is followed in a few hours to days by muscle weakness, mainly in muscles innervated by the upper portion of the plexus. The pain subsides as the weakness appears. The muscles most frequently affected are the deltoid and teres minor (axillary nerve), supraspinous and infraspinous (suprascapular nerve), and serratus anterior muscles. The lesion is often bilateral but asymmetric. Most cases involve the right plexus. MRI of the cervical spine and axillary area is normal. EMG and somatosensory evoked potentials confirm the diagnosis. The prognosis is excellent; most patients recover within 2 years. Treatment consists of analgesics in the acute painful phase. A short course of steroids has a favorable effect on the pain. Physical therapy assists rehabilitation of the patient.

References

Kline DG, Hackett ER, Happel LH. Surgery for lesions of the brachial plexus. Arch Neurol 1986; 43:170.

Mumenthaler M, Narakas A, Gilliatt RW. Brachial plexus disorders. In: Dyck PJ, Thomas PK, Lambert EH, Bunge R, eds. Peripheral neuropathy. 2nd ed. Philadelphia: WB Saunders, 1984:1383.

Cornblath DR, Chaudhry V. Brachial neuritis. In: Johnson R T, Griffin JW, eds. Current therapy in neurologic disease. 4th ed. St. Louis: Mosby; 1993.

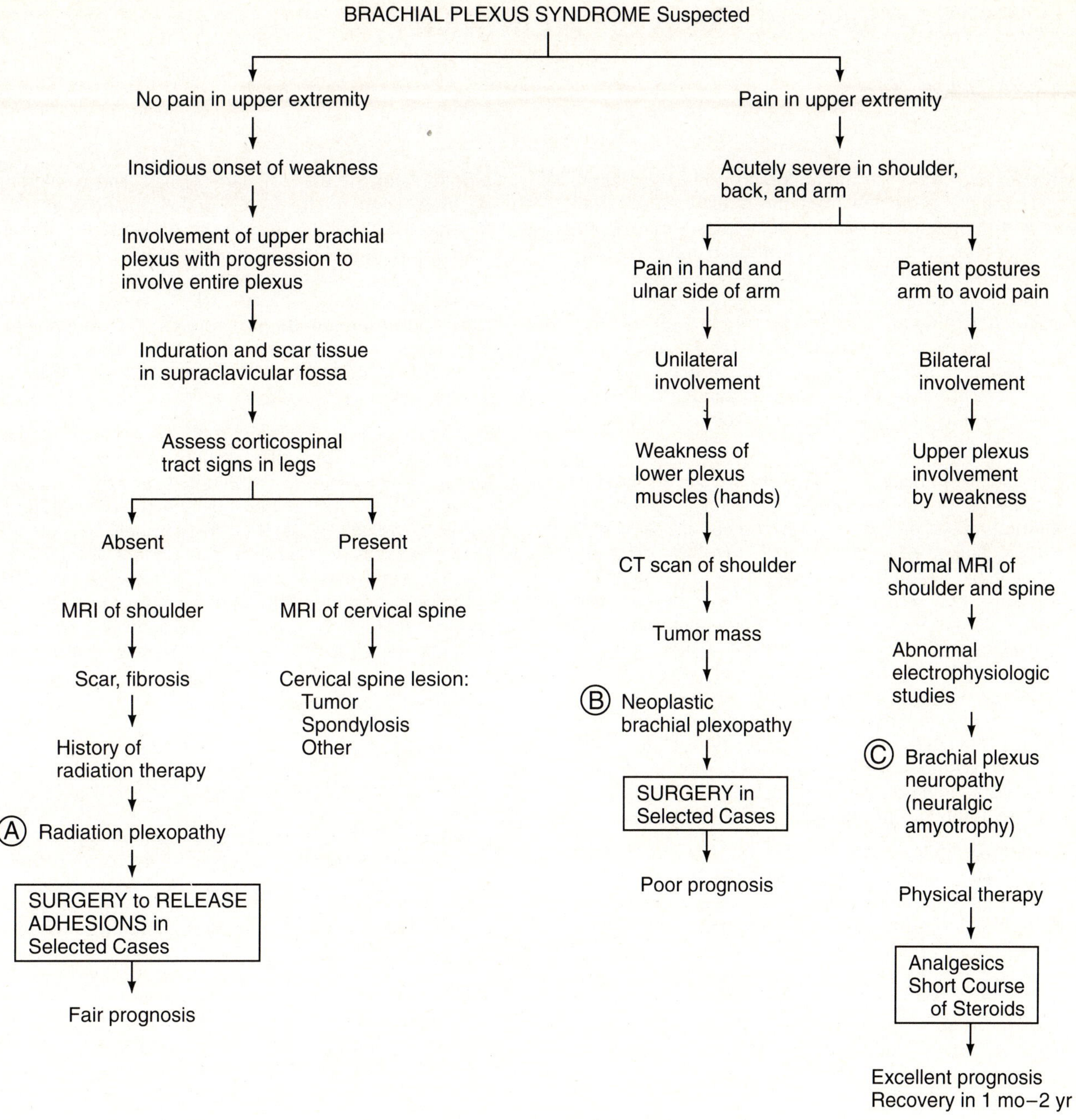

BRACHIAL PLEXUS SYNDROME Suspected
No pain in upper extremity
Pain in upper extremity
Insidious onset of weakness
Acutely severe in shoulder, back, and arm
Involvement of upper brachial plexus with progression to involve entire plexus
Induration and scar tissue in supraclavicular fossa
Assess corticospinal tract signs in legs
Absent
Present
MRI of shoulder
MRI of cervical spine
Scar, fibrosis
Cervical spine lesion: Tumor Spondylosis Other
History of radiation therapy
A Radiation plexopathy
SURGERY to RELEASE ADHESIONS in Selected Cases
Fair prognosis
Pain in hand and ulnar side of arm
Patient postures arm to avoid pain
Unilateral involvement
Bilateral involvement
Weakness of lower plexus muscles (hands)
Upper plexus involvement by weakness
CT scan of shoulder
Normal MRI of shoulder and spine
Tumor mass
Abnormal electrophysiologic studies
B Neoplastic brachial plexopathy
C Brachial plexus neuropathy (neuralgic amyotrophy)
SURGERY in Selected Cases
Physical therapy
Poor prognosis
Analgesics Short Course of Steroids
Excellent prognosis Recovery in 1 mo−2 yr

LUMBOSACRAL PLEXUS SYNDROME

Carlos A. Garcia, M.D.

By virtue of its position in the abdomen, the lumbosacral plexus is usually protected from direct external trauma. However, compression or damage of the plexus may occur during abdominal surgery; after prolonged labor or prolonged maintenance of the lithotomy position; or as a result of spontaneous retroperitoneal bleeding, as seen during anticoagulation therapy. Neoplastic infiltration of the plexus and radiation effects are also emerging as important etiologic factors. Diabetes mellitus continues to be the most important cause of lumbosacral plexopathy. Idiopathic (cryptogenic) plexopathy is not as common as its counterpart in the brachial plexus.

A. Idiopathic lumbosacral plexus neuropathy is rare. It usually begins with acute severe pain in either the femoral (upper plexus) or sciatic (lower plexus) distribution. This disorder occasionally involves both portions of the plexus. The pain is followed by weakness, areflexia, and sensory deficits in the predominantly affected (upper or lower) nerves. The upper portion of the plexus is most often affected. There are no sphincter abnormalities. MRI of the pelvis is normal. A prolonged nerve conduction time, electromyography (EMG), and somatosensory evoked potentials may confirm the diagnosis. The prognosis is excellent, with recovery within 1 year in most cases. Therapy should be directed toward the relief of pain in the acute phase and rehabilitation of the motor deficit later.

B. Lumbosacral plexopathy in cancer is characterized by an insidious onset of radicular pelvic or leg pain. Unlike the pain of traumatic disc disease, the pain is persistent and progressive and the patient cannot find a position in which symptoms are relieved. Weeks to months later, numbness, paresthesias, and weakness develop. These are frequently unilateral and affect the lower (L4-S1) plexus in 75% of patients, the upper (L1-L4) plexus in 31%, and the entire (L1-S3) plexus in 18%. Edema of the lower extremity and a rectal mass are found in some patients. MRI of the pelvis often shows the tumor mass and reveals hydronephrosis. The tumors most frequently associated with the syndrome are colorectal tumors, sarcomas, breast lesions, and lymphomas.

C. Radiation plexopathy often follows radiation of the pelvis area as a part of treatment in cancers of the uterus, cervix, ovaries, lymph nodes, and testicles and other organs. The disease begins as an insidious painless weakness of both extremities but in an asymmetric distribution. No involvement of the bladder, no rectal masses, and no edema are associated with the syndrome. MRI of the spine and pelvis is normal. EMG shows myokymic discharges. In most patients the disorder progresses slowly, eventually resulting in significant or severe disability. No effective therapy is available at present.

References

Jaeckle KA, Young DF, Foley KM. The natural history of lumbosacral plexopathy in cancer. Neurology 1985; 35:8.

Thomas JE, Cascino IL, Earle JD. Differential diagnosis between radiation and tumor plexopathy of the pelvis. Neurology 1985; 35:1.

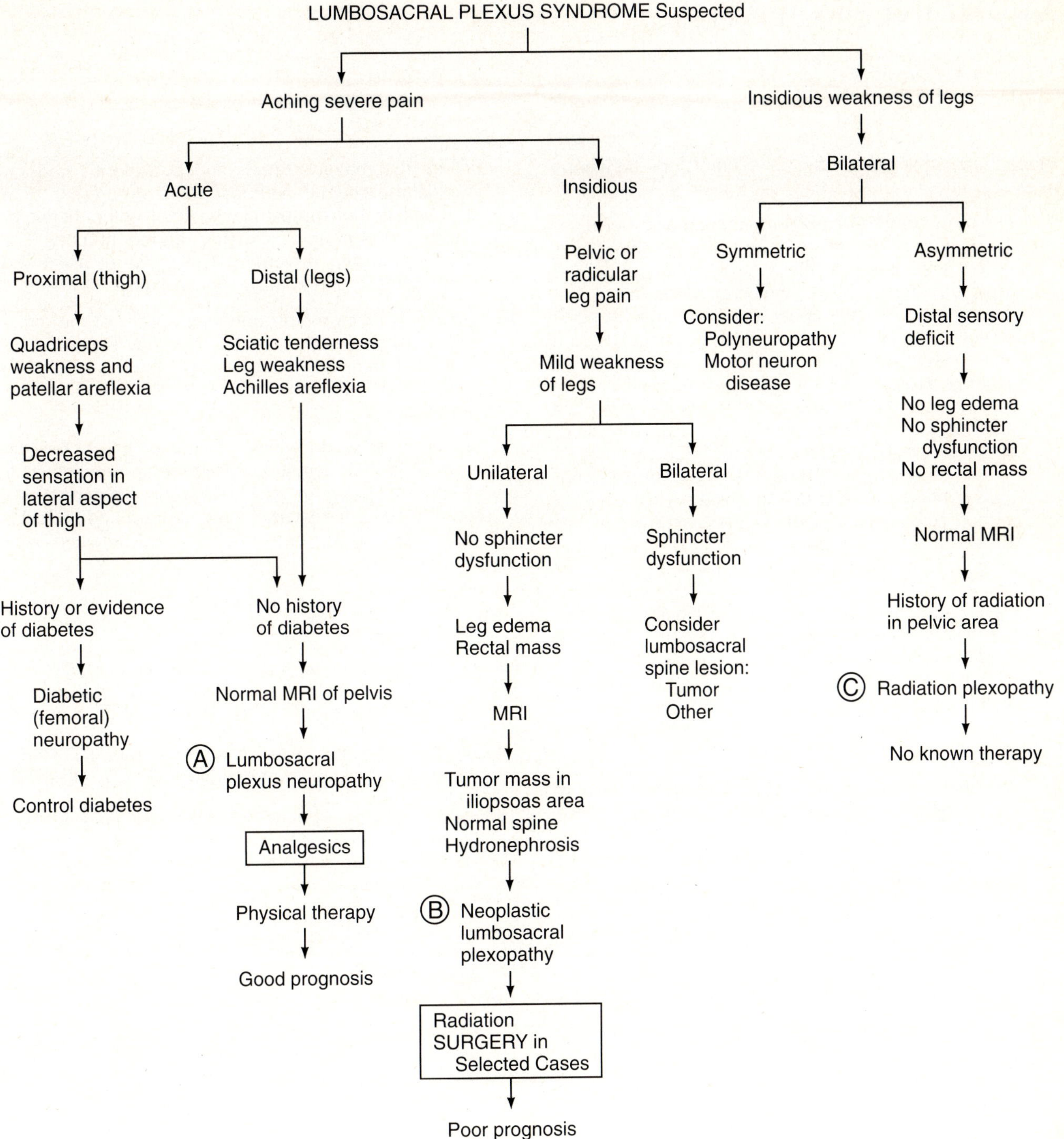

LUMBOSACRAL PLEXUS SYNDROME Suspected
Aching severe pain
Insidious weakness of legs
Acute
Insidious
Bilateral
Proximal (thigh)
Distal (legs)
Pelvic or radicular leg pain
Symmetric
Asymmetric
Quadriceps weakness and patellar areflexia
Sciatic tenderness
Leg weakness
Achilles areflexia
Mild weakness of legs
Consider:
Polyneuropathy
Motor neuron disease
Distal sensory deficit
Decreased sensation in lateral aspect of thigh
Unilateral
Bilateral
No leg edema
No sphincter dysfunction
No rectal mass
History or evidence of diabetes
No history of diabetes
No sphincter dysfunction
Sphincter dysfunction
Normal MRI
Diabetic (femoral) neuropathy
Normal MRI of pelvis
Leg edema
Rectal mass
Consider lumbosacral spine lesion:
Tumor
Other
History of radiation in pelvic area
Control diabetes
A Lumbosacral plexus neuropathy
MRI
C Radiation plexopathy
Analgesics
Tumor mass in iliopsoas area
Normal spine
Hydronephrosis
No known therapy
Physical therapy
B Neoplastic lumbosacral plexopathy
Good prognosis
Radiation
SURGERY in Selected Cases
Poor prognosis

MONONEUROPATHY

Carlos A. Garcia, M.D.

Mononeuropathies may affect the cranial or peripheral nerves.

A. The most common cranial mononeuropathy involves the seventh cranial nerve. If no cause is found, this is called Bell's palsy. In these cases, facial paralysis is frequently acute and of undetermined etiology. The paralysis involves the upper and lower face. Approximately 10% of patients are diabetics and 10% are hypertensive. Complete recovery occurs in 80% of patients. Prognostic indicators for a delayed or only partial recovery include age >45 years, complete paralysis with increased tearing, retroauricular pain, decreased taste, and electromyographic evidence of severe denervation 10 days after the onset of symptoms. A short course of steroids seems to be beneficial in most cases. Facial paralysis associated with herpes zoster oticus is called Ramsay Hunt syndrome, and the prognosis for recovery from the facial paralysis is poor. Isolated cranial nerve paralysis involving the third and sixth cranial nerves may be seen in diabetic patients; it is of acute onset and ischemic in origin. Third nerve palsy is associated with ptosis, oculomotor palsy, ocular pain, and sparing of the pupil. Diabetes mellitus is a frequent associated factor. In sixth nerve palsy, diplopia is a common complaint. The prognosis for both lesions is usually good.

B. The acute painful onset of quadriceps weakness may be caused by an ischemic lesion of the femoral nerve in diabetic patients. The patellar reflex may be absent and there may be early atrophy of the quadriceps muscles. Other causes of ischemic neuropathies include rheumatoid arthritis and polyarteritis nodosa. Vascular ischemic neuropathies may present as a multiple mononeuropathy with involvement of two or more nerves in an asymmetric random manner. The distribution may also be that of a diffuse distal and symmetric sensorimotor polyneuropathy.

C. Acute, painless motor mononeuropathy of the radial nerve (wrist drop) in adults may be due to lead intoxication. The neurologic symptoms are often associated with abdominal pain, constipation, and anemia.

D. Acute or subacute sensory mononeuropathy may be produced by a herpes zoster-varicella virus infection (shingles). The virus infects the root and nerve trunk and causes a dermatomal vesicular rash and radicular pain. The cranial nerve most commonly affected is the trigeminal.

References

Karnes W. Diseases of the seventh cranial nerve. In: Dyck PJ, Thomas PK, Lambert EH, Bunge R, eds. Peripheral neuropathy. 2nd ed. Philadelphia: WB Saunders, 1984:1266.

Niparko JK, Mattox DE. Bell's palsy. In: Johnson RT, Griffin JW, eds. Current therapy in neurologic disease. 4th ed. St. Louis: Mosby, 1993.

Thomas PK. Clinical features and differential diagnosis. In: Dyck PJ, Thomas PK, Lambert EH, Bunge R, eds. Peripheral neuropathy. 2nd ed. Philadelphia: WB Saunders, 1984:1169.

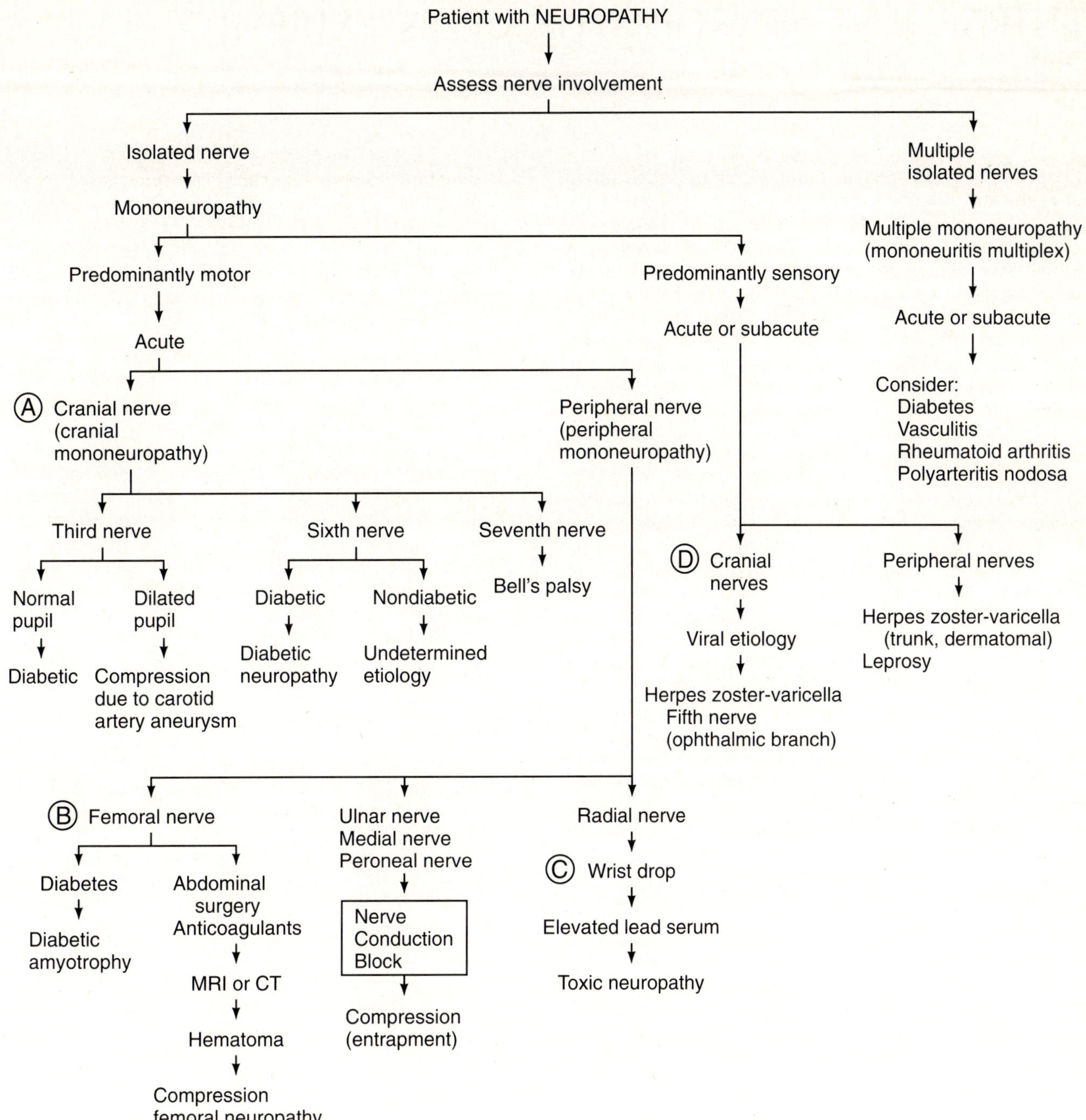

Patient with NEUROPATHY
Assess nerve involvement
Isolated nerve
Mononeuropathy
Multiple isolated nerves
Multiple mononeuropathy (mononeuritis multiplex)
Predominantly motor
Predominantly sensory
Acute or subacute
Acute
Acute or subacute
Consider:
Diabetes
Vasculitis
Rheumatoid arthritis
Polyarteritis nodosa
A Cranial nerve (cranial mononeuropathy)
Peripheral nerve (peripheral mononeuropathy)
Third nerve
Sixth nerve
Seventh nerve
D Cranial nerves
Peripheral nerves
Normal pupil
Dilated pupil
Diabetic
Nondiabetic
Bell's palsy
Viral etiology
Herpes zoster-varicella (trunk, dermatomal)
Leprosy
Diabetic
Compression due to carotid artery aneurysm
Diabetic neuropathy
Undetermined etiology
Herpes zoster-varicella
Fifth nerve (ophthalmic branch)
B Femoral nerve
Ulnar nerve
Medial nerve
Peroneal nerve
Radial nerve
Diabetes
Abdominal surgery
Anticoagulants
C Wrist drop
Diabetic amyotrophy
MRI or CT
Nerve Conduction Block
Elevated lead serum
Hematoma
Compression (entrapment)
Toxic neuropathy
Compression femoral neuropathy

ENTRAPMENT NEUROPATHY: UPPER EXTREMITY

Carlos A. Garcia, M.D.

Peripheral nerves may be compressed or squeezed in anatomically vulnerable areas such as the surface of the extremities or as they pass through narrow channels. The compression may be external or may be caused by a proliferation of abnormal adjacent tissue. In most instances of entrapment neuropathy, there are predisposing risk factors (e.g., chronic malnutrition, diabetes, alcoholism, rheumatoid arthritis, renal failure, dysthyroidism). Most compressive and entrapment neuropathies are painful, are acute in onset, and carry a good prognosis if the injurious agent is removed. In other cases, the onset is insidious and is produced by repeated minor trauma. Only the most common types are discussed below.

A. Most patients with carpal tunnel syndrome complain that they wake up because of either unilateral or bilateral pain and numbness in the hands that may be relieved by shaking the hands. The pain may come in bouts and often spreads to the arms and shoulders. Weakness and atrophy of hand muscles may appear later. The examiner may reproduce the pain by forced flexion of the wrist. When the carpal ligament is tapped, the patient may feel an electric current radiating down the fingers (Tinel sign). The diagnosis is confirmed in nerve conduction studies by the finding of prolonged distal latencies in the median nerve. Perform a complete electrophysiologic evaluation, including nerve conduction velocity (NCV) tests on other nerves and electromyography, to rule out polyneuropathies or other causes of paresthesia and weakness and wasting of hand muscles. In each case, a hand splint for use at night may relieve the symptoms. Steroid injections into the carpal tunnel may help. Surgical decompression may be needed if these two forms of therapy fail. The main differential diagnosis of the syndrome, as seen in the algorithm, is thoracic outlet syndrome. This syndrome is usually unilateral, with decreased sensation in the ulnar nerve distribution above the wrist.

B. Ulnar entrapment neuropathy may occur at different levels, but most commonly at the elbow. The main complaint is numbness of the fourth and fifth fingers. Weakness of the hand muscles may be seen later in the course. Examination shows decreased sensation in the ulnar distribution, including the medial surface of the arm and hand. Weakness and atrophy are seen in the hypothenar eminence and in the first dorsal interosseous muscle. Difficulty with flexion of the fourth and fifth digits occurs at the metacarpophalangeal joint. A claw hand may be seen in advanced cases. The diagnosis is confirmed by NCV studies demonstrating conduction block at the elbow. Surgical decompression is needed in most cases.

References

Stewart JD, Aguaijo AJ. Compression and entrapment neuropathies. In: Dyck PJ, Thomas PK, Lambert EH, Bunge R, eds. Peripheral neuropathy. 2nd ed. Philadelphia: WB Saunders, 1984:1435.

Wilbourn AJ, Sweeny PJ. Entrapment neuropathy. In: Johnson R, ed. Current therapy in neurologic disease. 3rd ed. Philadelphia: BC Decker, 1990:380.

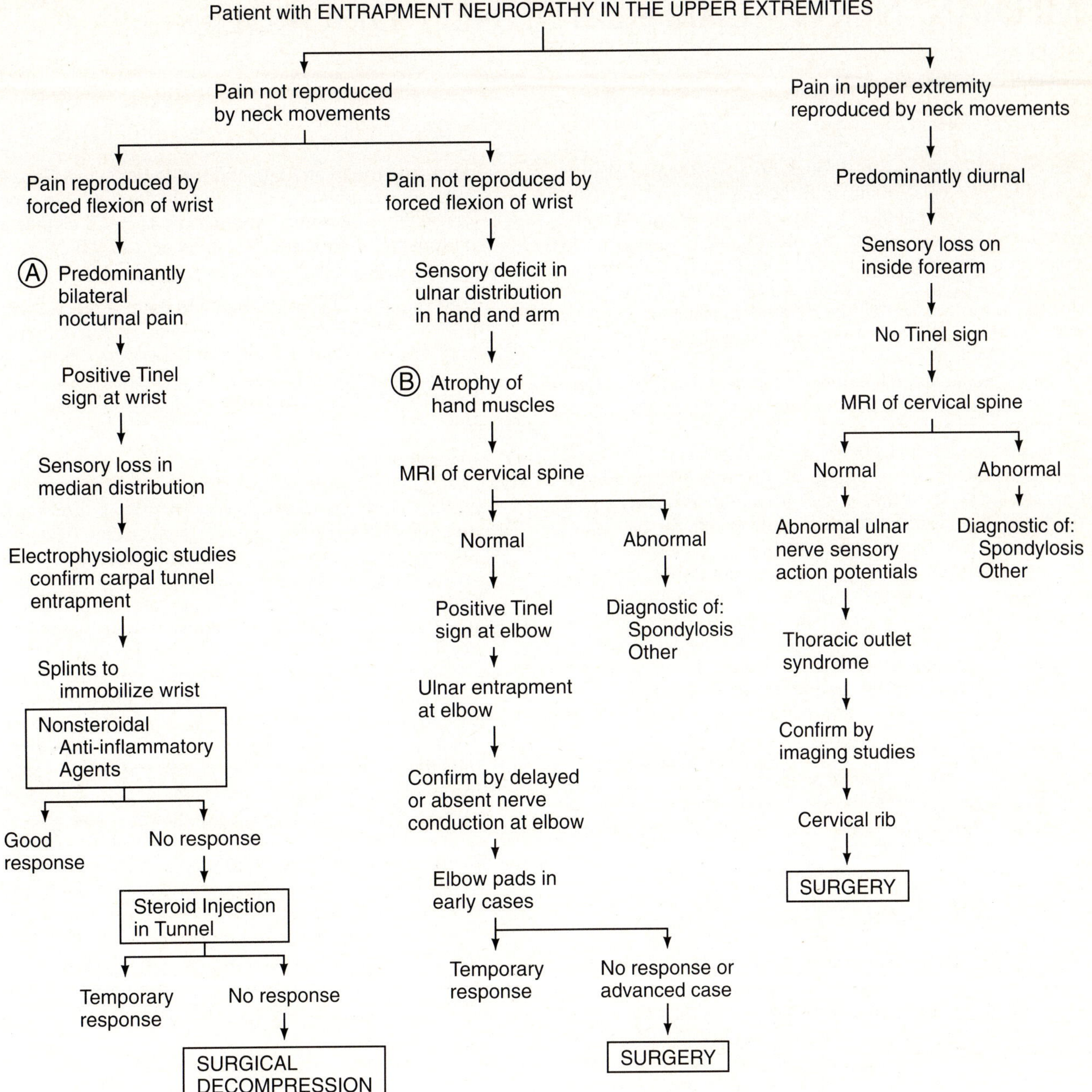

Patient with ENTRAPMENT NEUROPATHY IN THE UPPER EXTREMITIES
Pain not reproduced by neck movements
Pain in upper extremity reproduced by neck movements
Pain reproduced by forced flexion of wrist
Pain not reproduced by forced flexion of wrist
Predominantly diurnal
A Predominantly bilateral nocturnal pain
Sensory deficit in ulnar distribution in hand and arm
Sensory loss on inside forearm
Positive Tinel sign at wrist
B Atrophy of hand muscles
No Tinel sign
Sensory loss in median distribution
MRI of cervical spine
MRI of cervical spine
Electrophysiologic studies confirm carpal tunnel entrapment
Normal
Abnormal
Normal
Abnormal
Splints to immobilize wrist
Positive Tinel sign at elbow
Diagnostic of: Spondylosis Other
Abnormal ulnar nerve sensory action potentials
Diagnostic of: Spondylosis Other
Nonsteroidal Anti-inflammatory Agents
Ulnar entrapment at elbow
Thoracic outlet syndrome
Good response
No response
Confirm by delayed or absent nerve conduction at elbow
Confirm by imaging studies
Steroid Injection in Tunnel
Elbow pads in early cases
Cervical rib
Temporary response
No response
Temporary response
No response or advanced case
SURGERY
SURGICAL DECOMPRESSION
SURGERY

MEDIAN NERVE (CARPAL TUNNEL) DISORDERS

Leon A. Weisberg, M.D.

The median nerve passes through the carpal tunnel. This is bounded by carpal bones and the transverse carpal ligament (flexor retinaculum). The median nerve may be compressed as a result of (1) local tissue swelling, as in pregnancy, hypothyroidism, acromegaly, or tenosynovitis; or (2) tunnel narrowing, as in arthritis, connective tissue disorders, tumors, or fracture deformity. The median nerve may be damaged in patients whose work involves prolonged, repetitive wrist motion (e.g., carpenters, typists, butchers, truckers, jackhammer operators). Clinical criteria for diagnosis of carpal tunnel syndrome (CTS) include (1) aching pain in the hand, wrist, or arm that develops at night or after repetitive hand or wrist movement and is relieved by hand shaking or discontinuation of activity that precipitates pain; (2) paresthesia with impaired sensation in the median nerve distribution; (3) weakness in the hand and wrist such as difficulty opening jars or gripping objects between the thumb and index finger, and motor dysfunction of the hand due to weakness of the abductor pollicis and opponens pollicis; (4) autonomic disturbances, including dry skin and loss of hair pattern over the fingers; and (5) symptoms reproduced with forced wrist flexion (Phalen sign) or tapping over the median nerve at the wrist (Tinel sign).

A. In many patients, CTS findings are characteristic; in some, however, clinical features are atypical. Suspect CTS in patients with wrist and hand pain, hand paresthesias and numbness, and hand clumsiness and weakness. In mild cases of CTS, patients report hand and wrist pain and intermittent hand numbness or paresthesias, but there are no abnormal examination findings, and the Tinel and Phalen signs are absent.

B. Failure to reproduce sensory disturbances with the Tinel and Phalen tests does not exclude CTS. If neurologic signs and symptoms are confined to the median nerve distribution, perform diagnostic studies to exclude conditions that compress the median nerve and simulate CTS. Investigate the wrist (fracture, bone or joint disease), neck (cervical radiculopathy), and thorax (cervical rib, lung apex mass) with radiographic studies. Perform endocrine (diabetes, acromegaly, hypothyroidism), hematologic (coagulation disorders), and rheumatologic and serologic (Lyme disease) tests. Assess nerve conduction velocity (NCV) in other nerves to determine whether there is generalized peripheral neuropathy. Not all cases of median nerve dysfunction are due to CTS.

C. If no specific cause is defined and there is electromyographic (EMG) and NCV evidence of CTS, initiate appropriate therapy. If electrophysiologic studies are normal, consider a therapeutic trial to confirm CTS, because a few CTS patients have normal EMG/NCV tests.

D. Once the diagnosis is established, begin treatment if symptoms interfere with daily activities. Therapeutic agents (diuretics, systemic corticosteroids, nonsteroidal anti-inflammatory agents, pyridoxine) have not proved effective in CTS but are often used. Noninvasive (nonsurgical) treatment includes activity modification and use of a ventrally applied wrist splint at night and during activities that exacerbate symptoms. Employ this strategy if there is no motor deficit. With a wrist splint, improvement is expected within 2 to 3 weeks. If this treatment is ineffective, perform local steroid injections into the carpal tunnel. If symptoms initially respond to local injection but recur, repeat the injection. Surgical resection of the transverse carpal ligament is indicated if nonsurgical techniques are ineffective or if there is motor weakness with evidence of thenar muscle atrophy. After successful surgery, pain relief is usually immediate; however, motor improvement may take 3 to 6 months. After surgery, a wrist dressing and splint are worn for 2 to 3 weeks. For bilateral CTS, surgery on both hands at the same time may incapacitate patients for several days but avoids a second operation. Patients who have had CTS on one side are at increased risk of contralateral CTS.

References

Dawson DM, Hallett M, Millender LH. Entrapment neuropathies. 2nd ed. Boston: Little, Brown, 1990:25.
Phalen GS. Reflections on 21 years' experience with the carpal tunnel syndrome. JAMA 1970; 212:1365.

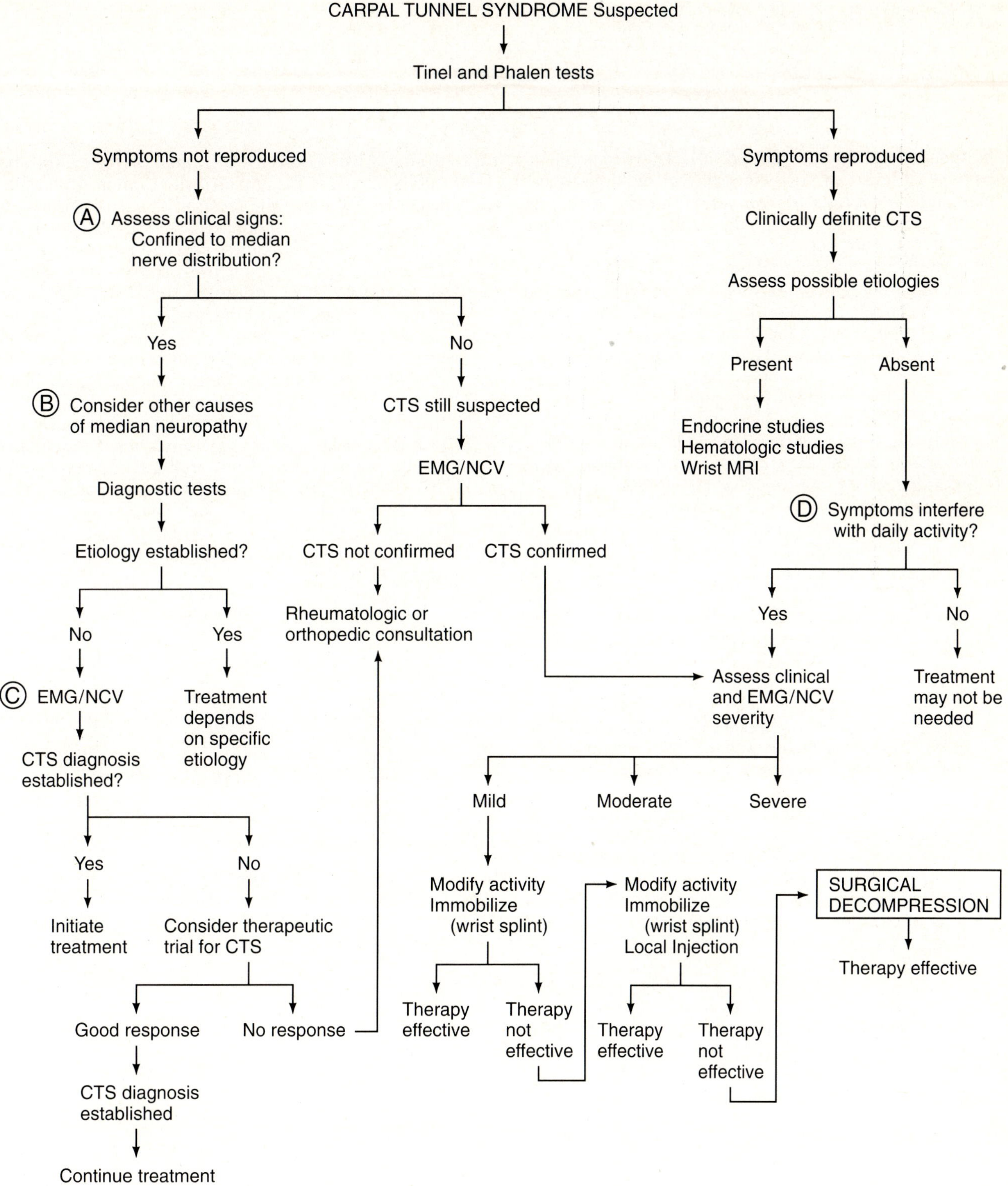

CARPAL TUNNEL SYNDROME Suspected
Tinel and Phalen tests
Symptoms not reproduced
Symptoms reproduced
A Assess clinical signs: Confined to median nerve distribution?
Clinically definite CTS
Assess possible etiologies
Yes
No
Present
Absent
B Consider other causes of median neuropathy
CTS still suspected
Endocrine studies
Hematologic studies
Wrist MRI
Diagnostic tests
EMG/NCV
D Symptoms interfere with daily activity?
Etiology established?
CTS not confirmed
CTS confirmed
No
Yes
Yes
No
C EMG/NCV
Treatment depends on specific etiology
Rheumatologic or orthopedic consultation
Assess clinical and EMG/NCV severity
Treatment may not be needed
CTS diagnosis established?
Yes
No
Mild
Moderate
Severe
Initiate treatment
Consider therapeutic trial for CTS
Modify activity Immobilize (wrist splint)
Modify activity Immobilize (wrist splint) Local Injection
SURGICAL DECOMPRESSION
Good response
No response
Therapy effective
Therapy not effective
Therapy effective
Therapy not effective
Therapy effective
CTS diagnosis established
Continue treatment

ULNAR NEUROPATHY

Carlos A. Garcia, M.D.

The ulnar nerve may be affected in isolation (mononeuropathy) or as part of polyneuropathy or multiple mononeuropathy. Most isolated ulnar lesions are due to entrapment or compressions. Knowledge of the trajectory of the nerve and its surrounding structures is important to an understanding of the different ulnar syndromes. The ulnar nerve can be compressed or traumatized at the axilla but usually in conjunction with the median and radial nerve. Isolated compressions of the ulnar nerve by the head of a sleeping partner can occur at the medial aspect of the arm. The nerve travels in the elbow behind the medial epicondyle through the ulnar groove, and 2 cm distally passes through the cubital tunnel. The roof of this tunnel is formed by the aponeurosis of the flexor carpi ulnaris muscle. Most ulnar nerve entrapments occur at these two areas. Most lesions at the groove are stretch or compressive in nature. By contrast, most cubital tunnel lesions are caused by external compression or entrapments. The combination of all these mechanisms can occur in one patient, the so-called cubital tunnel syndrome.

A. The clinical manifestations of lesions at the level of the cubital tunnel consist of numbness and tingling of the fourth and fifth digits and the medial border of the palm. Some patients may notice wasting of the intrinsic hand muscles, and some may complain of pain at the elbow. Weakness of abduction and adduction of the fingers and weakness of the fourth and fifth fingers at the metacarpophalangeal joint, along with wasting of the intrinsic hand muscles, produce a claw hand. Electrophysiologic studies may show a focal demyelination (conduction block) in only half of the patients. In the other half the predominant lesion is axonal and electromyography (EMG) is less precise. Treatment consists of elbow protectors, a brief trial of nonsteroidal anti-inflammatory agents, and surgical intervention if the symptoms are progressive. Surgical procedures include medial epicondylectomy, tunnel decompression, and nerve transposition. Surgical procedures do not improve the symptoms in some patients, and in a few may accentuate or produce an axonal loss, probably an ischemic event caused by stripping of the blood vessels at the time of the surgery.

B. Ulnar neuropathy associated with skin lesions should suggest leprosy. A skin biopsy may disclose the acid-fast organism.

C. Compressive lesions of the ulnar nerve below the cubital tunnel in the arm are rare. Compression again becomes an important cause in the wrist and hand. Lesions here are produced by repeated pressure caused by bicycle handles, pressure tools, or the use of canes or crutches. Fractures, arthritis, and tumors also produce ulnar lesions in the hand. The ulnar nerve enters the hand through Guyon's canal where the nerve bifurcates and gives origin to the superficial terminal branch and the deep motor branch. The deep motor branch innervates the hypothenar muscles and then innervates the third and fourth lumbricales muscles, all the interossei, the abductor pollicis, and part of the flexor pollicis brevis muscles. Four clinical syndromes result from wrist and hand compressions. The most common syndrome is caused by compression of the deep terminal branch before it supplies the branches of the hypothenar muscles. This produces a pure motor deficit of all the ulnar-innervated muscles of the hand.

D. When the nerve is compressed just proximal to or in Guyon's canal, there is a mixed motor and sensory deficit. The weakness affects all the ulnar-innervated muscles of the hand; the sensory deficit consists of loss of sensation in the distal hypothenar palmar areas and the palmar surfaces of the ulnar-innervated fingers.

E. The second most common compression is that of the deep branch after it supplies the branches of the hypothenar muscles. This produces a pure motor deficit of all the ulnar-innervated hand muscles except those of the hypothenar eminence.

F. The least common compression occurs in the superficial terminal branch in or just distal to Guyon's canal. It produces a pure sensory deficit of the distal palmar hypothenar area and palmar surfaces of the ulnar-innervated fingers.

References

Stewart JD, Aguayo AJ. Compression and entrapment neuropathies. In: Dyck PJ, Thomas PK, Lambert EH, Bunge R, eds. Peripheral neuropathy. 2nd ed. Philadelphia: WB Saunders, 1984:1435.

Wilbourn AJ, Sweeny PJ. Entrapment neuropathies. In: Johnson R, ed. Current therapy in neurologic disease. 3rd ed. Philadelphia: BC Decker, 1990:380.

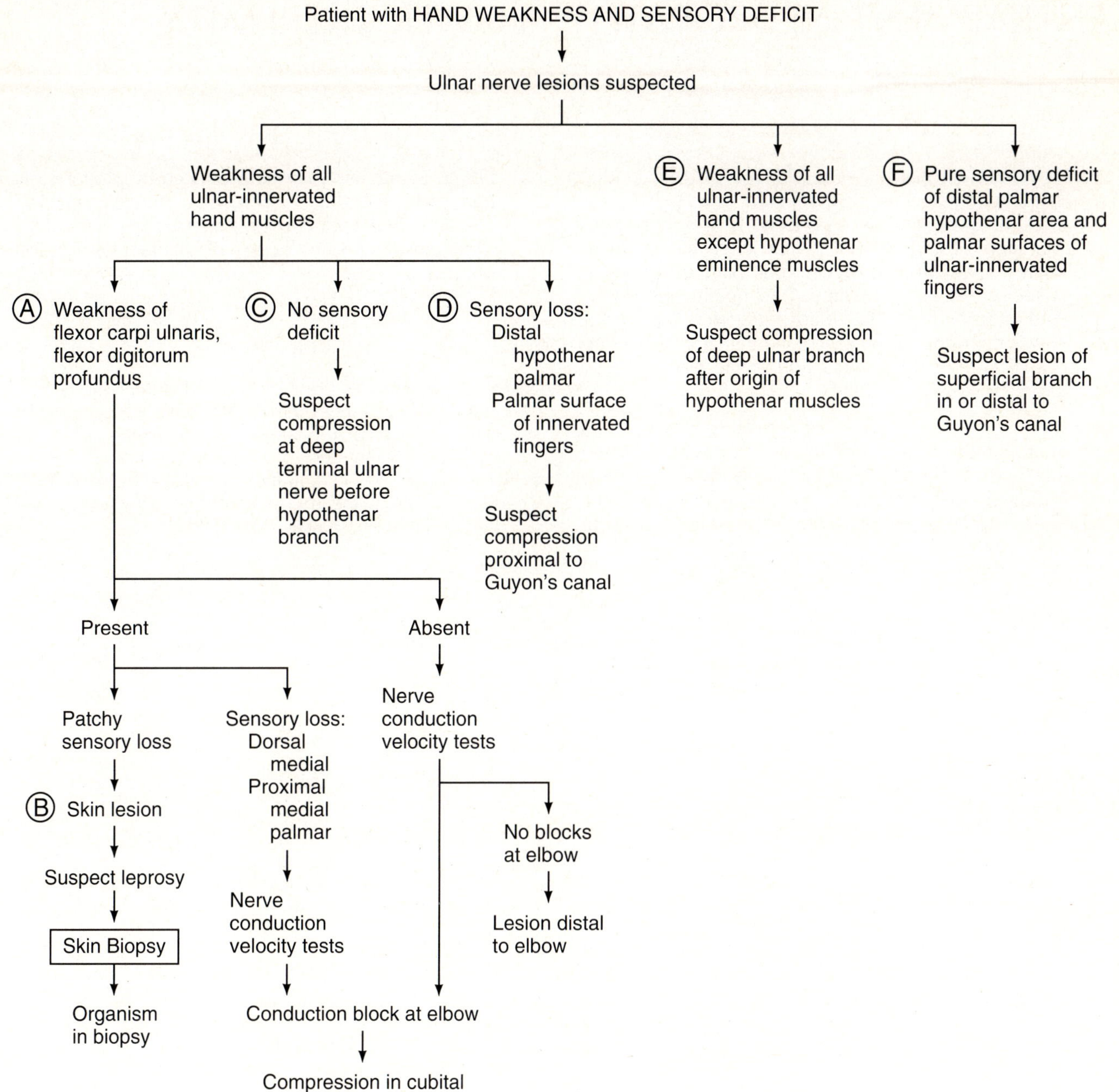

Patient with HAND WEAKNESS AND SENSORY DEFICIT
Ulnar nerve lesions suspected
Weakness of all ulnar-innervated hand muscles
E Weakness of all ulnar-innervated hand muscles except hypothenar eminence muscles
F Pure sensory deficit of distal palmar hypothenar area and palmar surfaces of ulnar-innervated fingers
A Weakness of flexor carpi ulnaris, flexor digitorum profundus
C No sensory deficit
D Sensory loss: Distal hypothenar palmar Palmar surface of innervated fingers
Suspect compression of deep ulnar branch after origin of hypothenar muscles
Suspect lesion of superficial branch in or distal to Guyon's canal
Suspect compression at deep terminal ulnar nerve before hypothenar branch
Suspect compression proximal to Guyon's canal
Present
Absent
Patchy sensory loss
Sensory loss: Dorsal medial Proximal medial palmar
Nerve conduction velocity tests
B Skin lesion
Suspect leprosy
No blocks at elbow
Nerve conduction velocity tests
Skin Biopsy
Lesion distal to elbow
Conduction block at elbow
Organism in biopsy
Compression in cubital canal, ulnar groove

ENTRAPMENT NEUROPATHY: LOWER EXTREMITY

Carlos A. Garcia, M.D.

A. Femoral neuropathy (see p 211 and 214) in nondiabetic patients occurs predominantly during anticoagulant therapy and is produced by a spontaneous hematoma compressing the nerve in the iliac compartment. The onset is acute and painful. There is associated severe weakness of the quadriceps muscle and patellar areflexia. A tomographic scan of the pelvis confirms the presence of a hematoma. Conservative treatment or evacuation of the clot seems to produce the same results.

B. Common peroneal nerve entrapment is manifested by foot drop due to weakness of dorsiflexion and eversion of the foot. There is sensory loss in the anterolateral surface of the lower part of the leg and dorsum of the foot. The compression occurs at the fibular neck or fibular tunnel and may be produced by plaster casts, tight high boots, leg crossing, or prolonged squatting. Therapy consists of conservative management and, if symptoms are severe, the use of leg braces (ankle-foot orthosis).

References

Stewart JD, Aguayo AJ. Compression and entrapment neuropathies. In: Dyck PJ, Thomas PK, Lambert EH, Bunge R, eds. Peripheral neuropathy. 2nd ed. Philadelphia: WB Saunders, 1984:1435.

Wilbourn AJ, Sweeny PJ. Entrapment neuropathy. In: Johnson R, ed. Current therapy in neurologic disease. 3rd ed. Philadelphia: BC Decker, 1990:380.

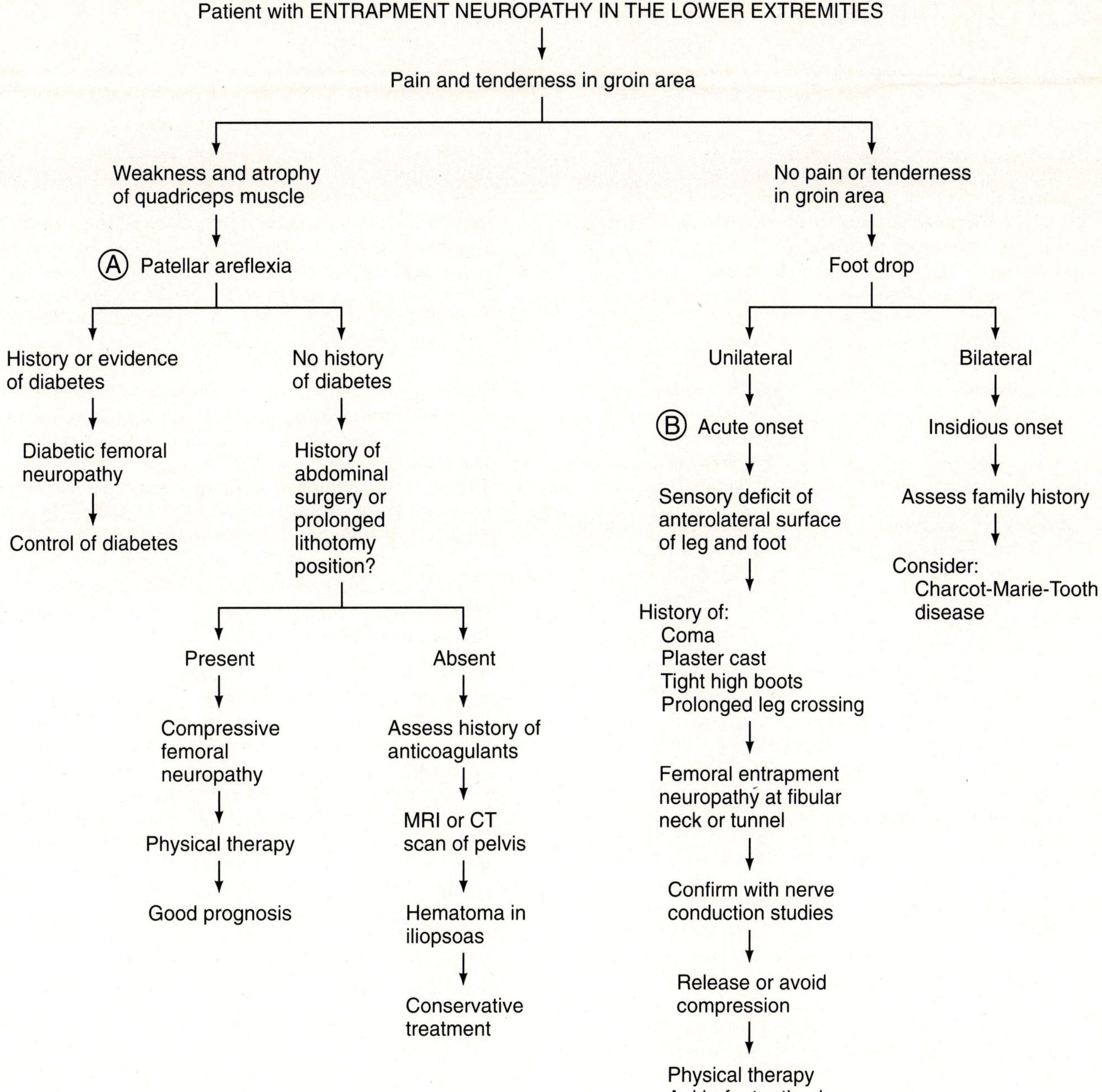

Patient with ENTRAPMENT NEUROPATHY IN THE LOWER EXTREMITIES
Pain and tenderness in groin area
Weakness and atrophy of quadriceps muscle
No pain or tenderness in groin area
A Patellar areflexia
Foot drop
History or evidence of diabetes
No history of diabetes
Unilateral
Bilateral
Diabetic femoral neuropathy
History of abdominal surgery or prolonged lithotomy position?
B Acute onset
Insidious onset
Control of diabetes
Sensory deficit of anterolateral surface of leg and foot
Assess family history
Present
Absent
Consider: Charcot-Marie-Tooth disease
Compressive femoral neuropathy
Assess history of anticoagulants
History of:
Coma
Plaster cast
Tight high boots
Prolonged leg crossing
Physical therapy
MRI or CT scan of pelvis
Femoral entrapment neuropathy at fibular neck or tunnel
Good prognosis
Hematoma in iliopsoas
Confirm with nerve conduction studies
Conservative treatment
Release or avoid compression
Physical therapy
Ankle-foot orthosis

MOTOR NEURON DISEASE

Carlos A. Garcia, M.D.

Motor neuron disease (MND) is a degenerative, relentlessly progressive disease of unknown etiology. The disease affects the motor neurons of the brain (upper motor neurons [UMNs]) with secondary degeneration of the corticobulbar and corticospinal tracts. It also affects the motor neurons of the spinal cord and brain stem (lower motor neurons [LMNs]).

Most cases (95%) of MND are sporadic, but some familial cases have been reported. These latter occur in younger patients; there is a greater female predominance and a more fulminant course. A higher incidence of this disease in younger people (especially associated with parkinsonian features and dementia) has been described in certain Pacific regions (e.g., Guam, Mariana Islands).

A. Progressive degeneration of the LMNs in the spinal cord and the brain stem results in motor weakness associated with severe atrophy and fasciculations (amyotrophy), decreased tone, and hyporeflexia. When the LMNs of the brain stem are involved, the symptoms include difficulty in swallowing and disturbed speech (dysarthria). On examination the tongue appears atrophic and shows fasciculations. There is weakness of the nasopharyngeal muscles manifested by a failure to elevate the palate (progressive bulbar palsy). Progressive degeneration of motor neurons in the brain results in spasticity, hyperreflexia, and present Babinksi sign or pseudobulbar palsy.

B. The disease can be classified by the type of symptoms and the distribution of the weakness. (1) Progressive bulbar palsy (see A.) may be the first manifestation of MND, with a rapid course and death within 3 years after onset of symptoms. Most patients die because of swallowing (aspiration) and respiratory muscle involvement. (2) In pseudobulbar palsy, the lesion involves the corticobulbar tracts rather than the bulbar nuclei. The tongue is not atrophic but spastic; there are no fasciculations of the tongue and there is hyperreflexia of the jaw reflex. There may be associated outbursts of crying or laughing in the absence of any obvious provoking factors (emotional incontinence), owing to involvement of the corticobulbar fibers. Pseudobulbar palsy may be seen in combination with LMN findings or in isolation; both are frequent components of MND. (3) In progressive muscular atrophy (PMA), there are signs of LMN involvement, which may begin in the upper or lower extremities. This disorder is frequently distal and is manifested by evidence of wasting and fasciculation in association with weakness of the hands and legs. The disorder may also begin in the lower extremities, involving the feet rather than the hips. There is no evidence of sensory involvement and usually no sphincter disturbance. PMA may begin in the legs and spread to the arms. There may be bulbar involvement that causes swallowing and respiratory difficulty. It appears that PMA is the most slowly progressive of the motor neuron disturbances. This involvement of the anterior horn cells of the motor neuron type may be seen in young patients with proximal muscle involvement and a family history of the disease; this disorder is called Kugelberg-Welander disease. (4) In primary lateral sclerosis, there may be predominant signs of UMN disease as manifested by weakness and spasticity of the arms and legs with associated hyperreflexia and a present Babinski sign. There are no accompanying sensory impairments and no sphincter disturbances. There is usually no bulbar involvement with this form of the disease. (5) In amyotrophic lateral sclerosis, there is evidence of both UMN and LMN disturbances, manifested by weakness and wasting with accompanying fasciculations involving the arms and legs. There are also findings of spasticity, hyperreflexia, and bilateral Babinski signs. The lack of both sphincter involvement and sensory impairment usually helps to differentiate this from other spinal cord lesions and demyelinating disease. This disorder often involves the bulbar muscles.

C. The diagnosis of MND may be difficult in its early phase because there are no biologic markers of the disease and no confirmatory neuroradiographic studies. The diagnosis is established by clinical and electrical diagnostic studies. Nerve conduction velocities are normal, but the electromyogram (EMG) shows evidence of widespread denervation in both the upper and lower extremities. If there are UMN findings, a posterior fossa lesion can be excluded with CT/MRI. If this is negative, examination of CSF for abnormal immunoglobulins helps exclude multiple sclerosis. If the patient with UMN involvement has accompanying sensory loss, consider the existence of a cavity within the central portion of the cord (syringomyelia) in younger patients and cervical spondylosis in older patients. However, some patients with cervical spondylosis may have no sensory deficit. This diagnosis can be excluded with appropriate diagnostic studies, including myelography and MRI. Other causes of motor neuron involvement include thyroid dysfunction and certain toxins (including organic and inorganic compounds), which can usually be excluded by appropriate diagnostic studies. There is no treatment for MND. Management of these patients includes the following: (1) confirm the diagnosis with the highest degree of certainty; (2) support respiratory function and consider tracheostomy; (3) provide alimentation, including a nasogastric tube; and (4) control secretions to avoid aspiration pneumonia. MND is a fatal disorder. Appropriate family counseling is crucial.

Reference

Clawson LL, Rothstein JD, Kuncl RW. Amyotrophic lateral sclerosis. In: Johnson R, Griffin JW, eds. Current therapy in neurologic disease. 4th ed. St. Louis: Mosby, 1993.

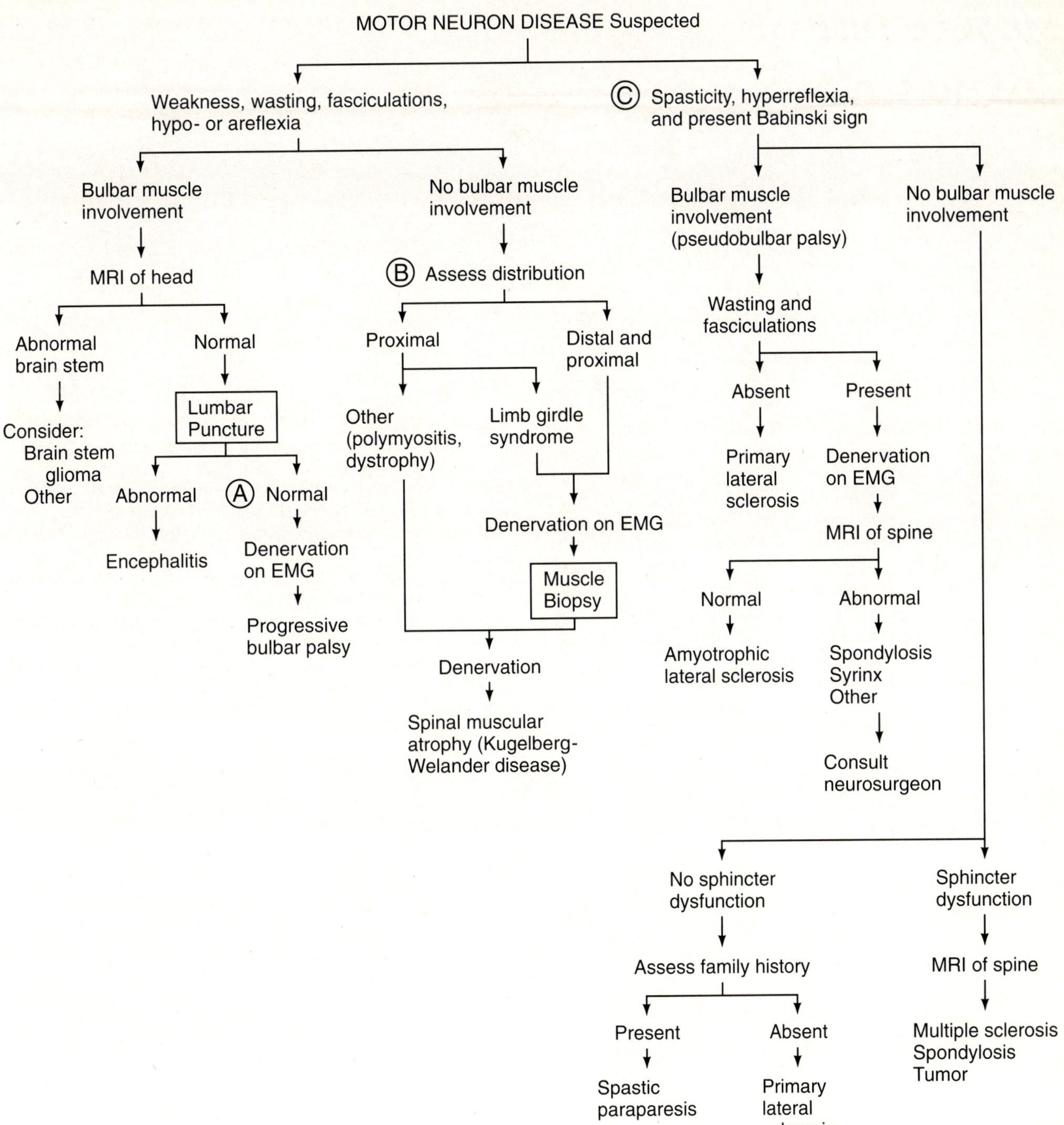

MOTOR NEURON DISEASE Suspected
Weakness, wasting, fasciculations, hypo- or areflexia
C Spasticity, hyperreflexia, and present Babinski sign
Bulbar muscle involvement
No bulbar muscle involvement
Bulbar muscle involvement (pseudobulbar palsy)
No bulbar muscle involvement
MRI of head
B Assess distribution
Wasting and fasciculations
Abnormal brain stem
Normal
Lumbar Puncture
Proximal
Distal and proximal
Absent
Present
Consider: Brain stem glioma Other
Abnormal
A Normal
Other (polymyositis, dystrophy)
Limb girdle syndrome
Primary lateral sclerosis
Denervation on EMG
Encephalitis
Denervation on EMG
Denervation on EMG
MRI of spine
Progressive bulbar palsy
Muscle Biopsy
Normal
Abnormal
Denervation
Amyotrophic lateral sclerosis
Spondylosis Syrinx Other
Spinal muscular atrophy (Kugelberg-Welander disease)
Consult neurosurgeon
No sphincter dysfunction
Sphincter dysfunction
Assess family history
MRI of spine
Present
Absent
Multiple sclerosis Spondylosis Tumor
Spastic paraparesis
Primary lateral sclerosis

MUSCLE DISEASE

MYOPATHY

Carlos A. Garcia, M.D.

The term myopathy is nonspecific and too generic, and should be avoided except early in the evaluation of symptoms before a definitive diagnosis is confirmed. Involvement of the facial, ocular, and bulbar muscles and the distribution of the muscles affected provide clues to the disease process. Make a pedigree of the family and examine close relatives of the affected person to detect subtle signs. The inheritance pattern (when available), the distribution of the weakness, and the progression of the symptoms in time will lead the clinician to the diagnosis and orient the work-up. Determination of muscle enzymes (creatine kinase), electrodiagnostic studies (including ischemic exercise when necessary), single fiber electromyography, and a muscle biopsy may be necessary to confirm the diagnosis. The clinical evaluation and tests should preferably be done by an expert in neuromuscular disorders to avoid repetition of invasive procedures. Muscle tissue should be sampled from an adequate muscle, and a portion of the fresh muscle should be freshly snap frozen for further biochemical analysis or blotting to detect DNA deletions.

The attached algorithm is an oversimplified overview of a few of the most common muscle disorders. Further details can be found in other chapters.

References

Brooke MH. A clinician's view of neuromuscular diseases. 2nd ed. Baltimore: Williams & Wilkins, 1986.

Ciafaloni E, Ricci E, Shanske S, et al. MELAS: Clinical features, biochemistry, and molecular genetics. Ann Neurol 1992; 31:391.

Dalakas M. Polymyositis, dermatomyositis, and inclusion body myositis. N Engl J Med 1991; 325:1487.

DiMauro S. Mitochondrial encephalomyopathies. Brain Pathol 1992; 2:111.

DiMauro S, Bonilla E, Faviani M, et al. Mitochondrial myopathies. Ann Neurol 1985; 17:521.

Griggs RC, Karpati G. The pathogenesis of dermatomyositis. Arch Neurol 1991; 48:21.

Haerer AF. DeJong's the neurological examination. 5th ed. Philadelphia: JB Lippincott, 1992.

Mastaglia FL, Ojeda VJ. Inflammatory myopathies. Part 1. Ann Neurol 1985; 17:215.

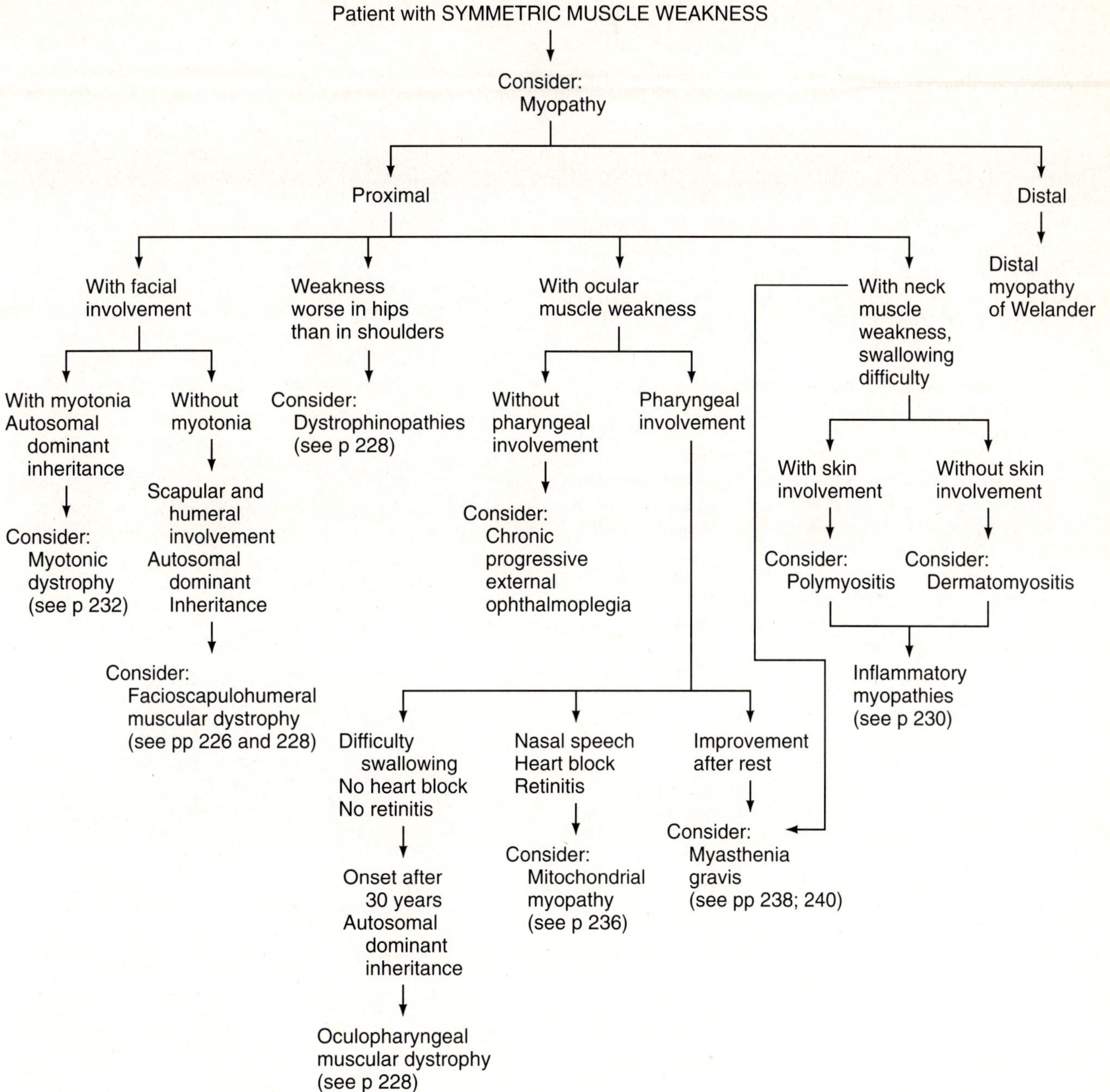

Patient with SYMMETRIC MUSCLE WEAKNESS
Consider:
Myopathy
Proximal
Distal
With facial involvement
Weakness worse in hips than in shoulders
With ocular muscle weakness
With neck muscle weakness, swallowing difficulty
Distal myopathy of Welander
With myotonia Autosomal dominant inheritance
Without myotonia
Consider: Dystrophinopathies (see p 228)
Without pharyngeal involvement
Pharyngeal involvement
With skin involvement
Without skin involvement
Consider: Myotonic dystrophy (see p 232)
Scapular and humeral involvement Autosomal dominant Inheritance
Consider: Chronic progressive external ophthalmoplegia
Consider: Polymyositis
Consider: Dermatomyositis
Consider: Facioscapulohumeral muscular dystrophy (see pp 226 and 228)
Difficulty swallowing No heart block No retinitis
Nasal speech Heart block Retinitis
Improvement after rest
Inflammatory myopathies (see p 230)
Onset after 30 years Autosomal dominant inheritance
Consider: Mitochondrial myopathy (see p 236)
Consider: Myasthenia gravis (see pp 238; 240)
Oculopharyngeal muscular dystrophy (see p 228)

DYSTROPHIC MYOPATHY

Carlos A. Garcia, M.D.

The muscular dystrophies (MDs) are a special group of degenerative diseases of muscle, some of which are due to gene abnormalities (deletions, mutations). The diseases are hereditary and progressive and are classified according to the inheritance pattern, the muscles affected, and the age at onset. They are of insidious onset and variable but usually have a slow progressive course, with contractures of joints developing as muscles become atrophic.

A. Duchenne's MD (pseudohypertrophic), the most common dystrophy of childhood, is an X-linked inherited disease with a high incidence of spontaneous mutations. DNA analysis has shown that 65% of Duchenne's patients have deletion mutations of the dystrophin gene, which is in the p21 region of the X chromosome. Dystrophin is the protein product of this gene. The disease affects boys at about 4 years of age. There is often a history of slow motor development (slow to walk), and the parents have noticed that the child is clumsy, walks on his toes, falls frequently, and has difficulty getting up from the floor. Examination shows a husky child with enlarged (pseudohypertrophic) calves and proximal muscle weakness. When sitting on the floor, the child gets up by turning around and propelling himself up by using his hands against his legs (Gowers' syndrome). The creatine kinase (CK) level is usually elevated into the thousands, and electromyography (EMG) shows a myopathic pattern. Muscle biopsy shows dystrophic changes and absent dystrophin by fluorescent immunohistochemistry. The disease is progressive, and the child becomes wheelchair bound at about 12 years of age. Physical therapy and braces may keep the patient active longer. The heart is involved (fibrosis) by the disease process. Death from cardiorespiratory failure occurs in the early 20s. Contractures are common in atrophic muscles once the child is chairbound. There is often intellectual retardation. Carriers of the disease may be identified (female relatives of the patient) by DNA analysis. Carriers may be asymptomatic or may have proximal muscle weakness (so-called manifesting carriers.)

B. Becker's MD is a benign form of Duchenne's MD with the same inheritance pattern, a later onset (5 to 10 years), and survival into the fifth decade. No intellectual or cardiac involvement is seen. In Becker's MD the dystrophin in the muscle biopsy is decreased or abnormal. Duchenne's and Becker's MD, manifesting carriers of Duchenne's, and a few other rare muscle disorders produced by deficiency or abnormalities of dystrophin are grouped under the term "dystrophinopathies."

C. Limb girdle MD is inherited as an autosomal recessive trait. The age at onset varies but is generally in the second or third decade. The disease affects the hip girdle muscles first and then the shoulder muscles. Progression is slow and insidious without intellectual or cardiac involvement. Physical therapy and braces may keep the patient ambulatory a few years longer.

D. Congenital MD is an autosomal recessive inherited disease seen at birth (floppiness) or in early life. Contractures of joints are common, and weakness and atrophy of the muscles are frequent and prominent. Release of contractures by physical therapy or surgery and braces facilitates management of these patients.

E. Facioscapulohumeral MD is an autosomal dominant inherited disease. It may present early in life (infantile form) with a rapid progression of weakness and contractures, or may begin later, in the 20s or 30s, with a slow progression. Relatives may relate that the patient sleeps with his eyes open (orbicularis oculi muscle weakness), and the patient reports difficulty in whistling and drinking through a straw. The facial weakness may be a prominent feature or minimal and

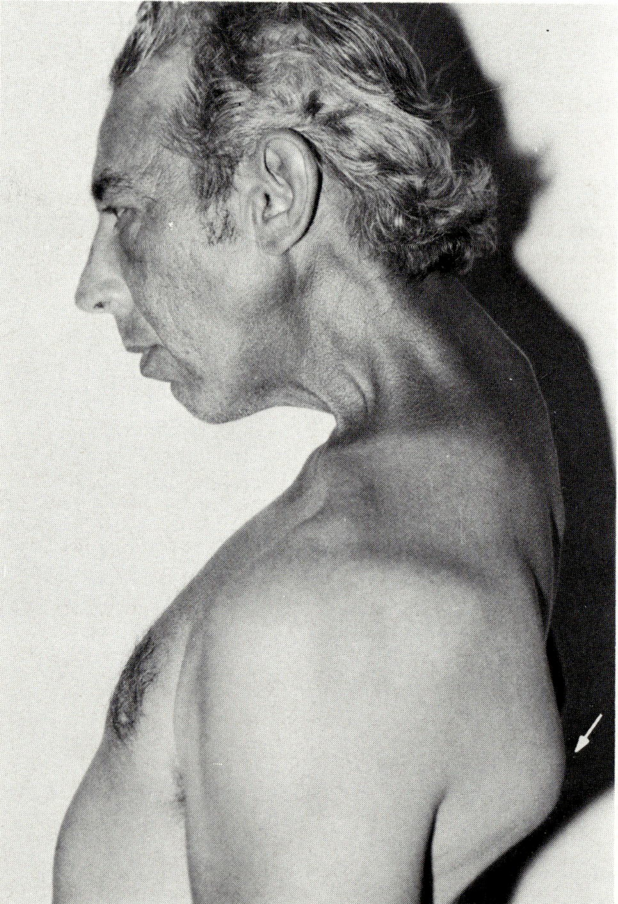

Figure 1 Weakness and atrophy of the neck muscle (swan neck) and winging of the scapula (*arrow*), as seen in facioscapulohumeral MD.

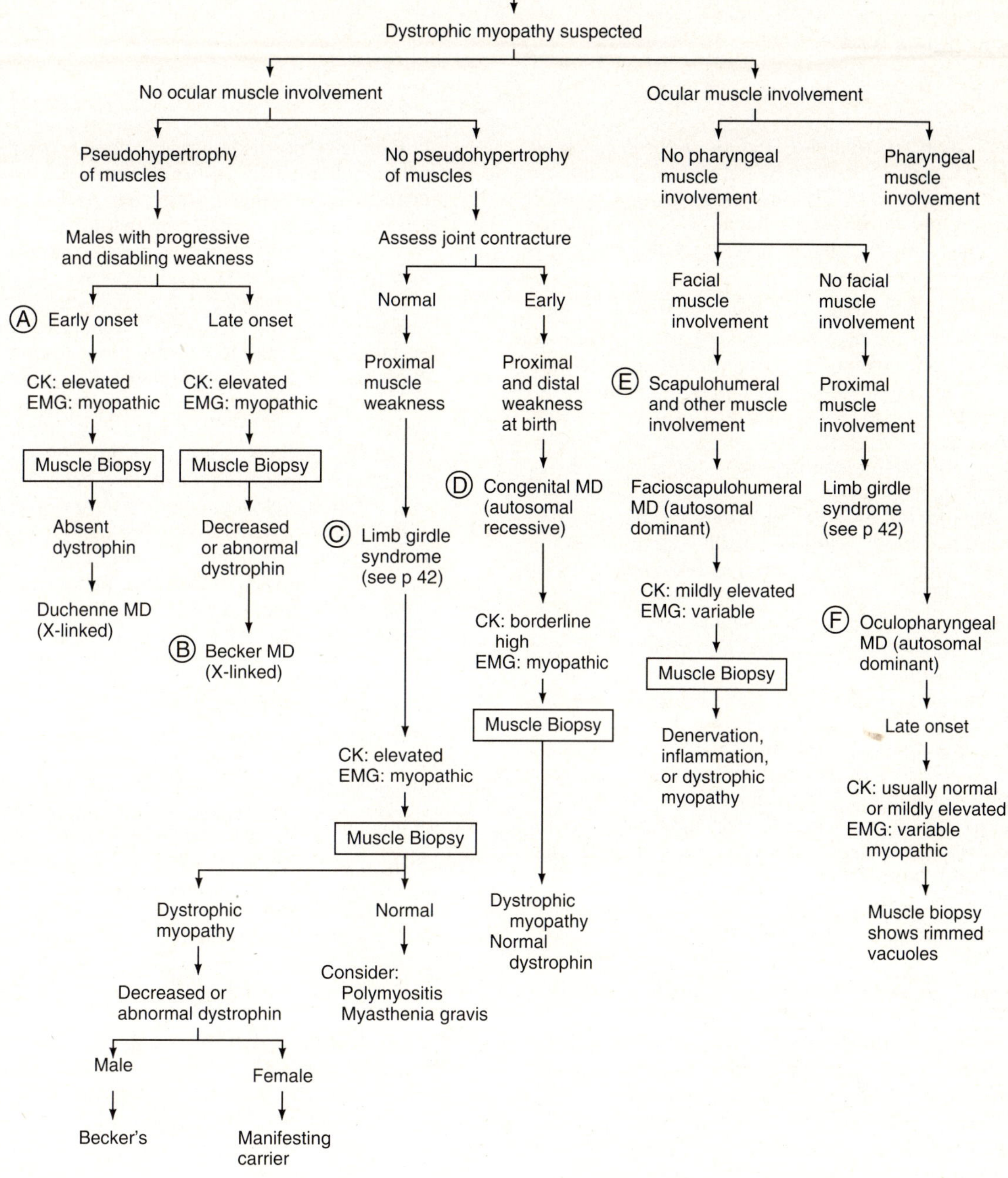

is associated with atrophy and weakness of the biceps and triceps (humeral) and scapular (winging) muscles (Fig. 1). The hip muscles also are often affected. Physical therapy retards or avoids contractures.

F. Oculopharyngeal MD is an autosomal dominant inherited disease with a late onset of symptoms, usually in the 40s or 50s. The disease is manifested by slowly progressive ptosis and extraocular muscle weakness. However, diplopia is rare. The patient also complains of difficulty swallowing (predominantly meat and bread, but all solids). Patients frequently adapt to this impediment and live a normal life span.

There are other less common types of muscular dystrophies that are not discussed here. See "Myotonic Syndromes" for a discussion of myotonic dystrophy.

References

Brooke MH. A clinician's view of neuromuscular diseases. 2nd ed. Baltimore: Williams & Wilkins, 1986.

Hoffman EP, Arahata K, Bonilla E, et al. Dystrophinopathy in isolated cases of myopathy in females. Neurology 1992; 42:967.

Hoffman EP, Kunkel LM. Dystrophin abnormalities in Duchenne (Becker) muscular dystrophy. Neurology 1989; 2:1019.

INFLAMMATORY MYOPATHIES

Carlos A. Garcia, M.D.

The inflammatory myopathies include a heterogeneous group of diseases characterized by necrosis and an inflammatory reaction of muscle. The myositis may be produced by a known infectious agent (bacteria, viruses, fungi, parasites), but in most cases no specific etiologic agent is found (idiopathic myositis).

A. The patient complains of acute painful weakness, usually localized to one thigh or calf. Examination reveals a red, swollen, tender area. There often are systemic signs of infection. Obtain blood cultures and carry out a muscle biopsy. Most cases of pyomyositis are produced by *Staphylococcus aureus* and *Streptococcus* and are secondary to a focus elsewhere. Suspect drug addiction with injection (Talwin) as an important factor. Mycotic infections can be identified by muscle biopsy and are usually due to *Candida albicans,* which is seen in immunosuppressed patients or drug addicts. If no systemic symptoms are detected and the symptoms are bilateral and symmetric, suspect a viral etiology (coxsackie) and obtain acute and convalescence serum. Sarcoidosis is a rare form of myositis; this diagnosis is established by finding noncaseating granulomas in the muscle biopsy specimen. When the patient presents with diffuse myalgia and has a history of recent travel to tropical areas or recent consumption of raw meats, suspect parasitic diseases, such as cysticercosis (eosinophilia in blood), trichinosis (gastrointestinal symptoms and periorbital edema), or toxoplasmosis (skin rash and lymphadenopathy). These specific types of myositis are very rare; if they are suspected, consult an infectious disease specialist.

B. Idiopathic inflammatory myositis includes a group of disorders of unknown etiology that are due to disturbances of immunoregulation. The clinical features vary according to the age of the patient, associated diseases, and involvement or noninvolvement of the skin (see Table 1). In pure polymyositis (PM) the predominant symptom is proximal symmetric muscle weakness (see p 38), which may be acute in onset or slowly progressive. Muscle pains and tenderness may be seen in acute cases but are not features in the insidious type. Neck muscle weakness and dysphagia are common and important features that may help to differentiate the disease from other myopathies. The extraocular muscles are not involved. PM is a cell-mediated disease manifested by partial invasion of non-necrotic muscle cells by cytotoxic lymphocytes. This type of presentation is most common in adult patients. When the skin is involved, the disorder is called dermatomyositis (DM) and there is an erythematous rash on the face, neck, and chest. The rash on the face has a butterfly distribution around the nose and a heliotrope discoloration and edema of the eyelids. There may be an erythematous rash on the dorsal surfaces of the elbows, knees, and ankles and over the knuckles (Gottron sign), which may be associated with periungual telangiectasias. The skin on the extremities is edematous, tense, and inelastic. Skin ulcerations in the acute phase of the disease, and subcutaneous calcifications later in the course, are seen in juvenile DM. Humoral-mediated damage to blood vessels initiates the angiopathy (vasculitis) that produces the characteristic muscle biopsy finding of perifascicular atrophy (Fig. 1). Adult DM may be associated with malignant tumors and is usually seen in male patients >50 years of age. Carcinomas of the lung and gastrointestinal tract are seen in males, and carcinomas of the breast and ovary in females. DM may precede discovery of the tumor by several months or a few years. Systemic cancer is rare in juvenile DM and in pure PM. Approximately 20% of cases of DM-PM are associated with connective tissue disorders (e.g., systemic lupus erythematosus, systemic sclerosis, rheumatoid arthritis, Sjögren's syndrome, polyarteritis nodosa, mixed connective tissue disorders). Some medications (e.g., penicillamine, procainamide, hydralazine) have been associated with PM-DM.

Diagnosis of PM-DM is based on four criteria: (1) predominantly or exclusively proximal, usually symmetric, muscle weakness progressing over weeks or months, with or without myalgia and with or without compatible dermatologic features; (2) biopsy evidence

TABLE 1 Classification of DM-PM

Childhood and juvenile dermatomyositis
Infantile polymyositis
Adult polymyositis
Adult dermatomyositis
DM and PM associated with malignancy
DM and PM associated with connective tissue disorder
Drug-induced DM-PM
Miscellaneous types

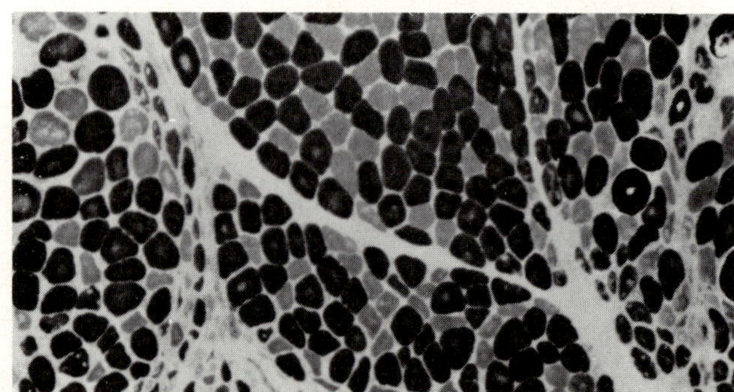

Figure 1 Microphotograph showing perifascicular atrophy in a case of dermatomyositis (ATPase stain pH 9.4, magnification 10×).

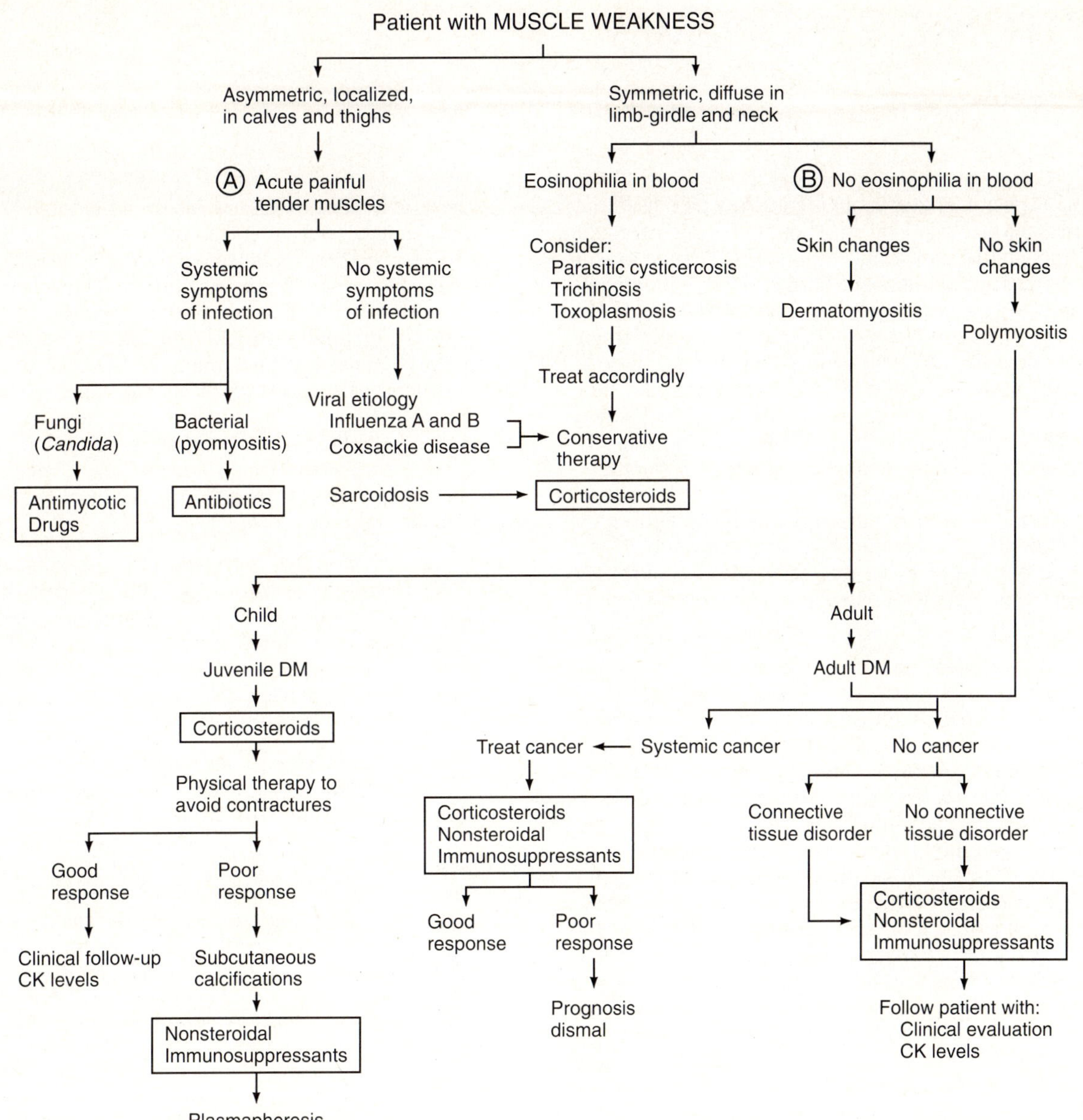

of muscle fiber necrosis, regeneration, and mononuclear cellular infiltrate (perivascular and intrafascicular), with or without perifascicular atrophy; (3) elevated serum creatine kinase (CK) (MM isoenzyme), aldolase, or myoglobin levels; and (4) multifocal electromyographic changes of myopathy (small, short duration, polyphasic motor unit potentials), with or without increased insertional activity and spontaneous potentials. A definitive diagnosis requires positive findings on all four criteria. A probable diagnosis requires three of the criteria. A muscle biopsy may not always show abnormalities even under the best circumstances because of the focal patchy nature of the inflammatory lesion.

Treatment consists of corticosteroid immunosuppression with a daily dose of 60 to 80 mg prednisone for 6 to 8 weeks, with gradual reduction of the dose and addition of nonsteroidal immunosuppressive drugs (azathioprine, cyclophosphamide) if no response is seen. Plasmapheresis and other forms of treatment such as cyclophosphamide (Cytoxan) IV Ig, have been used with mixed response.

References

Dalakas M. Polymyositis, dermatomyositis, and inclusion body myositis. N Engl J Med 1991; 325:1487.

Griggs RC, Karpati G. The pathogenesis of dermatomyositis. Arch Neurol 1991; 48:21.

Mastaglia FL, Ojeda VJ. Inflammatory myopathies. Part 1. Ann Neurol 1985; 17:215.

MYOTONIC SYNDROMES

Carlos A. Garcia, M.D.

Myotonia is characterized by an involuntary painless delay in the relaxation of skeletal muscles, either after forceful contraction (active myotonia) or after percussion of the muscle (percussion or mechanical myotonia). Stiffness, the main complaint, is worse early in the day or after inactivity; it improves after exercise (in contrast to the pattern of fatigability-myasthenia). Myotonia is aggravated by cold. When asked to make a forceful fist and then open the hand rapidly, patients with myotonia flex the wrist and slowly extend the fingers in a dystonia-like posturing (Fig. 1). Percussion of the thenar eminence produces a dimple in the muscle and abduction of the thumb with slow postcontraction relaxation. In generalized myotonia, patients have difficulty opening the eyes after closing them tightly. The family history, age of onset, and associated features are important factors with which to differentiate the myotonias.

A. Myotonic dystrophy (DM-1) is the most common of the myotonias and the most common of all dystrophies in adults. The disease is inherited in an autosomal dominant pattern with a variable clinical expression and variable age of onset (20 to 50 years). The genetic abnormality is due to an unstable fragment of DNA on chromosome 19. The copy number of extra copies of this fragment (the trinucleotide AGC) correlates well with the severity of the disease. Most patients consult the physician late in the disease and complain mainly of weakness of the hands or legs. The examination reveals ptosis, lack of facial expression, atrophy of the temporal and masseter muscles, and opened mouth (myopathic facies). The speech is fast, short, and dysarthric. There is distal weakness and atrophy of the hands, arms, feet, and legs, together with premature baldness, cataracts, and refraction problems. The disease is associated with diabetes and gonadal dysfunction. Low testosterone levels have been found.

There is hypersomnia and often cardiac involvement (arrhythmias). Treatment consists of physical therapy and testosterone replacement in males. Myotonia is rarely a complaint but in some patients may be an important symptom; it responds temporarily to phenytoin or tocainide HCl (Tonocard). Procainamide should be used with caution because of the heart disorders. Children born of affected females may be affected at birth (congenital myotonic dystrophy) but present with floppiness, myopathic facies, difficulty in sucking and swallowing, and respiratory impairment. The myotonia appears later in life and is associated with mental retardation.

B. A rare myotonic-atrophic disorder seen in young adults or children is associated with hyperhidrosis and deformity of the feet. There is generalized and constant myokymia and heat intolerance. Isaac's syndrome, neuromyokymia, stiff-man syndrome, and other names have been given to this obscure disorder; it responds to phenytoin, 300 mg/day.

C. Myotonia congenita is a myotonic disorder associated with hypertrophy of muscles. The disease is diagnosed early in life and affects most muscles, including ocular and facial muscles and those of the extremities. The inheritance pattern is autosomal recessive but in a few families is autosomal dominant. There are no associated endocrinopathies and no baldness or cataracts, and the heart is not affected. The myotonia responds to tocainide HCl. A rare form of congenital myotonia is associated with dwarfism and ocular abnormalities; this is chondrodystrophic myotonia (Schwartz-Jampel disease).

D. A rare form of myotonia not associated with changes in muscle size is seen early in life and is precipitated by cold. Cold also produces a generalized weakness sometimes associated with hypokalemia, known as paramyotonia congenita (Eulenburg's disease).

E. Myotonia can be produced by some medications. Clofibrate causes stiffness and myotonia. Also, some insecticides and monocarboxylic aromatic acids may produce myotonia. Pseudomyotonia is observed in hypothyroidism in older patients, and electrophysiologically in some glycogenoses of muscle and in some peripheral neuropathies.

References

Brooke MH. A clinician's view of neuromuscular diseases. 2nd ed. Baltimore: Williams & Wilkins, 1986.

Buxton J, Shelbourne P, Davis J, et al. Detection of an unstable fragment of DNA specific to individuals with myotonic dystrophy. Nature 1992; 355:547.

Harper PS. Myotonic dystrophy. 2nd ed. Philadelphia: WB Saunders, 1989.

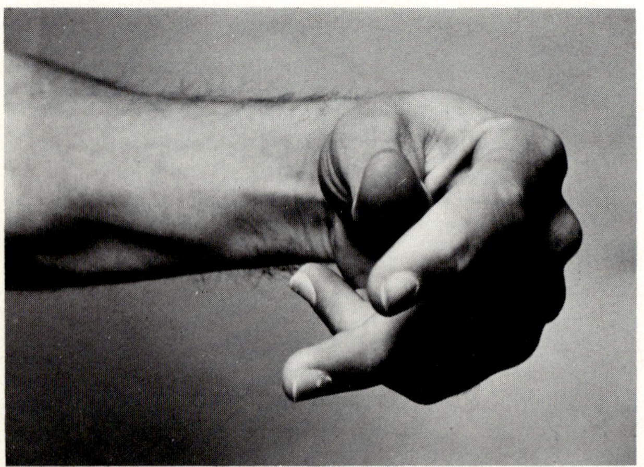

Figure 1 Contraction myotonia seen when the patient is trying to open his hand after making a forceful fist.

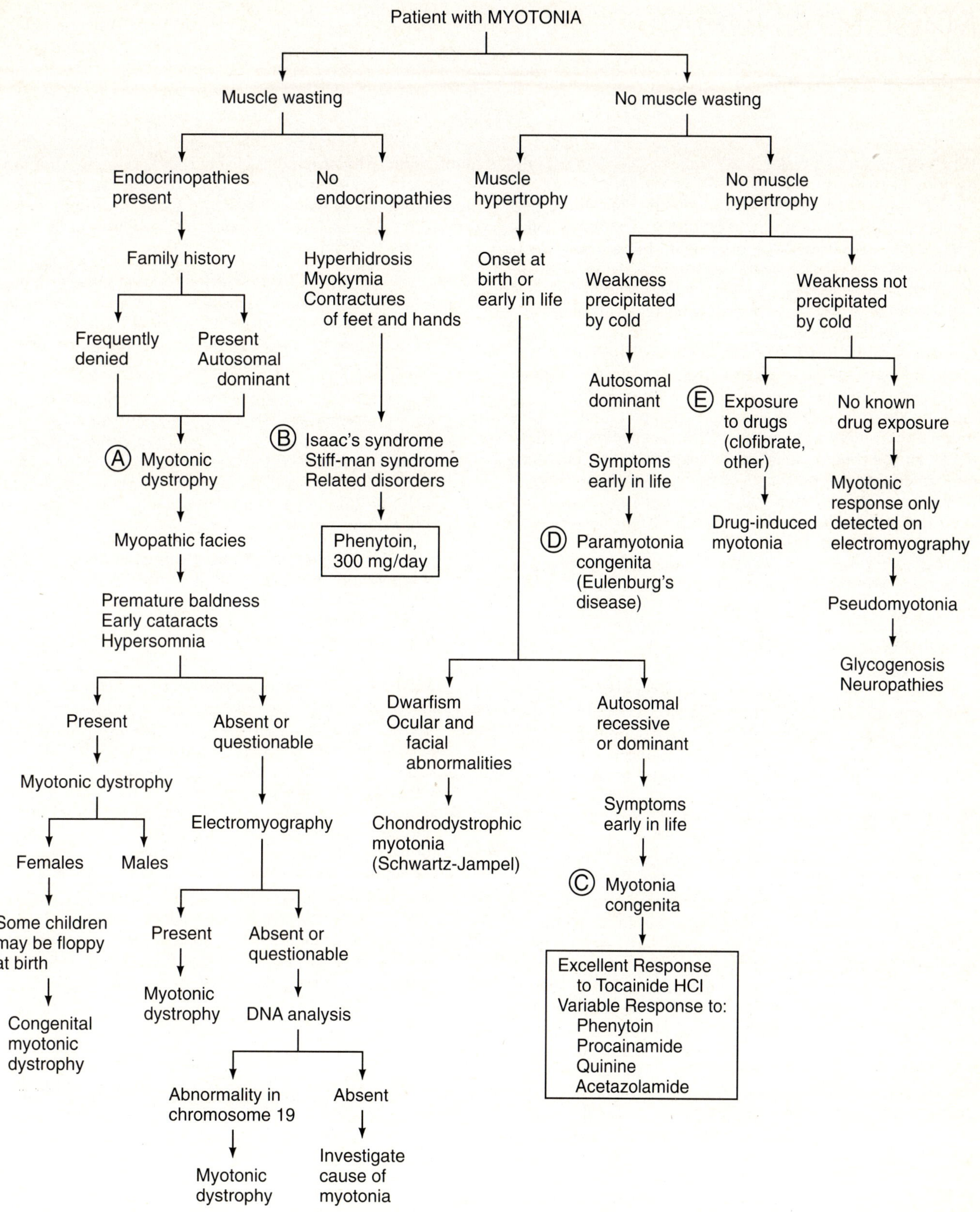

Patient with MYOTONIA
Muscle wasting
No muscle wasting
Endocrinopathies present
No endocrinopathies
Muscle hypertrophy
No muscle hypertrophy
Family history
Hyperhidrosis
Myokymia
Contractures of feet and hands
Onset at birth or early in life
Weakness precipitated by cold
Weakness not precipitated by cold
Frequently denied
Present Autosomal dominant
A Myotonic dystrophy
B Isaac's syndrome
Stiff-man syndrome
Related disorders
Autosomal dominant
E Exposure to drugs (clofibrate, other)
No known drug exposure
Phenytoin, 300 mg/day
Symptoms early in life
Drug-induced myotonia
Myotonic response only detected on electromyography
Myopathic facies
D Paramyotonia congenita (Eulenburg's disease)
Pseudomyotonia
Premature baldness
Early cataracts
Hypersomnia
Glycogenosis
Neuropathies
Present
Absent or questionable
Dwarfism
Ocular and facial abnormalities
Autosomal recessive or dominant
Myotonic dystrophy
Electromyography
Chondrodystrophic myotonia (Schwartz-Jampel)
Symptoms early in life
Females
Males
C Myotonia congenita
Some children may be floppy at birth
Present
Absent or questionable
Excellent Response to Tocainide HCI
Variable Response to:
Phenytoin
Procainamide
Quinine
Acetazolamide
Congenital myotonic dystrophy
Myotonic dystrophy
DNA analysis
Abnormality in chromosome 19
Absent
Myotonic dystrophy
Investigate cause of myotonia

MYOGLOBINURIA

Carlos A. Garcia, M.D.

When there is acute disintegration of muscle with accompanying necrosis (rhabdomyolysis), myoglobin, one of the protein constituents of muscle, is released into the blood and then into the urine (myoglobinuria). The terms rhabdomyolysis and myoglobinuria have been used interchangeably to describe these phenomena. When rhabdomyolysis occurs, there is a characteristic syndrome. This includes intense myalgias, fever, widespread weakness so that the patient is unable to walk, and swelling and tenderness of the limbs. The weakness usually involves the arms and legs, but the respiratory muscles may be involved in severe cases. There is a marked elevation of the blood creatine kinase (CK) level. Electromyography (EMG) shows myopathic potentials; muscle biopsy specimens show acute muscle necrosis. In most cases the urine becomes dark owing to the presence of myoglobin. Other conditions, including porphyria (the urine does not react with benzidine, the CK level is normal, and the Watson-Schwartz test is positive) and hemoglobinuria (the serum haptoglobin level is low and CK is normal) cause pigment deposition and discoloration of the urine. In most cases of myoglobinuria the urine is discolored. However, it is possible to detect small amounts of myoglobin in the serum by radioimmunossay techniques when the urine does not appear discolored because the amount of myoglobin released from the muscle is too small to be seen on routine inspection of urine color. The major complication of myoglobinuria is that this substance accumulates in the kidneys to cause acute renal failure (anuria, azotemia, acidosis, hyperkalemia, hypercalcemia). In any patient with unexplained acute renal failure, suspect myoglobinuria. Carry out a CK determination and a radioimmunoassay for myoglobin.

What triggers these events of rhabdomyolysis in muscles? Over 50 different causes have been described and may be divided into genetic (metabolic) abnormalities of muscle (phosphorylase deficiency, carnitine palmitoyl transferase deficiency) and responses to certain drugs (succinylcholine, halothane) that cause biochemical abnormalities in muscle because the patient has a genetic impairment of the capacity to metabolize these drugs. The sporadic cases have been related to intense muscle exertional activity. This is most common in untrained athletes who perform vigorous exertion. The disorder may also occur following seizures or after the muscle has been crushed (an extremity is caught under heavy weight in an accident or the patient is in coma and remains fixed in one position). Occlusion of a major artery may cause ischemia, and this may trigger rhabdomyolysis. This condition may occur in alcoholics and heroin addicts, possibly because of depression of muscle metabolism. The three most common causes of myoglobinuria are alcohol abuse, muscle crush, and excessive activity. Primary muscle disorders (e.g., McArdle's disease) are rare causes of myoglobinuria.

A. In patients with acute renal failure of unexplained cause, perform a CK determination and a radioimmunoassay for myoglobin. If these are positive, treatment is directed toward preserving renal function. This includes promotion of diuresis with mannitol; since anuria is present, dialysis may be needed.

B. Search for causes of myoglobinuria: alcohol or heroin abuse; other drugs, including halothane and succinylcholine; metabolic factors, including hypothermia, acidosis, carbon monoxide, and hyperthermia; mechanical factors, including crush injury and ischemia of limbs; and exertional factors, including seizures or other intense exercise.

C. After the patient recovers from this episode, regaining strength and normal renal function, perform a full muscle evaluation, including muscle biopsy, to determine whether there is a metabolic muscle disorder of lipid or glycogen metabolism. This requires careful histochemical and biochemical analysis of muscle. Inherited recurrent myoglobinuria has been shown to be related to phosphorylase, phosphofructokinase, phosphoglycerate kinase, phosphoglyceromutase, and lactate dehydrogenase. These enzymes are involved in glycogenolysis and glycolysis. Carnitine palmitoyl transferase is involved in fatty acid transport and has been associated with myoglobinuria. Mitochondrial DNA deletions have been seen in some cases of inherited recurrent myoglobinuria. Rarely, myoglobinuria may result from acute polymyositis or occur in the course of Duchenne's muscular dystrophy. This muscle evaluation may be carried out after patients recover from the acute illness, or possibly should be reserved for those who have a second episode or recurrent episodes of myoglobinuria.

References

Gabow PA, Kaehny WD, Kelleher SP. The spectrum of rhabdomyolysis. Medicine 1982; 61:141.

Hno K, Tanaka M, Sahashi K, et al. Mitochondrial DNA deletions in inherited recurrent myoglobinuria. Ann Neurol 1991; 29:364.

Rowland LP. Myoglobinuria. Can J Neurol Sci 1984; 11:1.

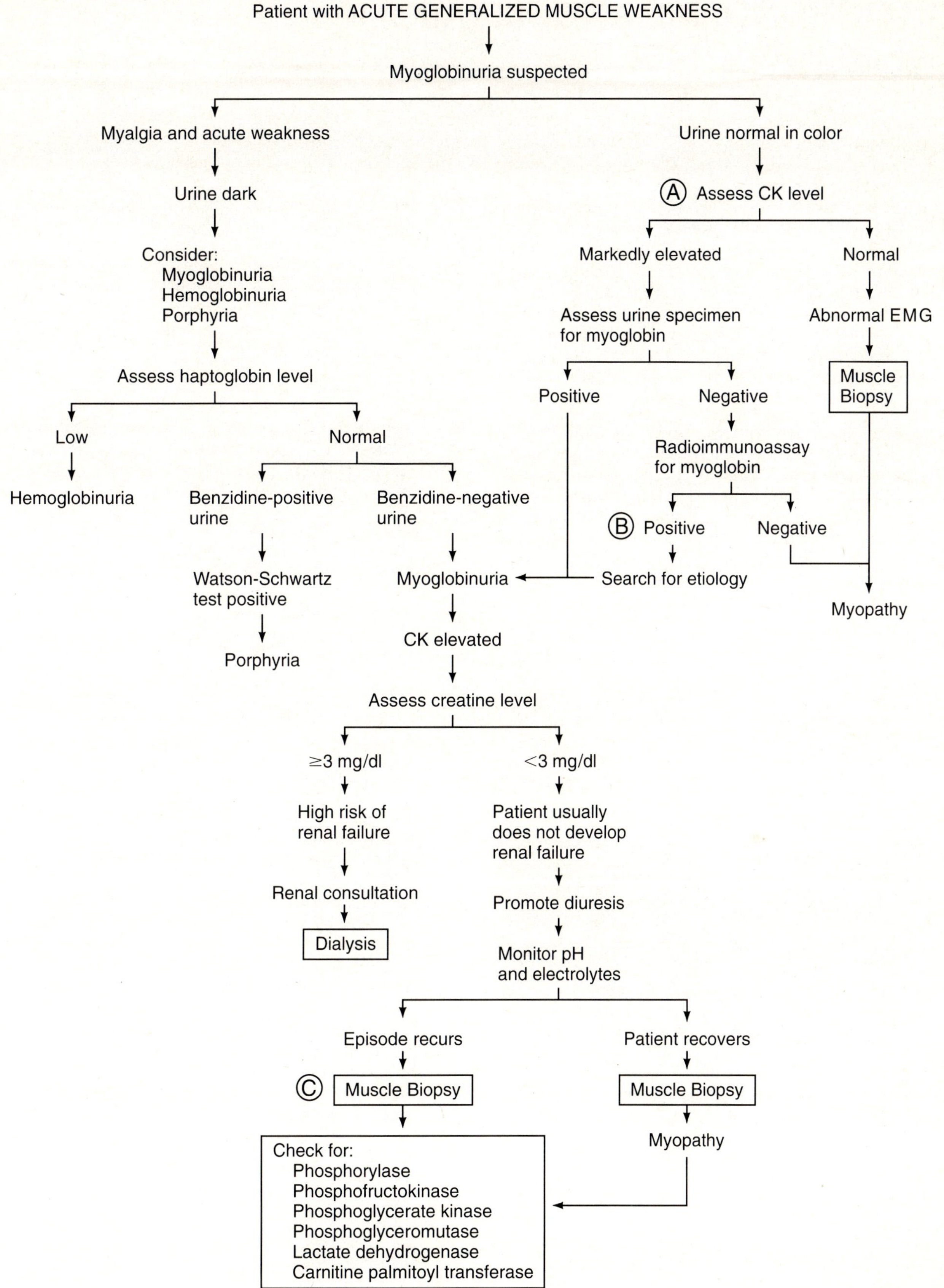

Patient with ACUTE GENERALIZED MUSCLE WEAKNESS
Myoglobinuria suspected
Myalgia and acute weakness
Urine normal in color
Urine dark
A Assess CK level
Consider:
Myoglobinuria
Hemoglobinuria
Porphyria
Markedly elevated
Normal
Assess urine specimen
for myoglobin
Abnormal EMG
Assess haptoglobin level
Positive
Negative
Muscle
Biopsy
Low
Normal
Radioimmunoassay
for myoglobin
Hemoglobinuria
Benzidine-positive
urine
Benzidine-negative
urine
B Positive
Negative
Watson-Schwartz
test positive
Myoglobinuria
Search for etiology
Myopathy
Porphyria
CK elevated
Assess creatine level
≥3 mg/dl
<3 mg/dl
High risk of
renal failure
Patient usually
does not develop
renal failure
Renal consultation
Promote diuresis
Dialysis
Monitor pH
and electrolytes
Episode recurs
Patient recovers
C Muscle Biopsy
Muscle Biopsy
Myopathy
Check for:
Phosphorylase
Phosphofructokinase
Phosphoglycerate kinase
Phosphoglyceromutase
Lactate dehydrogenase
Carnitine palmitoyl transferase

MITOCHONDRIAL AND METABOLIC MYOPATHY

Carlos A. Garcia, M.D.

Mitochondrial and metabolic myopathies constitute a rare and heterogeneous group of inherited disorders of muscle, some of which can affect other systems. The clinical presentation is variable, and muscle biopsy shows mitochondrial abnormalities of storage material. Biochemical analysis of muscle confirms the diagnosis in most cases. Large-scale deletions have been described in Kearns-Sayre syndrome, and point mutations of mitochondrial DNA have been found in Leber's optic neuropathy, MERF, MELAS, and multisystem disorders.

A. Kearns-Sayre syndrome is seen predominantly in males, with an onset before 20 years of age, and is characterized by ophthalmoplegia, pigmentary degeneration of the retina, and heart block. Patients frequently have cerebellar dysfunction and increased CSF protein. Muscle biopsy shows ragged red fibers with abnormal mitochondria (enlarged) containing paracrystalline inclusions on electron microscopy (Fig. 1).

B. Chronic progressive external ophthalmoplegia has a varied presentation. There is an insidious onset of ophthalmoplegia without retinal degeneration. Proximal muscle weakness may occur and heart block may be present. CNS involvement (cerebellar and corticospinal tract dysfunction) may be seen. The muscle biopsy specimen shows ragged red fibers with paracrystalline inclusions. The disease may begin at different ages, from young adulthood to the fourth or fifth decade.

C. Myoclonus epilepsy with ragged red fibers (MERF) is a rare familial syndrome manifested predominantly by CNS symptoms, including myoclonus, generalized seizures, and ataxia. Muscle biopsy examination shows ragged red fibers.

D. Mitochondrial myopathy, encephalopathy, lactic acidosis, and strokelike episodes (MELAS) are characteristics of a rare disease that presents after the first year of life with episodic vomiting, seizures, and cerebral damage. There is no ophthalmoplegia, and muscle biopsy shows abnormal mitochondria.

E. Carnitine deficiency is a rare disorder of muscle characterized by progressive proximal muscle weakness with an onset in childhood or young adulthood. No specific clinical features are seen. The muscle biopsy specimen shows excessive lipid accumulation, and muscle biochemical analysis demonstrates a deficiency of carnitine. Prednisone, carnitine replacement, and a high carbohydrate diet have proved beneficial for this condition. Systemic carnitine deficiency is seen in early life and is manifested by acute episodes of encephalopathy associated with hepatic dysfunction. A partial response to carnitine therapy has been demonstrated.

F. The most common form of glycogen storage disease type II (Pompe's disease) is the infantile form. It is an autosomal recessive inherited disorder manifested by floppiness and visceromegaly. Muscle biopsy shows a vacuolar myopathy with excessive glycogen storage in the muscle fibers. Biochemical analysis shows a deficiency in acid maltase (a lysosomal enzyme). Juvenile and adult forms may be seen. In the juvenile form, children present with proximal muscle weakness that is the same as that seen in the dystrophic myopathies and spinal muscular atrophy. Biopsy and biochemical analysis of muscles confirm the diagnosis. The adult form may present with a slowly progressive myopathy, but respiratory failure is a common presentation. No satisfactory treatment has been found except for symptomatic management. A rare form of glycogenosis (McArdle's disease) may present in young adults with muscle pains and cramps and exercise intolerance. An ischemic exercise test shows no elevation of lactic acid, and muscle biopsy and histochemical tests confirm the deficiency of myophosphorylase.

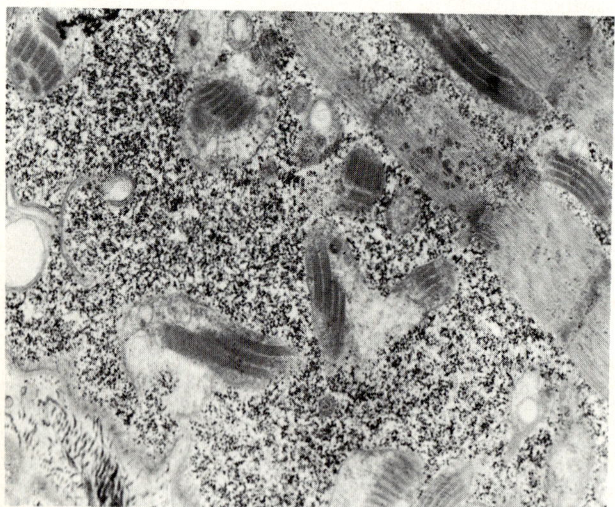

Figure 1 Electron micrograph showing paracrystalline inclusions within abnormal mitochondria in skeletal muscle (65,000×).

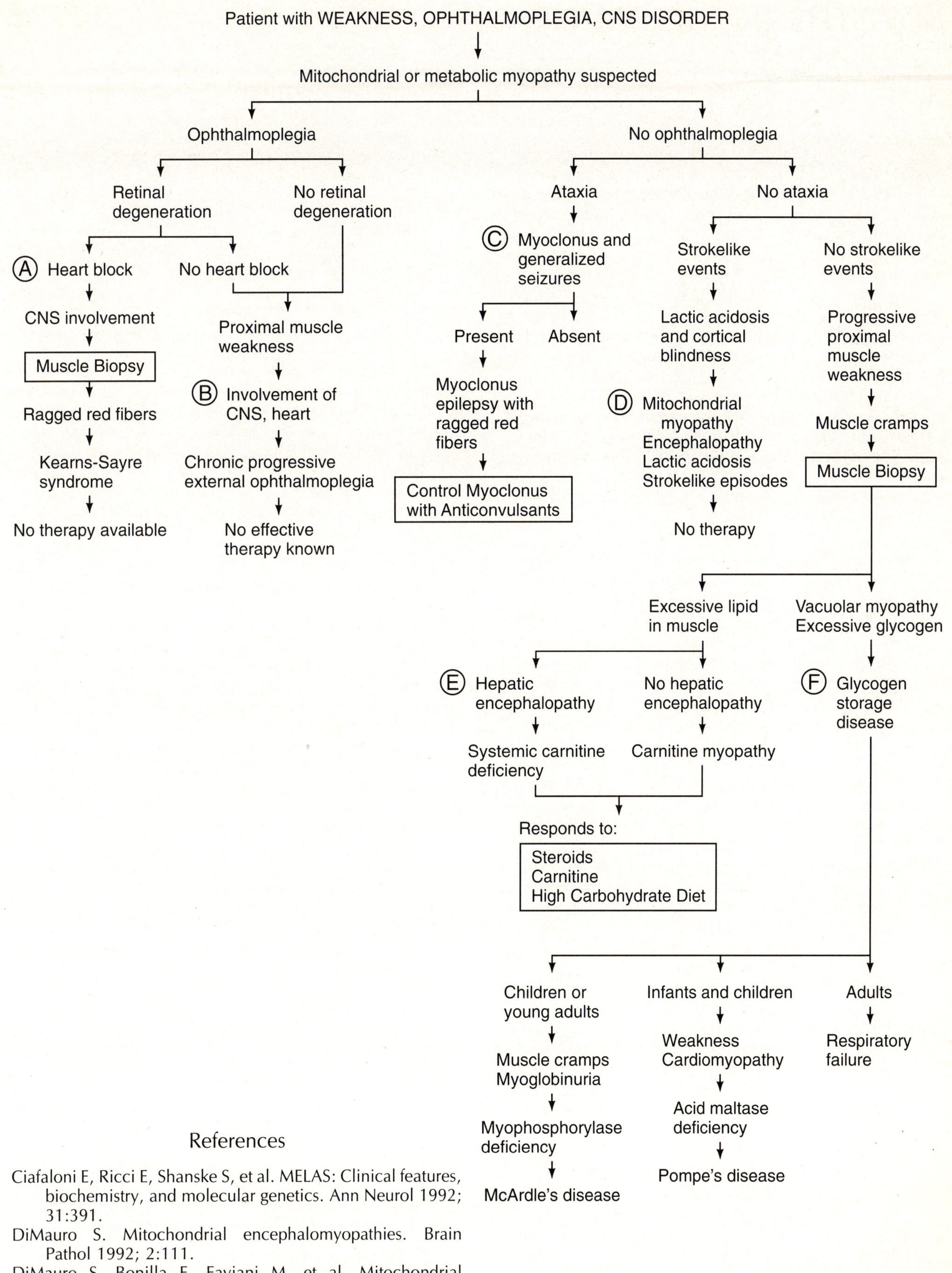

References

Ciafaloni E, Ricci E, Shanske S, et al. MELAS: Clinical features, biochemistry, and molecular genetics. Ann Neurol 1992; 31:391.

DiMauro S. Mitochondrial encephalomyopathies. Brain Pathol 1992; 2:111.

DiMauro S, Bonilla E, Faviani M, et al. Mitochondrial myopathies. Ann Neurol 1985; 17:521.

MYASTHENIC DISORDERS

Carlos A. Garcia, M.D.

The myasthenic disorders are a group of diseases that involve defects in neuromuscular transmission and are characterized clinically by fatigue. The group includes two autoimmune diseases, myasthenia gravis (MG) and the Eaton-Lambert syndrome, and some congenital myasthenic syndromes. Botulism also affects neuromuscular transmission.

MG is caused by a reduction in the number of acetylcholine receptors (AChR) due to the presence of antibody to AChR. It is characterized by fatigue with a rapid restoration of strength after rest. The fatigue affects the most active muscles. In nearly 50% of patients, ptosis or diplopia is the first symptom. The disease remains localized to the ocular muscles (ocular myasthenia) in 16% of patients. Generalized symptoms occur in most patients within 1 year. The disease onset is usually slow and insidious but may be acute, with generalized weakness and even respiratory failure (myasthenic crisis), usually precipitated by stress or infections.

A. If weakness is not evident at the time of examination, try to reproduce the weakness by fatiguing the muscles. Ask the patient to look up; the eyelids will droop slowly in myasthenic patients. Ask the patient to count, and listen for a nasal change in the voice of myasthenic patients. Ask the patient to sit or squat and get up several times, and observe the progressive difficulty in performing the task in myasthenic patients. Once there is objective evidence of weakness, perform a Tensilon (edrophonium chloride) test. Inject 2 mg (0.2 ml) of short-acting anticholinesterase intravenously. If no side effects occur, continue the injection very slowly until a positive response (increased strength) is obtained or 10 mg (1.0 ml) has been injected. Atropine sulfate (0.6 mg) should be available to inject in case the patient shows excessive tearing, sweating, nausea, and vomiting. Patients with MG show a dramatic and transient (lasting 5 minutes) improvement in strength within 30 to 60 seconds (positive Tensilon test). If there is no change in strength, the test is considered negative. If there is no objective weakness at the time of the examination and the fatigue is not reproduced, the Tensilon test is of no value and an electrophysiologic test may be required. This involves repetitive supramaximal nerve stimulation, which produces decremental contractions of the stimulated muscle in MG and differentiates the disease from the Eaton-Lambert syndrome.

B. Neuromuscular "jitters" and blocking in single fiber electromyography also help to confirm the diagnosis of MG. In 90% of myasthenic patients, AChR antibodies are found in serum. However, remember that the percentage of elevated antibodies is lower in pure ocular MG and that the titers in serum correlate loosely with the severity of the disease. Also, false-positive antibodies are found in first-degree relatives of myasthenic patients, in elderly patients with other immune disease, in patients with rheumatoid arthritis treated with penicillamine, and in myasthenic patients in remission.

C. Thymomas are found in 15% of myasthenic patients. However, thymic abnormalities are seen in 70% to 80% of myasthenic patients. Thymosin is a thymic hormone that seems to initiate and perpetuate the immune response against the AChR. Consequently, thymectomy should be performed as soon as the presence of a thymoma is established. Controversy still exists over the timing in nonthymomatous myasthenia and in pure ocular MG. In patients with thymoma, there is no sex predilection and no HLA antigen association. In patients without thymoma and onset before age 40, there is a female preponderance and an increased association with HLA-A1, B8, and WRW3 antigens. In patients with no thymoma and onset of MG after age 40, there is a male preponderance and an increased association with HLA-A3, B7, and DRW2 antigens.

D. Besides thymectomy, treatment consists of relief of symptoms with anticholinesterase drugs and immunosuppressive therapy. Pyridostigmine (Mestinon), 60 mg every 4 hours, may be used as a temporary measure to prevent aspiration in patients with bulbar symptoms. Alternate-day corticosteroid therapy, beginning with a low dose (20 mg prednisone) and with a slow rise to 80 to 100 mg, is beneficial in most patients. The initial low dose avoids the exacerbation of myasthenic symptoms seen when high doses are used immediately. Nonsteroidal immunosuppressive drugs such as azathioprine (Imuran) may be used as adjuvants when no response is obtained. Plasmapheresis produces rapid but short-lived improvement and is indicated in a myasthenic crisis or as an adjuvant in patients taking immunosuppressive therapy. The term myasthenic crisis is used when the patient goes into respiratory failure because of weakness of the intercostal muscles, diaghragm, and laryngeal muscles. In these cases the patient must be intubated; anticholinesterase therapy is discontinued and plasmapheresis carried out. The therapy previously outlined is reestablished after the patient is stabilized. IV immunoglobulin has been used with good response in some patients.

E. Botulism is produced by food intoxication due to the exotoxin of *Clostridium botulinum*. Symptoms occur within 36 hours after ingestion of contaminated food and consist of anorexia, nausea, and vomiting followed by blurred vision and diplopia, bulbar symptoms, and generalized weakness. Dilated and unreactive pupils differentiate the disease from MG. Therapy consists of IV injection of trivalent antiserum.

F. Eaton-Lambert syndrome is a rare autoimmune disease attributable to a reduction in the amount of acetylcholine released from the nerve terminal. The disease is characterized by proximal (predominantly hip) muscle weakness associated with dry mouth and a metallic

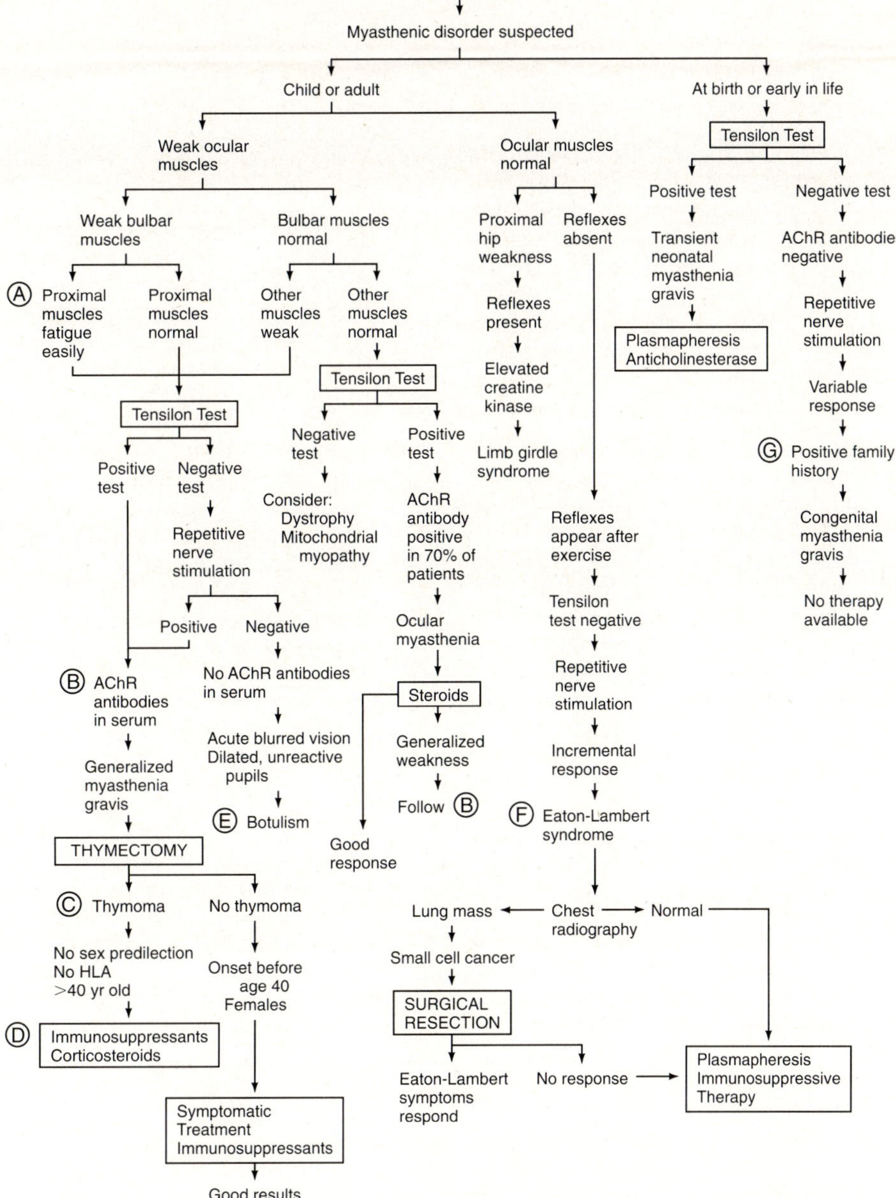

taste in the mouth. The extraocular muscles are frequently spared. Impotence often occurs. Reflexes are absent but reappear after exercise. The disease is often associated with small cell carcinoma of the lung. Treatment consists of eradication of the tumor when present. The disease responds to corticosteroid therapy, nonsteroidal immunosuppressants, and plasmapheresis.

G. Congenital myasthenic syndromes are characterized by ocular muscle weakness since birth, difficulty in chewing and swallowing, and fatigue in infancy. The disorders are familial. No immune mechanism is involved. AChR antibody levels are not elevated and there is no response to thymectomy or immunosuppressive therapy. The syndromes may be caused by a defect in acetylcholine synthesis, acetylcholinesterase deficiency, or an end-plate AChR deficiency. These disorders should be differentiated from the transient neonatal MG seen in children born to myasthenic mothers, who respond to plasmapheresis and anticholinesterase. In transient neonatal MG the symptoms subside within 4 weeks.

References

Engel AG. Myasthenia gravis and myasthenic syndromes. Ann Neurol 1984; 16:519.

Swift TR. Disorders of neuromuscular transmission other than myasthenia gravis. Muscle Nerve 1981; 4:334.

Verma PK, Oger JJF. Seronegative generalized myasthenia gravis: Low frequency of thymic pathology. Neurology 1992; 42:586.

AUTOIMMUNE MYASTHENIA GRAVIS: MANAGEMENT

Carlos A. Garcia, M.D.

The management of autoimmune myasthenia gravis should be directed toward improving the symptoms with anticholinesterase medications and suppressing the production of antibodies against acetylcholine (ACh) receptors by means of immunosuppressive therapy. Treatment should be individualized to each patient according to the severity of the symptoms and the response to therapy. The overview given here is based on hypothetical situations, is oversimplified, and should be used only as a guideline to be modified and adapted to each patient.

A. Mestinon (pyridostigmine bromide) is an active cholinesterase inhibitor that facilitates neuromuscular transmission by inhibiting the destruction of ACh by cholinesterase. It is available in 60-mg tablets, syrup containing 60 mg per teaspoonful (5 ml), Timespan 180-mg tablets, and 2-ml ampules for injection. Mestinon should be used as needed to improve the symptoms (e.g., 60-mg tablets 30 to 45 minutes before meals in patients with predominantly chewing and swallowing difficulty; every 2 or 3 hours for respiratory difficulty). Use the parenteral form to supplement the oral dose pre- and postoperatively, during labor, and in myasthenic crisis. Supplement Mestinon with other medications when the clinical response is not good in spite of high doses or when side effects occur frequently (abdominal cramps, diarrhea, nausea, weakness). Mestinon is still the first line of therapy.

B. Thymectomy is still a controversial issue. It should be performed in all patients with thymomas detected by imaging studies and also in all patients with generalized myasthenia gravis regardless of age who do not respond adequately to anticholinesterase therapy. It may be beneficial in some cases of pure ocular myasthenia. Respiratory, bulbar, and generalized symptoms should be controlled before thymectomy by Mestinon or plasmapheresis. Adequate response to thymectomy may take a few months to several years, depending on the severity and duration of the disease before surgery.

C. Plasmapheresis produces a good and fast but temporary improvement of the myasthenic symptoms. It is ideally used in myasthenic crisis and in conjunction with other therapy. It may be used before thymectomy to improve respiratory and bulbar symptoms. Plasmapheresis should be performed daily or every other day for five sessions and ideally should replace the blood volume approximately 2500 ml per session in adult patients.

D. Prednisone improves symptoms in most patients with ocular and generalized myasthenia. Use it only when the symptoms do not respond to Mestinon. It can be started pre- or post-thymectomy according to the response to Mestinon. Begin with 20 mg every other day with increments of 10 mg every third dose to reach 80 or 100 mg or remission of myasthenic symptoms. An initial low dose with progressive increments will reduce the exacerbation of symptoms that can occur when a high dose is given at the beginning of treatment. Use a daily dose in severe cases and a high initial dose if the patient is under close supervision for the first 2 weeks. Tapering of steroids should begin 3 to 6 months after the myasthenic symptoms have improved. Keep in mind all the side effects of high-dose steroids (e.g., diabetes mellitus, hypertension, osteoporosis, aseptic necrosis of the head of the femur). While the patient is on steroids, supplement the calcium intake with one 500-mg tablet daily and supplement the potassium intake with one K-Lyte tablet a day.

E. Azathioprine (Imuran) (2 mg/kg/day) may be used as an adjuvant therapy in myasthenic patients who have had thymectomy, are on Mestinon and prednisone, and have not responded adequately. Advise women of reproductive age of the possible teratogenic effects of the medication. Other immunosuppressants such as cyclosporin and cyclophosphamide have been used with mixed results.

F. IV immunoglobulin (IgG) has been tried in some myasthenic patients, with mixed results. The use of this expensive therapy should wait until controlled studies show good results.

References

Engel AG. Myasthenia gravis and myasthenic syndromes. Ann Neurol 1984; 16:519.

Swift TR. Disorders of neuromuscular transmission other than myasthenia gravis. Muscle Nerve 1981; 4:334.

Verma PK, Oqer JJF. Seronegative generalized myasthenia gravis: Low frequency of thymic pathology. Neurology 1992; 42:586.

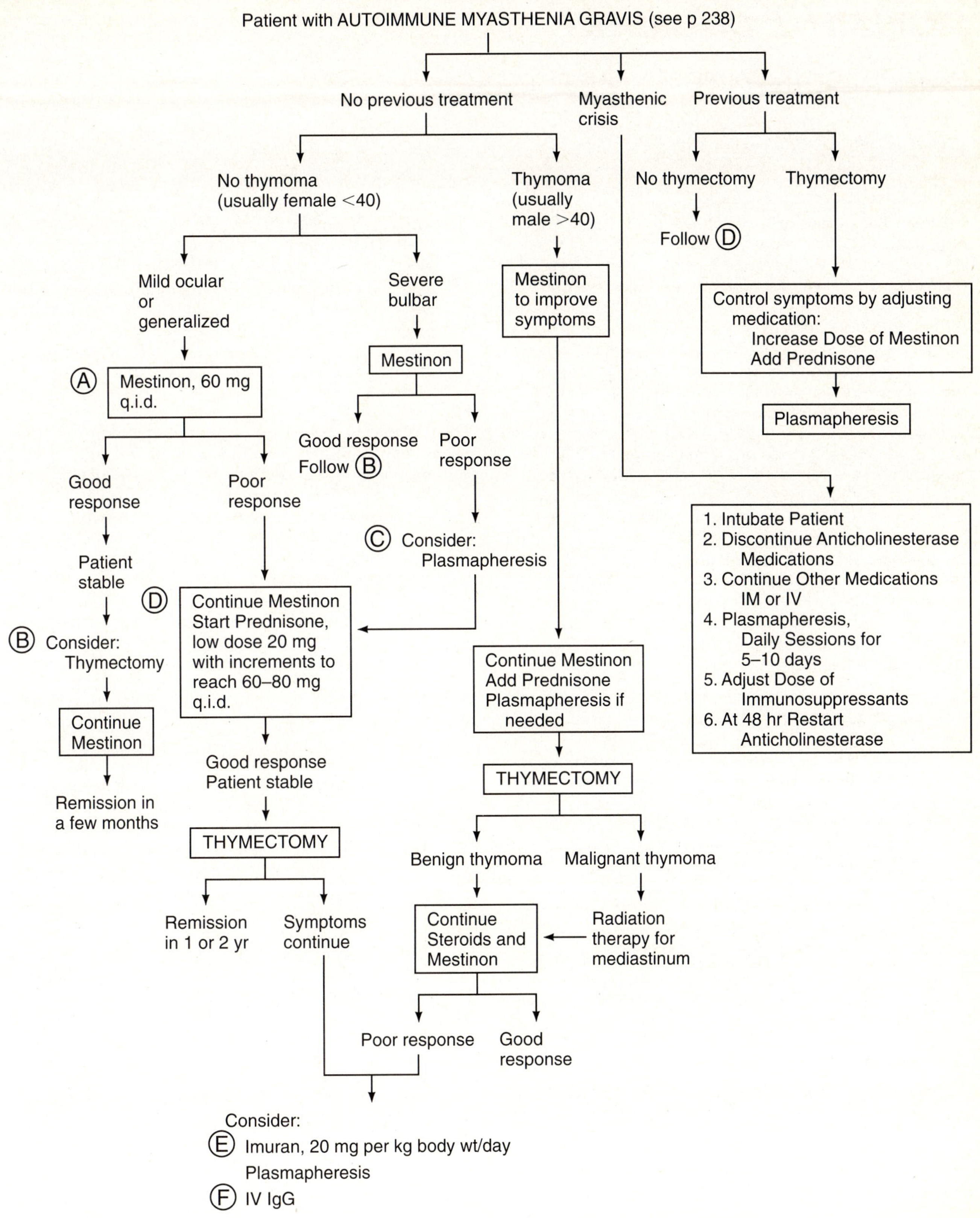

Patient with AUTOIMMUNE MYASTHENIA GRAVIS (see p 238)

No previous treatment
Myasthenic crisis
Previous treatment

No thymoma (usually female <40)
Thymoma (usually male >40)
No thymectomy
Thymectomy

Mild ocular or generalized
Severe bulbar
Mestinon to improve symptoms
Follow (D)
Control symptoms by adjusting medication:
Increase Dose of Mestinon
Add Prednisone

(A) Mestinon, 60 mg q.i.d.
Mestinon
Plasmapheresis

Good response
Poor response
Good response Follow (B)
Poor response

Patient stable
(C) Consider: Plasmapheresis
1. Intubate Patient
2. Discontinue Anticholinesterase Medications
3. Continue Other Medications IM or IV
4. Plasmapheresis, Daily Sessions for 5–10 days
5. Adjust Dose of Immunosuppressants
6. At 48 hr Restart Anticholinesterase

(B) Consider: Thymectomy
(D) Continue Mestinon Start Prednisone, low dose 20 mg with increments to reach 60–80 mg q.i.d.

Continue Mestinon
Continue Mestinon Add Prednisone Plasmapheresis if needed

Remission in a few months
Good response Patient stable

THYMECTOMY
THYMECTOMY

Remission in 1 or 2 yr
Symptoms continue
Benign thymoma
Malignant thymoma

Continue Steroids and Mestinon
Radiation therapy for mediastinum

Poor response
Good response

Consider:
(E) Imuran, 20 mg per kg body wt/day
Plasmapheresis
(F) IV IgG

MOVEMENT DISORDERS

PARKINSON-LIKE SYMPTOMS

Leon A. Weisberg, M.D.

Patients who present with symptoms of idiopathic Parkinson's disease (coarse, slow, high-amplitude resting tremor; impaired postural stability; rigidity; bradykinesia) should be evaluated for other disorders to exclude "secondary" parkinsonism. Perform diagnostic studies to exclude structural brain lesions such as neoplasm, subdural hematoma, normal-pressure hydrocephalus, and multi-infarct arteriosclerotic parkinsonism. Exclude other degenerative disorders with parkinsonian features (e.g., olivopontocerebellar degeneration, progressive supranuclear palsy, striatonigral degeneration); this is usually possible by reviewing other associated neurologic findings. The diagnosis of idiopathic parkinsonism is established by clinical findings and there is no definitive laboratory test to confirm it. Diagnosis may be definitively established by autopsy findings, including loss of dopamine-producing neurons of the substantia nigra and the presence of Lewy bodies. Patients do not usually have parkinsonian symptoms until there is an 80% loss of striatal dopamine content. In 90% of parkinsonian patients, there is a response to dopaminergic medication; failure to respond to this medication suggests a condition that may simulate idiopathic parkinsonism.

A. Obtain a history of psychiatric drug use (antipsychotic and antidepressant medications). A parkinsonian syndrome has been reported in patients with an occupational history of manganese exposure. In patients who survive carbon monoxide poisoning, parkinsonian symptoms may result from necrotic basal ganglia lesions. Exposure to neurotoxin MPTP (*N*-methyl-4-phenyl-tetrahydropyridine) may cause parkinsonian syndrome. This toxin is a substance produced in the synthesis of synthetic heroin that is illegally attempted by "street chemists." MPTP may cause a parkinsonian syndrome and this deficit may not be reversed despite treatment with high-dose dopaminergic agents.

B. New cases of postencephalitic parkinsonism resulting from the encephalitis epidemic of 1918 are not usually seen today. Other forms of viral encephalitis may cause parkinsonism. Jakob-Creutzfeldt disease may cause Parkinson-like symptoms, usually with dementia and myoclonic jerks; this diagnosis is suggested by characteristic periodic EEG abnormalities and confirmed by brain biopsy findings (spongiform encephalopathy). Serologic and CSF examination findings are used to diagnose neurosyphilis, which is a possible cause of parkinsonism.

C. CT and MRI are usually normal in idiopathic parkinsonism. Because patients with other neurologic disorders may present with parkinsonian features (basal ganglia neoplasm, normal-pressure hydrocephalus), CT/MRI should be performed. CT/MRI may show posterior fossa atrophy in cerebellar and olivopontocerebellar degeneration, or midbrain atrophy in progressive supranuclear palsy. In patients with parkinsonian symptoms, an abnormal serum calcium level or CT evidence of basal ganglia calcification should prompt careful evaluation for parathyroid hormone abnormalities.

D. Wilson's disease may present with parkinsonian features. Abnormal liver function studies and slit lamp evidence of Kayser-Fleischer rings are diagnostic of Wilson's disease. In patients with evidence of hepatic dysfunction who develop parkinsonian symptoms but in whom there is no slit lamp findings, or other laboratory evidence of Wilson's disease (normal ceruloplasmin and normal urine copper levels), consider nonwilsonian hepatolenticular basal ganglia degeneration. If Huntington's disease is suspected and antipsychotic drugs are used to control the abnormal behavior manifested by these patients, drug-induced parkinsonism may develop as a side effect. Rigidity is seen in patients with juvenile Huntington's disease.

E. The finding of atypical clinical features of parkinsonism and poor response to dopaminergic medications should suggest an alternative diagnosis to idiopathic parkinsonism. Impaired upward gaze is not uncommon in elderly patients with Parkinson's disease, but vertical (upward and downward) gaze paresis suggests progressive supranuclear palsy. These patients also show axial dystonia and rigidity, pseudobulbar palsy, and frontal lobe signs. Progressive supranuclear palsy is frequently confused with parkinsonism, but this condition does not respond to dopaminergic medication, in contrast to a good response in idiopathic parkinsonism. If patients with parkinsonian symptoms also have cerebellar disturbances (dysarthria, limb and gait dysmetria and ataxia), this suggests olivopontocerebellar degeneration. Parkinsonian features may develop in a later stage of Alzheimer's or Jakob-Creutzfeldt disease. The finding of postural hypotension before initiation of dopaminergic drug therapy in patients with parkinsonian symptoms suggests the possibility of Shy-Drager syndrome. If there are parkinsonian symptoms without tremor and the patient does not respond to dopaminergic medication, consider striatonigral degeneration; this condition can be diagnosed only on the basis of autopsy findings.

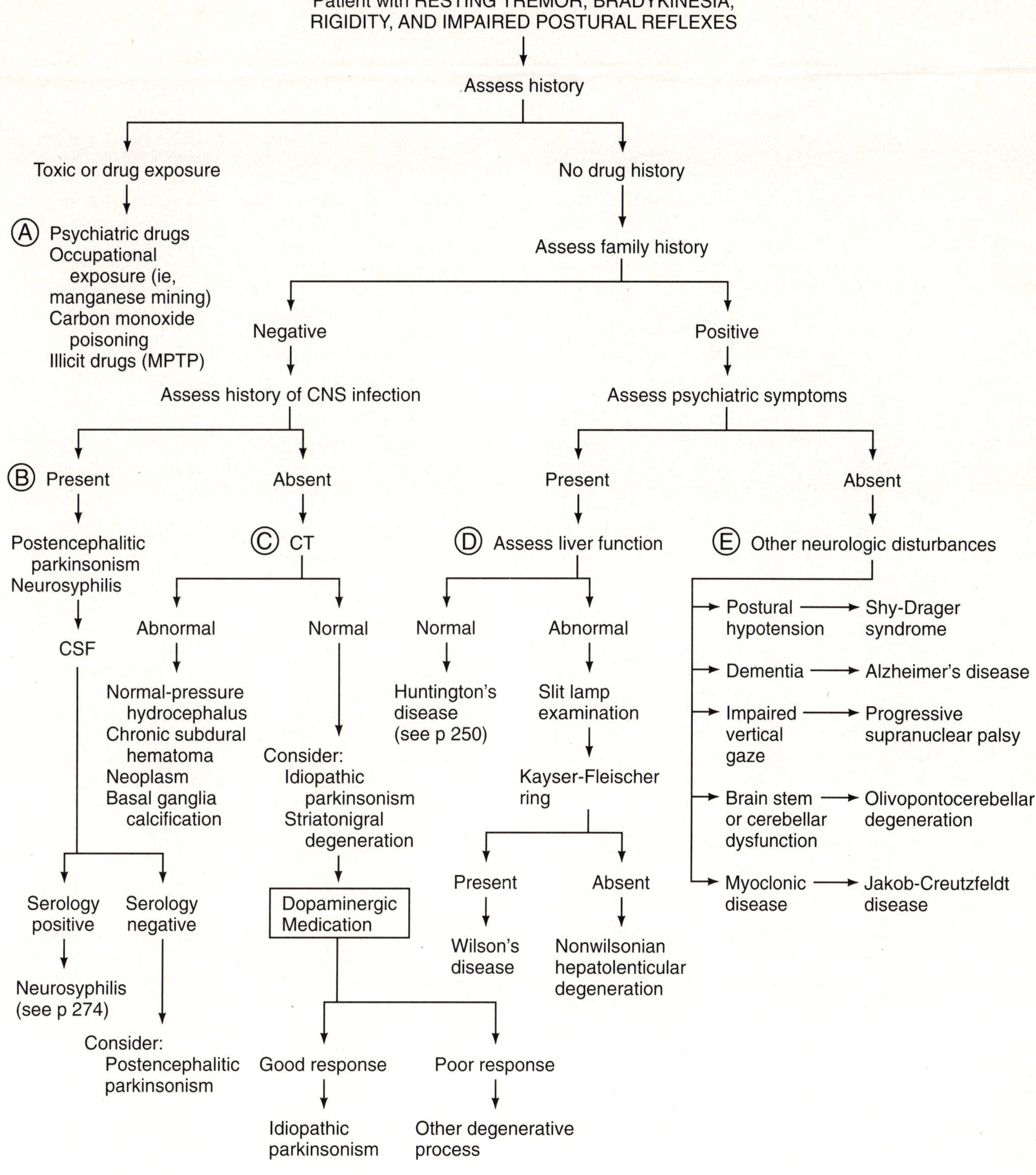

References

Jankovic J. Progressive supranuclear palsy: Clinical and pharmacologic update. Neurol Clin North Am 1984; 2:473.

Polinsky RJ. Multiple system atrophy: Clinical aspects, pathophysiology and treatment. Neurol Clin North Am 1984; 2:487.

PARKINSONISM: TREATMENT STRATEGIES

Leon A. Weisberg, M.D.

When patients with idiopathic parkinsonism become symptomatic, there is 80% loss of striatal dopamine content with relative preservation of brain acetylcholine content. Treatment is designed to restore the neostriatal dopamine-acetylcholine balance. Most idiopathic parkinsonian patients initially respond to dopaminergic medication, and this initial response is sometimes used for diagnostic purposes. In the early stages of parkinsonism, symptoms may not be functionally disabling. The decision to begin treatment should be carefully considered, because early therapy with dopaminergic medication does not alter disease progression but may cause these drugs to be less effective when symptoms become more functionally disabling at a later stage. In addition, evidence is emerging that dopaminergic medication may actually exacerbate disease progression. Symptoms of parkinsonism may be divided into two types: (1) a predominantly resting tremor and (2) predominantly impaired postural stability, usually with rigidity and bradykinesia. Patients in the second group are more functionally impaired than those in the first.

A. For tremor, anticholinergic drugs (trihexyphenidyl HCl [Artane], benztropine mesylate [Cogentin]) are efficacious. Side effects may include dry mouth, visual blurring, palpitations, tachycardia, dizziness, difficult urination, constipation, increased intraocular pressure, confusional states, and psychoses.

B. For patients with postural impairment, dopaminergic drugs are used. This is accomplished with Sinemet, a combination of levodopa (L-dopa) and a peripheral dopa decarboxylase inhibitor (carbidopa). This combination drug is most effective in preventing peripheral (systemic) side effects (nausea, vomiting, postural hypotension) but does not reduce CNS side effects (confusion, psychoses, hallucinations, dyskinesias). Initiate treatment with Sinemet 25/100 (25 mg dopa decarboxylase inhibitor and 100 mg L-dopa), one-half tablet twice daily. Increase the dose by one-half tablet every third day and monitor clinical improvement. Increase the dose slowly to ensure that the patient has achieved maximal clinical effect at that particular dose. Use the lowest dosage to accomplish symptomatic functional relief without causing toxicity. To avoid toxicity, it may be necessary to use a dosage that does not achieve maximal clinical improvement. As the dose is increased, the time interval of medication administration should initially be every 4 hours but this may vary, depending on the rate at which the dopaminergic effect wears off. Some patients have a short (1 to 2 hours) response and others have a response of long duration. If CNS toxicity develops, reduce the dosage. Most patients initially respond to dopaminergic drugs; one third continue to respond and two thirds show declining clinical response with a significant decline in the drug's effect after 5 years. Amantadine (100 mg twice daily) may be used to potentiate the effect of Sinemet; this synergistic action rapidly diminishes within several months.

C. The side effects of dopaminergic medication may be divided into those that are drug related and those due to disease progression. Nausea is less severe with Sinemet than with L-dopa alone. If Sinemet 25/100 is used (high carbidopa–to–L-dopa ratio) rather than Sinemet 10/100 or 25/250, nausea may be further minimized. If nausea persists, use trimethobenzamide HCl (Tigan) or hydroxyzine pamoate (Vistaril), but avoid prochlorperazine maleate (Compazine), as this drug may exacerbate parkinsonism. Orthostatic hypotension may be minimized by using Sinemet 25/100; other techniques to avoid this complication include use of support stockings, having the patient rise slowly and sit before standing, and administration of mineralocorticoid medication. Treat the agitation and confusion caused by dopaminergic drug effect with a lowered Sinemet dosage. If confusion persists, use selected neuroleptic antipsychotic drugs such as thioridazine HCl (Mellaril), which are less likely to exacerbate parkinsonism. To achieve best clinical response and minimize side effects, administer Sinemet with small snacks. Sinemet taken on an empty stomach increases the potential for nausea; if it is taken with meals of high protein content, this may reduce medication effectiveness.

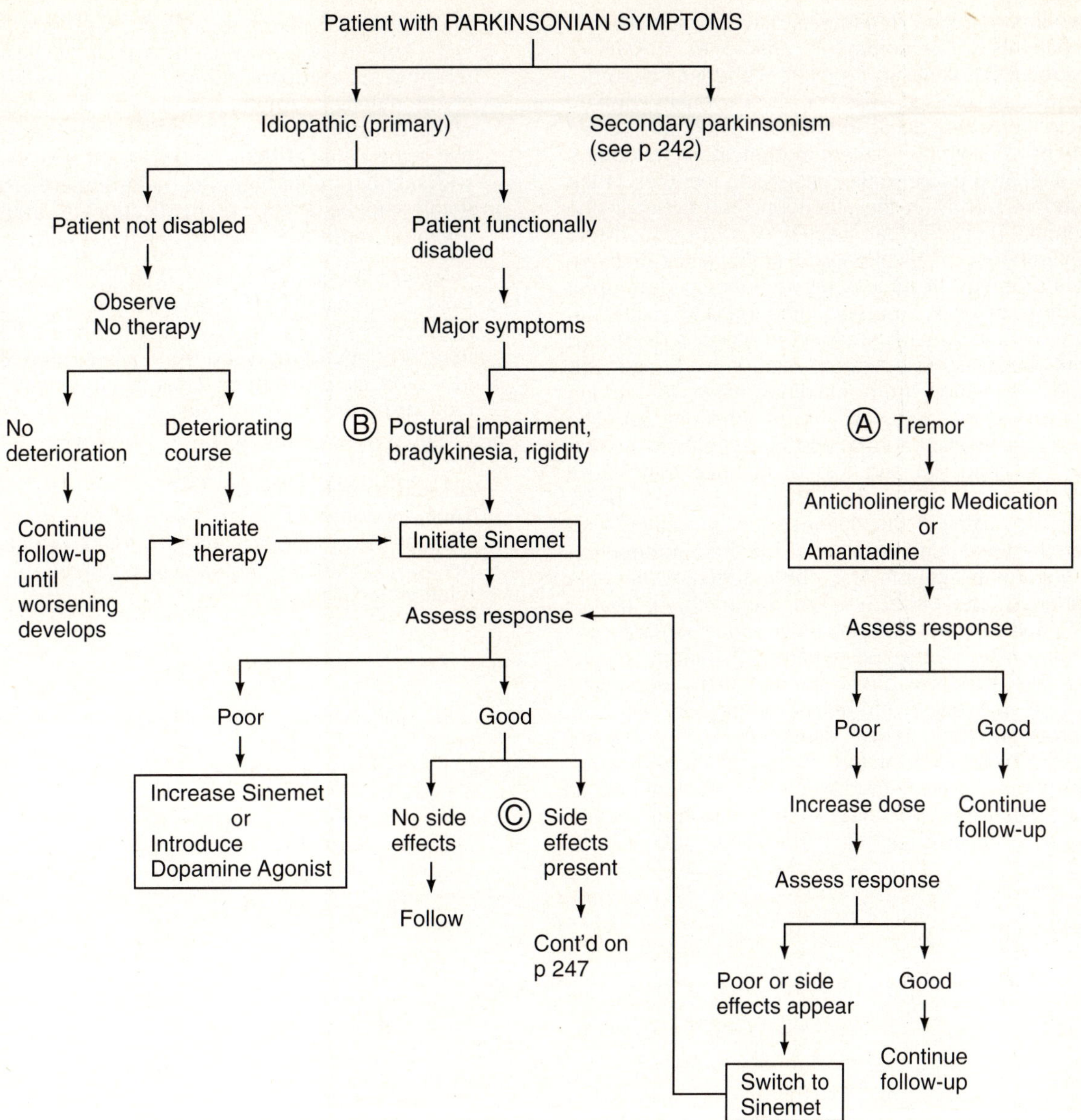

Patient with PARKINSONIAN SYMPTOMS

Idiopathic (primary)

Secondary parkinsonism
(see p 242)

Patient not disabled

Patient functionally
disabled

Observe
No therapy

Major symptoms

No
deterioration

Deteriorating
course

B Postural impairment,
bradykinesia, rigidity

A Tremor

Continue
follow-up
until
worsening
develops

Initiate
therapy

Initiate Sinemet

Anticholinergic Medication
or
Amantadine

Assess response

Assess response

Poor

Good

Poor

Good

Increase Sinemet
or
Introduce
Dopamine Agonist

No side
effects

C Side
effects
present

Increase dose

Continue
follow-up

Follow

Assess response

Cont'd on
p 247

Poor or side
effects appear

Good

Switch to
Sinemet

Continue
follow-up

D. Levodopa-induced dyskinesias may develop in 75% of patients, most commonly after 3 to 5 years of treatment. Dyskinesias correlate with medication duration and dosage. Clinical parkinsonian disease fluctuations may occur in both untreated and treated patients. A common pattern of clinical fluctuations is for untreated parkinsonian patients to feel well in the morning, poorly in the afternoon, and better in the evening. These fluctuations may occur in response to dopaminergic medication and are a major management problem. In some cases, dyskinesias develop at the time of peak dose concentration. Other fluctuations include an early wearing-off effect, a decreased peak effect, akinesia with no relation to dosage, and rapid fluctuation from maximal effect to sudden wearing off or "freezing" (on-off phenomena). The rapid change from normal postural stability to sudden freezing (akinesia) and loss of balance may cause patients to fall. When this happens, they may break their hip. Clinical fluctuations may be treated with more frequent administration of Sinemet, introduction of dopamine agonists (e.g., bromocriptine mesylate [Parlodel], pergolide mesylate [Permax]), or use of sustained-release carbidopa-levodopa preparations. Parkinsonism spares postsynaptic dopamine receptors, and therefore direct stimulation by dopamine agonists may effectively reduce symptoms. The most appropriate time to use dopamine agonists is not settled, but they probably should be started when Sinemet is associated with clinical fluctuations or when the disease worsens. Dopamine agonists are less effective than L-dopa but cause fewer side effects.

Their potential toxicities include gastrointestinal effects, hypotension, psychiatric symptoms, vasospasm resulting in acroparesthesias, angina pectoris, and erythromelalgia. Another management strategy used when dopaminergic medication becomes less effective is the "drug holiday"; however, this is associated with marked exacerbation of parkinsonian symptoms. If this can be accepted, medication is often better tolerated and more effective when started again.

E. Selegiline (deprenyl) and vitamin E are antioxidants used to halt pathologic disease progression. Deprenyl is a selective monoamine oxidase B inhibitor, and this may offer neuroprotection by blocking production of free radicals and reducing the neurotoxicity of free radicals on the brain. The dosage is 5 mg twice daily. It is not clear whether this drug also causes symptomatic improvement, but this is probable because deprenyl acts to potentiate the CNS dopaminergic effects. There is some evidence that early treatment with deprenyl slows disease progression and delays the need to introduce symptomatic treatment with dopaminergic agents.

References

Boshes B. Sinemet and the treatment of parkinsonism. Ann Intern Med 1981; 94:364.

Burton K, Calne D. Pharmacology of Parkinson's disease. Neurol Clin 1984; 2:461.

Koller WC, Giron LT. Selegiline: Selective MAO-type B inhibitor. Neurology 1990; 40(Suppl 3):61.

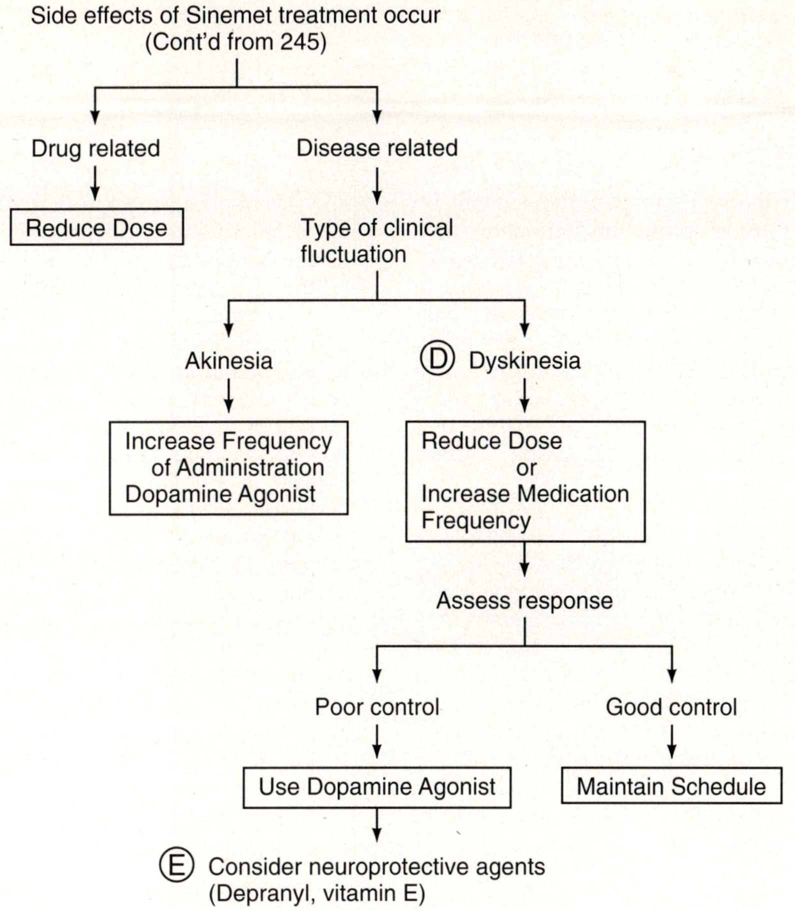

Side effects of Sinemet treatment occur
(Cont'd from 245)
Drug related
Disease related
Reduce Dose
Type of clinical
fluctuation
Akinesia
D Dyskinesia
Increase Frequency
of Administration
Dopamine Agonist
Reduce Dose
or
Increase Medication
Frequency
Assess response
Poor control
Good control
Use Dopamine Agonist
Maintain Schedule
E Consider neuroprotective agents
(Depranyl, vitamin E)

TREMOR

Leon A. Weisberg, M.D.

Tremor consists of rhythmic oscillating movements by agonist and antagonist muscles (pronation-supination, flexion-extension, abduction-adduction) around a fixed axis. The movements are equal in amplitude and frequency in both directions. The rhythmic character of the movement differentiates tremor from other abnormal involuntary movements. Tremor is classified as resting, sustentional (posture maintenance), or intentional, depending on when it is maximally present. It is worsened by anxiety and lessened by sedative medication and relaxation. Tremor disappears during sleep.

A. Resting tremor occurs in parkinsonism. It consists of movements of hands and fingers (3 to 5 cycles per second) resembling the act of manipulating a pill between the fingers (pill-rolling tremor). Tremor may be present initially on only one side but it later involves both sides. If resting tremor is due to parkinsonism, other neurologic signs (bradykinesia, rigidity, impaired postural reflexes) are present. Other movements that may simulate resting tremor include fasciculations (arrhythmic individual muscle fiber contractions that do not move the joint) and shivering movements. In segmental myoclonus (e.g., palatal myoclonus), rhythmic movements simulating tremor may occur. Palatal myoclonus *persists* during sleep; tremor disappears during sleep.

B. Postural tremor becomes prominent as the patient uses various muscle groups to sustain an antigravity posture. This tremor usually involves the upper extremities but may include the head; lower extremities are rarely involved. It may involve phonation muscles, causing voice tremor; it is noted when patients are under stress or fatigued. Postural tremor of the upper extremities is noticed when the arms are held outstretched in front of the patient. Postural tremor of the upper extremities must be differentiated from asterixis (see p 290). This condition results from failure to sustain wrist dorsiflexion position. Since amplitude rates of both phases of movement are unequal in asterixis, this is not a true tremor. Asterixis is seen in patients with metabolic encephalopathy (hepatic, renal, respiratory) and, less commonly, drug intoxication (phenytoin, metrizamide) and structural midbrain lesions.

C. Normal individuals show a low-amplitude tremor 6 to 12 Hz in frequency. This is most prominent when the patient holds both hands outstretched horizontally with the fingers abducted and fully extended. This is a form of physiologic tremor. The tremor due to lithium or valproic acid (Depakote) is similar in pattern, but the amplitude is coarser than that in physiologic tremor. Factors precipitating postural tremor include physiologic states (anxiety, fatigue, exercise), drugs (caffeine, adrenergic agonists, valproic acid, lithium), and metabolic disorders (thyrotoxicosis, pheochromocytoma, hypoglycemia). In patients with postural tremor involving the upper extremities and head and with no identified etiologic factors, consider essential tremor. This is referred to as "familial" if the family history is positive, or "senile" if it develops in an elderly person. Essential tremor is reduced in amplitude by alcohol, diazepam (Valium), propranolol (Inderal), or primidone (Mysoline). Essential tremor initially presents as a distal postural upper extremity tremor. It is most prominent at the end of goal-directed motor movement and is not associated with other cerebellar or extrapyramidal signs. It may become progressively more severe, interfering with handwriting, holding cups, and manipulating tools and utensils. Tremor that is prominent on posture maintenance is not due to parkinsonism; however, sustention tremor may be seen in parkinsonism.

D. Tremor that is most prominent in voluntary movement and posture maintenance indicates cerebellar dysfunction. These patients perform poorly on finger-to-nose and heel-to-shin tests. The tremor manifests as rhythmic, coarse, side-to-side motion during intentional motor activities. Tremor must be differentiated from ataxia (breakdown in performance of coordinated motor tasks) and dysmetria (missing the target). If tremor is unilateral, consider a structural (midbrain, cerebellar) lesion; if bilateral, consider spinocerebellar degeneration, Wilson's disease, multiple sclerosis, toxins, metabolic conditions (thyroid), and infection (measles or other exanthematous disorders).

E. Postural and intention tremor may occur in certain polyneuropathies as a result of impaired proprioception. If proprioception is intact, tremor may be related to muscle fatigue due to anterior horn cell disease, motor polyneuropathy, or subtle weakness of upper motor neuron origin.

References

Hern JEC. Tremor. Br Med J 1984; 288:1072.
Koller WC. Diagnosis and treatment of tremors. Neurol Clin North Am 1984; 2:499.

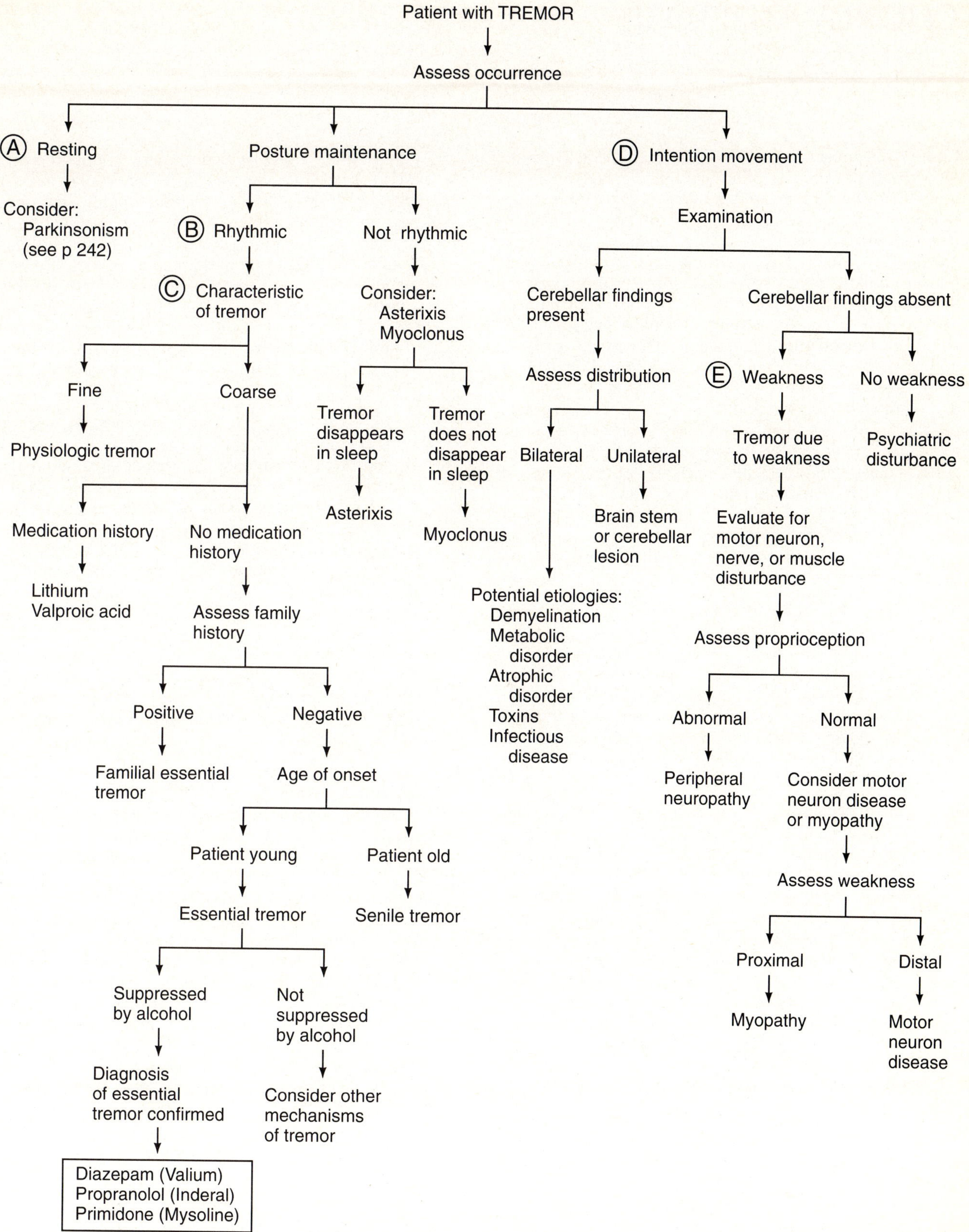

Patient with TREMOR
Assess occurrence

A Resting
Posture maintenance
D Intention movement

Consider:
Parkinsonism
(see p 242)

B Rhythmic
Not rhythmic

Examination

C Characteristic
of tremor

Consider:
Asterixis
Myoclonus

Cerebellar findings
present

Cerebellar findings absent

Fine
Coarse

Tremor
disappears
in sleep

Tremor
does not
disappear
in sleep

Assess distribution

E Weakness
No weakness

Physiologic tremor

Asterixis

Myoclonus

Bilateral
Unilateral

Tremor due
to weakness

Psychiatric
disturbance

Medication history
No medication
history

Brain stem
or cerebellar
lesion

Evaluate for
motor neuron,
nerve, or muscle
disturbance

Lithium
Valproic acid

Assess family
history

Potential etiologies:
Demyelination
Metabolic
disorder
Atrophic
disorder
Toxins
Infectious
disease

Assess proprioception

Positive
Negative

Abnormal
Normal

Familial essential
tremor

Age of onset

Peripheral
neuropathy

Consider motor
neuron disease
or myopathy

Patient young
Patient old

Assess weakness

Essential tremor
Senile tremor

Proximal
Distal

Suppressed
by alcohol

Not
suppressed
by alcohol

Myopathy

Motor
neuron
disease

Diagnosis
of essential
tremor confirmed

Consider other
mechanisms
of tremor

Diazepam (Valium)
Propranolol (Inderal)
Primidone (Mysoline)

CHOREA-ATHETOSIS

Leon A. Weisberg, M.D.

Choreic movements are semipurposeful, hyperactive motor movements that are fast, short-lived, and arrhythmic. They include facial grimaces, shoulder shrugs, and finger twitches. Patients with chorea have difficulty maintaining fixed postures so that they cannot maintain a handshake or grasp. They initially have a firm grasp, but this is rapidly relaxed (milkmaid's grasp). If the tongue is extended with the mouth open, it may dart in and out (serpent's tongue). Muscle tone in choreic patients is usually hypotonic, but some young patients with juvenile Huntington's chorea appear rigid. Athetosis refers to slow writhing movements of outstretched extremities; the distal fingers are extended and abducted, the wrist is flexed, and the forearm is pronated. Athetosis is a slow form of chorea; these movements later evolve into dystonic movements. Most patients have both chorea and athetosis. Most patients with chorea are hypotonic and hyperkinetic, as contrasted with parkinsonian patients, who are hypertonic and bradykinetic. High-potency antipsychotic neuroleptic drugs are antidopaminergic and may induce parkinsonism; they are therefore effective in treating chorea.

A. In suspected cases of chorea, consider other dyskinesias. Tics (habit spasms) are stereotypic, repetitive, semipurposeful, sudden movements; they may be single or multiple. The most common tics are eyelid blinks, facial grimaces, and shoulder jerks (see p 254). Myoclonus consists of rapid, nonpurposeful, random jerks of extremities. Dystonia is a slow turning or twisting movement resulting in abnormal body positions (see p 252).

B. Chorea developing in childhood may be associated with rheumatic fever (Sydenham's chorea). Findings include elevations in erythrocyte sedimentation rate and antistreptolysin O titer and cardiac abnormalities (carditis). The major cause of death in Sydenham's chorea is cardiovascular. Sydenham's chorea usually remits in several months and recurs in one third of cases. Chorea may be suppressed by sedative drugs (reserpine, tetrabenazine, clonazepam) or antidopaminergic neuroleptic medication (e.g., haloperidol [Haldol]). Chorea is treated when functionally or socially disabling, but some cases may be mild and require no medication. Wilson's disease may also present with chorea in childhood.

C. In adults with chorea, consider Huntington's disease and Wilson's disease. Detection of a Kayser-Fleischer ring on slit lamp eye examination is diagnostic of Wilson's disease, indicating deposition of copper in the corneal layer. This ring must be present for neurologic symptoms to be attributed to Wilson's disease. In Wilson's disease, laboratory abnormalities include low ceruloplasmin level, abnormal liver function profile, and elevated urinary copper content. Wilson's disease is inherited as an autosomal recessive disorder and is due to an abnormality in copper metabolism. Neurologic and hepatic dysfunction respond to penicillamine therapy. Huntington's disease is inherited as autosomal dominant, so that disease is manifested in one parent. Neurobehavioral disorders (depression, psychosis, dementia) may be manifestations of Huntington's disease. Chorea may be controlled with phenothiazines (haloperidol), but dementia is progressive and not affected by phenothiazines.

D. If the onset of chorea is focal (hemichorea, hemiballismus) and sudden, consider a vascular disorder (hemorrhage, ischemia). If the onset is focal and insidious, consider a neoplasm (metastases, glioma) or focal encephalitis (toxoplasmosis). Lesions causing chorea may be in the caudate nucleus. Hemiballistic movements result from lesions in the subthalamic nucleus. Hemiballismus is a violent type of hemichorea; most patients have a combined form of hemiballismus-hemichorea. Lesions in the caudate, striatum, lenticular nucleus, thalamus, and subthalamus may cause hemiballismus-hemichorea. Chorea has also been associated with hyperglycemia, phenytoin toxicity, neuroleptic drugs (even though these are the most common drugs used for treatment), multiple sclerosis, head trauma, and neurodegenerative disease.

E. Chorea in adults has multiple possible causes. It may develop in elderly patients who have no neurobehavioral disturbances and a negative family history (senile chorea). Chorea may occur with neurobehavioral symptoms in patients with systemic lupus erythematosus; this diagnosis is established by laboratory studies. Some patients with chorea show abnormal red blood cells (acanthocytosis); these may have polyneuropathy and retinitis pigmentosa. This condition is due to absence of beta-lipoprotein; serum lipid levels are reduced. Chorea may develop in pregnant women or women taking contraceptive drugs; it is self-limited and remits at termination of pregnancy or after medication is stopped. Metabolic disorders and medications may cause chorea. Chorea may result from encephalitis; CSF analysis establishes this etiology.

References

Dewy RB, Jankovic J. Hemiballism-hemichorea. Arch Neurol 1989; 46:862.

Duvoisin RC. Chorea. Semin Neurol 1982; 2:351.

Nauseida PA, Grossman BJ, Kaller WC, et al. Sydenham chorea: An update. Neurology 1980; 30:331.

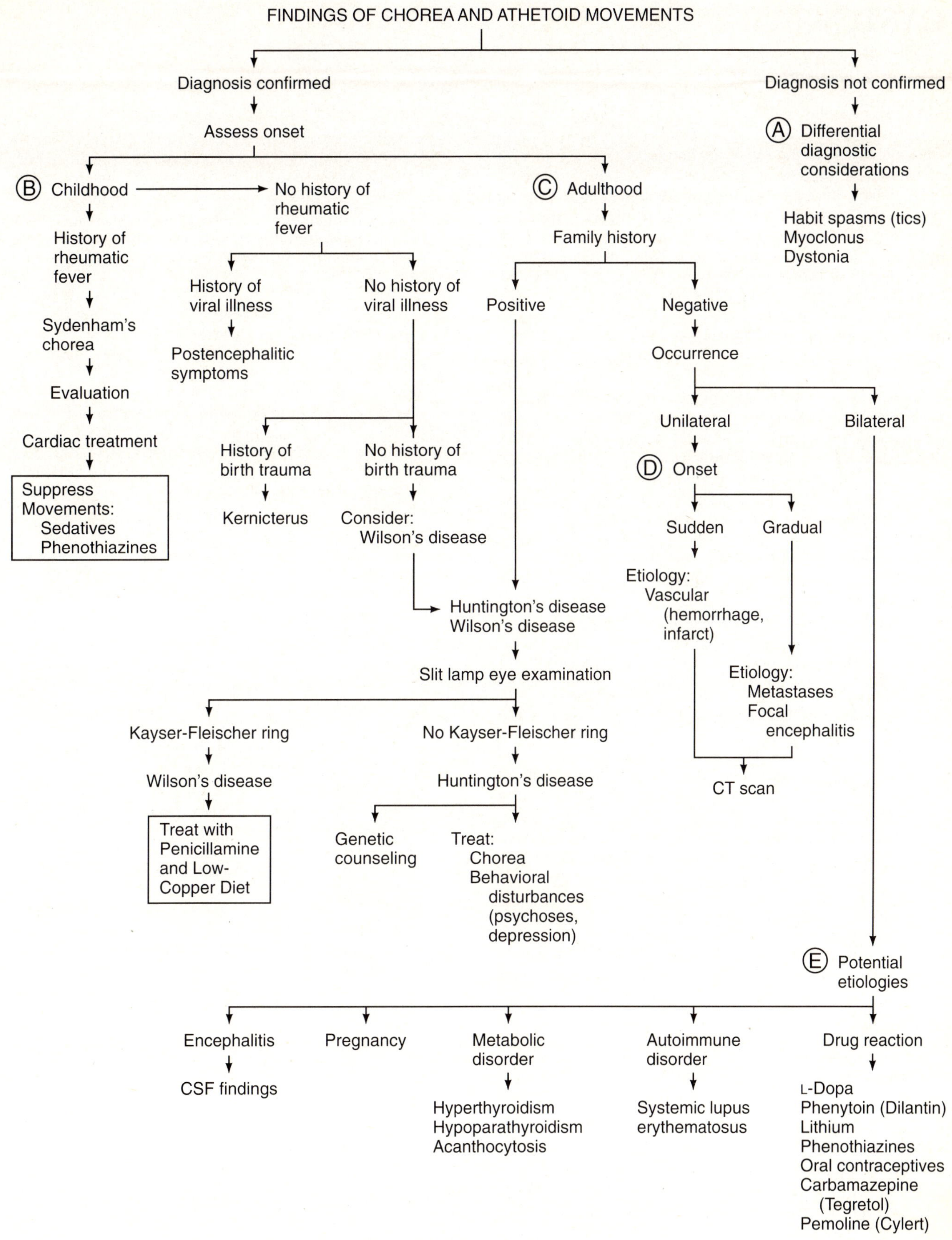

FINDINGS OF CHOREA AND ATHETOID MOVEMENTS
Diagnosis confirmed
Assess onset
B Childhood
History of rheumatic fever
Sydenham's chorea
Evaluation
Cardiac treatment
Suppress Movements:
Sedatives
Phenothiazines
No history of rheumatic fever
History of viral illness
Postencephalitic symptoms
No history of viral illness
History of birth trauma
Kernicterus
No history of birth trauma
Consider: Wilson's disease
C Adulthood
Family history
Positive
Huntington's disease
Wilson's disease
Slit lamp eye examination
Kayser-Fleischer ring
Wilson's disease
Treat with Penicillamine and Low-Copper Diet
No Kayser-Fleischer ring
Huntington's disease
Genetic counseling
Treat:
Chorea
Behavioral disturbances (psychoses, depression)
Negative
Occurrence
Unilateral
D Onset
Sudden
Etiology:
Vascular (hemorrhage, infarct)
Gradual
Etiology:
Metastases
Focal encephalitis
CT scan
Bilateral
Diagnosis not confirmed
A Differential diagnostic considerations
Habit spasms (tics)
Myoclonus
Dystonia
E Potential etiologies
Encephalitis
CSF findings
Pregnancy
Metabolic disorder
Hyperthyroidism
Hypoparathyroidism
Acanthocytosis
Autoimmune disorder
Systemic lupus erythematosus
Drug reaction
L-Dopa
Phenytoin (Dilantin)
Lithium
Phenothiazines
Oral contraceptives
Carbamazepine (Tegretol)
Pemoline (Cylert)

DYSTONIA

Leon A. Weisberg, M.D.

Dystonia is one of the hyperkinetic movement disorders. It consists of simultaneous contractions of agonist and antagonist muscle groups, resulting in sustained and twisting involuntary movements (head, neck, trunk, or extremity). The muscle contractions may last several seconds or minutes. They result in repetitive twisting movements of a single group of muscles or may involve the entire neck or trunk or an entire limb. Dystonic postures are usually infrequent and intermittent initially and later may become more frequent and prolonged. Dystonia may be sustained, causing postures that result in limb contractures or joint deformities. Dystonias may be misdiagnosed as hysterical conversion reactions because of the unusual body postures. Dystonic movements are usually slow (but may be rapid), repetitive, and patterned, as contrasted with choreic movements (which are random, rapid, and semipurposeful) and myoclonic movements (which are rapid, jerking, and nonpurposeful). Some patients with severe neck pain may maintain the neck in a fixed twisted position to simulate dystonia; conversely, some patients with initial signs of dystonia may describe a sensation of the neck pulling to one side with accompanying stiffness. Because of the neck pain and stiffness reported by some dystonia patients, they are sometimes evaluated initially by orthopedists. In patients with suspected neck dystonia, carefully assess possible accompanying signs of cervical radiculopathy or myelopathy.

A. The most common pattern of dystonia involves the neck (spasmodic torticollis). This is often drug-induced (caused by phenothiazines), but in most cases no etiology is identified. Acute drug-induced dystonia is treated with anticholinergic medication, usually with rapid and complete clinical response; however, tardive drug-induced dystonia may be resistant to treatment. Spasmodic torticollis most commonly develops as an isolated finding in patients during the third to fifth decades of life. There is sustained neck muscle contraction involving the sternocleidomastoid, trapezius, and scalene muscles. This pulls the head backward (retrocollis) or toward one side (torticollis). There is sustained head deviation intermixed with relaxation. Dystonia may occur at rest or in association with specific voluntary motor activity (action dystonia). For example, dystonia may occur only during specific motor activity: this is seen with writing (writer's cramp), playing a musical instrument, or typing.

B. Treat drug-induced dystonia reactions with anticholinergic medication. Initially use low doses; increase the dose until dystonia is controlled or side effects develop. If anticholinergic drugs are ineffective, muscle relaxation drugs of the diazepam (Valium) type are given. Injection of botulin toxin directly into involved dystonic muscles has been effective in focal dystonia. For disabling dystonias not medically controlled, surgery (thalamotomy) has been advocated, but the benefits of this procedure have not been established. Patients learn that dystonia can be intensified by certain activities (walking, writing, changing body position). It can be relieved by rest, hypnosis, sensory tricks, and counterpressure (placing one hand on the chin to prevent torticollis).

C. If dystonia is insidious in onset, consider Wilson's disease. Perform a slit lamp examination looking for a Kayser-Fleischer ring, which indicates copper deposition in the cornea and is always present if there is a CNS disturbance due to Wilson's disease. Obtain any family history of hereditary neurologic diseases, including dystonia musculorum deformans. In this disorder, which begins in childhood, there is first sustained plantar flexion and inturning of one foot (equinovarus deformity). Dystonia may later spread to the upper extremities (flexed elbow, flexed wrist), and may become bilateral and involve the trunk and neck. This may result in dystonic postures due to sustained muscle contractions (torticollis, tortipelvis, kyphosis, scoliosis). The end result may be contractures and fixed joint deformities, and patients may be unable to walk, stand, or sit.

D. Focal or segmental dystonia may be the initial symptom of neurologic disorders, with other signs developing later (dystonia musculorum deformans, Wilson's or Huntington's disease), or these may remain monosymptomatic. Focal dystonias may be manifested as writer's cramp; patients develop spasms interfering with the fine coordinated movements necessary for writing, drawing, and manipulating tools or utensils. Eyelids may be involved in blepharospasm (involuntary closing of the eyelids); this eyelid dystonia may be severe enough to interfere with vision. Dystonia may involve the laryngeal muscles, to cause spasmodic dysphonia that interferes with speaking. Craniocervical dystonia is a segmental dystonia involving blepharospasm combined with facial, oromandibular, lingual, pharyngeal, laryngeal, and cervical muscle dystonia. If the onset of dystonia is before age 20, it frequently becomes generalized; if the onset is after age 20, it usually remains localized. If the onset is sudden and unilateral, it may be due to a basal ganglia (usually putaminal) infarct or hemorrhage. Dystonia may be drug-related, especially in patients who received phenothiazines. Dystonia that develops in childhood is usually inherited, whereas adult-onset dystonia is generally sporadic.

References

Fahn S. Torsion dystonia: Clinical spectrum and treatment. Semin Neurol 1982; 2:316.

Fahn S. High dosage anticholinergic therapy in dystonia. Neurology 1983; 33:1255.

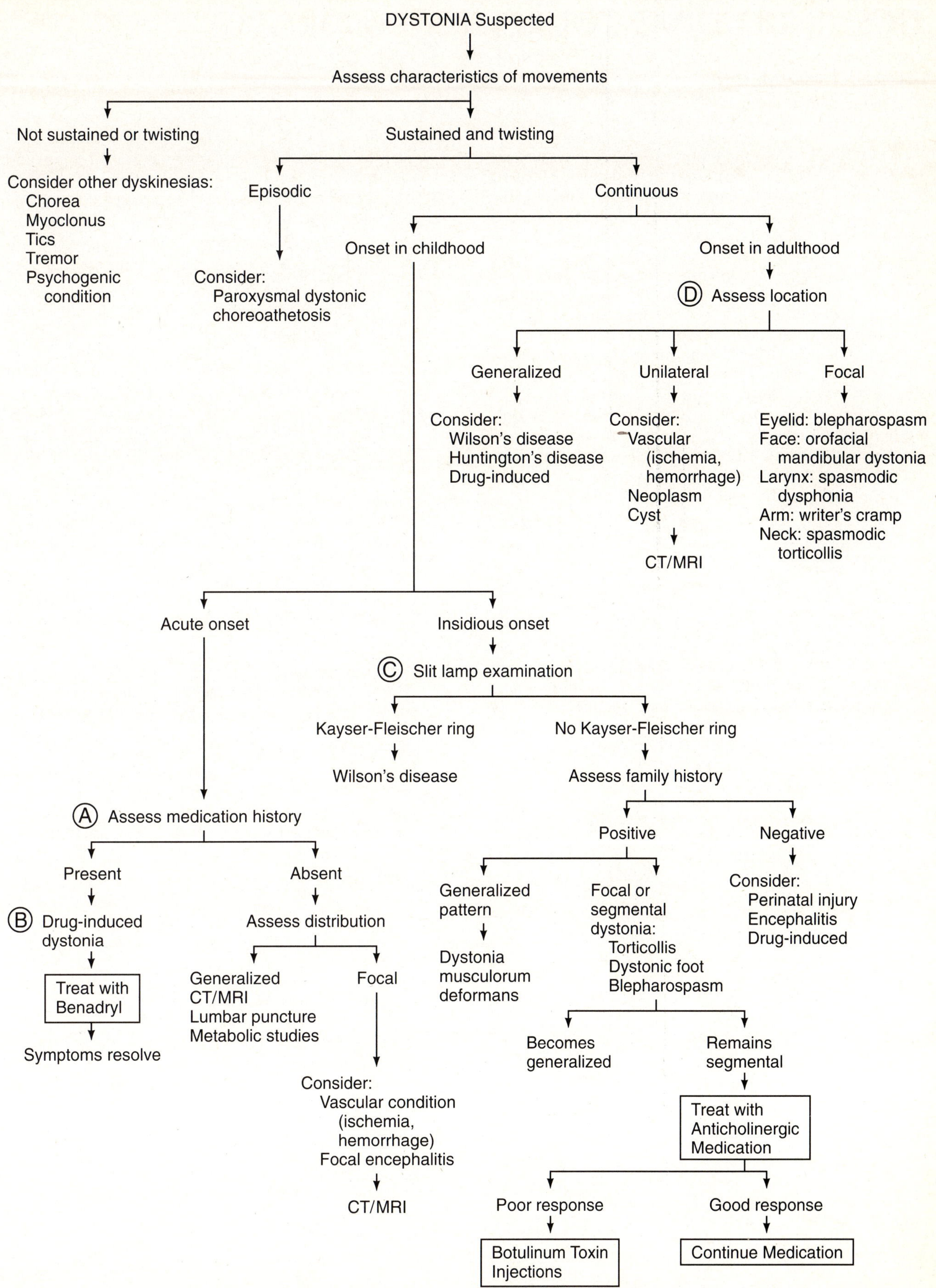

DYSTONIA Suspected
Assess characteristics of movements

Not sustained or twisting
Sustained and twisting

Consider other dyskinesias:
Chorea
Myoclonus
Tics
Tremor
Psychogenic
condition

Episodic
Continuous

Consider:
Paroxysmal dystonic
choreoathetosis

Onset in childhood
Onset in adulthood

D Assess location

Generalized
Unilateral
Focal

Consider:
Wilson's disease
Huntington's disease
Drug-induced

Consider:
Vascular
(ischemia,
hemorrhage)
Neoplasm
Cyst

CT/MRI

Eyelid: blepharospasm
Face: orofacial
mandibular dystonia
Larynx: spasmodic
dysphonia
Arm: writer's cramp
Neck: spasmodic
torticollis

Acute onset
Insidious onset

C Slit lamp examination

Kayser-Fleischer ring
No Kayser-Fleischer ring

Wilson's disease
Assess family history

Positive
Negative

Generalized
pattern

Focal or
segmental
dystonia:
Torticollis
Dystonic foot
Blepharospasm

Consider:
Perinatal injury
Encephalitis
Drug-induced

Dystonia
musculorum
deformans

A Assess medication history

Present
Absent

B Drug-induced
dystonia

Assess distribution

Treat with
Benadryl

Generalized
CT/MRI
Lumbar puncture
Metabolic studies

Focal

Symptoms resolve

Consider:
Vascular condition
(ischemia,
hemorrhage)
Focal encephalitis

CT/MRI

Becomes
generalized
Remains
segmental

Treat with
Anticholinergic
Medication

Poor response
Good response

Botulinum Toxin
Injections
Continue Medication

TICS (INCLUDING TOURETTE'S SYNDROME)

Leon A. Weisberg, M.D.

Motor tics are sudden, patterned, stereotyped dyskinesias. They may be simple, rapid, short-lived motor movements involving isolated body regions (shoulder shrug, eyelid blink) or complex tics consisting of rapid head, trunk, or limb movements (touching, scratching, obscene gesturing). Tics are sudden, purposeless, unprovoked, and unpredictable. Stress, suggestion, or noise may exacerbate them. Patients may have periods without tics, which may then suddenly break through to occur in prolonged bursts. Tics may migrate from one region to another or remain localized within one region and be of one motor pattern. Three features are characteristic of tics and do not occur in other dyskinesias: (1) an irresistible urge to move occurs immediately before tics, and tension is relieved by performing the motor act of the tics; (2) voluntary suppression of tics for relatively long periods is followed by a breakthrough burst of motor tics; and (3) tics occur during all sleep stages (both REM and non-REM sleep).

A. Tics must be differentiated from other hyperkinetic movement disorders, including myoclonus, chorea, and dystonia. Myoclonus consists of rapid, stereotyped, focal jerking movements that are frequently precipitated by sensory input and cannot be suppressed. These are usually not present during sleep, except sleep myoclonus and palatal myoclonus. Chorea consists of continuous and unpredictable semipurposeful movements. Dystonia has a twisting and sustained muscle contraction pattern. Tics may persist in sleep; chorea and dystonia disappear in sleep. Mannerisms may be difficult to differentiate from tics. These mannerisms are usually seen in childhood and later disappear in adolescence.

B. Tourette's syndrome (TS) is the most important condition to consider in patients with tics. In TS, the age of onset is usually 5 to 10 years and most patients are boys. The initial tic is usually a simple motor type (e.g., shoulder shrugs, eyelid blinking, neck extensions). These may be single or may occur in rapid succession. Tics may spontaneously resolve but recur several months later. Vocal tics develop later, consisting of grunting, barking, guttural noises, crying sounds, sniffing, snorting, hissing, or a noisy breathing pattern. Coprolalia (use of obscene words) is the most characteristic involuntary vocalization. TS patients may have speech disorders, including stuttering and echolalia (repeating speech of others).

C. The diagnosis of TS is established on a clinical basis. Important factors to consider include gender, age when tic first developed, and the presence of persistent fluctuating motor or vocal tics. Tics not related to TS occur commonly in children. The *transient* childhood variety are usually single motor tics but may be of two types; these resolve spontaneously within several weeks or months. *Chronic* and persistent childhood tics are also common. In both transient and chronic tics, the motor pattern is simple and stereotyped; vocal tics do not develop. Their presence is highly suggestive of TS.

D. TS tics may fluctuate in severity and frequency. Remissions may occur for 6 months. Treatment with haloperidol (Haldol) is effective. First, use a low dose (0.5 mg bid), which may be increased to 4 to 6 mg daily. Pimozide (Orap) may be given as an initial dose of 1 mg per day and increased to 10 to 20 mg daily in adults. Monitor the ECG to avoid any cardiotoxic effect of this drug.

E. Differential considerations for TS include Sydenham's chorea, juvenile Huntington's chorea, dystonia, Wilson's disease, drug-induced (stimulants, anticonvulsants, dopaminergic drugs, phenothiazines) dyskinesias, and psychiatric disorders. Blood studies and neurologic and mental status examinations should exclude these disorders. CNS stimulant medication (e.g., methylphenidate [Ritalin]) used to treat an "attention deficit disorder" may precipitate tics.

References

Butler IJ. Tourette's syndrome. Neurol Clin North Am 1984; 2:571.

Shapiro AK, Shapiro ES. Tourette's syndrome: Clinical aspects, treatment and etiology. Semin Neurol 1982; 2:373.

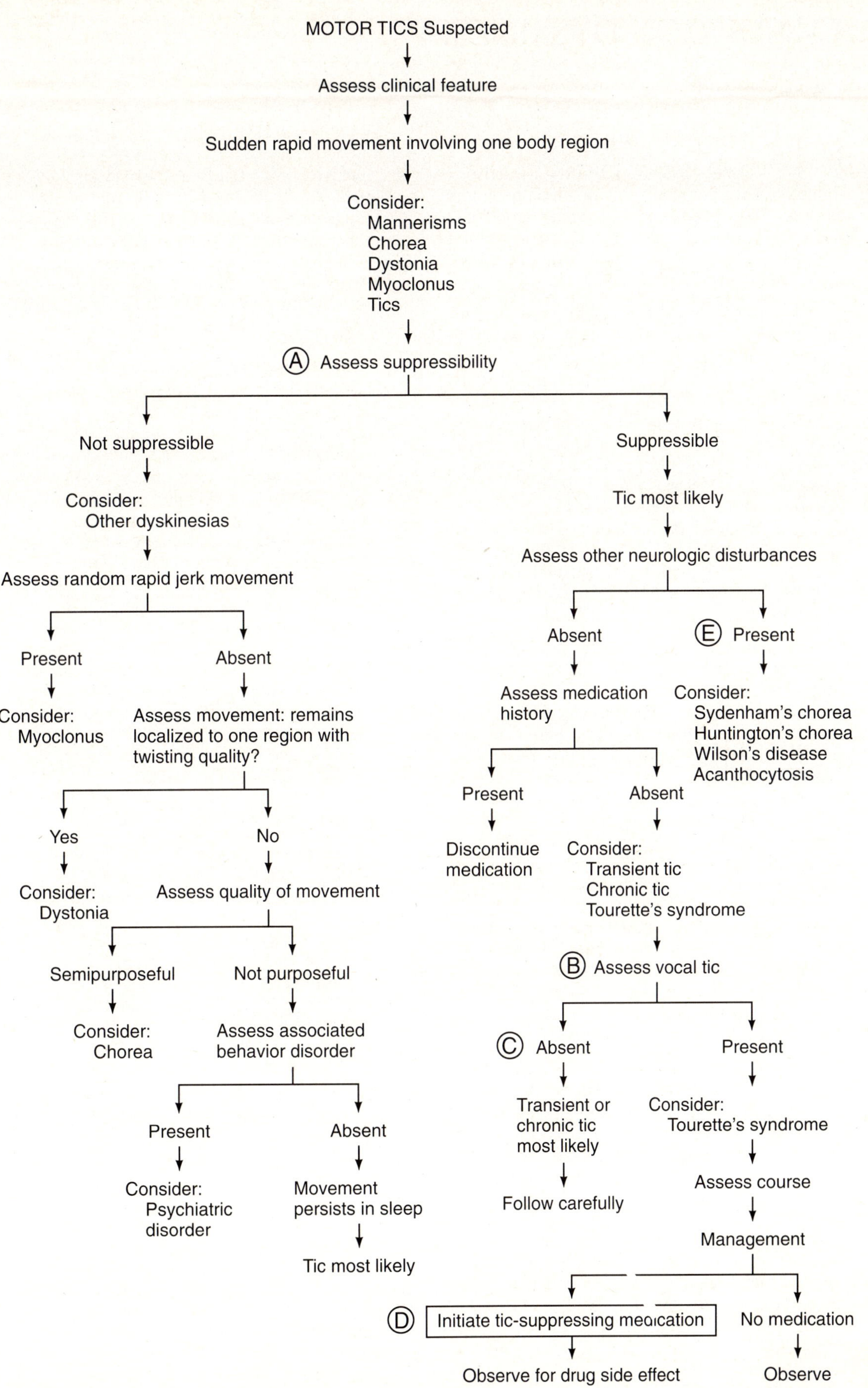

MOTOR TICS Suspected
Assess clinical feature
Sudden rapid movement involving one body region
Consider:
Mannerisms
Chorea
Dystonia
Myoclonus
Tics
A Assess suppressibility
Not suppressible
Suppressible
Consider:
Other dyskinesias
Tic most likely
Assess random rapid jerk movement
Assess other neurologic disturbances
Present
Absent
Absent
E Present
Consider:
Myoclonus
Assess movement: remains localized to one region with twisting quality?
Assess medication history
Consider:
Sydenham's chorea
Huntington's chorea
Wilson's disease
Acanthocytosis
Yes
No
Present
Absent
Consider:
Dystonia
Assess quality of movement
Discontinue medication
Consider:
Transient tic
Chronic tic
Tourette's syndrome
Semipurposeful
Not purposeful
B Assess vocal tic
Consider:
Chorea
Assess associated behavior disorder
C Absent
Present
Present
Absent
Transient or chronic tic most likely
Consider:
Tourette's syndrome
Consider:
Psychiatric disorder
Movement persists in sleep
Follow carefully
Assess course
Tic most likely
Management
D Initiate tic-suppressing medication
No medication
Observe for drug side effect
Observe

DRUG-INDUCED DYSKINESIAS

Leon A. Weisberg, M.D.

Dyskinesias may result from antipsychotic drugs because of their dopamine receptor antagonism. Dopamine receptors are classified as D-1 (presynaptic, stimulate adenylate cyclase when activated) or D-2 (postsynaptic, inhibit adenylate cyclase). D-2 receptor affinity correlates with potent antipsychotic and dyskinetic effects.

A. Acute dyskinesias may develop within several days after initiating neuroleptic medication. These drugs are dopamine-blocking agents. Dyskinesias include torticollis, facial grimacing, and oculogyric crisis. Spasmodic torticollis causes painful neck contractions; laryngeal and pharyngeal dystonias cause respiratory difficulties. Acute dyskinesias may be incorrectly diagnosed as seizures (altered consciousness and abnormal EEG), tetanus (spasms involve lumbar muscles, resulting in opisthotonos of jaw muscles to produce trismus), or a hysterical reaction (movements are not stereotyped). Dyskinesias are treated with antihistamines (diphenhydramine) or anticholinergics (benztropine, biperiden). After initiation of treatment, the dyskinesia usually resolves rapidly.

B. Akathisia is defined as motor restlessness. It is not characterized by abnormal involuntary movements but rather by an irresistible urge for constant body motion. Patients cannot sit still and they appear agitated. Akathisia usually develops within 3 months after neuroleptic therapy is begun but may develop as a delayed complication. This motor restlessness may also occur in association with parkinsonian features. Akathisia is believed due to blockade of the mesolimbic dopamine system. It is sometimes difficult to differentiate the agitated condition of psychotic patients from drug-related akathisia; however, psychotic agitation usually improves after neuroleptic treatment. If akathisia is mild and not bothersome to the patient, no change in neuroleptic medication is warranted; reducing the dose or using alternative antipsychotic medication may ameliorate the condition. Treatment with anticholinergic medication is utilized if akathisia symptoms are disturbing to the patient.

C. Drug-related (secondary) parkinsonism occurs in 10% of patients receiving neuroleptic drugs, developing within 3 months of initiation of the medication. It is caused by nigrostriatal postsynaptic D-2 receptor blockade. Dopaminergic drugs may not be effective in reversing parkinsonian symptoms because dopamine receptors are blocked by phenothiazine drugs. Tremor is usually a prominent drug-related parkinsonian manifestation, but functional disability from neuroleptic-induced parkinsonism is usually only mild. Symptoms may decrease spontaneously with time and may resolve within several months after the neuroleptic drug is discontinued. Treatment with anticholinergic drugs is helpful but usually not necessary from a functional disability perspective.

D. Delayed-onset (tardive) dyskinesias may develop in patients receiving high-dose neuroleptic therapy of long duration. Symptoms may be noticed when the dose is reduced or the drug discontinued. Symptoms usually resolve within 12 weeks, but some resolve more slowly and others not at all. If the drug is reinstituted at the former dosage level, dyskinesia may disappear. Manifestations of dyskinesia include chewing movements, rapid tongue protrusions, puckering of lips, eyelid blinking, grunting sounds, choking, and irregular respiratory movements. Some patients develop tardive dystonia or tics. The mechanism of the dystonia or tics is believed similar to that of tardive dyskinesia, and treatment is with dopamine-depleting drugs. Of those who receive neuroleptic medication, older patients (especially women) with preexisting brain injury and patients previously treated with anticholinergics are at greatest risk for tardive dyskinesia. The clinical manifestations of tardive dyskinesia are similar to those of chorea. It is probable that their mechanism is via a chronic dopamine receptor blockade resulting in receptor site supersensitivity. This is caused by increased activity of D-2 dopamine receptors with decreased activity of cholinergic and gamma-aminobutyric acid (GABA) receptors. Treatment has included (1) cholinomimetic drugs (deanol, lecithin, physostigmine); (2) GABA agonists (baclofen, valproic acid, diazepam); (3) an increase of neuroleptic drug dosage, which acts to reduce dyskinesia but worsens dopamine receptor blockade; and (4) dopamine-depleting drugs (reserpine).

E. Alternative diagnostic considerations in tardive dyskinesias include (1) focal perioral tremor (rabbit syndrome), which occurs in idiopathic parkinsonism or with neuroleptic drugs and responds to anticholinergics; (2) habit spasm unrelated to neuroleptics, which requires no treatment; (3) mannerisms of schizophrenia, which may persist even after treatment with neuroleptics; (4) Huntington's disease, in which psychosis develops initially and chorea may develop later despite treatment with neuroleptic drugs, which are usually effective in suppressing chorea; and (5) tardive dystonia with slow, writhing movements of the face, neck, and mouth that respond to anticholinergics.

References

Black JL, Richelson E, Richardson JW. Antipsychotic agents: A clinical update. Mayo Clin Proc 1985; 60:777.

Scheife RT, Growden JH. Treating tardive dyskinesia. Semin Neurol 1982; 2:305.

Smith JM, Baldessarini RJ. Changes in prevalence, severity and recovery in tardive dyskinesia with age. Arch Gen Psychiatry 1980; 37:1368.

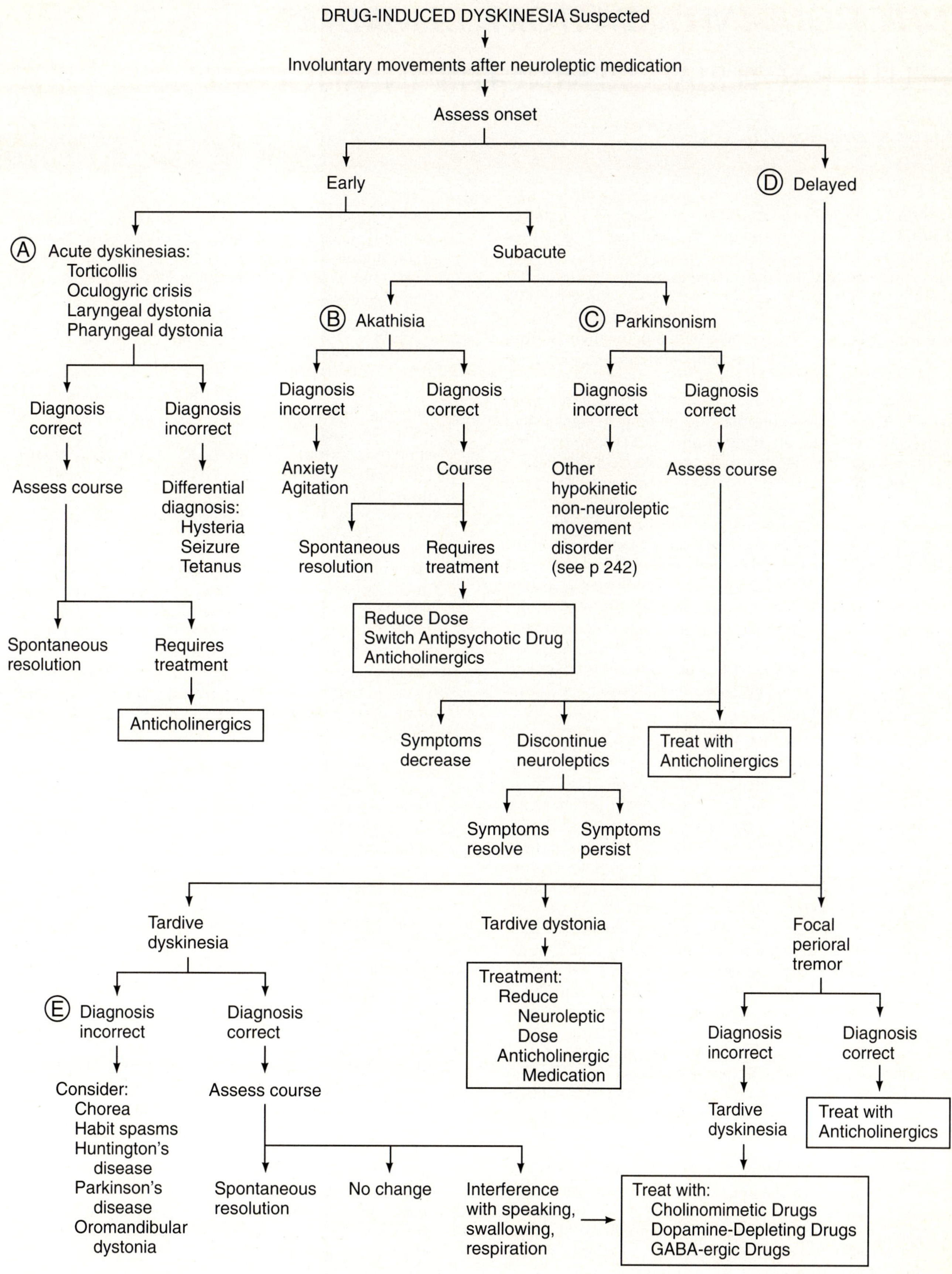

DRUG-INDUCED DYSKINESIA Suspected
Involuntary movements after neuroleptic medication
Assess onset
Early
D Delayed
A Acute dyskinesias:
Torticollis
Oculogyric crisis
Laryngeal dystonia
Pharyngeal dystonia
Subacute
B Akathisia
C Parkinsonism
Diagnosis correct
Diagnosis incorrect
Diagnosis incorrect
Diagnosis correct
Diagnosis incorrect
Diagnosis correct
Assess course
Differential diagnosis:
Hysteria
Seizure
Tetanus
Anxiety
Agitation
Course
Other hypokinetic non-neuroleptic movement disorder (see p 242)
Assess course
Spontaneous resolution
Requires treatment
Spontaneous resolution
Requires treatment
Reduce Dose
Switch Antipsychotic Drug
Anticholinergics
Anticholinergics
Symptoms decrease
Discontinue neuroleptics
Treat with Anticholinergics
Symptoms resolve
Symptoms persist
Tardive dyskinesia
Tardive dystonia
Focal perioral tremor
E Diagnosis incorrect
Diagnosis correct
Treatment:
Reduce Neuroleptic Dose
Anticholinergic Medication
Diagnosis incorrect
Diagnosis correct
Consider:
Chorea
Habit spasms
Huntington's disease
Parkinson's disease
Oromandibular dystonia
Assess course
Tardive dyskinesia
Treat with Anticholinergics
Spontaneous resolution
No change
Interference with speaking, swallowing, respiration
Treat with:
Cholinomimetic Drugs
Dopamine-Depleting Drugs
GABA-ergic Drugs

INFECTIOUS-INFLAMMATORY DISORDERS

ACUTE BACTERIAL MENINGITIS IN ADULTS

Leon A. Weisberg, M.D.

Bacterial meningitis is an acute or subacute infectious-inflammatory process involving the meninges. This causes CSF pleocytosis. When a patient presents with symptoms suggesting meningitis, the clinician must determine (1) whether meningitis is present; (2) if so, the probable etiology; and (3) whether meningeal inflammatory reaction is causing pleocytosis associated with a parenchymal brain lesion (e.g., cerebral infarction, abscess, subdural or epidural empyema).

Suspect acute bacterial meningitis in patients with fever, headache, photophobia, and meningeal signs. Most patients present with an acute course, but *Listeria* or Lyme meningitis may present in a subacute pattern, and tuberculous meningitis may be subacute or chronic. In some elderly, alcoholic, or immunosuppressed patients, meningeal symptoms and signs may be absent or difficult to demonstrate. In these patients, suspicion of meningitis must be high and CSF examined even if clinical meningeal signs are few. The diagnosis of infectious meningitis is established by findings of CSF pleocytosis with positive studies for a causal infectious agent. In general, patients with viral meningitis appear less severely ill than those with bacterial meningitis. Maintain a high index of suspicion for bacterial meningitis, because morbidity and mortality may be high if treatment is delayed.

A. In patients with suspected meningitis without papilledema, altered consciousness, or focal signs, lumbar puncture (LP) is indicated; CT precedes LP if these signs are present. Rarely, LP may disturb intracranial pressure dynamics and precipitate herniation. Meningitis is a life-threatening acute infection, and failure to perform a timely LP is a greater risk than deterioration due to an untimely LP. If you suspect meningitis, perform LP immediately! Do not wait for CT or MRI; these are useful only to exclude structural brain disease that may complicate meningitis. Papilledema in a patient with suspected meningitis suggests a complicating process (abscess, empyema, brain swelling, infarct, hydrocephalus). In patients with suspected meningitis who also have papilledema and focal neurologic signs, CT/MRI should precede LP. In patients with headache and meningeal signs, meningitis and subarachnoid hemorrhage (SAH) are likely diagnoses that can be differentiated only by CSF findings.

B. In bacterial meningitis, CSF contains polymorphonuclear leukocytes (PMLs); fluid appears cloudy. Pleocytosis may be minimal or absent in leukopenic patients or the early stage of meningococcal meningitis. Mixed (PMLs and lymphocytes) pleocytosis occurs in partially treated bacterial meningitis. PML pleocytosis may occur as an inflammatory response in cerebral infarction, hemorrhage, neoplasm, abscess,

and migraine or after status epilepticus. In these conditions, CSF sugar level is normal and bacteriologic studies are negative. These patients have neurologic signs of an underlying lesion as well as meningeal signs.

C. Determine the CSF sugar level. Normally, it is two thirds of the blood sugar level; it should never be <45 mg/dl when blood sugar is normal. A reduced sugar level is seen in bacterial, tuberculous, fungal, syphilitic, sarcoid, and neoplastic meningitis and rarely in SAH. The sugar level is normal in viral (except herpes simplex and mumps) meningitis and partially treated bacterial meningitis. An elevated protein level is a nonspecific disease marker indicating blood-brain barrier impairment. In bacterial meningitis, protein is often >100 mg/dl.

D. Sediment of freshly centrifuged CSF should undergo microscopic examination, including Gram stain, acid-fast stain, India ink preparation, and wet smear for fungi and amebae. CSF Gram stains are positive in 90% of patients with acute bacterial meningitis. Special studies may be needed to identify *Listeria*. Bacteriologic cultures may detect potential infectious etiologies, and antibiotic sensitivities may be determined.

E. Counterimmunoelectrophoresis (CIE) or latex particle agglutination studies identify capsular antigens in certain strains of *Meningococcus, Haemophilus influenzae,* and *Streptococcus pneumoniae.* These may be positive even if the Gram stain and cultures are negative. They are especially valuable in partially treated bacterial meningitis.

F. Treat bacterial meningitis with IV antibiotics for 10 to 14 days. Give ampicillin initially; use chloramphenicol in penicillin-allergic patients. Change antibiotics later if indicated by culture and sensitivity results. For gram-negative meningitis, use third-generation cephalosporins. Other types of antibiotics are indicated in head trauma because *Staphylococcus* may occur, or in ear infections because *Proteus* and *Pseudomonas* are common. Because cerebral edema and inappropriate secretion of antidiuretic hormone may complicate meningitis, avoid overhydration. Measures to reduce intracranial hypertension (mannitol, hyperventilation) and cerebral edema may be necessary. Increasing evidence indicates the value of giving corticosteroids before antibiotic therapy. With antibiotic therapy, patients should become afebrile and meningeal signs disappear. CSF Gram stain and bacterial culture become negative rapidly. The sugar level becomes normal; cellular response decreases with lymphocytes being predominant. Examine CSF

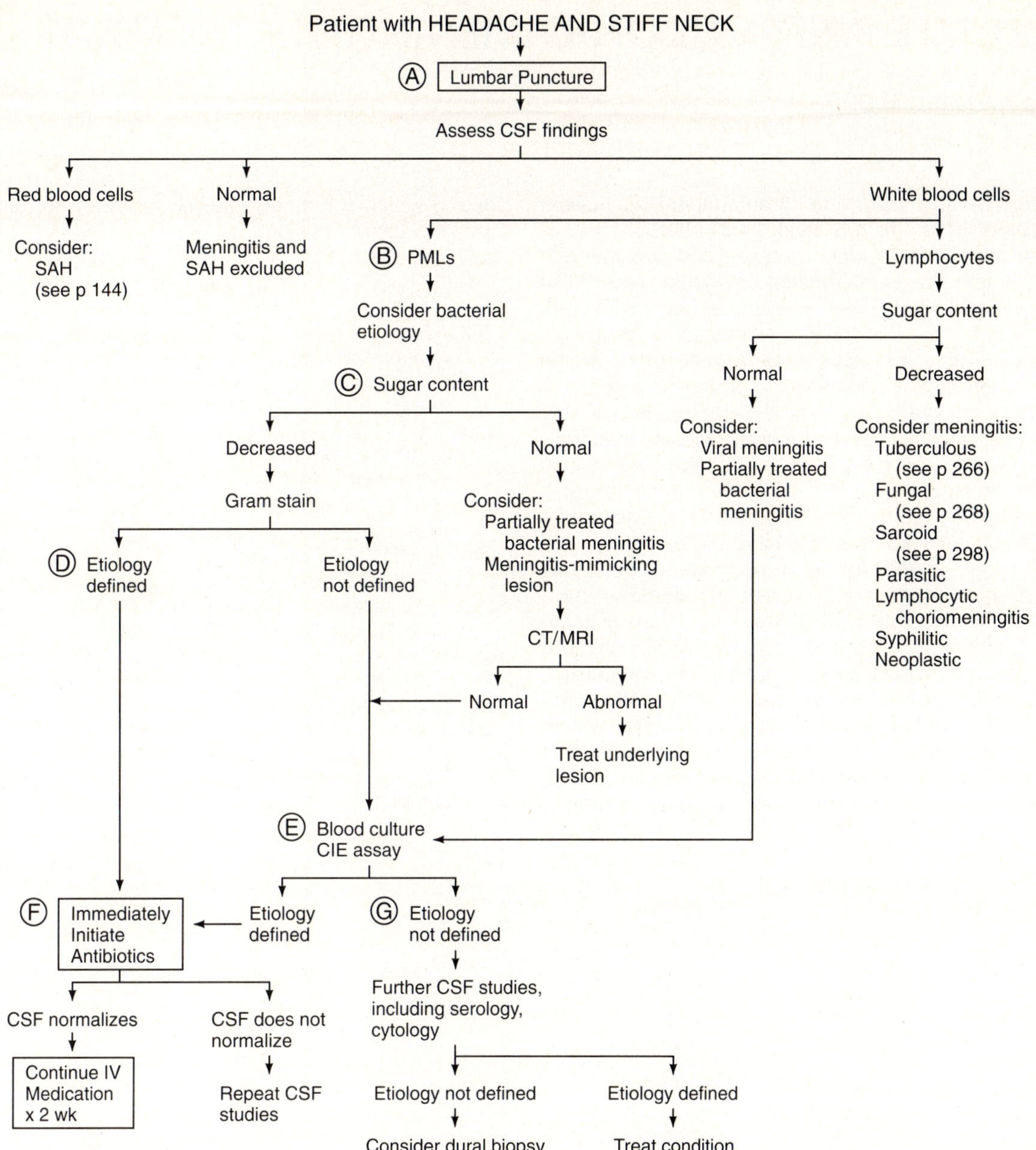

24 to 48 hours after initiating therapy and when concluding therapy to confirm that CSF is sterile. After 2 weeks of antibiotics, CSF may still contain several hundred white blood cells; however, if CSF is sterile, no further LP or antibiotics are needed. If meningitis recurs, consider a parameningeal infection source (sinusitis, mastoiditis, osteomyelitis), basilar skull fracture with dural tear, or CSF leak (usually due to a cribriform plate defect).

G. In patients with pleocytosis and negative bacteriologic studies, perform several cytologic studies for neoplastic cells. Granulomatous (sarcoid) conditions may cause meningitis; diagnosis may require meningeal (dural) biopsy. CT/MRI contrast studies may show densely enhancing basal meninges (see p 298). Serologic studies exclude syphilitic meningitis. If there is predominantly lymphocytosis with normal glucose content, consider partially treated bacterial meningitis, sarcoid, Lyme disease, HIV disease, leptospirosis, neoplastic meningitis, parameningeal infection, or tuberculous or fungal meningitis. If sugar is decreased, also consider lymphocytic choriomeningitis, mumps, or *Listeria* meningitis.

References

Bolan G, Barza M. Acute bacterial meningitis in children and adults. Med Clin North Am 1985; 69:231.

Shelton MM, Marks WA. Bacterial meningitis: An update. Neurol Clin North Am 1990; 8:605.

Swartz MN, Dodge PR. Bacterial meningitis—a review of selected aspects. N Engl J Med 1965; 272:725, 842, 954, 1001.

SUBACUTE AND CHRONIC MENINGITIS IN ADULTS

Carlos A. Garcia, M.D.

Most patients with subacute or chronic meningitis present with a history of headaches, neck pain, photophobia, or signs of increased intracranial pressure and general malaise. Some may have intermittent low-grade fever. The symptoms usually have been present for several days to several weeks. The neurologic examination frequently shows papilledema and signs of meningeal irritation (stiff neck and photophobia) and no focal neurologic deficit. The medical history is important; inquire about trips abroad that may have allowed the patient to acquire parasitic infections such as cysticercosis and malaria. Ask about factors that cause immunosuppression (e.g., extended use of steroids, transplant surgery, and [most important] risk factors for AIDS). Obtain serologic tests for HIV, Lyme disease, and parasites; draw blood for viral antibodies and Lyme disease. A chest x-ray film may reveal granulomas, tumor, or other infections. CT or MRI will rule out a mass effect to allow for a safe lumbar puncture. Send CSF for chemistries, protein, and cultures of aerobic and anaerobic organisms, cytology, VDRL, and determination of antigens for parasites. Repeated lumbar puncture may be needed to obtain CSF for further specific tests. The clinical features, imaging studies, and CSF studies will allow a definitive diagnosis in most cases. However, there are a few subacute meningitides in which a definite diagnosis cannot be made; most follow a benign course.

References

Bell WE. Treatment of fungal infections of the central nervous system. Ann Neurol 1981; 9:417.

Finkel MG, Halperin JJ. Nervous system Lyme borreliosis tevistes. Arch Neurol 1992; 49:102.

Garcia CA, Weisberg LA, Lacorte WSJ. Cryptococcal intracerebral mass lesions: CT pathologic considerations. Neurology 1985; 35:731.

Halperin JJ. Neurological complication of Lyme disease. Neurol Chronicle 1992; 1:1.

Holmes MD, Brant-Zawadski MM, Simon RP. Clinical features of meningovascular syphilis. Neurology 1984; 34:553.

Merritt HH, Adams RD, Solomon HC. Neurosyphilis. New York: Oxford University Press, 1946.

MGH Case Records (Case 32-1991). A 35 year old man with changed mental status and multiple intracerebral lesions. N Engl J Med 1991; 325:414.

White M, Cirrincione C, Blevins A, Armstrong D. Cryptococcal meningitis: Outcome in patients with AIDS and patients with neoplastic disease. J Infect Dis 1992; 165:960.

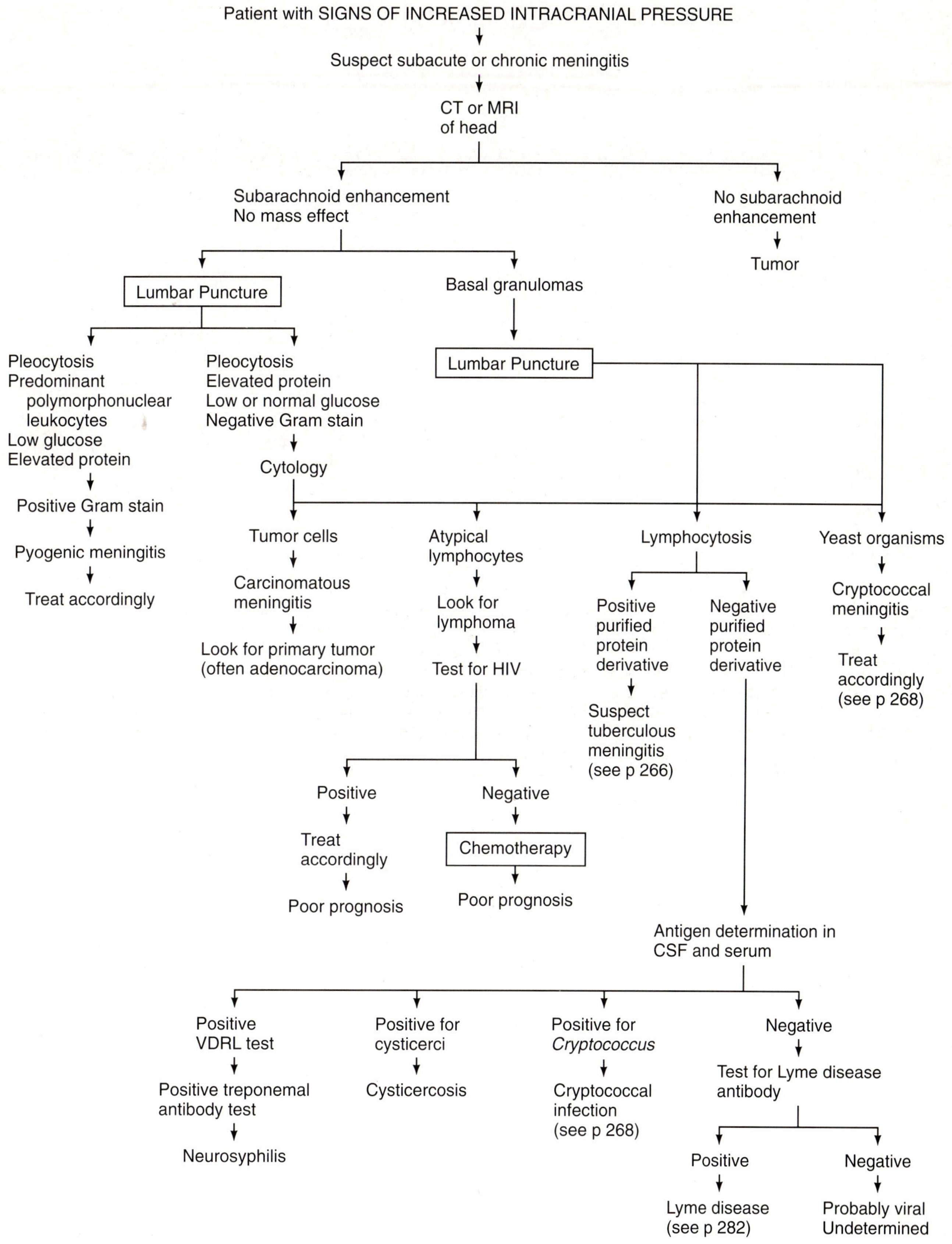

Patient with SIGNS OF INCREASED INTRACRANIAL PRESSURE

Suspect subacute or chronic meningitis

CT or MRI
of head

Subarachnoid enhancement
No mass effect

No subarachnoid
enhancement

Tumor

Lumbar Puncture

Basal granulomas

Lumbar Puncture

Pleocytosis
Predominant
  polymorphonuclear
  leukocytes
Low glucose
Elevated protein

Pleocytosis
Elevated protein
Low or normal glucose
Negative Gram stain

Positive Gram stain

Cytology

Lymphocytosis

Yeast organisms

Pyogenic meningitis

Treat accordingly

Tumor cells

Atypical
lymphocytes

Positive
purified
protein
derivative

Negative
purified
protein
derivative

Cryptococcal
meningitis

Carcinomatous
meningitis

Look for
lymphoma

Suspect
tuberculous
meningitis
(see p 266)

Treat
accordingly
(see p 268)

Look for primary tumor
(often adenocarcinoma)

Test for HIV

Positive

Negative

Treat
accordingly

Chemotherapy

Poor prognosis

Poor prognosis

Antigen determination in
CSF and serum

Positive
VDRL test

Positive for
cysticerci

Positive for
Cryptococcus

Negative

Positive treponemal
antibody test

Cysticercosis

Cryptococcal
infection
(see p 268)

Test for Lyme disease
antibody

Neurosyphilis

Positive

Negative

Lyme disease
(see p 282)

Probably viral
Undetermined

FOCAL INTRACRANIAL BACTERIAL DISEASE

Leon A. Weisberg, M.D.

Patients with cerebritis-abscess may present with focal signs and intracranial hypertension but no systemic infectious manifestations (this may simulate intracranial neoplasm) or focal neurologic and meningeal signs with evidence of systemic infection. Systemic signs (fever, peripheral leukocytosis, elevated erythrocyte sedimentation rate) indicate that an infectious source of focal brain suppuration is active and has not been adequately treated. If a patient with cerebritis abscess has meningeal signs, rupture of the cerebritis abscess into the subarachnoid or ventricular spaces is the probable explanation. Meningeal signs may indicate transtentorial or tonsillar herniation.

A. If a patient is suspected of harboring CNS infection (meningitis, empyema, cerebritis abscess) and has papilledema, CT/MRI should precede lumbar puncture (LP) because there is a risk of precipitating transtentorial herniation in these lesions. Uncomplicated meningitis does *not* cause papilledema. If systemic infection and neurologic signs develop, LP may be performed carefully if CT/MRI is not readily available. Be prepared to treat herniation symptoms. CSF abnormalities in meningitis are usually diagnostic, whereas in cerebritis abscess they are nonspecific and do not usually provide positive bacteriologic data on which to base an antibiotic regimen.

B. CT/MRI is extremely sensitive in demonstrating epidural or subdural empyema. Use radiography to assess potential contiguous sources of infection (orbit, sinus, ear, eye, mastoid). Treat these disorders with antibiotics and surgical drainage.

C. If the clinical findings suggest an infectious-inflammatory condition and CT/MRI shows an intracerebral lesion, differentiate vascular disorders (vasculitis, venous sinus thrombosis) from cerebritis abscess. Vascular conditions produce characteristic angiographic findings. In cerebritis abscess, CT shows a hypodense lesion with ri..g enhancement (Fig. 1). The completeness and thickness of ring enhancement correlate with the degree of encapsulation in cerebritis abscess. If CT/MRI shows a thick ring-enhancing lesion, this probably represents an encapsulated abscess (a walled-off collection of pus within brain parenchyma). Surgical evacuation is frequently necessary at this stage because antibiotic penetration through the thick abscess capsule is poor.

D. CT/MRI findings are not always specific enough to differentiate cerebritis (focal suppurative process with no or incomplete encapsulation) from abscess (encapsulated suppurative lesion). If multiple lesions are present, treat with IV antibiotics and corticosteroids. During treatment of patients with cerebritis abscess, serial CT/MRI may show its resolution if the antibiotic is appropriate for the infectious source and there is adequate penetration of the capsule wall. This healing process with normalization of CT/MRI results may take several months after completion of a routine 6- to 8-week course of antibiotics.

The standard antibiotic regimen for brain abscess is penicillin and chloramphenicol. Penicillin is given at a total daily dose of 24 million units IV every 4 hours; it is effective against gram-positive bacteria. Chloramphenicol is given at a daily dose of 6 to 8 g, 1.5 to 2 g every 6 hours. This is effective against some gram-positive bacteria and certain anaerobes but unreliable against *Enterobacter*. Metronidazole in a daily dose of 2 g, 0.5 g every 6 hours, is effective against obligate anaerobic bacteria that may occur in sinus and ear infections. For gram-negative bacilli causing ear infection, third-generation cephalosporins (cefotaxime, ceftizoxime) are effective. For *Enterobacter*, extended-spectrum penicillins (mezlocillin, piperacillin) are effective.

E. If CT/MRI shows a single lesion, it is best to assess whether this represents cerebritis or early abscess formation, but this is usually not possible on the basis of CT/MRI characteristics. Both of these conditions are treated initially with antibiotics and corticosteroids. Continue medical therapy if the patient remains clinically stable or improves; however, if clinical deterioration occurs, surgical drainage is necessary. If clinical and CT/MRI findings indicate that resolution has occurred, surgery may be avoided. If the abscess capsule is thick, surgery is necessary, because antibiotic penetration into this type of lesion is poor.

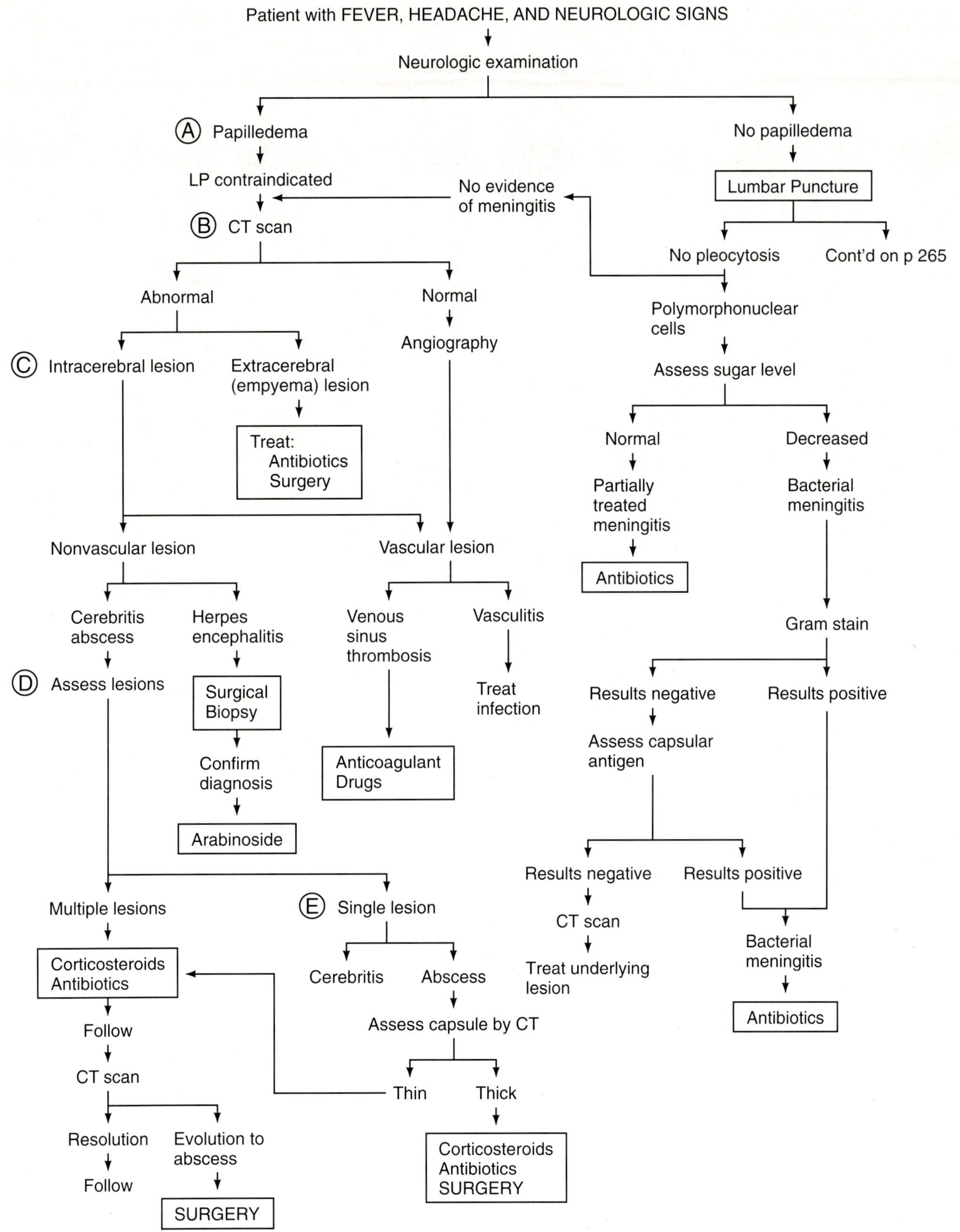

Patient with FEVER, HEADACHE, AND NEUROLOGIC SIGNS
Neurologic examination
A Papilledema
No papilledema
LP contraindicated
No evidence of meningitis
Lumbar Puncture
B CT scan
No pleocytosis
Cont'd on p 265
Abnormal
Normal
Polymorphonuclear cells
C Intracerebral lesion
Extracerebral (empyema) lesion
Angiography
Assess sugar level
Treat:
Antibiotics
Surgery
Normal
Decreased
Nonvascular lesion
Vascular lesion
Partially treated meningitis
Bacterial meningitis
Cerebritis abscess
Herpes encephalitis
Venous sinus thrombosis
Vasculitis
Antibiotics
D Assess lesions
Surgical Biopsy
Treat infection
Gram stain
Confirm diagnosis
Anticoagulant Drugs
Results negative
Results positive
Arabinoside
Assess capsular antigen
Multiple lesions
E Single lesion
Results negative
Results positive
Corticosteroids Antibiotics
Cerebritis
Abscess
CT scan
Follow
Assess capsule by CT
Treat underlying lesion
Bacterial meningitis
CT scan
Thin
Thick
Antibiotics
Resolution
Evolution to abscess
Corticosteroids
Antibiotics
SURGERY
Follow
SURGERY

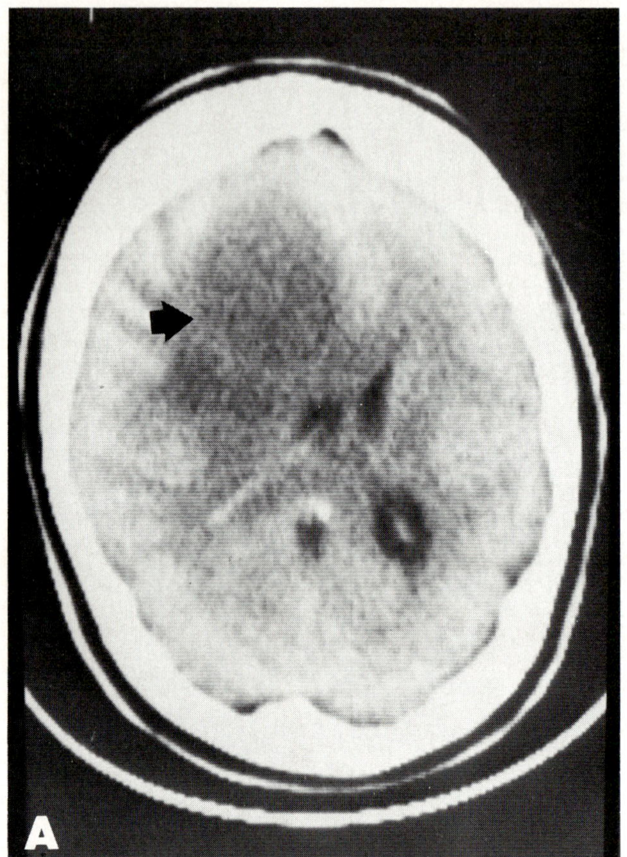
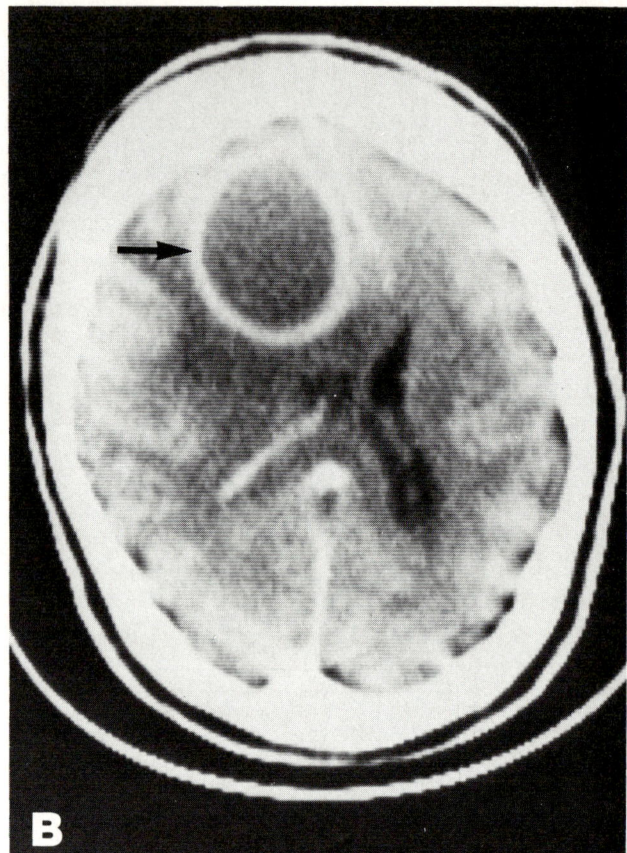
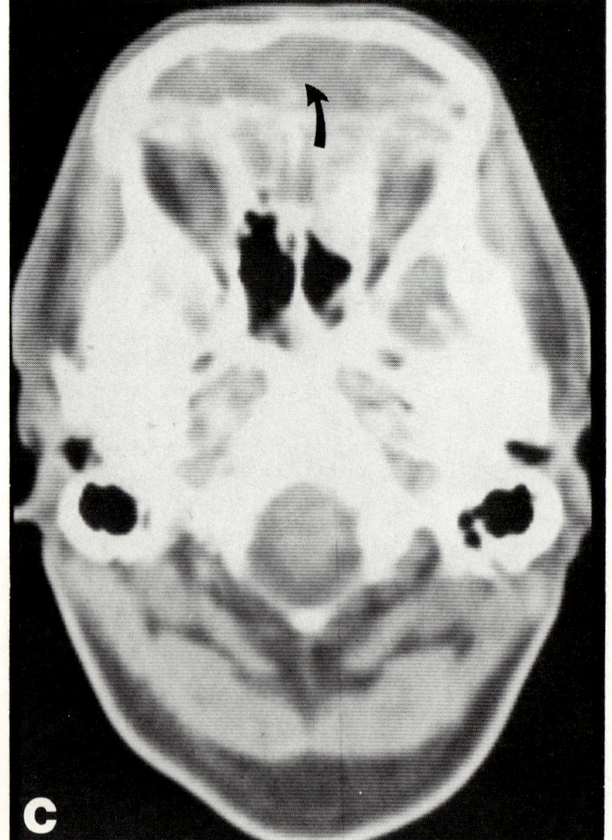

Figure 1 CT scan shows a large hypodense lesion *(A)* with peripheral ring enhancement *(B)* consistent with brain abscess in a patient with frontal sinusitis *(C)*.

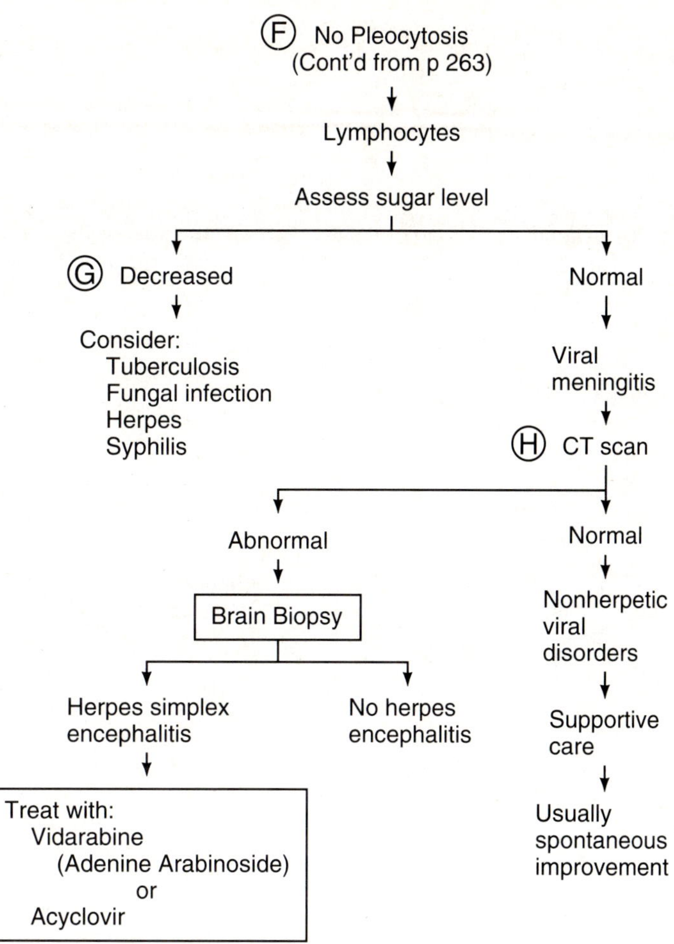

F. If a patient has focal neurologic and meningeal signs and CT shows no abnormality, CSF examination is needed. Polymorphonuclear CSF pleocytosis indicates a bacterial process; lymphocytic pleocytosis indicates a nonbacterial process. Glucose content may be reduced in nonviral disorders, and investigation for an infectious agent should reveal the cause of the pleocytosis.

G. Viral CNS infections cause lymphocytic pleocytosis. Herpes simplex encephalitis is the only viral process that results in CT/MRI abnormalities (hypodense lesions in one or both temporal lobes). EEG may show unitemporal or bitemporal spike discharges. Begin acyclovir therapy if the diagnosis is considered highly probable on the basis of clinical findings or is confirmed by brain biopsy (see p 270).

H. Other infectious processes (tuberculous, fungal, syphilitic) cause meningitic reaction; diagnosis is established by CSF findings. These conditions may produce CT/MRI abnormalities if vascular occlusion or arteritis causes cerebral infarction due to arteritis or if granulomatous tissue reaction (tuberculoma, syphilitic gumma) results in focal mass lesion. The vascular changes due to inflammatory arteritis are detected by angiography.

References

Britt RH, Enzmann DR, Yeager AS. Neuropathological and computerized tomographic findings in experimental brain abscess. J Neurosurg 1981; 55:590.

Heineman HS, Braude AL, Osterholm JL. Intracranial suppurative disease: Early presumptive diagnosis and successful treatment without surgery. JAMA 1971; 218:1542.

Miller MH. Sinusitis-induced subdural empyema. Neurology 1983; 33:123.

Weisberg LA. Nonsurgical management of focal intracranial infection. Neurology 1981; 31:575.

TUBERCULOUS MENINGITIS

Carlos A. Garcia, M.D.

Tuberculous meningitis is a subacute CNS infection that develops from a primary focus in the lungs, kidneys, or bones. In some patients there may be no evidence of active systemic tuberculosis; however, most immunologically competent patients have positive skin tests and evidence of some type of chest lesion consistent with active or inactive tuberculosis. The meningeal exudate tends to concentrate around the base of the brain as a fibrinous mononuclear exudate (lymphocytic pleocytosis in CSF) and may cause cranial nerve involvement and severe arteritis with secondary ischemic brain lesions (Fig. 1). Untreated tuberculous meningitis is invariably fatal. Early diagnosis and rapid treatment are essential in controlling the disease.

A. The symptoms of tuberculous meningitis are those found in any meningitis. They include headache, confusion, behavioral disturbances, and lethargy. Symptoms are insidious in onset (subacute), developing over several weeks. All these symptoms may be preceded by general malaise and nocturnal low-grade fever. On examination there may be signs of meningeal irritation (e.g., stiff neck, photophobia, miosis). Signs of increased intracranial pressure can be confirmed by the finding of papilledema. Owing to basilar meningitis, there may also be cranial nerve involvement, causing ocular muscle weakness, facial paralysis, and reduced hearing.

B. Tuberculous meningitis may present as acute hemiplegia, coma, or some other sudden neurologic deterioration. Any of these symptoms produced by ischemia may occur during the course of the disease. The cerebral infarcts found on CT are caused by severe arteritis of large vessels at the base of the brain. Focal neurologic deficit may also be due to tuberculomas.

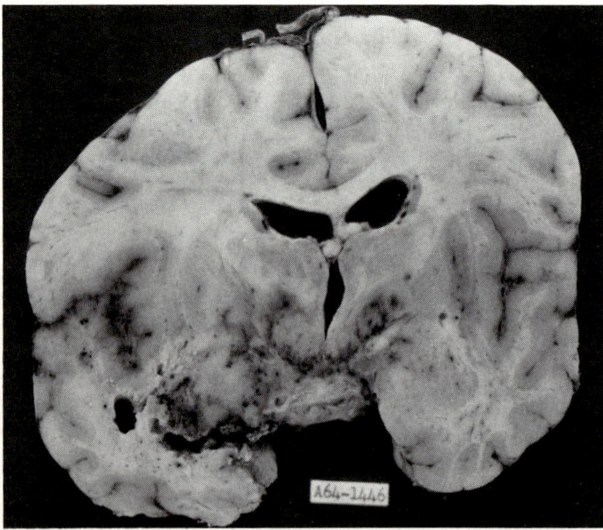

Figure 1 Coronal section of the brain in tuberculous meningitis showing fibrinous exudate occupying the basal and insular meninges.

The focal symptoms in tuberculomas are more insidious and suggest intracranial tumors. Cerebral tuberculomas are usually multiple and are easily detected on CT. The most common site of tuberculomas is the cerebellum. These may shrink with antituberculous medicine, but some may require surgical excision.

C. The chest x-ray view may be diagnostic of pulmonary tuberculosis. In adults the chest x-ray view may not show active pulmonary disease. A tuberculin skin test (intermediate strength) should be done and is frequently positive, but it takes 1 or 2 days to obtain the final reading. In rare patients with tuberculous meningitis (especially those who are immunologically compromised), the skin test may be negative.

D. Perform lumbar puncture when there is the slightest clinical suspicion of tuberculous meningitis. In uncomplicated meningitis, CSF pressure and protein content are elevated, sugar content is low, and there is a lymphocytic pleocytosis. Polymorphonuclear pleocytosis is usually associated with complicated meningitis, especially with cerebral infarcts. Acid-fast organisms, seen on direct smears, are present in only 10% of initial samples. CSF cultures are positive in 90% of cases but require 3 to 6 weeks for completion. The best yield is obtained if a large amount of CSF is used for cultures. Latex particle agglutination, enzyme-linked immunosorbent assay, or radioimmunoassay test of CSF are new, simple, and rapid tests that require small amounts of fluid and seem promising. The specific antituberculous treatment is variable, depending on the case, and should be initiated when there is the slightest suspicion of tuberculous meningitis and before confirmation of the diagnosis. Treatment consists of isoniazid, 300 mg/day, in combination with ethambutol, 15 mg/kg/day, and rifampin, 600 mg/day, for 4 months followed by isoniazid and rifampin for another 4 months. Treatment with isoniazid should continue for 2 years; monitor the response by clinical neurologic examination and CSF studies. Toxic effects of isoniazid can be prevented with pyridoxine. Ethambutol may impair color vision. Corticosteroid therapy in combination with antituberculosis therapy has been used early in the disease to prevent meningeal fibrosis. The treatment may vary with time and the development of new antibiotics. Consult an infectious disease specialist. There is recent evidence that tuberculous meningitis is being diagnosed more frequently in AIDS patients. There is also recent evidence of an increased number of "atypical" or antibiotic resistant organisms.

References

Goldman KP. A new diagnostic test for tuberculous meningitis. Tubercle 1985; 66:157.

Kennedy DG, Fallon RJ. Tuberculous meningitis. JAMA 1979; 41:264.

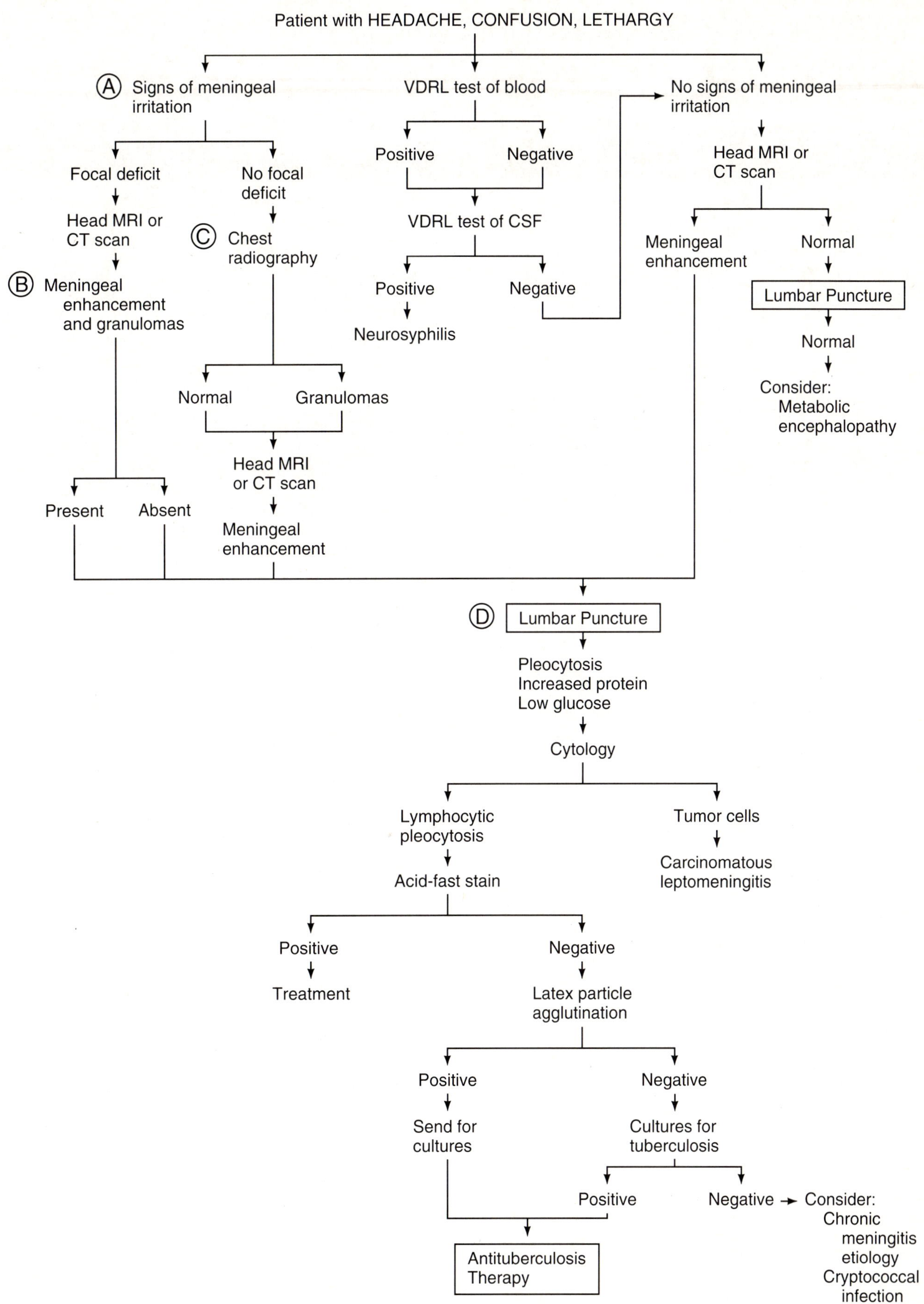

Patient with HEADACHE, CONFUSION, LETHARGY
A Signs of meningeal irritation
VDRL test of blood
No signs of meningeal irritation
Focal deficit
No focal deficit
Positive
Negative
Head MRI or CT scan
Head MRI or CT scan
C Chest radiography
VDRL test of CSF
Meningeal enhancement
Normal
B Meningeal enhancement and granulomas
Positive
Negative
Lumbar Puncture
Normal
Granulomas
Positive
Neurosyphilis
Normal
Present
Absent
Head MRI or CT scan
Consider: Metabolic encephalopathy
Meningeal enhancement
D Lumbar Puncture
Pleocytosis
Increased protein
Low glucose
Cytology
Lymphocytic pleocytosis
Tumor cells
Acid-fast stain
Carcinomatous leptomeningitis
Positive
Negative
Treatment
Latex particle agglutination
Positive
Negative
Send for cultures
Cultures for tuberculosis
Positive
Negative
Consider: Chronic meningitis etiology Cryptococcal infection
Antituberculosis Therapy

CRYPTOCOCCAL INFECTION OF THE CENTRAL NERVOUS SYSTEM

Carlos A. Garcia, M.D.

Cryptococcus neoformans is a yeast form of fungus. It is usually harbored in soil and the droppings of birds, especially pigeons. The primary focus of this infection is in the lungs. Cryptococcal meningitis is the most common mycotic CNS infection and is the most common CNS infection in AIDS patients in some areas of the United States.

A. Over 50% of patients with cryptococcal infections are immunosuppressed (AIDS, organ transplants, chronic dialysis, long-term corticosteroid therapy, diabetes). The symptoms in this CNS disease are nonspecific, insidious (weeks to months), and variable. Some patients may present with signs of intracranial hypertension (e.g., headache, neck pain, diplopia). In these the neurologic examination may show papilledema and lateral rectus muscle weakness. Other patients may present with dementia and no meningeal signs or with focal deficits, including paraparesis, hemiparesis, and cerebellar deficits.

B. The CNS lesion is usually secondary to a primary pulmonary focus. This lesion may be detected on chest radiography.

C. MRI or CT of the head may show hydrocephalus, diffuse edema, or focal enhancing (granulomas) or nonenhancing round hypodense (gelatinous pseudocysts) lesions.

D. The diagnosis is made by identifying the organism in the CSF. The lumbar puncture shows elevated pressure, increased protein content, low sugar content, and lymphocytic pleocytosis. Identification of the organism in the CNS is difficult; large amounts of the CSF may be needed. The encapsulated organisms may be seen with India ink preparations, and also in CSF cytology. Cryptococcal antigens in blood in the CSF may confirm the diagnosis of cryptococcal meningitis.

E. Treatment consists of systemic administration of amphotericin B, flucytosine, and miconazole. All these antifungal antimicrobials have a potential for causing hematopoietic and renal toxicity and should be administered by an experienced infectious disease specialist. Some of these medications should be given by an intrathecal route through direct lumbar punctures or an Ommaya reservoir. The prognosis is variable, but remission of the infection can be achieved in some patients.

References

Bell WE. Treatment of fungal infections of the central nervous system. Ann Neurol 1981; 9:417.

Garcia CA, Weisberg LA, Lacorte WSJ. Cryptococcal intracerebral mass lesions: CT pathologic considerations. Neurology 1985; 35:731.

White M, Cirrincione C, Blevins A, Armstrong D. Cryptococcal meningitis: Outcome in patients with AIDS and patients with neoplastic disease. J Infect Dis 1992; 165:960.

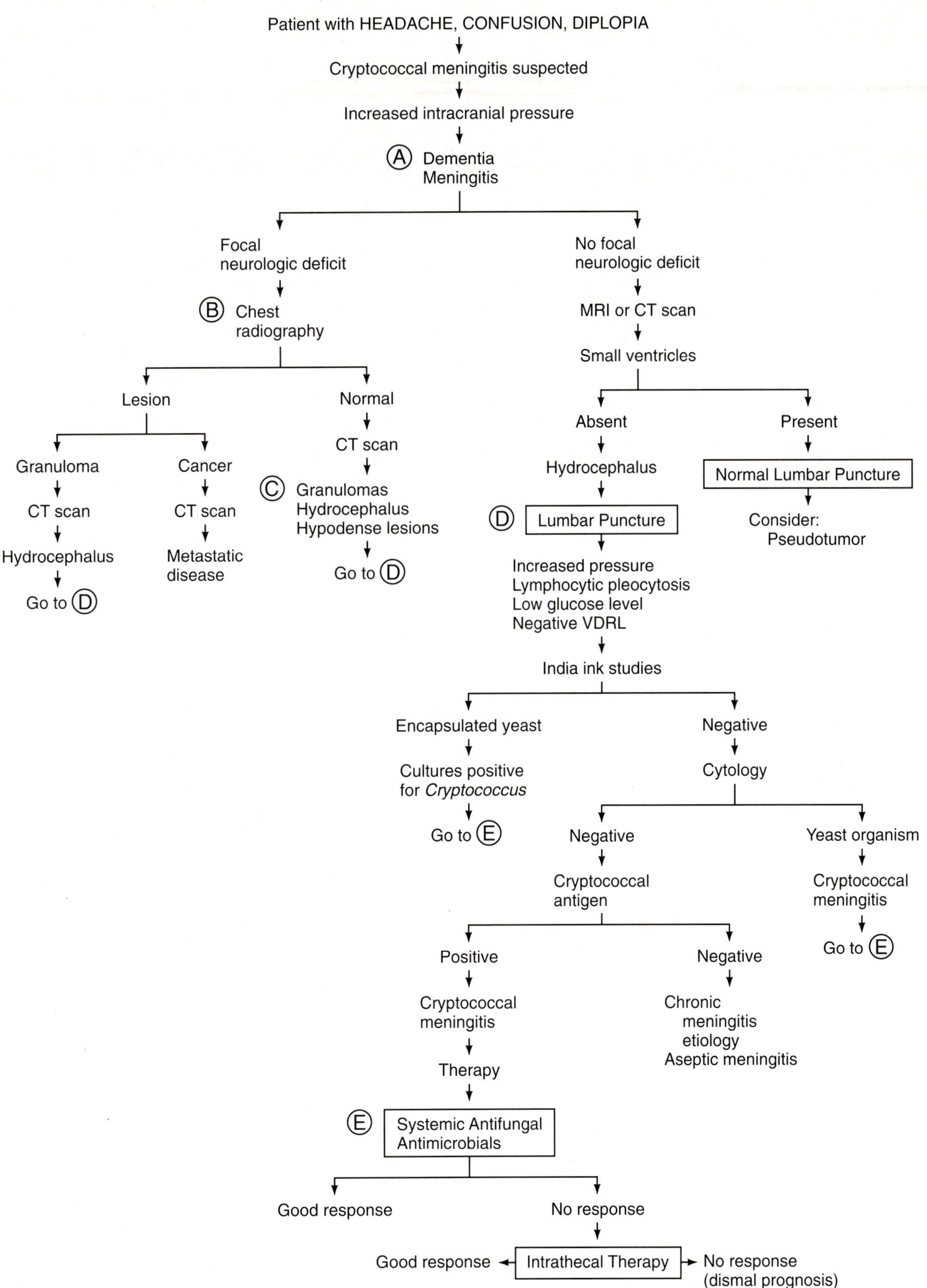

Patient with HEADACHE, CONFUSION, DIPLOPIA
Cryptococcal meningitis suspected
Increased intracranial pressure
A Dementia
Meningitis
Focal neurologic deficit
No focal neurologic deficit
B Chest radiography
MRI or CT scan
Small ventricles
Lesion
Normal
Absent
Present
Granuloma
Cancer
CT scan
Hydrocephalus
Normal Lumbar Puncture
C Granulomas Hydrocephalus Hypodense lesions
CT scan
CT scan
D Lumbar Puncture
Consider: Pseudotumor
Hydrocephalus
Metastatic disease
Go to D
Go to D
Go to D
Increased pressure
Lymphocytic pleocytosis
Low glucose level
Negative VDRL
India ink studies
Encapsulated yeast
Negative
Cultures positive for Cryptococcus
Cytology
Go to E
Negative
Yeast organism
Cryptococcal antigen
Cryptococcal meningitis
Positive
Negative
Go to E
Cryptococcal meningitis
Chronic meningitis etiology Aseptic meningitis
Therapy
E Systemic Antifungal Antimicrobials
Good response
No response
Good response
Intrathecal Therapy
No response (dismal prognosis)

ACUTE VIRAL ENCEPHALITIS

Leon A. Weisberg, M.D.

Encephalitis is defined as brain inflammation. This may be caused by multiple diverse microorganisms, including viruses, bacteria, fungi, and parasites. Acute viral encephalitis (AVE) is caused by a direct neuronal destructive effect of virus or white matter inflammation and demyelination triggered by a postviral immunologic process. Clinical features of AVE include acute or subacute onset of headache, fever, impaired mentation, and behavioral change or seizures. There may be focal neurologic signs, including aphasia, hemiparesis, homonymous hemianopia, and cranial nerve dysfunction. Meningeal signs are not common at the initial stages, but there is usually CSF lymphocytic pleocytosis. There is sufficient overlap among the clinical features of multiple diverse encephalitis disorders that an etiologic diagnosis of AVE is not usually possible on the basis of clinical features alone. As antiviral agents are developed, specific viral diagnosis of the AVE will become more important.

A. Herpes simplex type 1 encephalitis (HSE) is the most common cause of sporadic AVE in older children and adults. The patient need not have mucosal or skin vesicular eruptions. HSE causes hemorrhagic necrosis localized to orbitofrontal and temporal lobes. There may be uni- or bilateral cerebral hemispheric involvement. When it is localized to one temporal lobe, the clinical features of an expanding temporal lobe mass may result in uncal herniation. Focal neurologic signs are unusual in other types of AVE, which usually cause a diffuse encephalitic syndrome (altered consciousness, generalized seizures).

B. In HSE, CT may show a hypodense temporal lobe lesion with edema, hemorrhage, mass effect, and contrast enhancement; however, CT may be negative in 30% to 40% of biopsy-proven cases of HSE. If there is prominent ring enhancement, consider a brain abscess or neoplasm; this contrast-enhancing pattern is unlikely with HSE. MRI may be more sensitive than CT in detecting pathologic changes of HSE, perhaps showing earlier and more extensive temporal lobe changes. However, the superiority of MRI to CT has not been established at the present time.

C. EEG may show uni- or bilateral temporal lobe discharges in 80% of biopsy-proven cases of HSE, whereas in other forms of AVE EEG shows a diffuse slow wave pattern. The finding of bilateral temporal lobe discharges in HSE is associated with a poor prognosis because this indicates more extensive and advanced disease.

D. In HSE, CSF usually shows lymphocytic pleocytosis. Because HSE may cause hemorrhagic necrosis, red blood cells may be present. Protein content is usually elevated and sugar content sometimes low. Reduced sugar content is unusual with most forms of AVE except HSE and mumps. CSF studies for other causes of encephalitis are necessary, but with acute onset of encephalitis, the possibility of fungal, parasitic, or tuberculous disease is low. Herpes simplex virus (HSV) is rarely isolated from CSF, and detection of HSV antibodies or antigen has not been helpful in establishing the diagnosis of HSE. When the CSF findings are normal, HSE is extremely unlikely.

E. It is important to diagnose HSE as early as possible, because effective treatment exists for this type of AVE. The diagnosis is usually definitively established by brain biopsy findings. Morbidity and mortality rates of biopsy should be <2%. On the basis of clinical and neurodiagnostic findings, it should be possible to determine the appropriate biopsy site to include an actively involved brain region. However, if there are no localizing features, perform biopsy of a nondominant anterior inferior temporal lobe in a "blind" fashion. False-negative biopsy results occur in less than 5% of autopsy-proved cases, but are most common when biopsy is done in this "blind" manner necessitated by negative CT, MRI, and EEG findings. Depending on the results of immunofluorescent stains of the biopsy material, diagnosis of HSE may be immediately established so that treatment may be begun immediately after surgery. Brain biopsy may permit a specific pathologic diagnosis for conditions that may simulate the clinical and neurodiagnostic findings of HSE (e.g., glioma, metastases, toxoplasmosis, bacterial brain abscess).

F. Because early therapy of HSE is most effective, give acyclovir (30 mg/kg in three doses) initially if HSE is suspected before brain biopsy. If the patient shows clinical improvement, continue therapy for 10 days; biopsy may prove unnecessary. Acyclovir is more effective than vidarabine (15 mg/kg) and associated with a lower toxicity. If improvement does not occur with acyclovir, perform brain biopsy.

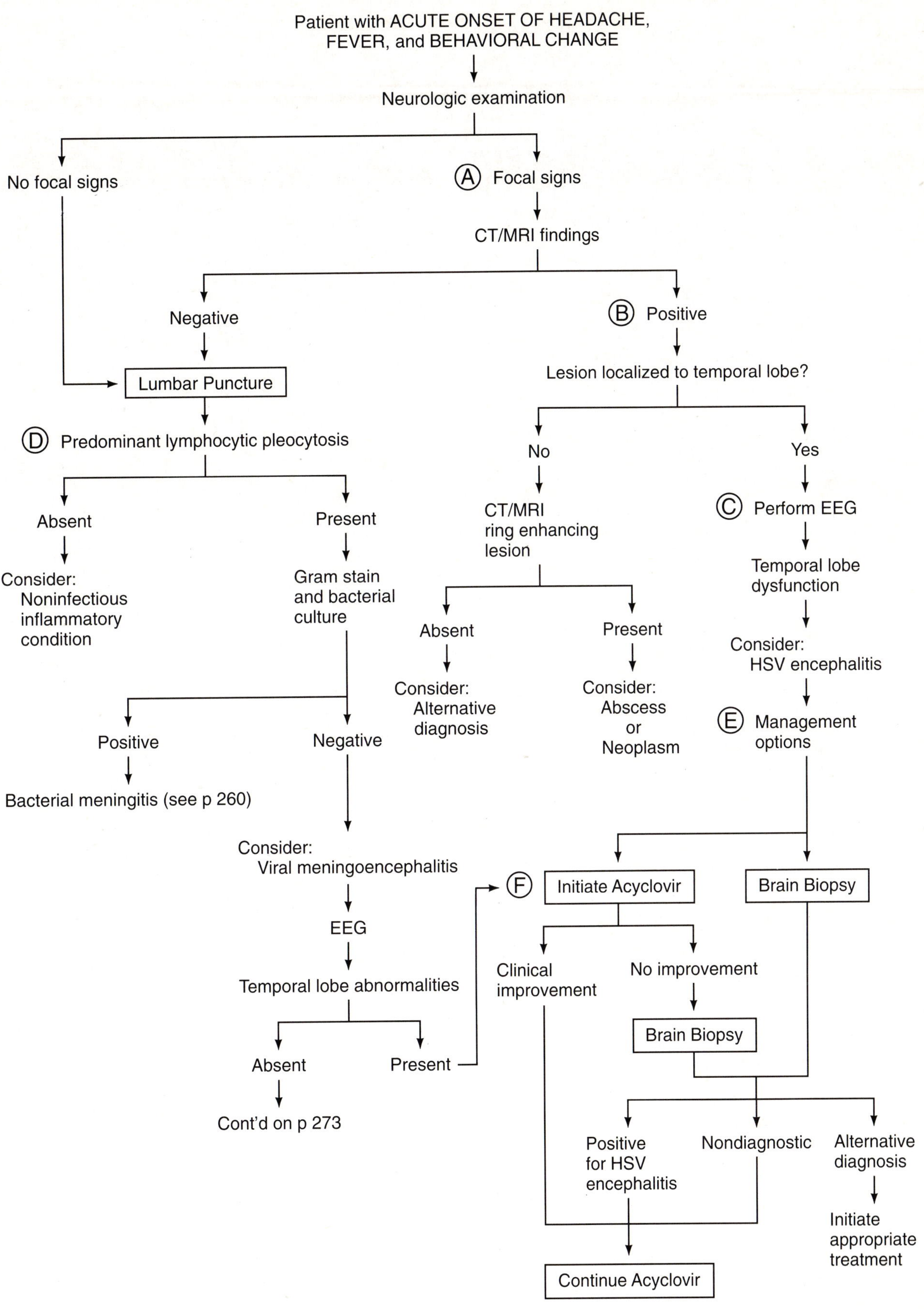

Patient with ACUTE ONSET OF HEADACHE, FEVER, and BEHAVIORAL CHANGE
Neurologic examination
No focal signs
A Focal signs
CT/MRI findings
Negative
B Positive
Lumbar Puncture
Lesion localized to temporal lobe?
D Predominant lymphocytic pleocytosis
No
Yes
Absent
Present
CT/MRI ring enhancing lesion
C Perform EEG
Consider: Noninfectious inflammatory condition
Gram stain and bacterial culture
Temporal lobe dysfunction
Absent
Present
Consider: HSV encephalitis
Positive
Negative
Consider: Alternative diagnosis
Consider: Abscess or Neoplasm
E Management options
Bacterial meningitis (see p 260)
Consider: Viral meningoencephalitis
F Initiate Acyclovir
Brain Biopsy
EEG
Temporal lobe abnormalities
Clinical improvement
No improvement
Absent
Present
Brain Biopsy
Cont'd on p 273
Positive for HSV encephalitis
Nondiagnostic
Alternative diagnosis
Initiate appropriate treatment
Continue Acyclovir

G. If CSF shows lymphocytic pleocytosis but there are no clinical or neurodiagnostic features to suggest HSE, investigate other etiologies. Arbovirus (arthropod-borne) and enterovirus are the most common epidemic forms of encephalitis. Serologic studies for arbovirus and enterovirus antibodies require acute and convalescent specimens; diagnosis of these forms of AVE is therefore established retrospectively after the time that acyclovir would be effective in HSE. Postinfectious encephalitis may result from measles or rubella. Varicella-zoster virus may cause prominent AVE with unique clinical features of cerebellar dysfunction. Epstein-Barr virus encephalitis may be suspected if there is a positive heterophile antibody titer. If vasculitis or collagen vascular disease is suspected, angiography may be necessary. Recurrent oral and genital ulcers and uveitis suggest Behçet's disease or Vogt-Koyanagi-Harada syndrome. HIV testing is mandatory in all patients with unexplained AVE even if there are no known risk factors for AIDS.

References

Anderson NE, Willoughby EW, Synek BJL. Brain biopsy in the management of focal encephalitis. J Neurol Neurosurg Psychiatry 1991; 54:1001.

Sawyer J, Ellner J, Ransohoff DF. To biopsy or not to biopsy in suspect herpes simplex encephalitis: A qualitative analysis. Med Decis Making 1988; 8:95.

Whitley RJ. Viral encephalitis. N Engl J Med 1990; 323:242.

Whitley RJ, Alford CA, Hirsch MS. Vidarabine versus acyclovir therapy in herpes simplex encephalitis. N Engl J Med 1986; 314:144.

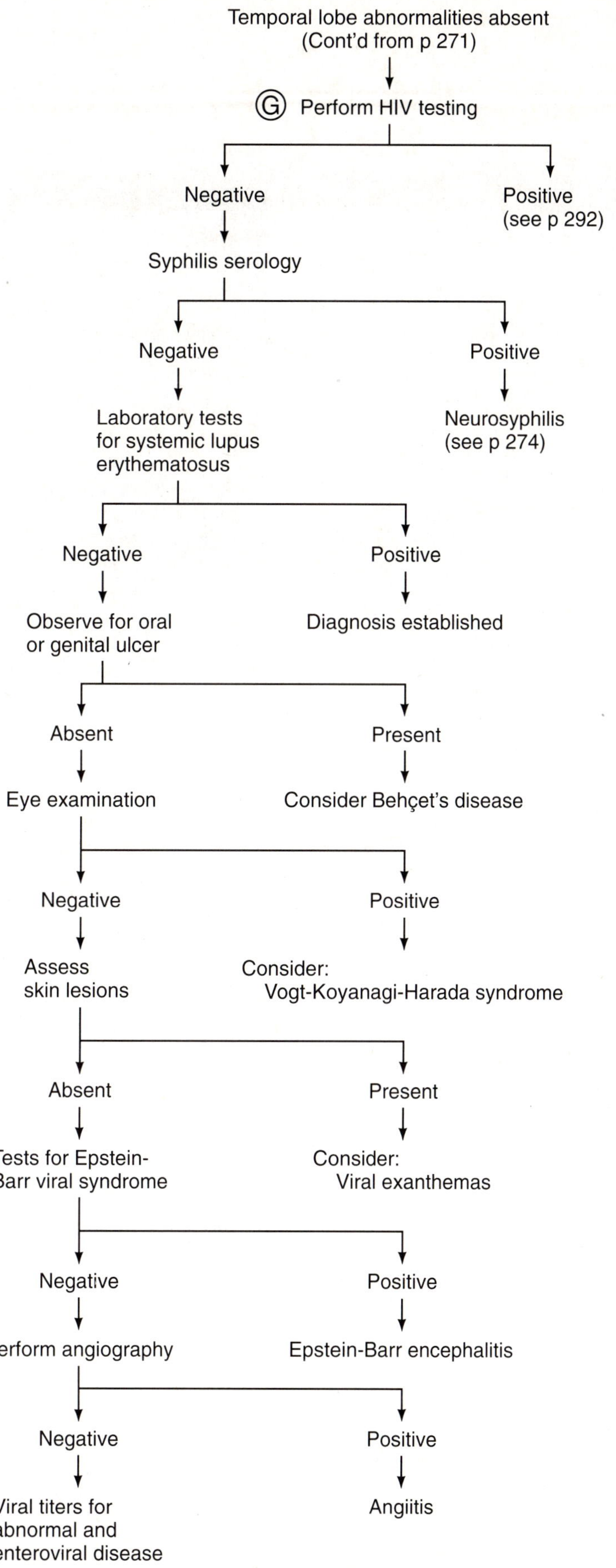

Temporal lobe abnormalities absent
(Cont'd from p 271)

G Perform HIV testing

Negative

Positive
(see p 292)

Syphilis serology

Negative

Positive

Laboratory tests
for systemic lupus
erythematosus

Neurosyphilis
(see p 274)

Negative

Positive

Observe for oral
or genital ulcer

Diagnosis established

Absent

Present

Eye examination

Consider Behçet's disease

Negative

Positive

Assess
skin lesions

Consider:
Vogt-Koyanagi-Harada syndrome

Absent

Present

Tests for Epstein-
Barr viral syndrome

Consider:
Viral exanthemas

Negative

Positive

Perform angiography

Epstein-Barr encephalitis

Negative

Positive

Viral titers for
abnormal and
enteroviral disease

Angiitis

NEUROSYPHILIS

Carlos A. Garcia, M.D.

Neurosyphilis is caused by invasion of *Treponema pallidum* into the CNS. The organism reaches the CNS within a few weeks to 18 months after the primary skin infection (chancre). The infection can produce intracranial or spinal lesions and may present with many different clinical features. However, there are two stages of neurosyphilis: asymptomatic (latent) and symptomatic. Symptomatic neurosyphilis may manifest as meningovascular syphilis and parenchymatous syphilis, which includes general paresis and tabes dorsalis. The incidence of syphilis has increased substantially in the last 10 years, predominantly in homosexuals, bisexuals, prostitutes, and patients who are HIV positive.

A. An asymptomatic or latent stage is discovered when a lumbar puncture is performed in a patient without CNS symptoms because of positive blood serology or during the course of investigation for other reasons. The infection may persist for years and then invade the brain tissue, or more often it may subside spontaneously. Early systemic dissemination of the treponeme has been documented before the development of a rash or secondary stage.

B. Secondary syphilis occurs 2 to 8 weeks after the primary infection and produces chronic meningitis at the base of the brain or in the spinal cord. The signs in the cord may be those of spinal arachnoiditis or "pachymeningitis cervicalis." The intracranial signs and symptoms are those of meningeal irritation, cranial nerve palsies, and vasculitis (endarteritis) of large or medium-sized vessels at the base of the brain (Heubner's arteritis), producing an ischemic brain lesion (ischemic stroke), usually in young individuals.

C. General paresis is produced by parenchymal (cerebral) invasion of the spirochete several years after the original infection (Fig. 1). The disease is manifested by progressive dementia, usually with personality change, memory dysfunction, grandiose ideation, seizures, tremors, and long tract signs, including a positive Babinski sign and an Argyll Robertson pupil (which accommodates but does not react to light).

D. Tabes dorsalis, another form of parenchymal neurosyphilis, may present with sharp stabbing pains in the legs or abdomen. The patient is ataxic and the bladder is hypotonic, with overflow incontinence. Some patients may have joint deformities (knees, ankles, and hips), which usually are painless and occur late in the disease (Charcot joints). Examination shows a positive Romberg sign, no vibratory and position sense, and an abnormal pupil. The pupil is usually irregular, small, and nonreactive to light but reactive to accommodation (Argyll Robertson pupil). Neurosyphilis and HIV infection should be included in the differential diagnosis of any neurologic disease.

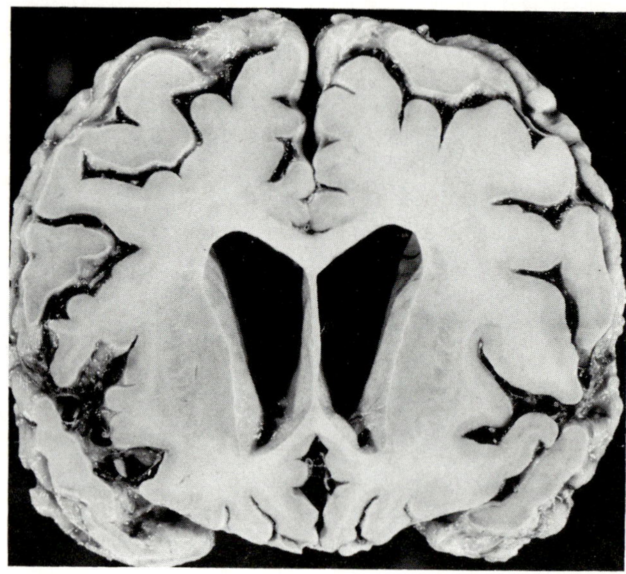

Figure 1 Coronal section of the brain showing thickened, edematous meninges; cortical atrophy; and hydrocephalus in paralytic dementia.

E. The CSF shows similar changes in any of the CNS manifestations of syphilis. These include lymphocytic pleocytosis (about 300 cells) with an elevated protein level (around 150 mg/dl) and a normal or borderline low glucose level. The diagnosis must be confirmed by demonstration of specific treponemal antibodies, using the treponemal immobilization (TPI) test and the fluorescent treponemal antibody absorption test (FTA-ABS). Treatment usually restores the CSF to normal. Reactivation of the disease is associated with pleocytosis and an increase in the treponemal antibody level. After treatment some patients may continue to show the presence of nonspecific reagin antibodies (VDRL slide test, highly sensitive but nonspecific).

F. Treatment consists of penicillin administration. Aqueous crystalline penicillin G, 2 million units IV every 4 hours for 10 days, seems to be the preferred and most effective therapy. However, some physicians give intramuscular injections of 2.4 million units of benzathine penicillin every week for 3 weeks. Tetracycline, 2 g/day for 30 days, or erythromycin, 1 g/day for 30 days, is an alternative choice in patients allergic to penicillin. In case of doubt regarding the diagnosis, CSF interpretation, or therapy, consult an infectious disease specialist or make inquiries of the Centers for Disease Control in Atlanta. Syphilis in HIV-infected patients is more aggressive and more difficult to treat, and a careful follow-up analysis of clinical and serologic tests is needed.

Patient with MENINGITIS, MYELOPATHY, POSITIVE BLOOD SEROLOGY
↓
Neurosyphilis suspected

HIV positive → Any neurologic symptom

No headache, irritability, meningeal signs → Assess blood serology
- Negative → (A) Lumbar Puncture → No cells / Normal protein / Positive VDRL and TPI tests → Latent neurosyphilis / Reactivated neurosyphilis
- Positive → Lumbar Puncture → Lymphocytic pleocytosis / Elevated protein / Normal or low glucose / Positive VDRL and TPI tests → Syphilitic meningitis

Headache, irritability, meningeal signs

Acute hemiplegia, aphasia, or seizures → CT scan → (B) Meningeal enhancement / Cerebral infarct → Lumbar Puncture → (E) Lymphocytic pleocytosis / Elevated protein / Normal or low glucose / Positive VDRL and TPI tests → Meningovascular syphilis

No hemiplegia, aphasia, or seizures

(C) Progressive dementia → Seizures / Aphasia → MRI or CT scan → Brain atrophy → Lumbar Puncture → Findings as in (E) → General paresis

No progressive dementia → (D) Recurrent abdominal pain / Ataxia / Optic atrophy / Loss of proprioception → Lumbar Puncture → Findings as in (E) → Tabes dorsalis

(F) Aqueous Crystalline Penicillin IV → Repeat Lumbar Puncture
- Normal CSF / Negative serology
- Abnormal CSF → Return to (F)

References

Holmes MD, Brant-Zawadski MM, Simon RP. Clinical features of meningovascular syphilis. Neurology 1984; 34:553.

Merritt HH, Adams RD, Solomon HC. Neurosyphilis. New York: Oxford University Press, 1946.

MGH Case Records (Case 32-1991). A 35 year old man with changed mental status and multiple intracerebral lesions. N Engl J Med 1991; 325:414.

TETANUS

Leon A. Weisberg, M.D.

Tetanus is caused by toxin produced by the anaerobe *Clostridium tetani*. The organism enters the body through infected wounds and then invades the spinal cord and brain stem. Tetanus toxin blocks spinal interneurons to cause stiffness and spasms. The clinical features of tetanus are due to blockade of inhibitory neurotransmitters in the spinal cord and brain stem. The earliest muscle spasm involves the thoracic and lumbar paraspinal muscles and results in opisthotonos. Spasms may involve the jaw (trismus or lockjaw), face (risus sardonicus), pharynx (dysphagia), or larynx (respiratory stridor) muscles. In focal tetanus, spasms may remain confined to the limb with the contaminated wound. Exercising the involved limb may provoke muscle spasms. In generalized tetanus, initial spasms involve the paraspinal muscles to cause intermittent opisthotonos so that the back appears arched off the bed. The spasms due to tetanus may be induced by excess sensory stimulation (e.g., loud noises).

A. The diagnosis of tetanus is established clinically. Patients have a contaminated wound and develop spasms that are initially mild and intermittent and later become more frequent, sustained, and severe. Tetanus toxin is produced in a contaminated anaerobic wound. The presence of a painful bite or wound with development of weakness and spasms (especially abdominal rigidity) suggests the neurotoxic effect of black widow spider venom rather than tetanus.

B. If a patient has muscle stiffness and is febrile but no wound is found, consider meningitis; perform lumbar puncture (LP). Hyperthermia, muscle hypertonia, autonomic instability (blood pressure fluctuations, cardiac arrhythmias, tachycardia), and altered consciousness may be caused by neuroleptic drugs. In malignant neuroleptic syndrome (MNS) the creatine kinase level is elevated; intense muscle breakdown may lead to myoglobinuria and renal failure. Muscle stiffness in MNS is treated with dantrolene (Dantrium) and bromocriptine (Parlodel).

C. If spasms are associated with peripheral nerve hyperexcitability (Trousseau or Chvostek sign, carpopedal spasm), consider tetany due to low serum calcium or magnesium content or alkalosis (precipitated by hyperventilation). Tetany responds to normalization of these electrolyte disturbances. If a patient has muscle rigidity and spasms without neuromuscular irritability, consider the stiff-man syndrome. This involves axial and proximal muscles but not jaw or facial muscles, in contrast to tetanus. This condition develops slowly and leads to joint deformities. Stiff-man syndrome may respond to diazepam.

D. If muscle stiffness and spasms are associated with upper motor neuron signs (clonus, Babinski sign) or decerebrate posturing, consider encephalomyelitis; perform CT, MRI, and LP. If consciousness is altered and there are spasms, consider seizures; perform EEG. Strychnine poisoning may cause spasms and convulsions; these may occur in drug addicts when street drugs are mixed with strychnine.

E. In tetanus, spasms usually become more severe. If complications are treated successfully, toxin is released from spinal and brain stem interneurons within 5 to 12 weeks; full recovery may occur when this happens. During the severe stage of clinical tetanus, place the patient in a quiet area of the intensive care unit (ICU) to reduce the frequency of stimulus-sensitive spasms. Treat seizures if they develop; prophylactic anticonvulsants are not warranted until seizures occur. Actively immunize patients with tetanus toxoid to avoid recurrence of tetanus, and provide passive immunization to bind any circulating toxin that has not yet reached the CNS. Because laryngeal spasm is a serious potential risk in tetanus patients and the clinical course of tetanus is usually prolonged, early tracheostomy is warranted to avoid respiratory complications; complete respiratory support is necessary. Use a central venous line for hyperalimentation; adequate parenteral alimentation avoids the development of a catabolic state with protein depletion and dehydration. Cardiac monitoring is essential to avoid sudden unexpected death due to autonomic abnormalities with cardiac arrhythmias and rapid blood pressure fluctuations. If cardiac sympathetic overdischarge occurs (hypertension, tachycardia), treat with beta-adrenergic blocking agents such as propranolol or labetalol. Muscle spasms due to generalized tetanus may be severe; suppress them with curare, given IV every 2 hours on a regular and continuing schedule. Less potent muscle relaxant agents (phenothiazines, diazepam, barbiturates) do not effectively control these tetanus spasms. If spasms are not controlled, muscle breakdown may occur, with resultant myoglobinuria. Meticulous skin care prevents decubitus ulcers. Low-dose subcutaneous anticoagulants prevent venous thrombosis and pulmonary embolism. With careful monitoring, mortality from tetanus should be low.

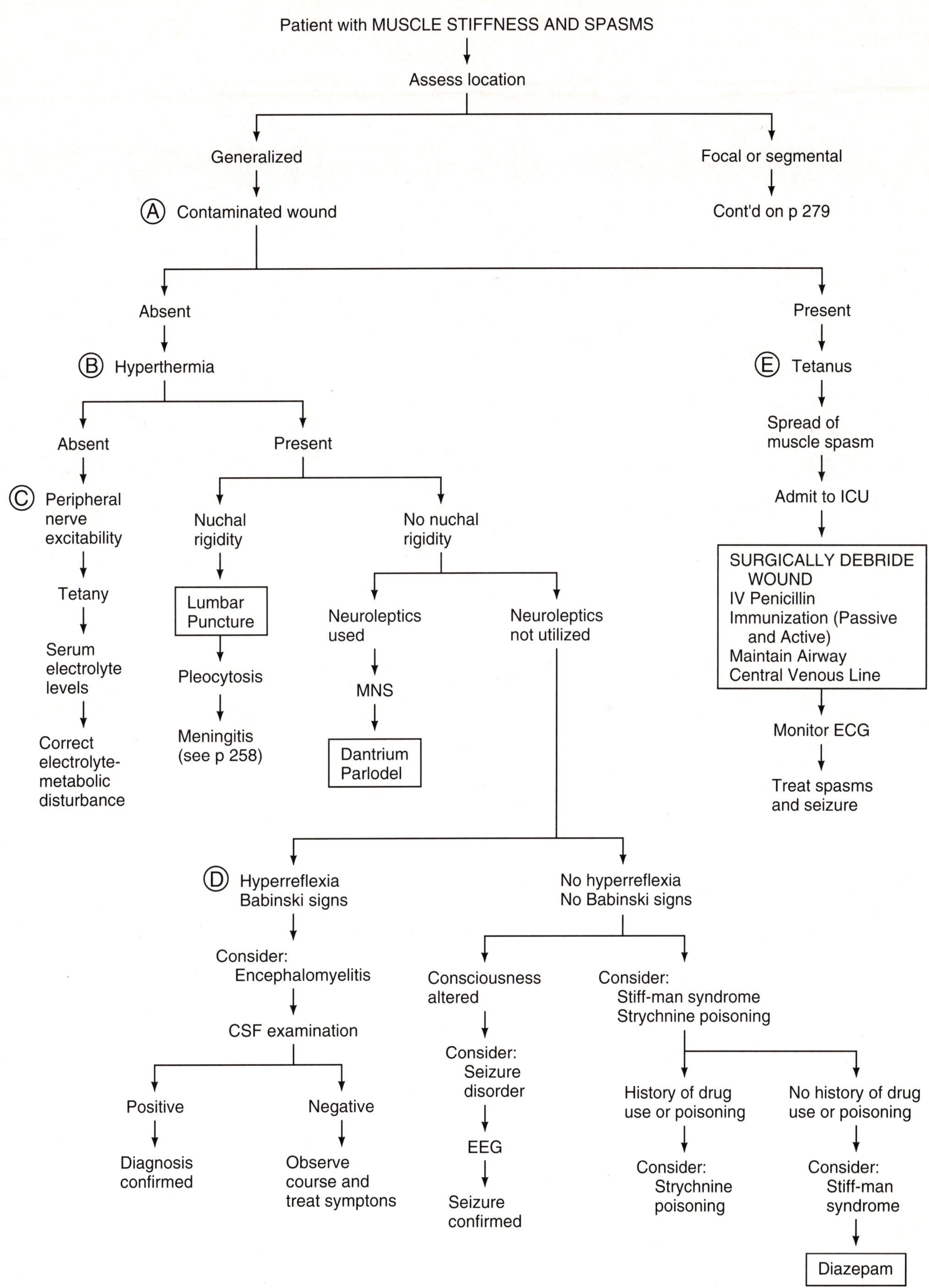

Patient with MUSCLE STIFFNESS AND SPASMS
Assess location
Generalized
Focal or segmental
A Contaminated wound
Cont'd on p 279
Absent
Present
B Hyperthermia
E Tetanus
Absent
Present
Spread of muscle spasm
C Peripheral nerve excitability
Nuchal rigidity
No nuchal rigidity
Admit to ICU
Tetany
Lumbar Puncture
Neuroleptics used
Neuroleptics not utilized
SURGICALLY DEBRIDE WOUND
IV Penicillin
Immunization (Passive and Active)
Maintain Airway
Central Venous Line
Serum electrolyte levels
Pleocytosis
MNS
Correct electrolyte-metabolic disturbance
Meningitis (see p 258)
Dantrium Parlodel
Monitor ECG
Treat spasms and seizure
D Hyperreflexia Babinski signs
No hyperreflexia No Babinski signs
Consider: Encephalomyelitis
Consciousness altered
Consider: Stiff-man syndrome Strychnine poisoning
CSF examination
Consider: Seizure disorder
History of drug use or poisoning
No history of drug use or poisoning
Positive
Negative
EEG
Consider: Strychnine poisoning
Consider: Stiff-man syndrome
Diagnosis confirmed
Observe course and treat symptons
Seizure confirmed
Diazepam

F. If focal muscle spasms occur, consider local tetanus. Examine the involved limb for an infected wound. If rhythmic spasms develop, consider focal seizures; perform EEG. If there are intermittent sustained and twisting focal movements, consider dystonia or hysterical conversion reaction. Observe carefully for contaminated wounds. Question the patient carefully about use of phenothiazine neuroleptic medication, including agents such as prochlorperazine (Compazine), a neuroleptic drug used as an antiemetic, which may cause dystonic spasms simulating tetanus.

References

Guze GH, Baxter LR. Neuroleptic malignant syndrome. N Engl J Med 1985; 313:163.

Weinstein L. Tetanus. N Engl J Med 1973; 289:1293.

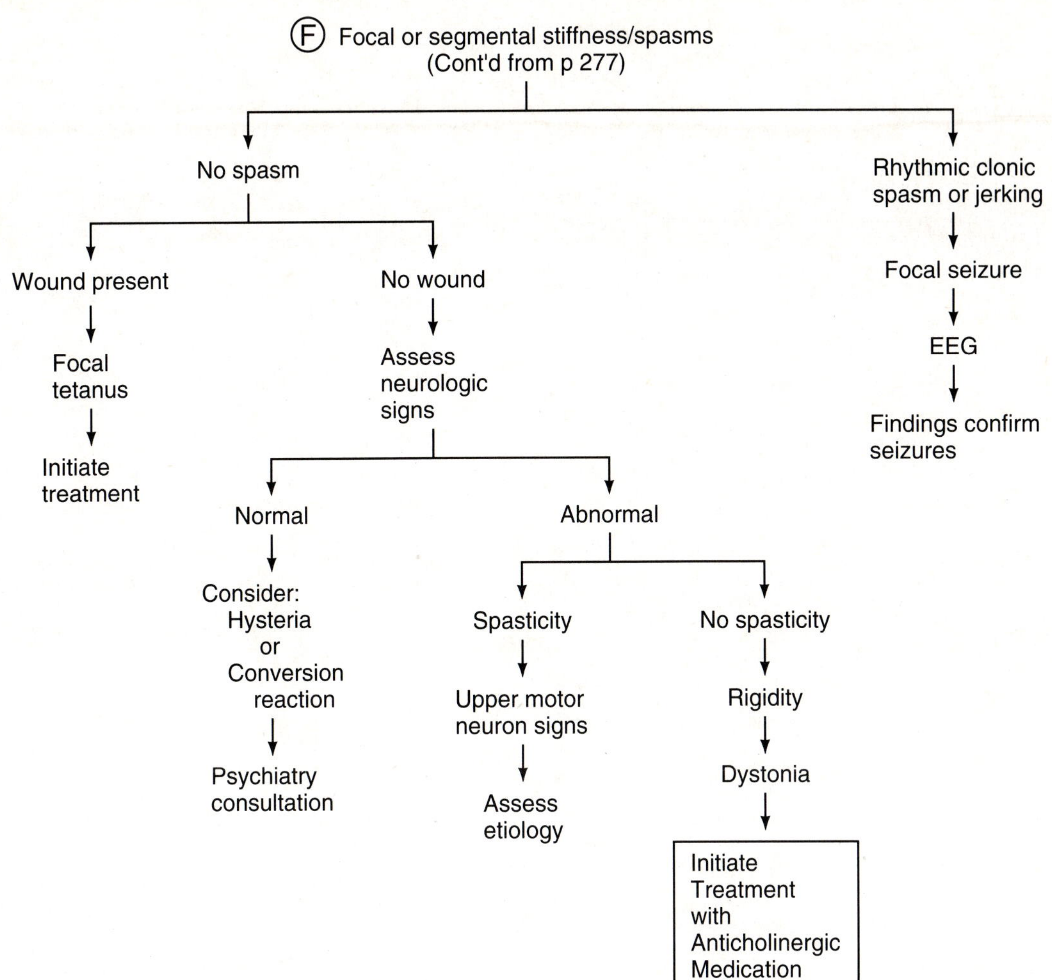

F Focal or segmental stiffness/spasms
(Cont'd from p 277)
No spasm
Rhythmic clonic spasm or jerking
Wound present
No wound
Focal seizure
Focal tetanus
Assess neurologic signs
EEG
Initiate treatment
Findings confirm seizures
Normal
Abnormal
Consider: Hysteria or Conversion reaction
Spasticity
No spasticity
Psychiatry consultation
Upper motor neuron signs
Rigidity
Assess etiology
Dystonia
Initiate Treatment with Anticholinergic Medication

RABIES

Carlos A. Garcia, M.D.

The rabies virus is a pleomorphic rhabdovirus that naturally infects wild carnivores. Human infection is acquired through infected saliva from animal bites. Dogs are frequent sources of infection in developing areas, but skunks, raccoons, foxes, bats, and cats are more important sources in the United States. The only means of human-to-human transmission described has been corneal transplantation. The virus travels from the site of inoculation to the CNS through the peripheral nerves by growth in perineurial cells and Schwann cells, or by retrograde axoplasmic flow.

A.	The incubation period varies from 14 days to 1 year, with a shorter time in deep bites of the neck and face. CNS symptoms are preceded by a prodromal stage of general malaise, fever, nausea, and vomiting. There are two forms of CNS rabies. A rare form is manifested by weakness of one extremity followed by ascending paralysis, similar to and frequently confused with the Guillain-Barré syndrome; this form is known as paralytic or "dumb" rabies.

B.	The most common form of rabies begins with agitation, anxiety, and confusion. There is also increased lacrimation, difficulty swallowing, excessive salivation, and laryngeal spasms (hydrophobia). This is the "furious" type of rabies. Both types progress to coma and seizures. The first stage of the disease may be confused with a psychiatric disorder. The late stage resembles any form of meningoencephalitis.

C.	The diagnosis may be confirmed by immunofluorescence of corneal smears and CSF studies that may show the virus after mouse inoculation. The disease is usually fatal 2 to 7 days after the onset of CNS symptoms. Only two human patients have been reported to have survived the disease.

D.	Immunization with human rabies immune globulin (RIG) and vaccination with human diploid cells rabies vaccine (HDCV) are important preventive measures after exposure to a rabid animal. Consult the Centers for Disease Control in Atlanta for further information.

References

Brownell B, Tomlinson AH. Virus diseases of the central nervous system. In: Adams JH, et al, eds. Greenfield's neuropathology. 4th ed. New York: John Wiley, 1985: 280.

Editorial. Rabies. Lancet, 1983; 1:967.

Fishbein DB, Arcangeli S. Rabies prevention in primary care: A four step approach. Postgrad Med 1987; 82:83.

Kauffman FH, Goldmann BJ. Rabies. Am J Emerg Med 1986; 4:525.

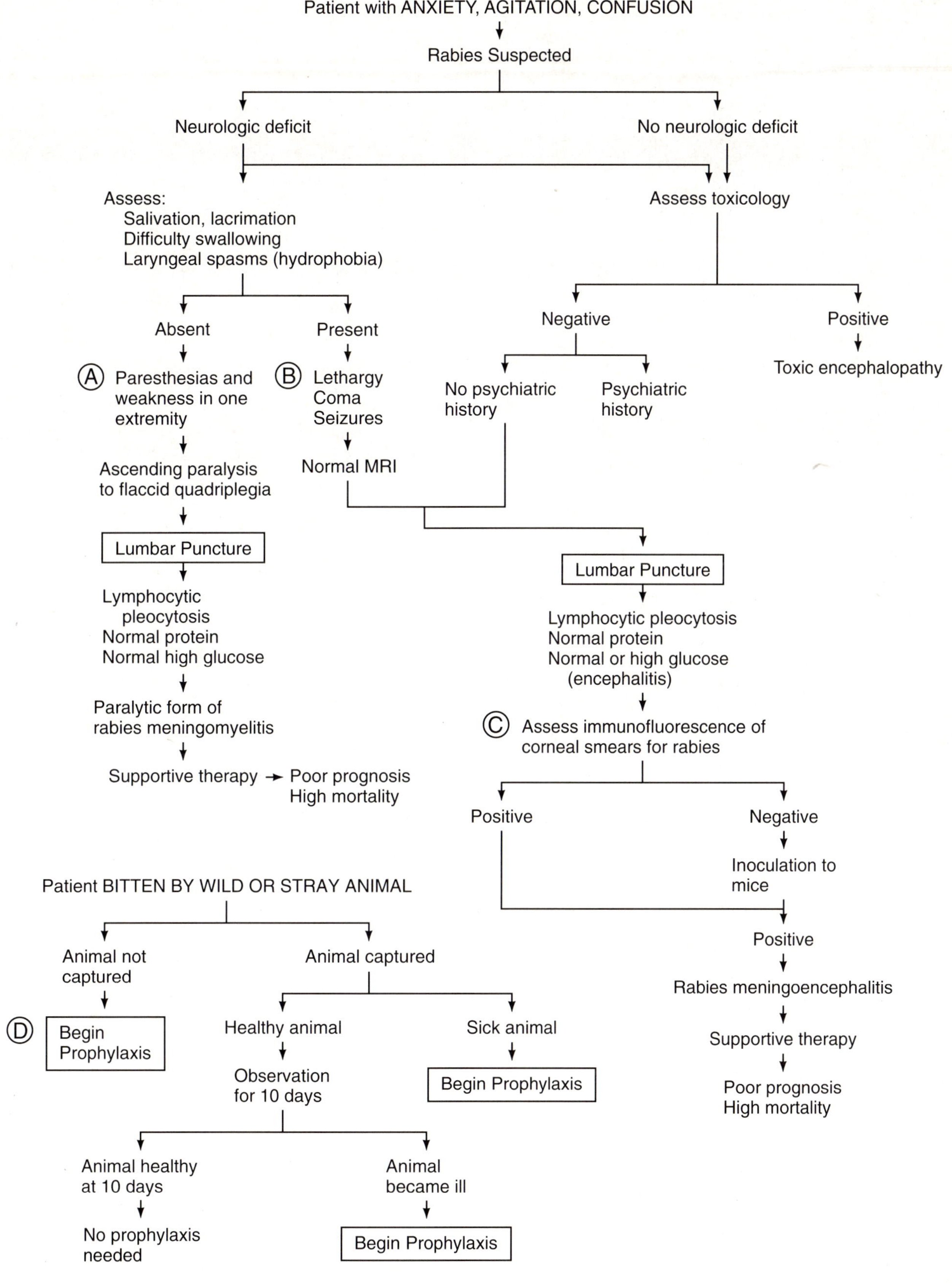

Patient with ANXIETY, AGITATION, CONFUSION
Rabies Suspected
Neurologic deficit
No neurologic deficit
Assess:
Salivation, lacrimation
Difficulty swallowing
Laryngeal spasms (hydrophobia)
Assess toxicology
Absent
Present
Negative
Positive
Toxic encephalopathy
A Paresthesias and weakness in one extremity
B Lethargy Coma Seizures
No psychiatric history
Psychiatric history
Ascending paralysis to flaccid quadriplegia
Normal MRI
Lumbar Puncture
Lumbar Puncture
Lymphocytic pleocytosis
Normal protein
Normal high glucose
Lymphocytic pleocytosis
Normal protein
Normal or high glucose
(encephalitis)
Paralytic form of rabies meningomyelitis
C Assess immunofluorescence of corneal smears for rabies
Supportive therapy
Poor prognosis High mortality
Positive
Negative
Inoculation to mice
Patient BITTEN BY WILD OR STRAY ANIMAL
Positive
Rabies meningoencephalitis
Animal not captured
Animal captured
Supportive therapy
D Begin Prophylaxis
Healthy animal
Sick animal
Poor prognosis High mortality
Observation for 10 days
Begin Prophylaxis
Animal healthy at 10 days
Animal became ill
No prophylaxis needed
Begin Prophylaxis

LYME DISEASE

Carlos A. Garcia, M.D.

Lyme disease, or Lyme borreliosis, is an infectious disease produced by the spirochete *Borrelia burgdorferi* acquired by inoculation through the skin by the hard-shelled tick (vector) *Ixodes dammini*. Lyme disease has similarities to syphilis. Lyme borreliosis begins at the site of the inoculation with an enlarging, target-like rash known as erythema migrans. This is the acute localized form of the disease. Dissemination of the organism may occur during the acute localized stage or later on in the acute disseminated stage, manifested by multifocal erythema migrans, acute arthritis, inflammation of cardiac and skeletal muscles, cardiac conduction abnormalities, meningoradiculitis, hepatitis, and encephalitis. Finally, there is the chronic disseminated form, which is usually insidious in onset or preceded by a mild acute phase manifested by chronic arthritis and peripheral and nervous system involvement.

Laboratory confirmation of the disease is difficult because the organisms are almost impossible to demonstrate, even in skin biopsy specimens during the acute phase. The organisms are also very difficult to culture. Most diagnosis is based on indirect serologic techniques (immunofluorescence, enzyme-linked immunosorbent assay) that indicate previous exposure to the organism and not an acute active disease. In some patients, anti-*B. burgdorferi* antibodies (ITAb) are trapped in immune complexes and may not be detected, giving false-negative results. Western blot and polymerase chain reaction (PCR) tests also have diagnostic drawbacks. At present, there is no single accurate diagnostic test to confirm active infection. Diagnosis of CNS infection is simpler and has been based on demonstration of intrathecal production of ITAb. This test has a specificity of 90% after VDRL-positive patients are eliminated. The antibodies remain high after successful treatment. The diagnosis of Lyme borreliosis should be based primarily on epidemiologic and clinical information.

A. Nervous system borreliosis can affect the CNS and peripheral nervous system (PNS). Lyme disease affecting the PNS may manifest as a cranial neuropathy, usually the seventh nerve (facial weakness), and may be associated with meningitis. Other cranial neuropathies may occur. Peripheral nerve involvement may present as a mononeuropathy multiplex, mononeuropathy, Guillain-Barré—like ascending paralysis (CSF pleocytosis), or brachial or lumbosacral plexopathy. Radiculoneuritis usually occurs in the dermatome of the bite site. Carpal tunnel syndrome has been associated with Lyme borreliosis. Nerve biopsies have confirmed a perivascular epi- and perineurial inflammatory infiltrate.

B. CNS lesions may present as lymphocytic meningitis (headache, photophobia, meningismus) in the acute disseminated phase of the illness. CSF shows lymphocytic pleocytosis associated with a normal glucose level and mild protein elevation. Parenteral antibiotic treatment is required.

C. Encephalomyelitis may present with alteration of sensorium and focal neurologic deficits localized to the spinal cord, brain stem, or optic nerves. Seizures are rare. MRI of the head shows white matter involvement. Some patients respond well to parenteral antibiotic therapy, but some may have persistent nonprogressive signs and symptoms.

D. Encephalopathy may present in some patients with alterations in memory and cognitive impairment even with a normal neurologic examination and normal CSF and MRI. The cause of the disorder is unknown. Symptoms improve after antibiotic therapy. Multiple sclerosis, amyotrophic lateral sclerosis, and Alzheimer-like disease have been blamed on Lyme borreliosis.

E. Oral antibiotics are usually effective for localized infection, but parenteral administration is required for CNS infections. Tetracyclines, penicillin and its derivatives, and third-generation cephalosporins are the ideal choices. If there is no CNS involvement, give doxycycline, 100 mg twice or three times a day for 2 or 3 weeks. Treat CNS invasion with ceftriaxone, 2 g/day for 2 to 4 weeks; cefotaxime, 2 g three times a day for 2 to 4 weeks; or penicillin, 20 million units IV for 2 to 4 weeks. Steroids may improve symptoms but may make subsequent eradication of the infection with antibodies more difficult.

References

Finkel MG, Halperin JJ. Nervous system Lyme borreliosis—revisited. Arch Neurol 1992; 49:102.

Halperin JJ. Neurological complications of Lyme disease. Neurol Chronicle 1992; 1:1.

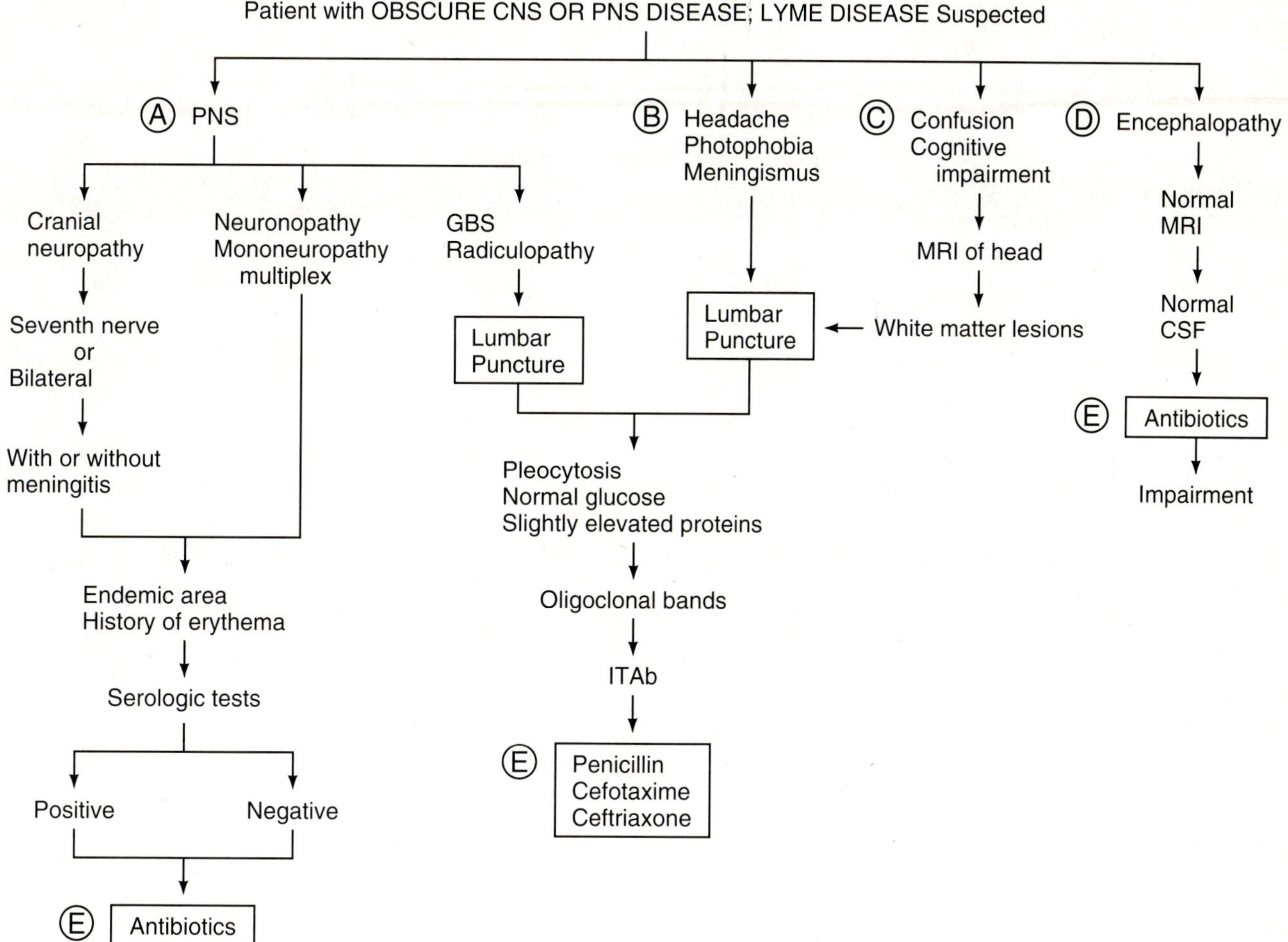

Patient with OBSCURE CNS OR PNS DISEASE; LYME DISEASE Suspected
A PNS
B Headache
Photophobia
Meningismus
C Confusion
Cognitive
impairment
D Encephalopathy
Cranial
neuropathy
Neuronopathy
Mononeuropathy
multiplex
GBS
Radiculopathy
Normal
MRI
Seventh nerve
or
Bilateral
MRI of head
Normal
CSF
With or without
meningitis
Lumbar
Puncture
Lumbar
Puncture
White matter lesions
E Antibiotics
Endemic area
History of erythema
Pleocytosis
Normal glucose
Slightly elevated proteins
Impairment
Serologic tests
Oligoclonal bands
Positive
Negative
ITAb
E Antibiotics
E Penicillin
Cefotaxime
Ceftriaxone

BENIGN (IDIOPATHIC) INTRACRANIAL HYPERTENSION

Leon A. Weisberg, M.D.

Benign intracranial hypertension (BIH) (pseudotumor cerebri, idiopathic intracranial hypertension) is characterized by symptoms (headache, nausea, vomiting, diplopia, visual obscurations) and signs (papilledema, abducens nerve paresis) of increased intracranial pressure (ICP). Patients have a normal mental state and no localizing neurologic signs. CSF examination is normal except for elevated opening pressure. If BIH is suspected but there are abnormalities of CSF content (pleocytosis, elevated protein, lowered sugar content), this suggests an alternative diagnosis (sarcoid, fungal, or neoplastic meningitis). Neurodiagnostic studies should be normal in BIH. Skull radiography may show an enlarged and eroded sella turcica due to the chronic effects of intracranial hypertension. There may be an empty sella syndrome due to BIH, but there are no visual or endocrine disturbances. In BIH, CT/MRI is usually normal. In some cases, CT/MRI may show small ventricles and basal cisterns possibly due to intracranial hypertension; however, this pattern is difficult to differentiate from the normal pattern of young patients. Since BIH usually occurs in young, otherwise healthy patients, it is not always possible to know if these small, slitlike ventricles are a normal variant or an abnormal finding due to intracranial hypertension. Enlarged ventricles (hydrocephalus) are not consistent with BIH. If this finding is noted, further diagnostic studies are necessary to determine the cause of hydrocephalus and the precise location of ventricular obstruction. If a patient has papilledema and other neurologic abnormalities on examination (e.g., hemiparesis, ataxia), the diagnosis is *never* BIH. In patients with suspected BIH, other intracranial lesions must be excluded by neurodiagnostic studies. Angiography is necessary to diagnose venous sinus thrombosis or dural vascular malformation.

A. In suspected cases of BIH, obtain an accurate CSF opening pressure measurement. A finding of elevated CSF pressure is necessary to confirm that BIH is active; normal pressure indicates that BIH is in remission or is not present. In 40% of patients with BIH, remission occurs after initial lumbar puncture (LP). The finding of normal CSF pressure in patients with funduscopic optic disc evidence of papilledema suggests the alternative diagnosis of pseudopapilledema (see p 112).

B. In BIH, the major threat is visual loss. There are visual symptoms (transient visual obscurations or diplopia) in 50% of patients. These may be transient (lasting approximately 30 seconds) and occur frequently throughout the day. Transient visual obscurations are due to optic nerve dysfunction, but their occurrence

does not predict subsequent visual loss. Diplopia is horizontal and maximal on far gaze; this results from abducens nerve paresis. This diplopia is a nonlocalizing effect of intracranial hypertension. Visual field examination shows enlarged blind spots; these do not cause visual symptoms. If ICP is not adequately lowered, visual acuity loss or visual field impairment (most commonly an inferior nasal quadrantanopia) may develop. These are due to optic nerve dysfunction caused by the intracranial hypertension. Better predictors and more sensitive tests of visual function include Goldmann perimetry and visual contrast sensitivity tests. It is possible to have optic nerve dysfunction even if visual acuity is 20/15; more sensitive tests of optic nerve function are therefore necessary if early treatment is to be initiated to prevent visual loss.

C. Recent or progressive visual loss due to BIH requires vigorous treatment. Perform alternate-day LP to remove 10 to 50 ml of CSF and lower CSF pressure to 120 mm H_2O; patient tolerance of repeated LP is low. Since most of these patients are obese, weight reduction is indicated, but often this is not accomplished rapidly enough to prevent visual loss and is not usually sustained even if initially successful. In addition, rapidly lost weight is soon regained and rapid weight loss may cause deleterious metabolic and electrolyte disturbances. To lower ICP, use carbonic anhydrase inhibitors such as acetazolamide (Diamox), in an initial dosage of 250 mg twice daily. The daily dose may be increased to a total of 2 to 3 g given in divided portions three or four times daily. Side effects, including paresthesias in extremities, taste alterations including a bitter metallic taste, gastrointestinal symptoms, and electrolyte disturbances, may limit the dosage of Diamox. If Diamox is not effective, prednisone may be given, 40 to 100 mg daily. This is continued for several weeks and then tapered during continued monitoring of visual function. Long-term corticosteroid administration may be dangerous, especially to the ocular system, because it may cause cataracts or glaucoma. Other potential corticosteroid-induced toxicities include weight gain, glucose intolerance, hypertension, osteoporosis, and hypothalamic-pituitary disturbances.

D. If visual loss persists, consider surgery. Lumbar-peritoneal diversionary shunts reduce ICP. Optic nerve sheath fenestration reduces direct pressure on the optic nerves but does not lower ICP or improve headache. *The major threat in BIH is visual loss.* In

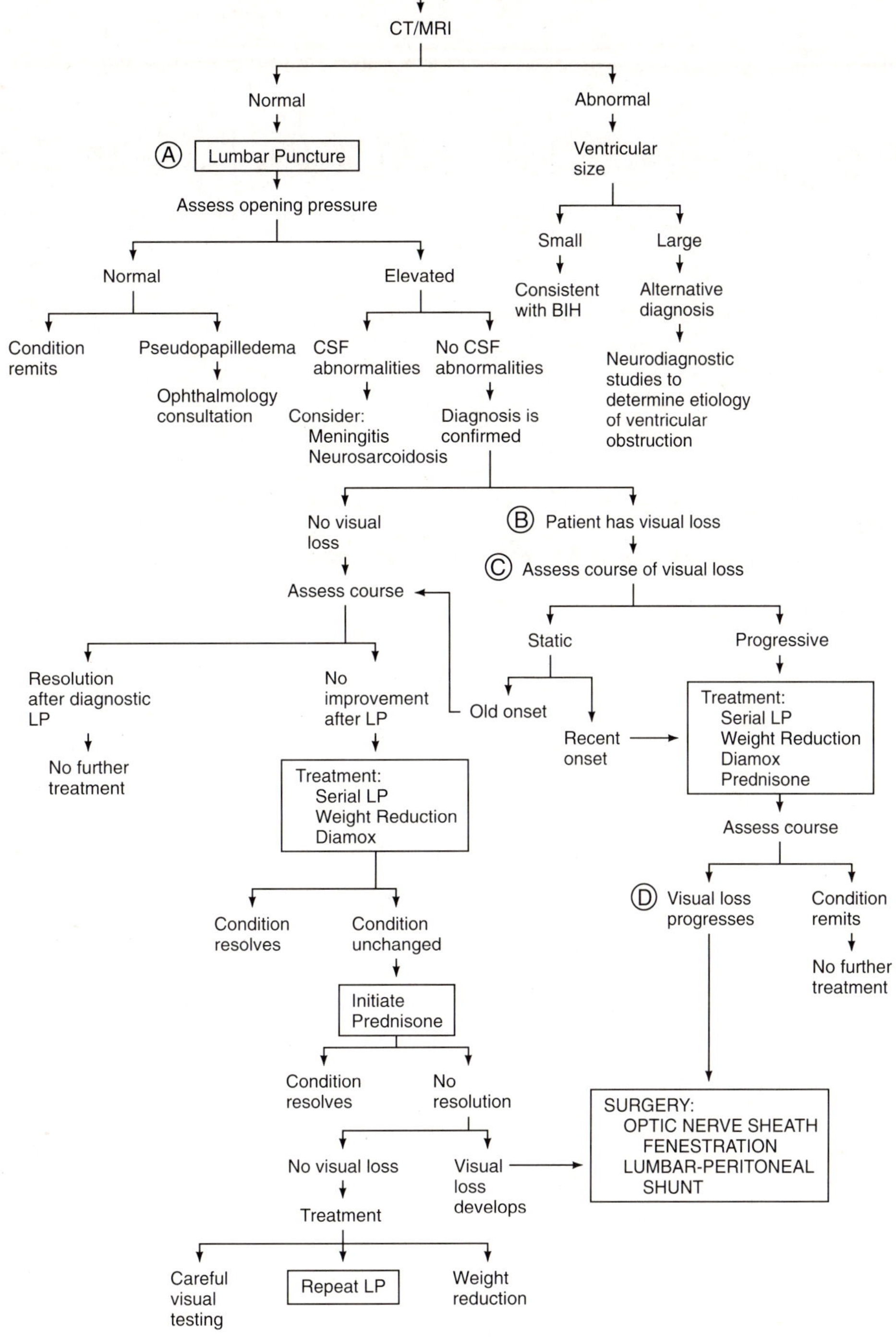

most cases, this develops slowly and progressively, but rarely it may occur rapidly. If CT/MRI is used, it is extremely unlikely that an intracranial mass lesion that presents with nonlocalized increased ICP to simulate BIH will fail to be detected. In some cases of BIH, angiography is necessary to exclude venous sinus thrombosis or vascular malformation, which may be difficult to detect with CT/MRI.

References

Wall M, George D. Idiopathic intracranial hypertension. Brain 1991; 114:155.

Wall M, Weisberg LA. Management of pseudotumor cerebri. In: Johnson R, ed. Current therapy in neurologic disease. Toronto: BC Decker, 1984:226.

Weisberg LA. Benign intracranial hypertension. Medicine 1975; 54:197.

NEUROLOGIC MANIFESTATIONS OF RENAL DISEASE

Leon A. Weisberg, M.D.

Neurologic disorders may result directly from uremia, but may also stem from metabolic disorders (hypocalcemia or hypercalcemia, hyponatremia, hypo-osmolality, hypertensive crisis, hepatic dysfunction [hepatorenal syndrome]). Manifestations of uremic encephalopathy include altered consciousness, slurred speech, gait imbalance, asterixis, myoclonus, and generalized hyperreflexia (sometimes with clonus and bilateral positive Babinski signs). As metabolic abnormalities resolve, the neurologic condition should also improve. If this does not occur, consider alternative diagnoses and perform neurodiagnostic studies.

A. In uremic encephalopathy there are diffuse, rather than focal, CNS signs. There may be intermittent confusion, dysarthria, ataxia, asterixis, action tremor, and myoclonus. Neurologic signs characteristically fluctuate throughout the day in patients with metabolic encephalopathy. Clinical features do not correlate with any specific laboratory abnormalities but do correlate with rapidity of onset of renal insufficiency. Focal neurologic signs suggest complicating pathologic disorders such as intracranial (subdural, intracerebral) hemorrhage due to coagulation or bleeding disorders, hypertensive crisis (see p 154) with hemorrhage or infarction, a focal infectious-inflammatory process secondary to impairment of the immunologic system, or an unusual neoplasm (lymphoma, sarcoma). If focal signs are present, perform neurodiagnostic studies. As is characteristic of metabolic encephalopathies, bilateral positive Babinski signs may be due to a metabolic disturbance; however, this explanation of Babinski signs should be accepted only after a negative neurodiagnostic evaluation for structural brain disease. CSF pleocytosis suggests infectious meningitis, but sterile pleocytosis may occur in azotemic patients without infectious-inflammatory meningitis.

B. Seizures are *late* complications of uremic encephalopathy. However, they may occur at an earlier stage if metabolic abnormalities are present (calcium, magnesium, or sodium disturbances; acidosis; hypo-osmolality) or if potentially neurotoxic drugs (penicillin, streptomycin) that depend on renal clearance are used. Uremic seizures are difficult to treat because of decreased antiepileptic drug binding by serum albumin. This leads to higher free drug levels at lower plasma levels. Phenobarbital and diazepam may increase sedation due to uremic encephalopathy.

C. Neuropathy occurs in patients with chronic renal failure. This may be asymptomatic at first, and the only findings may be impairment (loss) of ankle reflexes and distally impaired sensation in the feet and hands. Early symptoms of neuropathy are a burning sensation in the feet and the restless leg syndrome. This may progress to painful dysesthesias and inability to walk, which are worse at night. These are treated most effectively with clonazepam (Clonopin). After hemodialysis, neuropathy stabilizes or improves; neuropathy may worsen for several weeks after initiation of dialysis. Renal transplantation causes a decrease in the severity of neuropathy symptoms. Muscle cramps and myalgias are common in the legs and may occur in patients showing no evidence of neuropathy. These cramps-myalgias may reflect shifts of fluid and electrolytes in the muscles.

D. After dialysis, neurologic symptoms (headache, muscle cramps, agitation, seizures) may develop. These may occur immediately or up to 24 hours after dialysis. This disorder, which is self-limited and resolves within 24 hours, is called dialysis dysequilibrium syndrome and is due to rapid brain fluid and electrolyte compartment shifts. If symptoms do not resolve, neurodiagnostic studies are indicated to exclude an intracranial lesion or cerebral edema. Wernicke's syndrome may result from malnutrition and dialysis of water-soluble thiamine molecules across the dialysate membrane. Treat these patients with adequate multivitamin supplementation, which should include thiamine. Symptoms of headache, vomiting, altered consciousness, and seizures that do not rapidly resolve should raise the possibility of intracranial hemorrhage rather than dialysis dysequilibrium. This may relate to rapid fluid shifts, systemic hypertension, coagulation-bleeding disorders, or excessive use of heparin in the dialysis process.

E. Dementia with speech disturbance, myoclonus, and asterixis may develop in patients undergoing chronic hemodialysis. EEG shows diffuse slowing with interspersed synchronous triphasic phases. The etiology is related to trace metals (aluminum) in dialysate or aluminum-containing antacids used by these patients. Brain neoplasms, including sarcomas and lymphomas, occur with unusual frequency in patients who undergo renal transplantation. Unusual CNS opportunistic infections (fungal, parasitic) are related to the immunosuppressive effect of medication used by patients with chronic renal disorders.

References

Lederman RJ, Henry CE. Progressive dialysis encephalopathy. Ann Neurol 1978; 4:199.

Raskin NH, Fishman RA. Neurological disorders of renal failure. N Engl J Med 1976; 294:143, 204.

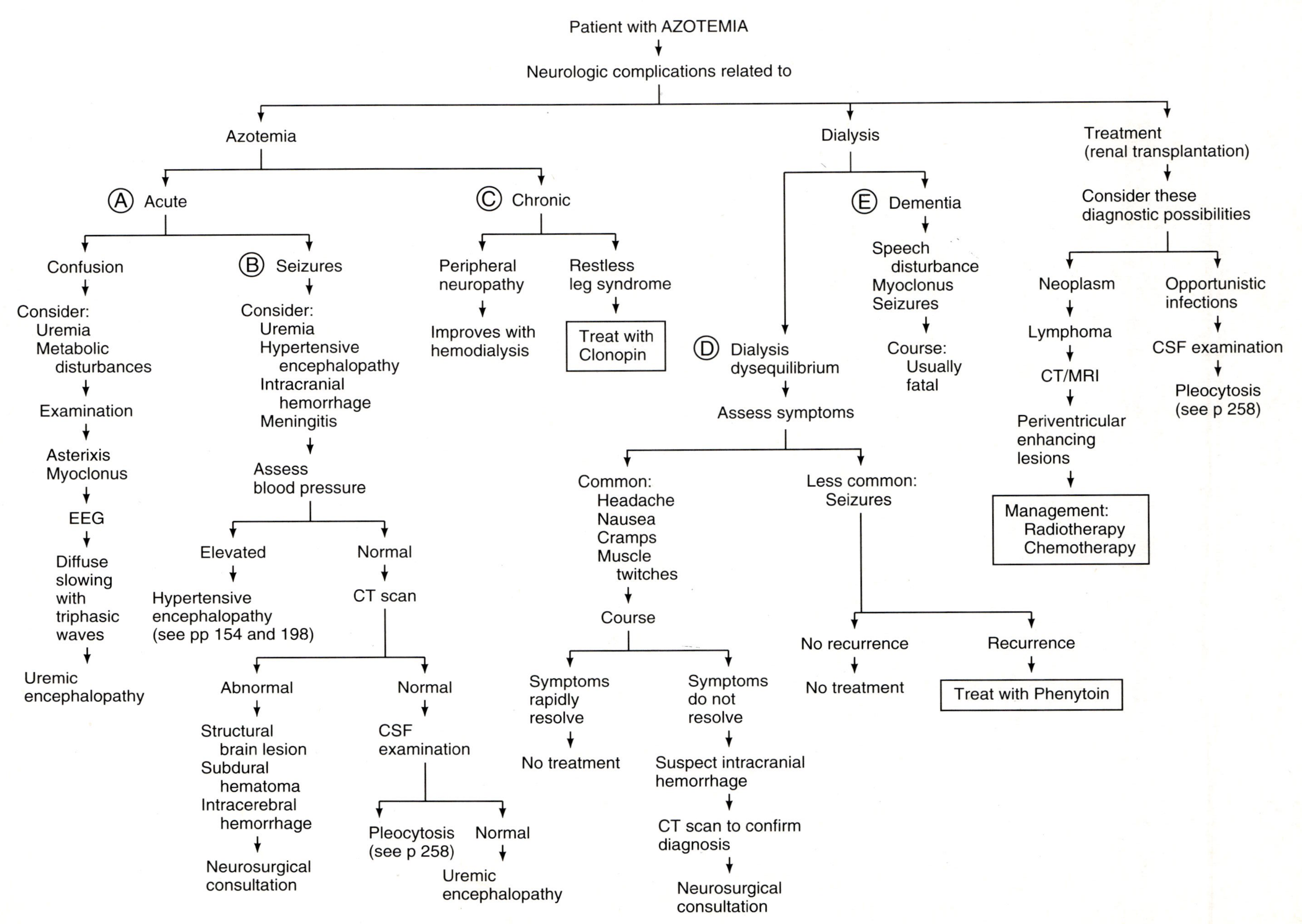

Patient with AZOTEMIA
Neurologic complications related to
Azotemia
Dialysis
Treatment (renal transplantation)
A Acute
C Chronic
E Dementia
Consider these diagnostic possibilities
Confusion
B Seizures
Peripheral neuropathy
Restless leg syndrome
Speech disturbance Myoclonus Seizures
Neoplasm
Opportunistic infections
Consider: Uremia Metabolic disturbances
Consider: Uremia Hypertensive encephalopathy Intracranial hemorrhage Meningitis
Improves with hemodialysis
Treat with Clonopin
D Dialysis dysequilibrium
Course: Usually fatal
Lymphoma
CSF examination
Examination
Assess blood pressure
Assess symptoms
CT/MRI
Pleocytosis (see p 258)
Asterixis Myoclonus
Periventricular enhancing lesions
EEG
Elevated
Normal
Common: Headache Nausea Cramps Muscle twitches
Less common: Seizures
Management: Radiotherapy Chemotherapy
Diffuse slowing with triphasic waves
Hypertensive encephalopathy (see pp 154 and 198)
CT scan
Course
No recurrence
Recurrence
Uremic encephalopathy
Abnormal
Normal
Symptoms rapidly resolve
Symptoms do not resolve
No treatment
Treat with Phenytoin
Structural brain lesion Subdural hematoma Intracerebral hemorrhage
CSF examination
No treatment
Suspect intracranial hemorrhage
Neurosurgical consultation
Pleocytosis (see p 258)
Normal
CT scan to confirm diagnosis
Uremic encephalopathy
Neurosurgical consultation

NEUROLOGIC MANIFESTATIONS OF ALCOHOLISM: ACUTE INTOXICATION AND WITHDRAWAL

Leon A. Weisberg, M.D.

A. Alcohol causes CNS depression. Symptoms of acute alcohol intoxication are caused by inhibition of cortical and subcortical neural structures. In nonalcoholics, acute intoxication symptoms may begin at 50 mg/dl. These include behavioral (pressured or slurred speech, inappropriate and irrational social conduct, decreased attention span) and motor (reduced coordination, slowed reaction time, impaired walking) disturbances. Neurologic signs include dysarthria, gait ataxia, motor incoordination, hyperactive reflexes, nystagmus, and impaired cognitive function. During intoxication, "blackouts" may occur; this term refers to lost memories (amnesia), not syncopal or "passing-out" episodes. Autonomic (sympathetic) nervous system overdischarge signs of acute alcohol intoxication include pupillary dilatation, tachycardia, and skin flushing. At blood levels of 250 to 500 mg/dl, CNS depression may occur; the signs include lethargy, hyporeflexia, respiratory slowing, bradycardia, and hypotension. Death from severe cardiovascular or respiratory depression may occur at blood alcohol levels >500 mg/dl. In chronic alcoholic patients, metabolic tolerance may develop so that acute intoxication signs are not seen until there are higher blood levels than would cause similar signs in nonalcoholic patients.

   If patients become agitated owing to alcohol's effect on the CNS, initially treat with chlordiazepoxide (Librium); other medications used include amobarbital (Amytal), hydroxyzine (Vistaril), or phenothiazines (Haldol). If consciousness is impaired, support respiratory and cardiovascular systems and correct any existing metabolic disturbances (hypomagnesemia, thiamine deficiency, dehydration, hypernatremia or hyponatremia). Gastric lavage may be used to remove unabsorbed alcohol but is usually not helpful because of rapid alcohol absorption by the stomach.

B. There are two reasons that alcoholic patients markedly reduce or cease alcohol consumption. Either they run out of money to purchase alcohol, or they develop an intercurrent illness (e.g., gastritis, pneumonia, pancreatitis) causing abdominal pain and vomiting (related to gastritis or pancreatitis) so that they can no longer drink. Early (minor) withdrawal syndrome, which includes irritable behavior and tremulousness, develops within several hours after the patient's last drink; tremulousness may persist for 24 to 48 hours. Symptoms include exaggerated physiologic tremor and signs of sympathetic overdischarge (tachycardia, pupillary dilatation, hypertension). This syndrome is self-limited and requires no treatment; patients may control these symptoms by having their usual morning alcoholic drink. Because this condition is benign, many sedative, neuroleptic, beta-adrenergic blocking, and calcium blocking drugs have been reported to be effective in its "cure" or termination. In reality, the syndrome usually resolves spontaneously without treatment.

   Acute delirium tremens (DT) is the major alcohol withdrawal syndrome. It occurs 4 to 28 days after an alcoholic patient stops drinking. It is important to differentiate this major withdrawal syndrome from the minor withdrawal syndrome or the syndrome of acute auditory hallucinosis. The latter occurs in patients with an otherwise clear sensorium and no tremor; it usually resolves spontaneously. DT consists of agitated (delirium) confusion, hallucinations (frequently visual or auditory type), tremulousness, and autonomic hyperactivity (fever, tachycardia, diaphoresis, blood pressure lability). Rarely, DT may be a malignant condition and patients may die secondary to circulatory collapse or overwhelming infection. Diagnostic studies are necessary to exclude complicating conditions such as subdural hematoma or meningitis. These should be performed if unusual clinical features of DT (focal neurologic signs, nuchal rigidity) are present. These patients with DT appear acutely agitated, are combative, and seem fearful of their hallucinations, showing signs of agitated psychoses. In certain cases, DT is confused with drug-induced toxic psychoses; therefore, perform drug toxicology tests in suspected DT patients. Treatment of DT consists of correction of dehydration and electrolyte imbalance, sedative medication (Librium, paraldehyde), and supplemental vitamins. Avoid neuroleptic medication in patients with DT; these drugs may cause cardiac toxicity, which may be a serious complication in patients with underlying cardiomyopathy. Alcohol withdrawal seizures do not usually require treatment because they are usually single and short-lived. They occur within 72 hours of cessation of drinking and usually before DT develops (see p 174).

C. Alcohol may cause CNS depression to result in coma. If focal neurologic signs are present, perform CT to exclude structural (traumatic, infectious-inflammatory, hemorrhagic) lesions. In alcoholic patients, focal neurologic signs may *never* be attributed to metabolic encephalopathy. If CT is negative, perform EEG to exclude status epilepticus as the cause of coma.

D. Alcohol-induced hypoglycemia may cause coma and seizures. Administer glucose with thiamine, because glucose alone may rapidly deplete already diminished thiamine reserves, and this thiamine deficiency in turn may cause cardiovascular collapse.

References

Victor M. The alcohol withdrawal syndrome. Ann NY Acad Med 1973; 215:210.

Victor M, Adams RD. The effect of alcohol on the nervous system. Res Publ Assoc Res Nerv Ment Dis 1953; 32:526.

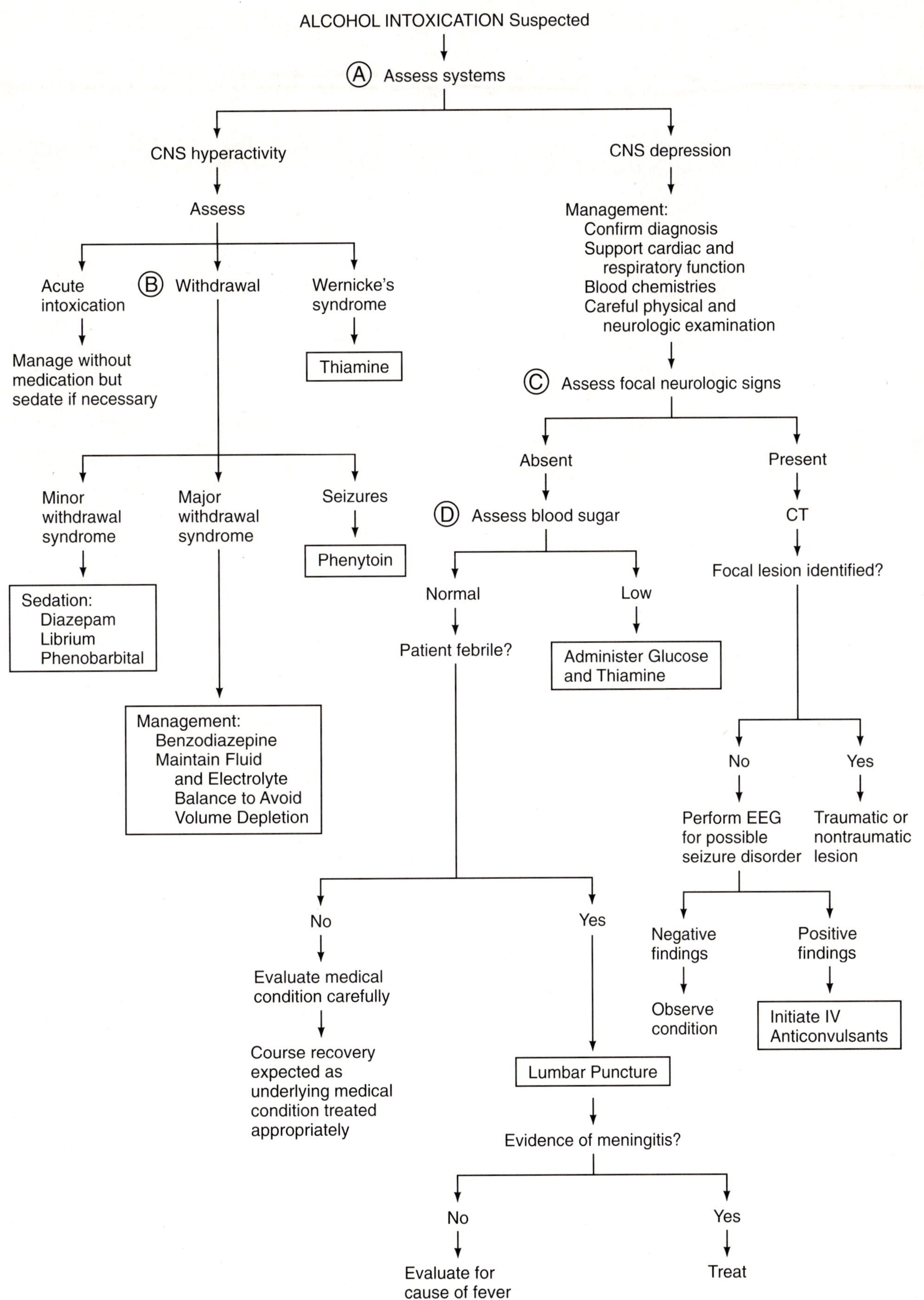

ALCOHOL INTOXICATION Suspected
A Assess systems
CNS hyperactivity
CNS depression
Assess
Management:
Confirm diagnosis
Support cardiac and
respiratory function
Blood chemistries
Careful physical and
neurologic examination
Acute intoxication
B Withdrawal
Wernicke's syndrome
Manage without medication but sedate if necessary
Thiamine
C Assess focal neurologic signs
Absent
Present
Minor withdrawal syndrome
Major withdrawal syndrome
Seizures
D Assess blood sugar
CT
Phenytoin
Sedation:
Diazepam
Librium
Phenobarbital
Normal
Low
Focal lesion identified?
Patient febrile?
Administer Glucose and Thiamine
Management:
Benzodiazepine
Maintain Fluid
and Electrolyte
Balance to Avoid
Volume Depletion
No
Yes
No
Yes
Evaluate medical condition carefully
Lumbar Puncture
Perform EEG for possible seizure disorder
Traumatic or nontraumatic lesion
Course recovery expected as underlying medical condition treated appropriately
Evidence of meningitis?
Negative findings
Positive findings
No
Yes
Observe condition
Initiate IV Anticonvulsants
Evaluate for cause of fever
Treat

NEUROLOGIC COMPLICATIONS OF ALCOHOLISM: CHRONIC (INCLUDING HEPATIC ENCEPHALOPATHY)

Leon A. Weisberg, M.D.

A. When acute changes in consciousness occur in an alcoholic patient, consider acute intoxication. To confirm this diagnosis, perform blood alcohol toxicology tests and exclude other clinical conditions, including acute delirium tremens (DT), Wernicke's syndrome, structural or infectious CNS processes, and systemic illness. Also, consider metabolic disorders, including hepatic encephalopathy. If eye movement abnormalities and gait ataxia are also present, this suggests Wernicke's syndrome due to vitamin B_1 (thiamine) deficiency. Eye movement abnormalities in Wernicke's syndrome include nystagmus (horizontal or vertical) or ocular palsies (lateral rectus paresis is most common). Ataxia is due to vestibular and cerebellar dysfunction. If the condition is not treated rapidly, neurologic sequelae, including profound memory impairment and ataxia, may persist.

B. If the patient shows coarse sustention tremor with symptoms and signs of sympathetic hyperactivity, consider major withdrawal syndrome (acute DT). These patients appear delirious and tremulous.

C. Hepatic encephalopathy is characterized by a confusional state accompanied by asterixis (see p 246) and other motor hyperactivity signs (tremor, myoclonus, hyperreflexia). EEG may show periodic triphasic slow waves. Hepatic encephalopathy is most common in patients with liver failure due to alcoholism, but may also result from other conditions that impair liver function. The clinical features of hepatic encephalopathy are due to toxic products accumulating in the brain, which may include ammonia, biogenic amines, false neurotransmitters, and excessive levels of gamma-aminobutyric acid compounds. The presence of hepatic encephalopathy correlates with an elevated arterial blood ammonia content. Treatment includes protein restriction and administration of lactulose, neomycin, or sorbitol to reduce the ammonia level.

D. Central pontine myelinolysis (CPM) is a demyelinating disorder often seen in alcoholics. It develops in association with rapidly corrected hyponatremic states. The clinical features include coma, pseudobulbar signs, and quadriparesis; these are due to demyelination involving the central-ventral pons. In some alcoholic patients, the direct metabolic effect of alcohol causes CNS depression that may result in coma and respiratory and cardiac collapse.

E. Chronic complications of alcoholism include cognitive, memory, and gait disorders. An amnestic syndrome with a prominent confabulatory response (Korsakoff's syndrome) occurs in alcoholic patients, usually in those who were initially diagnosed with Wernicke's syndrome. Alcohol may be directly toxic to brain cells and may cause brain cognitive impairment (alcoholic dementia). In chronic alcoholic patients, CT/MRI may show marked brain atrophy. This atrophy may be reversible if the patient complies with medical treatment, including cessation of alcohol and proper diet (multivitamin supplementation, protein repletion).

F. Gait impairment in alcoholics may result from several conditions (see p 48). In alcoholic peripheral neuropathy, there is axonal degeneration. Patients show a positive Romberg sign and have poor balance swing to proprioceptive dysfunction. This disorder usually improves after abstinence from alcohol. Alcoholic cerebellar degeneration causes truncal and gait ataxia, which is due to midline vermal (anterior and superior) cerebellar degeneration. This disorder develops gradually and may reverse after cessation of drinking. Alcohol may cause both acute necrotizing myopathy and chronic myopathy. Both result in proximal weakness with difficulty arising from a chair or climbing stairs. Necrotizing myopathy may result in myoglobinuria. Alcoholic patients may develop electrolyte disturbances such as hyponatremia, hypokalemia, and hypophosphatemia; this may also cause proximal muscle weakness.

References

Fraser CL, Arieff AI. Hepatic encephalopathy. N Engl J Med 1985; 313:865.

Victor M, Adams RD, Collins GH. The Wernicke-Korsakoff syndrome and related neurologic disorders due to alcoholism and malnutrition. 2nd ed. Philadelphia: FA Davis, 1989.

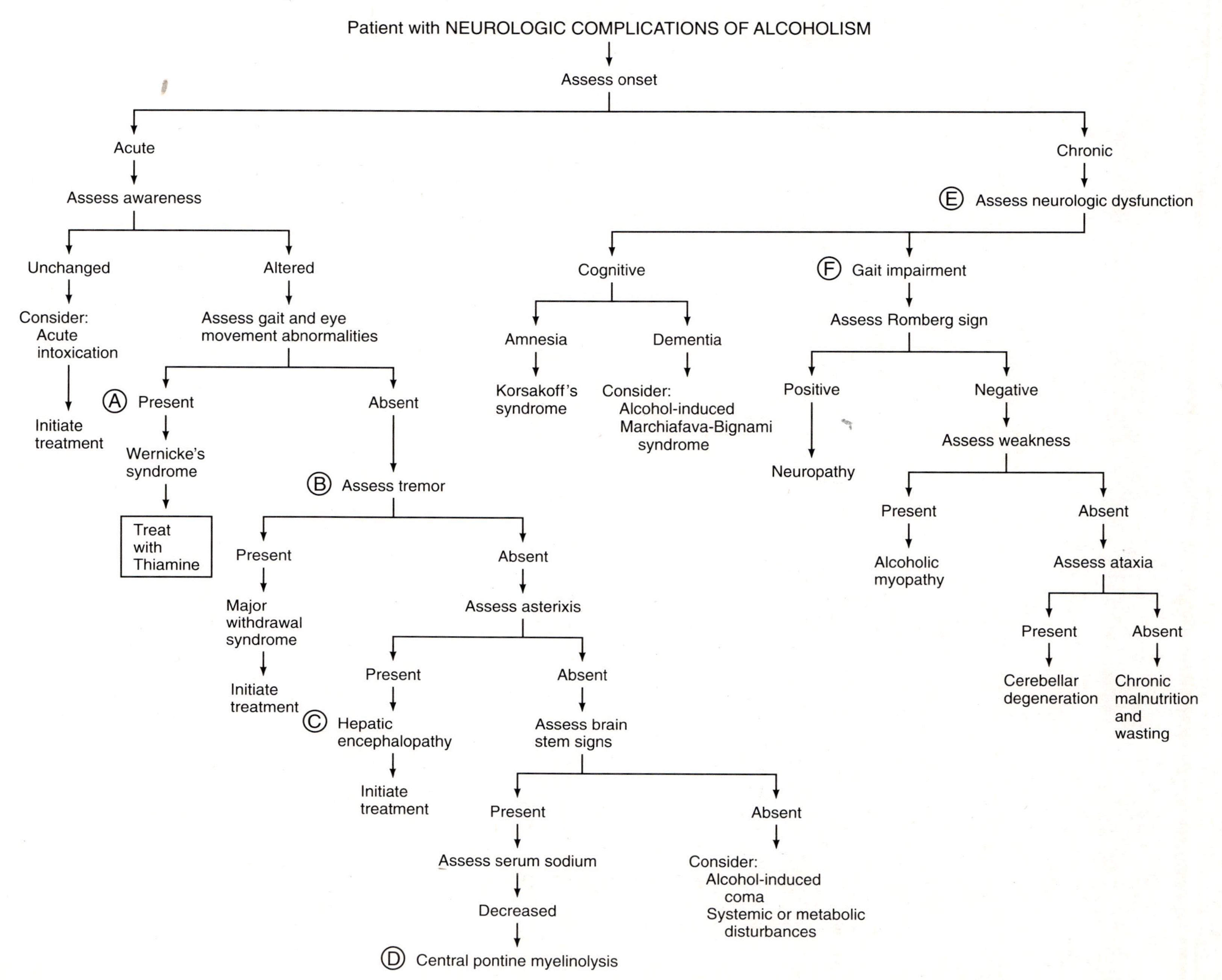

Patient with NEUROLOGIC COMPLICATIONS OF ALCOHOLISM
Assess onset
Acute
Chronic
Assess awareness
E Assess neurologic dysfunction
Unchanged
Altered
Cognitive
F Gait impairment
Consider: Acute intoxication
Assess gait and eye movement abnormalities
Amnesia
Dementia
Assess Romberg sign
Initiate treatment
A Present
Absent
Korsakoff's syndrome
Consider: Alcohol-induced Marchiafava-Bignami syndrome
Positive
Negative
Wernicke's syndrome
B Assess tremor
Neuropathy
Assess weakness
Treat with Thiamine
Present
Absent
Present
Absent
Major withdrawal syndrome
Assess asterixis
Alcoholic myopathy
Assess ataxia
Initiate treatment
Present
Absent
Present
Absent
C Hepatic encephalopathy
Assess brain stem signs
Cerebellar degeneration
Chronic malnutrition and wasting
Initiate treatment
Present
Absent
Assess serum sodium
Consider: Alcohol-induced coma Systemic or metabolic disturbances
Decreased
D Central pontine myelinolysis

CENTRAL NERVOUS SYSTEM MANIFESTATIONS OF HIV INFECTION

Leon A. Weisberg, M.D.

Patients with AIDS have abnormalities of the cell-mediated (lymphocyte) immune system. Immunologic incompetence may lead to the development of opportunistic infections and uncommon neoplasms (lymphoma, sarcoma). Systemic manifestations of AIDS include lymphadenopathy, fever, night sweats, weight loss, and pulmonary infections (including *Pneumocystis carinii,* tuberculosis, and fungal disorders). Neurologic complications occur in 40% of AIDS patients. HIV is neurotropic and may damage the subcortical (basal ganglia, thalamus) region.

A. There is evidence that asymptomatic, seropositive AIDS patients have CSF abnormalities (lymphocytic pleocytosis, elevated protein content, elevated gamma-globulin synthesis), but no cognitive impairment or other neurobehavioral abnormalities at this stage. In the early stages of HIV infection, patients may report memory and concentration disturbances; however, careful neuropsychological testing and routine mental status examination show no organic neurologic abnormalities. Consider depression as the possible cause of these memory and concentration difficulties. Suspect "pseudodementia" in these patients and evaluate them for depression or anxiety. Other HIV-positive patients have definite cognitive impairment, but previous use of alcohol, illicit drugs, or prescribed psychoactive medication may be implicated in these cognitive disturbances. If drug detoxification is achieved, there is often marked improvement in intellectual function. If cognitive improvement does not occur with drug detoxification and treatment of depression, perform full neurodiagnostic studies.

B. If an HIV-positive patient shows cognitive impairment that cannot be otherwise explained, has focal neurologic signs on examination, or develops seizures, perform neurodiagnostic studies. If a focal intracranial lesion is present, consider toxoplasmosis as the most likely diagnosis. CT usually shows evidence of single or multiple contrast-enhancing lesions. In unusual cases of toxoplasmosis, CT is normal, but MRI may be more sensitive and show a focal brain lesion. It is not usually possible to differentiate toxoplasmosis, lymphoma, tuberculosis, cryptococcosis, herpes simplex, neurosyphilis, and progressive multifocal leukoencephalopathy (PML) on the basis of CT or MRI characteristics. Certain features (location—cortical or subcortical; density—hypodense, hyperdense, mixed density, calcified; enhancement—absent or present; enhancement pattern—diffuse nodular, ring, periventricular) permit an educated guess at the pathologic nature of the visualized lesion. For example, if CT or MRI shows single or multiple discrete white matter subcortical hypodense nonenhancing lesions, con-

sider PML. These are presumed to represent PML, especially if repeat CT studies show progression to more extensive but similar-appearing white matter lesions. In most cases, it is inadvisable to base management decisions on CT/MRI patterns.

C. If CT or MRI shows no focal lesion, perform lumbar puncture. If CSF shows lymphocytic pleocytosis, evaluate patients for tuberculosis, cryptococcosis, herpes simplex, neurosyphilis, or cytomegalovirus (CMV) infection. If CSF shows lymphocytic pleocytosis but no specific cause is identified, consider AIDS-dementia syndrome (HIV encephalopathy). This is a subcortical dementia in which the intellectual-cognitive dysfunction is most pronounced in tasks requiring visual-motor coordination. These mental tasks (speed of processing information, motor functioning, abstract reasoning, visual-spatial skills) are most severely impaired in AIDS-dementia patients. Delirium and agitated psychotic states are uncommon in AIDS-dementia; their occurrence suggests drug withdrawal or toxic drug reaction. In patients with AIDS-dementia, motor dysfunction (ataxia, spasticity, clonus, Babinski signs) is present. CT, MRI, and EEG usually show no abnormalities in AIDS-dementia, but CT or MRI may show small, circumscribed, nonenhancing lesions in subcortical (thalamic, basal ganglia) regions. The course of AIDS-dementia consists of progressive deterioration and ultimately death from the systemic opportunistic infections. The drug AZT may slow viral replication in the CNS but does not halt CNS disease progression. Pathologic findings of AIDS-dementia include white matter pallor, demyelination, vacuolated tissue appearance, and multinucleated and foamy astrocytes and macrophages; these are most prominent within the subcortical region and there is relatively little gray matter involvement. CMV may cause an encephalitis similar to that seen in AIDS-dementia. In patients suspected of having AIDS-dementia, perform an eye examination to exclude CMV retinitis. Ganciclovir may be effective in CMV encephalitis and retinitis.

It is important to differentiate AIDS-dementia from HIV-1–related meningitis. The latter may develop early in asymptomatic HIV-seropositive patients or in patients with AIDS-related complex. Patients with HIV-1–related meningitis present with headache, meningeal signs, cranial neuropathies (most commonly, bilateral facial palsies), and signs of transient and reversible encephalopathy. CSF shows lymphocytic pleocytosis with elevated protein and gamma-globulin content. This disorder may resolve completely, and these patients do not necessarily later develop AIDS-dementia.

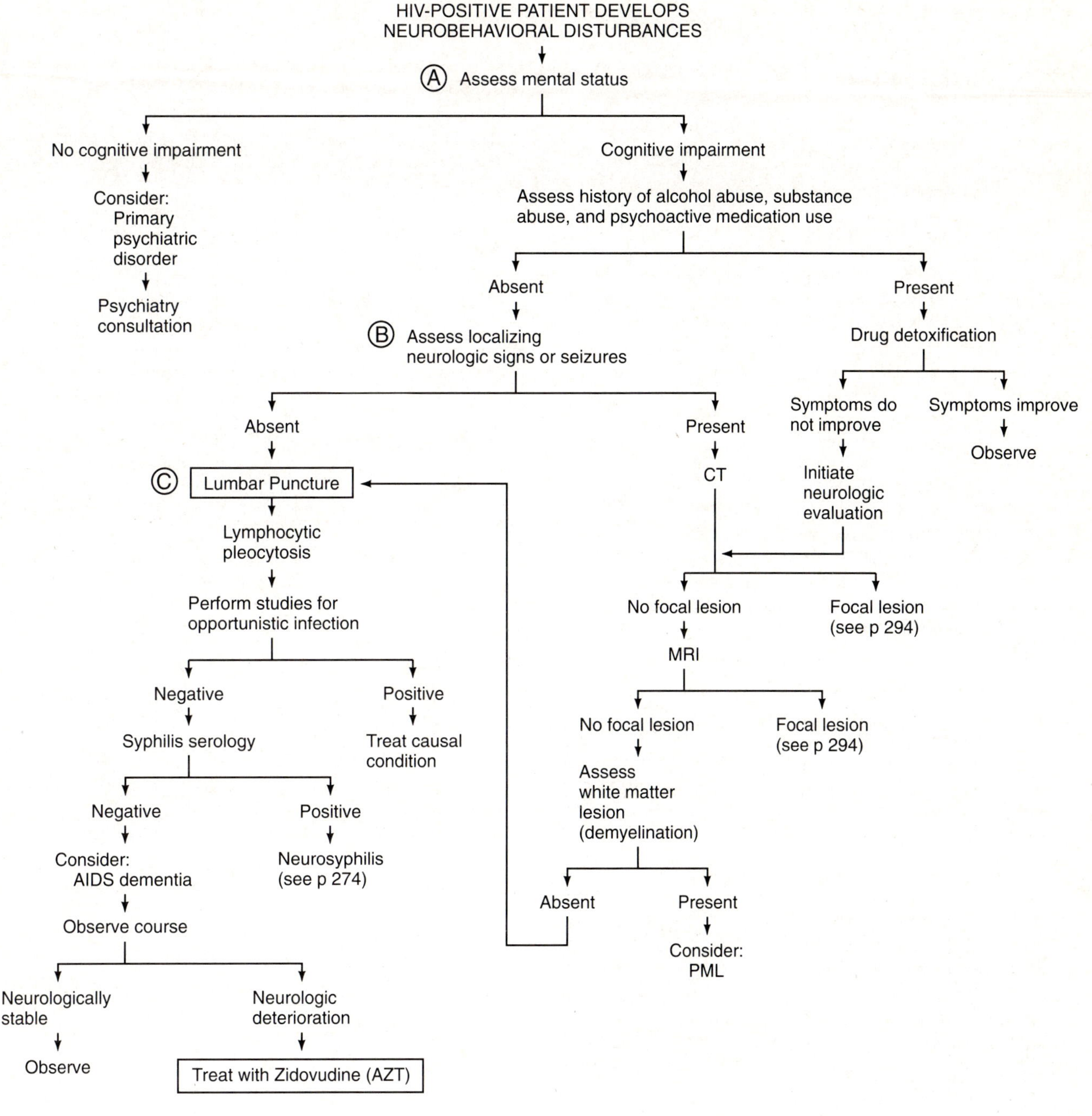

References

Levy RM, Bredesen DE, Rosenblum ML. Neurological manifestations of the acquired immunodeficiency syndrome (AIDS); experience at UCSF and review of the literature. J Neurosurg 1985; 62:475.

McArthur JC. Neurologic manifestations of AIDS. Medicine 1987; 66:407.

Navia BA, Price RW. AIDS-dementia complex. Ann Neurol 1986; 19:525.

Working Group of the American Academy of Neurology AIDS Task Force. Nomenclature and research case definitions for neurologic manifestation of human immunodeficiency virus-type 1 (HIV-1) infection. Neurology 1991; 41:778.

MANAGEMENT OF INTRACRANIAL MASS LESIONS IN HIV-POSITIVE PATIENTS

Leon A. Weisberg, M.D.

Intracranial mass lesions may develop in HIV-positive patients. These represent infectious-inflammatory and neoplastic conditions. Because these patients are immunocompromised, multiple concurrent opportunistic infections may coexist. Optimal management depends on diagnosing the underlying pathologic condition, but empiric therapy usually begins with the assumption that the focal intracranial lesion represents toxoplasmosis. This assumption is made because toxoplasmosis is the most common neurologic opportunistic condition occurring in HIV-positive patients. Clinical and neuroimaging (CT, MRI) features suggest the possibility of toxoplasmosis, but the pathologic and etiologic diagnosis cannot be established with absolute certainty unless biopsy confirmation is obtained. The risk of diagnostic error is further increased because AIDS patients may have multiple concurrent infections, and the lesion that is biopsy-proven may be only one of several underlying pathologic processes.

A. The location (cortical versus subcortical) and enhancement (CT or MRI) characteristics of the lesions may provide important diagnostic clues. Symmetric nonenhancing white matter lesions initially visualized in the posterior brain regions (parietal and occipital cortex, cerebellum) suggest progressive multifocal leukoencephalopathy (PML) (Fig. 1). The clinical findings of PML include dementia, blindness, and quadriparesis. PML is due to a papovavirus; treatment with antiviral drugs may be attempted, but there has

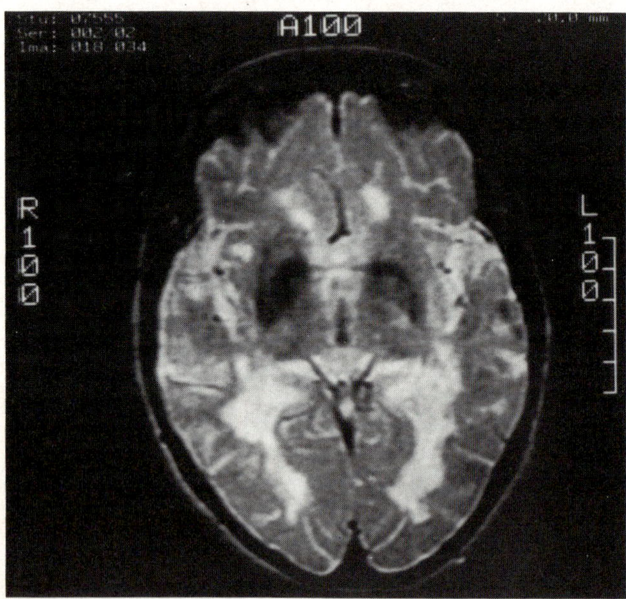

Figure 1   MRI shows multiple focal high-signal intensity lesions in the white matter surrounding the lateral ventricles. These are most prominent in the parietal-occipital region. This pattern is consistent with progressive multifocal leukoencephalopathy (PML).

been minimal success in arresting the progress of PML. Lymphoma and sarcoma show enhancing periventricular, cerebellar, basal ganglia, and thalamic lesions. These neoplasms are responsive to radiotherapy or chemotherapy. If CT shows ring or nodular enhancing cortical or subcortical lesions, consider an infectious-inflammatory process; toxoplasmosis is the most common pathologic condition in AIDS patients.

B. Toxoplasmosis occurs in 10% of AIDS patients. This is an obligate intracellular protozoan that may cause necrotic brain abscesses. These lesions may be single or multiple and are seen in cerebral hemispheric, subcortical, cerebellum, and brain stem regions. The initial lesion is commonly seen in the basal ganglia or thalamus. CT shows a hypodense, irregularly marginated lesion, sometimes with a small, central hyperdense portion. There is usually nodular or ring enhancement, but sometimes the hypodense lesion does not enhance. CSF may show lymphocytic pleocytosis with elevated protein and reduced sugar content; however, CSF serologic toxoplasmosis antibody tests do not have adequate sensitivity to establish this diagnosis. If CT-visualized lesions are consistent with toxoplasmosis, initiate empiric therapy, including pyrimethamine, 25 mg daily, and sulfadiazine, 6 to 8 g daily in four divided doses. Folinic acid, 5 to 10 mg daily, is used to reduce bone marrow suppression due to pyrimethamine. If there is a good clinical response within 2 to 4 weeks of initiation of therapy, continue this regimen. Perform follow-up CT within 3 weeks to determine whether the lesion size is decreasing. If toxoplasmosis is present, life-long maintenance therapy is needed. If a skin rash develops with empiric toxoplasmosis therapy, this reaction is most likely due to sulfadiazine; in this case, substitute clindamycin, 1.2 g every 6 hours. If patient's clinical condition does not improve, repeat CT/MRI. If there is increased mass effect, give dexamethasone, 4 mg every 6 hours, and continue empiric toxoplasmosis therapy. If CT/MRI shows new lesions, perform stereotactic biopsy of one of the new lesions.

C. Multicentric primary B cell CNS lymphoma may cause progressive dementia and focal neurologic signs. CT/MRI may show hyperdense, multifocal lesions, usually in the basal ganglia, thalamus, cerebellum, or periventricular white matter. They show dense contrast enhancement usually encircling the ventricular system. CSF examination rarely shows positive cytology for neoplastic cells in patients with this type of lymphoma. Chemotherapy or radiotherapy should not be carried out without previous biopsy confirmation of lymphoma. Cytomegalovirus (CMV) may cause encephalitis, which is clinically similar to several other

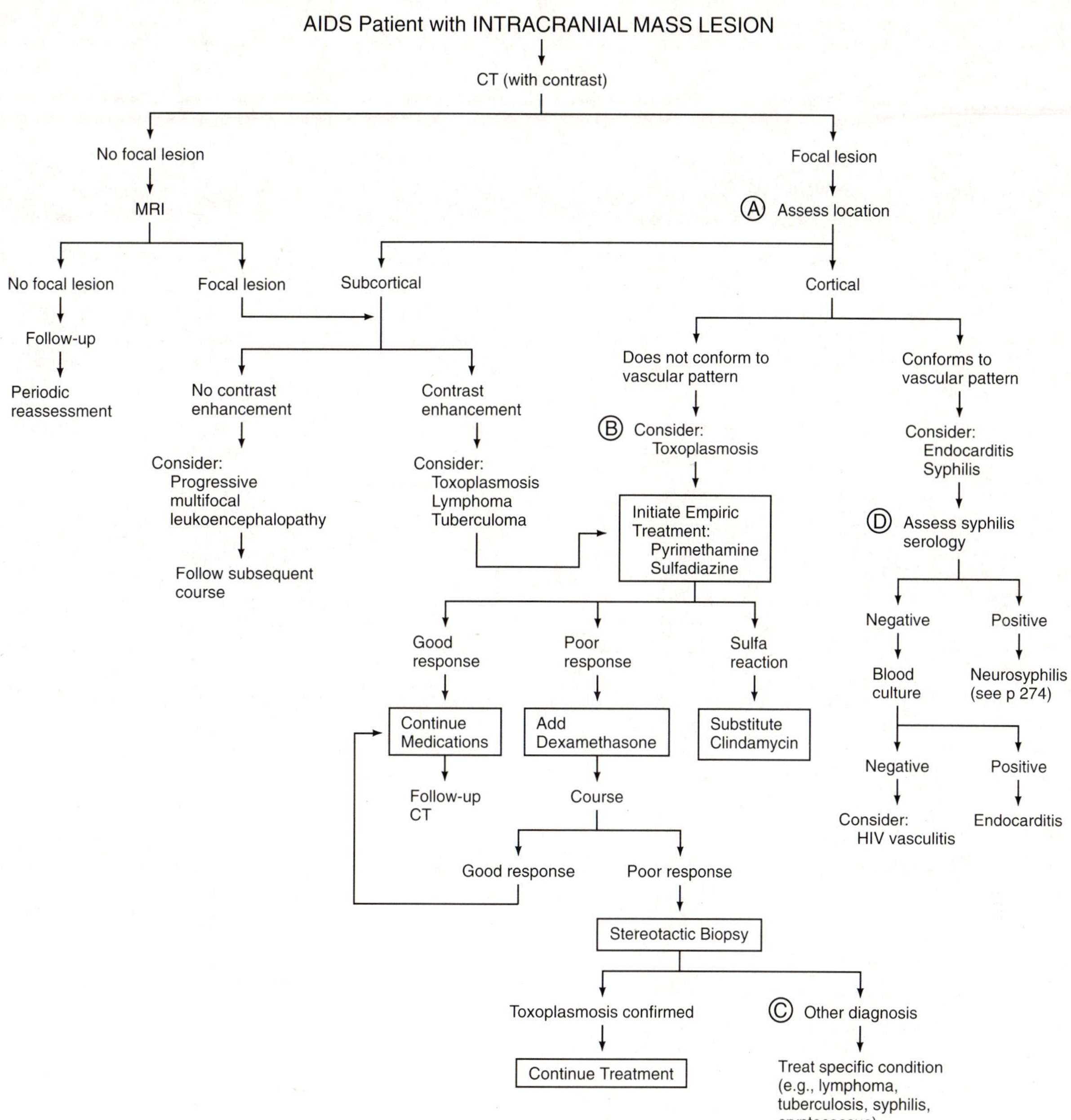

conditions, including AIDS-dementia encephalitis, toxoplasmosis, and lymphoma. Ophthalmologic examination in patients with CMV infection may show accompanying retinitis; this positive finding is diagnostic of CMV. Tuberculosis and *Cryptococcus* may cause focal intracranial lesions, but they usually cause meningitis, so that the diagnosis is established by CSF findings.

D. Patients with AIDS may develop vascular lesions. A cerebral ischemic lesion may suggest embolism from endocarditis (infectious or marantic) or HIV-related arteritis; intracranial hemorrhage may result from endocarditis or coagulopathy. Meningovascular syphilis may present with stroke syndromes. The time course to CNS infection in neurosyphilis is shortened in HIV-positive patients, and there have been reports of false-negative serology in patients with biopsy-proven neurosyphilis; however, this is rare. When ischemic stroke develops in an HIV-positive patient, neurosyphilis is the most likely cause. Also, carefully consider whether the patient may be a substance abuser, in which case drug-related ischemic stroke is the most likely diagnosis.

References

Haverkos H. Assessment of therapy for toxoplasmosis encephalitis. Am J Med 1987; 82:907.

Hochberg FH, Miller DC. Primary central nervous lymphoma. J Neurosurg 1988; 68:835.

Navia BA, Petito CK, Gold JW. Cerebral toxoplasmosis complicating the acquired immunodeficiency syndrome. Ann Neurol 1986; 19:224.

PERIPHERAL NERVOUS SYSTEM COMPLICATIONS OF AIDS

Leon A. Weisberg, M.D.

HIV is neurotropic, damaging both central and peripheral nervous systems. It is important to be aware of those HIV-related disorders that may cause motor or sensory disturbances. These may be due to spinal cord, nerve root, or peripheral nerve or muscle damage.

A. For patients with predominantly motor symptoms, consider the distribution of weakness: if proximal, consider myopathy; if HIV-related, consider AZT (zidovudine)-induced mitochondrial myopathy or HIV-induced myopathy. The clinical features of these two types of myopathies may be very similar, so differentiation is based on muscle biopsy findings. Both AZT-induced myopathy and HIV inflammatory myopathy show biopsy evidence of inflammatory changes. With AZT-related myopathy, biopsy findings include ragged-red fibers consistent with abnormal mitochondria; this change is not seen with HIV inflammatory myopathy. Many AIDS patients report myalgias (muscle pain and aches or cramps) without being weak or showing muscle wasting. In these patients, electromyography (EMG) shows no myopathic features. Treatment for myalgias includes nonsteroidal anti-inflammatory drugs or quinine.

B. With leg weakness only, suspect a spinal cord lesion. Perform neuroimaging studies to exclude a compressive cord lesion. It is unusual for such lesions to develop without sensory or autonomic findings. If a patient has leg weakness with associated neurobehavioral signs, consider AIDS-dementia syndrome (see p 292). Perform studies for vitamin B_{12} deficiency, which may cause myelopathy with distal leg sensory findings. If all studies fail to identify the cause of leg weakness, HIV-1–associated vacuolar myelopathy is the most likely diagnosis. This diagnosis can be suspected on the basis of clinical findings but cannot be confirmed without autopsy findings. Pathologic findings include a spinal cord vacuolar change, similar to the subcortical brain change seen in AIDS-dementia. If leg weakness is the only abnormal neurologic finding, consider spinal cord, peripheral nerve, or multiple nerve root (polyradiculopathy) lesions.

C. If there are both motor and sensory symptoms, distribution of these abnormalities should help delineate the underlying neurologic disorder. If the legs are involved, the arms are spared, and there is autonomic dysfunction, consider spinal cord or spinal root syndrome. Cytomegalovirus (CMV) may cause cauda equina polyradiculopathy with prominent sacral involvement. This may result in bladder, bowel, and sexual dysfunction. Sacral sensory disturbances strongly suggest a spinal cord lesion or radiculopathy. This pattern is not common in peripheral neuropathy.

D. If the hands and feet are initially involved (distal pattern), consider polyneuropathy. In early stages of HIV infection, acute demyelinating inflammatory neuropathy may develop. This may rapidly ascend and often results in cranial neuropathy (bilateral facial nerve paresis). This AIDS-related demyelinating inflammatory disorder may simulate Guillain-Barré (acute ascending inflammatory demyelinating) polyneuropathy and responds to plasmapheresis or IV immunoglobulins. This treatment may need to be repeated every several weeks if neurologic symptoms recur after an initial good response. Avoid corticosteroids, which may unmask latent tuberculosis or fungal disease in patients with HIV-related demyelinating neuropathy.

E. In the later stages of HIV infection, axonal polyneuropathy often develops. This may be due to a direct HIV effect on the peripheral nerve. Alternative etiologies include medication effect, metabolic disorders, and toxic factors. In most cases, the predominant neuropathic features are sensory disorders. These patients complain of burning, uncomfortable paresthesias in the feet, which are frequently exacerbated at night. If due to direct HIV effect, these symptoms would be expected to improve with AZT, but this is not usually the course. The alternative drug to AZT that is used to treat HIV infection is ddI, a potentially neurotoxic agent that may cause or worsen an existing neuropathy. Tricyclic antidepressants (amitriptyline [Elavil]), 25 to 50 mg at night, may relieve the sensory neuropathic symptoms, which may be severe and persistent enough to interfere with sleep.

References

Dalakas MC, Pezeshkpour GH. Neuromuscular diseases associated with human immunodeficiency virus infection. Ann Neurol 1988; 23(Suppl):S38.

Parry GJ. Peripheral neuropathy associated with human immunodeficiency virus infection. Ann Neurol 1988; 23(Suppl):S49.

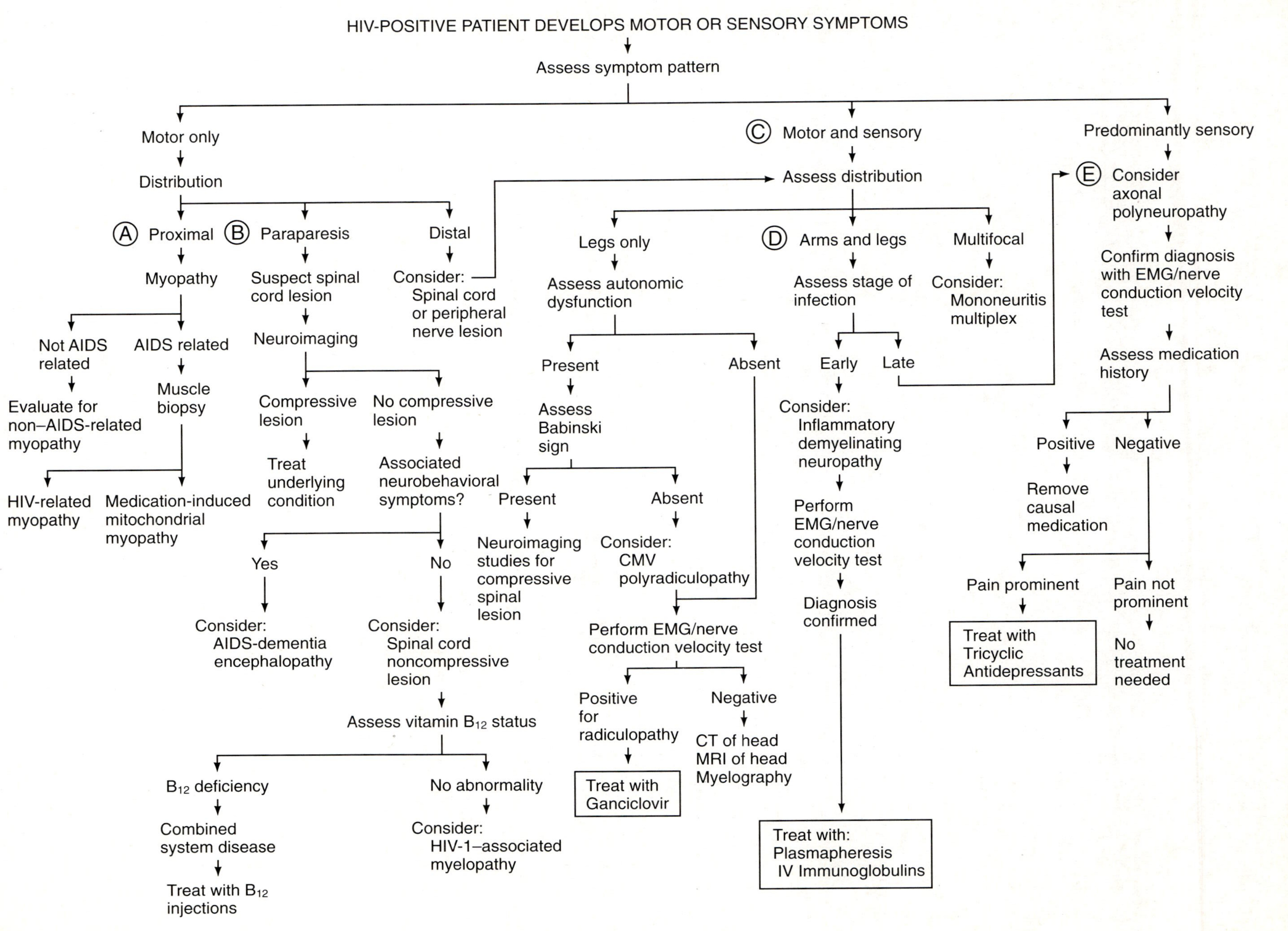

HIV-POSITIVE PATIENT DEVELOPS MOTOR OR SENSORY SYMPTOMS
Assess symptom pattern
Motor only
Distribution
A Proximal
Myopathy
Not AIDS related
Evaluate for non–AIDS-related myopathy
HIV-related myopathy
AIDS related
Muscle biopsy
Medication-induced mitochondrial myopathy
B Paraparesis
Suspect spinal cord lesion
Neuroimaging
Compressive lesion
Treat underlying condition
No compressive lesion
Associated neurobehavioral symptoms?
Yes
Consider: AIDS-dementia encephalopathy
No
Consider: Spinal cord noncompressive lesion
Assess vitamin B12 status
B12 deficiency
Combined system disease
Treat with B12 injections
No abnormality
Consider: HIV-1–associated myelopathy
Distal
Consider: Spinal cord or peripheral nerve lesion
C Motor and sensory
Assess distribution
Legs only
Assess autonomic dysfunction
Present
Assess Babinski sign
Present
Neuroimaging studies for compressive spinal lesion
Absent
Consider: CMV polyradiculopathy
Perform EMG/nerve conduction velocity test
Positive for radiculopathy
Treat with Ganciclovir
Negative
CT of head MRI of head Myelography
Absent
D Arms and legs
Assess stage of infection
Early
Late
Consider: Inflammatory demyelinating neuropathy
Perform EMG/nerve conduction velocity test
Diagnosis confirmed
Treat with: Plasmapheresis IV Immunoglobulins
Multifocal
Consider: Mononeuritis multiplex
Predominantly sensory
E Consider axonal polyneuropathy
Confirm diagnosis with EMG/nerve conduction velocity test
Assess medication history
Positive
Remove causal medication
Pain prominent
Treat with Tricyclic Antidepressants
Negative
Pain not prominent
No treatment needed
297

NEUROLOGIC MANIFESTATIONS OF SARCOIDOSIS

Leon A. Weisberg, M.D.

Sarcoidosis is defined as a "multisystem noncaseating granulomatous disorder of unknown etiology, most commonly affecting young adults and presenting most frequently with bilateral hilar lymphadenopathy, pulmonary infiltration, skin or eye lesions." Diagnosis is most secure when supported by histologic evidence of widespread noncaseating epithelioid cell granulomas in more than one organ, or a positive Kveim skin test. Biopsy sites include lymph nodes, skin or mucosal lesions, salivary glands, conjunctiva, liver, and pulmonary tissue. There may be an elevated blood level of angiotensin-converting enzyme. Neurologic involvement occurs in 5% of patients, usually in those with systemic manifestations; neurologic disturbances are rarely the initial or isolated symptom. If neurologic signs suggest neurosarcoidosis, a complete systemic evaluation or biopsy of involved neurologic tissue (muscle, peripheral nerve, dura, brain) may be necessary.

A. Cranial neuropathy is the most common clinical manifestation of neurosarcoidosis; it is believed due to granulomatous meningitis. CSF examination usually shows lymphocytic pleocytosis, high protein content, and low sugar content. Peripheral seventh nerve paresis is most common; the parotid glands may be enlarged. Eighth nerve involvement may cause hearing or equilibrium dysfunction. Extraocular motility disturbances are uncommon in sarcoidosis. If the pupils are unreactive with normal extraocular motility, the etiology is uveitis, not primary neurologic disease. Visual loss may be due to orbital sarcoid granuloma. A soft tissue orbital mass is demonstrated by CT/MRI; no specific CT/MRI patterns differentiate sarcoid from other orbital masses. Sarcoid may cause visual loss due to inflammatory optic neuritis. CT/MRI may show enlarged optic nerves in sarcoid optic neuritis. If the orbital or basal meningeal region is involved, CT/MRI may show a densely contrast-enhancing dural region. MRI is more sensitive than CT in demonstrating a thickened meningeal-dural pattern and enlarged optic nerves.

B. Sterile lymphocytic pleocytosis may occur with decreased sugar and elevated protein content in sarcoid meningitis. Order complete CSF studies to exclude infectious (tuberculous, fungal) or neoplastic meningitis. A diagnosis of granulomatous meningitis due to sarcoid may require meningeal biopsy. Always consider tuberculous and fungal infections in sarcoid patients, because these infections may develop especially in patients treated with corticosteroids.

C. Hydrocephalus is due to mass effect by an intracranial granulomatous lesion or infiltration of CSF pathways by granulomatous meningitis. Most severe cases of sarcoid-induced hydrocephalus occur because of aqueductal stenosis or fourth ventricular outlet obstruction. The diagnosis of hydrocephalus is established by CT/MRI. Meningeal or dural biopsy may be necessary to identify sarcoid granuloma as the cause. The appropriate treatment of hydrocephalus is a diversionary shunt.

D. Intracranial or intraspinal lesions are uncommon. They may be solitary or multiple. Suprasellar granulomas simulate pituitary neoplasms and may cause visual or endocrine dysfunction. Hyperprolactinemia and diabetes insipidus are due to hypothalamic involvement. Cortical granulomatous lesions may cause seizures. Posterior fossa lesions may cause cerebellar or brain stem signs and hydrocephalus. CT/MRI may demonstrate these mass lesions but do not permit differentiation from other infectious-inflammatory or neoplastic disorders. Sarcoid mass lesions decrease in size when treated with corticosteroids. If there is no response to corticosteroids, surgical removal or radiotherapy may be necessary. In rare cases, an intracranial sarcoid lesion develops in a patient with no systemic sarcoidosis manifestations; the diagnosis is established by surgical biopsy findings, and surgical removal of the lesion should be attempted.

E. Seizures may develop in patients with sarcoidosis and may be related to sarcoidosis vasculopathy. CT, MRI, and CSF may show no abnormalities; there may be no seizure-precipitating metabolic disturbance (e.g., hyponatremia, hypercalcemia). If neurodiagnostic studies show no active sarcoid, treat with anticonvulsants; do not give corticosteroids. If there is evidence of active neurosarcoidosis, begin treatment with prednisone, 40 to 60 mg daily. Continue this dose for 8 weeks and if there has been a good clinical response, slowly taper the dose. If symptoms recur, increase the dose to the level at which it was last effective and continue this dose for 8 weeks before attempting to taper again. Some patients require long-term therapy. If a patient neither improves nor worsens, consider increasing the prednisone dose. If a patient worsens despite 60 mg prednisone, increase the dose to 100 or 120 mg, or give methylprednisolone 500 mg IV four times daily. If there is improvement, switch to oral prednisone. For corticosteroid-resistant mass lesions, consider radiation therapy.

F. Nerve involvement may occur as symmetric sensorimotor polyneuropathy or mononeuropathy multiplex. Nerve biopsy may demonstrate granulomas. Myopathy is unusual in sarcoidosis; muscle biopsy may show granuloma even in patients without clinical weakness. Myopathy may develop as a side effect of corticosteroid medication, and it may not be possible to differentiate the cause of myopathy (sarcoid or corticosteroid-induced) without biopsy findings.

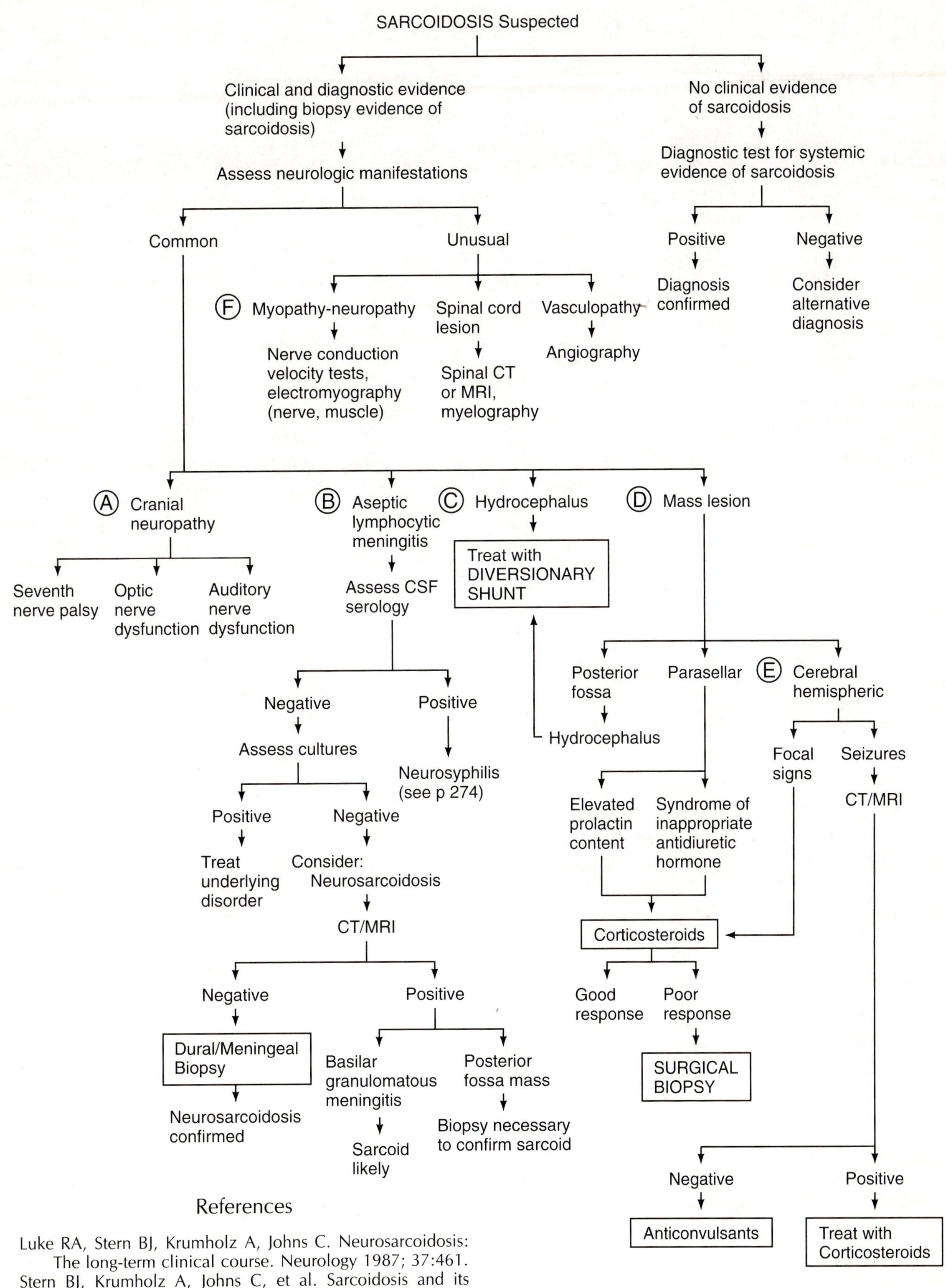

References

Luke RA, Stern BJ, Krumholz A, Johns C. Neurosarcoidosis: The long-term clinical course. Neurology 1987; 37:461.

Stern BJ, Krumholz A, Johns C, et al. Sarcoidosis and its neurological manifestations. Arch Neurol 1985; 42:909.

MULTIPLE SCLEROSIS: DIAGNOSIS AND MANAGEMENT

Carlos A. Garcia, M.D.

Multiple sclerosis (MS) is a disease of undetermined etiology characterized by focal destruction of CNS myelin in a disseminated and randomly distributed manner (Fig. 1). The disease is most common in young people and may present as a visual loss, motor weakness, sensory or cerebellar impairment, or spinal cord dysfunction. In two thirds of cases the disease is characterized by exacerbations and remissions; the remaining patients have a progressive course. In middle age the disease usually presents with a progressive myelopathy with spastic paraplegia. Paresthesias and weakness of one or more extremities are the initial presentation in half the cases. Visual impairment, fatigue, cerebellar deficit, and electric shock—like pains down the back and into the legs precipitated by flexion of the neck (Lhermitte sign) are frequent complaints. Acute transverse myelopathy, associated with blindness (Devic's disease) or without blindness, may be seen in young patients as the first manifestation or during the course of the disease.

Different clinical criteria for the diagnosis of MS, using terms such as definite, probable, and even "possible," have been delineated by different authors and by committees dealing with the disease in the hope of promoting standardized criteria to use as a baseline for therapy. The most reliable aspects of the disease are that the signs and symptoms are "scattered in time and space," are not explained by lesions other than demyelinating, and have a tendency toward remission. In a few patients the disease may be slowly progressive (primarily those with an onset in middle age).

A. There is no specific test to confirm the diagnosis of MS. CT scan may show lucent enhanced white matter lesions during the active phase of the disease, but the lesions become isodense during remission. MRI defines and identifies the demyelinating lesions in the cerebral hemisphere, brain stem, and spinal cord and detects asymptomatic lesions. MRI findings need to be correlated with the clinical features, CSF findings, and evoked responses.

B. Visual evoked responses (VER), brain stem auditory evoked potentials (BAEP), and short-latency somatosensory evoked potentials (SEP) may disclose asymptomatic lesions. None of these tests is diagnostic for demyelinating disease.

C. IgG synthesis in MS plaques has been demonstrated and may appear in the CSF as an oligoclonal band. This abnormal band has also been found in CNS infections and other diseases. Myelin basic protein may appear in the CSF, particularly at the time of relapse, but is a nonspecific feature of the disease. All these tests should be correlated with the clinical features and other tests.

D. The use of different therapeutic agents is controversial, as is evaluation of the disease. Corticosteroids seem to be effective in the acute phase. However, immunosuppressive agents continue to show very questionable benefits over placebo treatment.

Management should be directed toward preventing recurrences by the avoidance of stress, trauma, and systemic infections. Spasticity due to myelopathies can be partially controlled with baclofen (Lioresal) (10-mg tablets). Small doses (5 mg) should be used, and the dose increased as tolerated until sedation or weakness appears. Amantadine (Symmetrel) has controlled fatigue in some patients. Braces may be used to help ambulation and improve hand or finger control. A consulting urologist can help with control and prevention of urinary infections and with bladder control. Analgesics should be used when painful syndromes appear. In essence, the comfort and welfare of the patient should be the first priority of the treating physician.

References

Goodin DS. The use of immunosuppressive agents in the treatment of multiple sclerosis. Neurology 1991; 4:980.

Kaetsier JE, ed. Demyelinating diseases. In: Handbook of clinical neurology. Revised series 3. Vol 5. New York: Elsevier, 1985:47.

Lee KH, Hashimoto SA, Hoodge JP, et al. Magnetic resonance imaging of the head in the diagnosis of multiple sclerosis: A prospective 2 year follow-up with comparison of clinical evaluation, evoked potentials, oligoclonal banding, and CT. Neurology 1991; 4:657.

McFarlin DE, McFarland HF. Multiple sclerosis. Medical progress. N Engl J Med 1982; 307:1183, 1246.

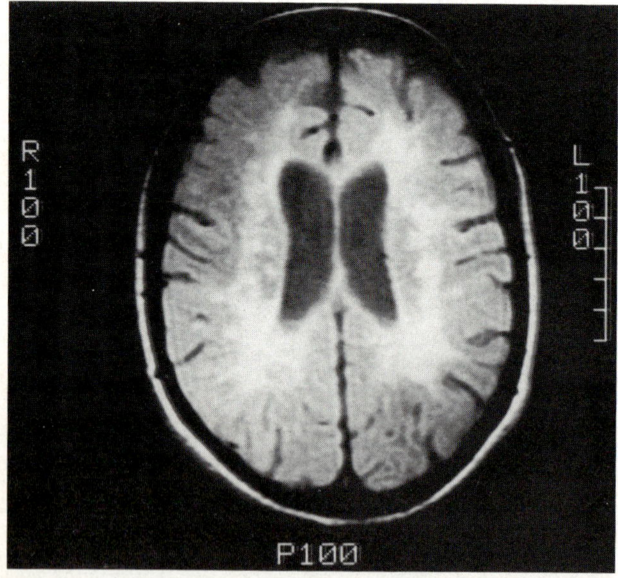

Figure 1 MRI shows high-signal (hyperintense) regions surrounding the lateral ventricles. This pattern is consistent with the diagnosis of multiple sclerosis.

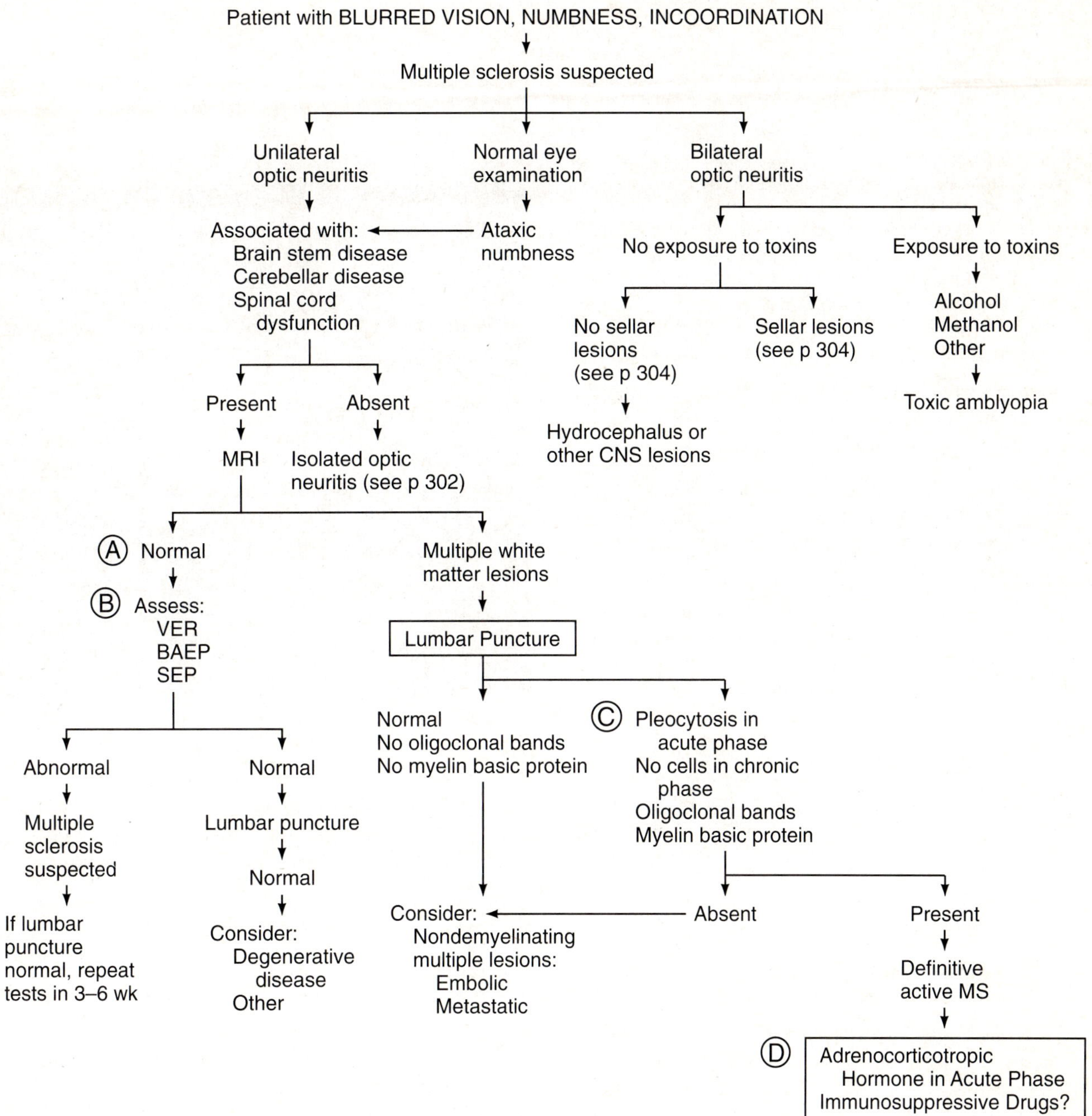

Patient with BLURRED VISION, NUMBNESS, INCOORDINATION

Multiple sclerosis suspected

Unilateral optic neuritis

Normal eye examination

Bilateral optic neuritis

Ataxic numbness

Associated with:
Brain stem disease
Cerebellar disease
Spinal cord dysfunction

No exposure to toxins

Exposure to toxins

Alcohol
Methanol
Other

No sellar lesions (see p 304)

Sellar lesions (see p 304)

Toxic amblyopia

Present

Absent

Hydrocephalus or other CNS lesions

MRI

Isolated optic neuritis (see p 302)

A Normal

Multiple white matter lesions

B Assess:
VER
BAEP
SEP

Lumbar Puncture

Abnormal

Normal

Normal
No oligoclonal bands
No myelin basic protein

C Pleocytosis in acute phase
No cells in chronic phase
Oligoclonal bands
Myelin basic protein

Multiple sclerosis suspected

Lumbar puncture

Normal

If lumbar puncture normal, repeat tests in 3–6 wk

Consider:
Degenerative disease
Other

Consider:
Nondemyelinating multiple lesions:
Embolic
Metastatic

Absent

Present

Definitive active MS

D Adrenocorticotropic Hormone in Acute Phase Immunosuppressive Drugs?

OPTIC NEURITIS

Carlos A. Garcia, M.D.

Optic neuritis is an acute demyelinating process that selectively affects the optic nerve. Controversy continues regarding optic neuritis and its relationship to multiple sclerosis (MS). Approximately half the cases are associated with MS and half are idiopathic. The importance of the controversy resides in the good prognosis if optic neuritis is a monophasic illness and the need to institute diagnostic tests and possibly therapy if it is an initial sign of MS.

A. Blurred vision or visual loss in one eye or both is the initial presenting sign in optic neuritis. This is accompanied by pain, usually behind the eye, which is exacerbated by touching or eye movement. The visual acuity decreases within days or weeks and is followed by progressive improvement in most patients. Eye examination shows reduced visual acuity, a centrocecal scotoma (area of blindness extending from the central fixation point to the blind spot), and an afferent pupillary defect in the involved eye. If visual loss occurs in a young male with a family history of visual loss, consider Leber's optic atrophy. Confirm this diagnosis by funduscopic and fluorescein angiographic findings.

B. In optic neuritis, funduscopy shows disc edema in 30% to 40% of patients. However, in retrobulbar neuritis the inflammation process and demyelination are behind the optic nerve head, and the disc initially may appear normal. In patients with visual loss in one eye and findings consistent with an optic nerve lesion, examine the visual fields carefully in the opposite eye for a superior temporal quadrant defect. This would indicate a chiasmal lesion. In patients with a possible chiasmal lesion, MRI and magnetic resonance angiography (MRA) will delineate a juxtasellar lesion.

C. With monocular and binocular blurred vision and disc edema, consider ischemic optic neuropathy. In elderly patients, strongly consider temporal arteritis as one cause of ischemic optic neuropathy.

D. The patient with optic neuritis is usually young and female. Visual acuity is impaired, especially color vision. If the disease is unilateral, light reactivity is lost in the involved eye. Funduscopy may show disc edema (papillitis), or findings may be normal (retrobulbar neuritis). Optic atrophy appears later (Fig. 1).

E. The work-up should include MRI of the orbit and sellar region (looking for an orbital or chiasmal lesion) and the head (looking for a demyelinating lesion). MRI may also detect intracranial demyelinating lesions. Evoked potentials—visual (VER), auditory (BAEP), and somatosensory (SSEP)—may show other areas of demyelination in the CNS. Lumbar puncture can be used to seek an elevated gamma globulin content (oligoclonal band) or myelin basic protein in MS.

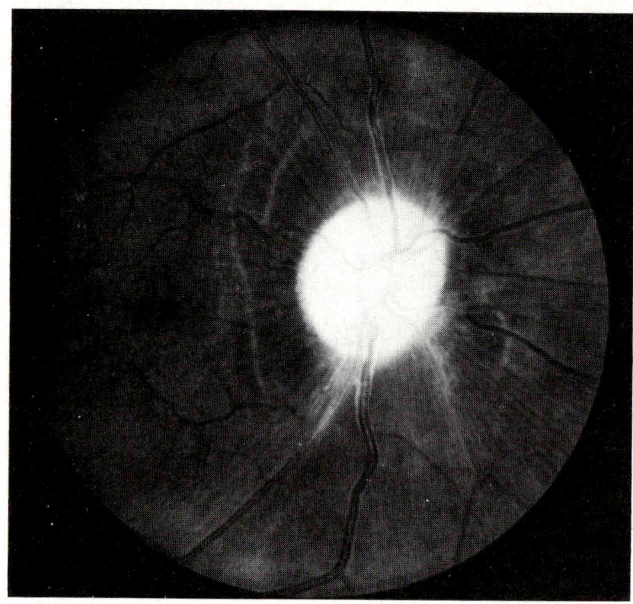

Figure 1 The optic disc appears pale with a reduced number of vessels. This is consistent with optic atrophy.

F. IV methylprednisolone speeds the recovery of visual loss optic neuritis. However, oral prednisone alone seems to be ineffective and increases the risk of new episodes.

G. Patients with isolated optic neuritis may have a recurrence in the same or the opposite eye. If neurologic signs consistent with MS develop in other portions of the nervous system, this usually occurs within 5 years after the initial episode of optic neuritis.

H. Certain cases of optic neuritis are associated with autoimmune disorders, including systemic lupus erythematosus. Optic neuritis may present before the patient shows systemic signs of lupus. Other patients (especially young women) present with optic neuritis and show laboratory evidence of an autoimmune disorder, but have no other clinical signs. It is important to recognize these autoimmune etiologies for optic neuritis because they are corticosteroid responsive, whereas optic neuritis due to MS does not respond to corticosteroids. Some patients require very high doses of steroids.

References

Beck RW, Cleary PA, Anderson MM, et al. A randomized controlled trial of corticosteroids in the treatment of acute optic neuritis. N Engl J Med 1992; 326:581.

Parkin PJ, Hierons R, McDonald WI. Bilateral optic neuritis: A long term follow-up. Brain 1984; 107:951.

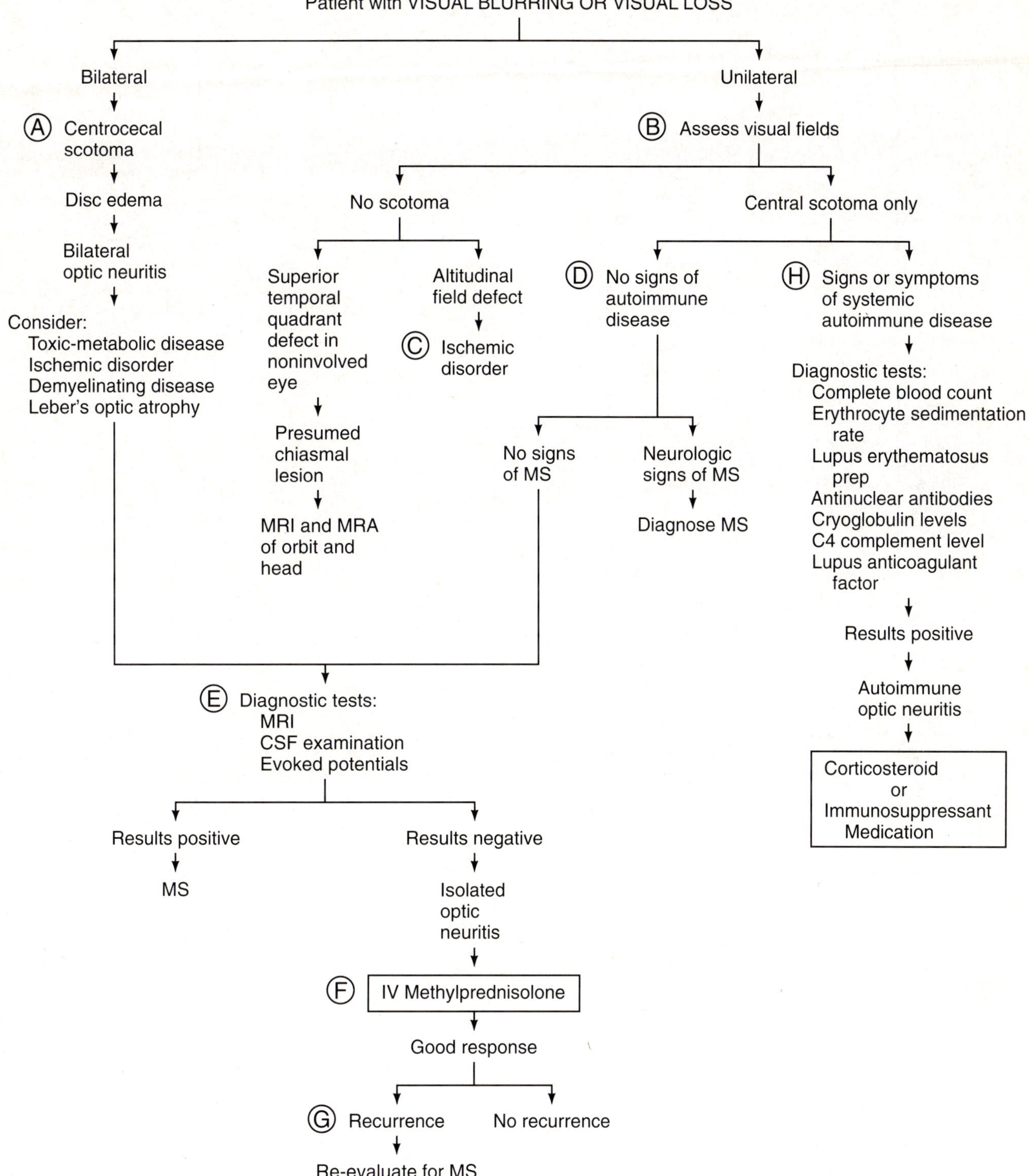

Patient with VISUAL BLURRING OR VISUAL LOSS
Bilateral
Unilateral
A Centrocecal scotoma
B Assess visual fields
Disc edema
No scotoma
Central scotoma only
Bilateral optic neuritis
Superior temporal quadrant defect in noninvolved eye
Altitudinal field defect
D No signs of autoimmune disease
H Signs or symptoms of systemic autoimmune disease
Consider:
Toxic-metabolic disease
Ischemic disorder
Demyelinating disease
Leber's optic atrophy
C Ischemic disorder
Presumed chiasmal lesion
No signs of MS
Neurologic signs of MS
Diagnostic tests:
Complete blood count
Erythrocyte sedimentation rate
Lupus erythematosus prep
Antinuclear antibodies
Cryoglobulin levels
C4 complement level
Lupus anticoagulant factor
MRI and MRA of orbit and head
Diagnose MS
Results positive
Autoimmune optic neuritis
E Diagnostic tests:
MRI
CSF examination
Evoked potentials
Corticosteroid or Immunosuppressant Medication
Results positive
Results negative
MS
Isolated optic neuritis
F IV Methylprednisolone
Good response
G Recurrence
No recurrence
Re-evaluate for MS

TEMPORAL (GIANT CELL) ARTERITIS

Leon A. Weisberg, M.D.

Temporal arteritis (TA) results in granulomas and arteritis within blood vessels, and these pathologic disturbances cause decreased ocular blood flow. TA may cause visual loss due to involvement of the posterior ciliary arteries, with resultant ischemic optic neuropathy; less commonly, the central retinal artery (CRA) is involved, resulting in retinal infarction.

A. TA rarely affects patients <50 years old; it is an important cause of blindness in older patients. When older patients present with visual symptoms, consider TA as a potentially preventable cause of visual loss.

B. Initial symptoms of TA may be visual loss or headache of recent onset. Visual loss is usually unilateral at first but later may become bilateral. It is important to begin evaluation early if TA is suspected. Visual deterioration may occur suddenly, without warning, and be irreversible. With ischemic optic neuropathy, examination findings include reduced visual acuity, scotomata, afferent pupillary defect, optic disc edema, and swelling. With CRA occlusion and infarction, unilateral visual loss may be total or altitudinal (involving the upper or lower field); the retina initially appears opaque and later becomes pale, and a cherry-red spot may be present. In younger patients with visual loss of sudden onset, consider optic neuropathies. These may be immune-mediated; associated with multiple sclerosis; a consequence of infectious and inflammatory disorders involving the paranasal sinuses, orbits, or basal meninges; or of unknown cause. If visual loss is not of sudden onset, consider compressive optic neuropathy (see p 62).

C. In patients >50 years old who have sudden unilateral visual impairment, check the erythrocyte sedimentation rate (ESR); TA rarely occurs without an elevated ESR. In patients >50 years old with sudden unilateral visual loss and elevated ESR, suspicion of TA is so high that corticosteroids are initiated without awaiting temporal artery biopsy. A delay in diagnosis may cause further visual loss, which may not be reversible even with corticosteroid treatment. Treat TA with prednisone, 80 to 100 mg daily. This should prevent further visual loss; headache improves, often within 48 hours.

In other patients suspected of TA, if visual loss is not sudden or if there is a headache of recent onset, perform temporal artery biopsy. Biopsy is positive in >90% of cases, but a negative biopsy does not exclude TA. A negative biopsy may result when skip lesions (areas of normal vessel alternating with arteritis and granulomas) occur or if the biopsy specimen is not long enough to include the representative lesions. If the initial biopsy is negative, consider contralateral temporal artery biopsy, even if that side is asymptomatic. If bilateral temporal artery biopsies are negative but ESR remains elevated, this may represent TA and corticosteroids should be given; however, consider nonarteritic ischemic optic neuropathy. Evaluate these patients for systemic disorders (hypertension, diabetes mellitus, cardiac disease, carotid artery disease) if nonarteritic optic neuropathy is suspected. Nonarteritic ischemic optic neuropathy does not respond to corticosteroids.

D. Continue prednisone at an initial dose of 60 to 80 mg for 4 to 8 weeks, then gradually taper over 6 to 12 months. Monitor visual function, ESR, and recurrence of headache or systemic symptoms. If any of these recur, increase the prednisone dose. Alternate-day corticosteroid therapy is not effective in TA.

E. If a patient with suspected TA presents with a headache of recent onset, investigate for other associated clinical features. Patients may have systemic symptoms (fever, anorexia, malaise), polymyalgia rheumatica (muscle aches usually involving proximal muscle groups), and jaw claudication. The temporal artery may be tender, nonpulsatile, and easily palpable. The scalp may be tender. Headache due to TA may be generalized rather than localized to one temporal region. If these symptoms and signs are present and ESR is elevated, begin prednisone without initially performing temporal artery biopsy. Systemic symptoms and headache usually resolve within 48 hours of initiating corticosteroids in patients with TA.

F. If systemic symptoms are absent and ESR is not elevated, consider other systemic or rheumatologic disorders as the cause of headache of recent onset.

References

Elliot DL, Watts WJ, Reuler JB. Management of suspected temporal arteritis: A decision analysis. Med Decis Making 1983; 3:63.

Hamilton CR, Shelley WM, Tumulty PA. Giant cell arteritis: Including temporal arteritis and polymyalgia rheumatica. Medicine 1971; 50:1.

Rosenfeld SI, Kosmorsky GS, Klingle TG. Treatment of temporal arteritis with ocular involvement. Am J Med 1986; 80:143.

TEMPORAL ARTERITIS Suspected

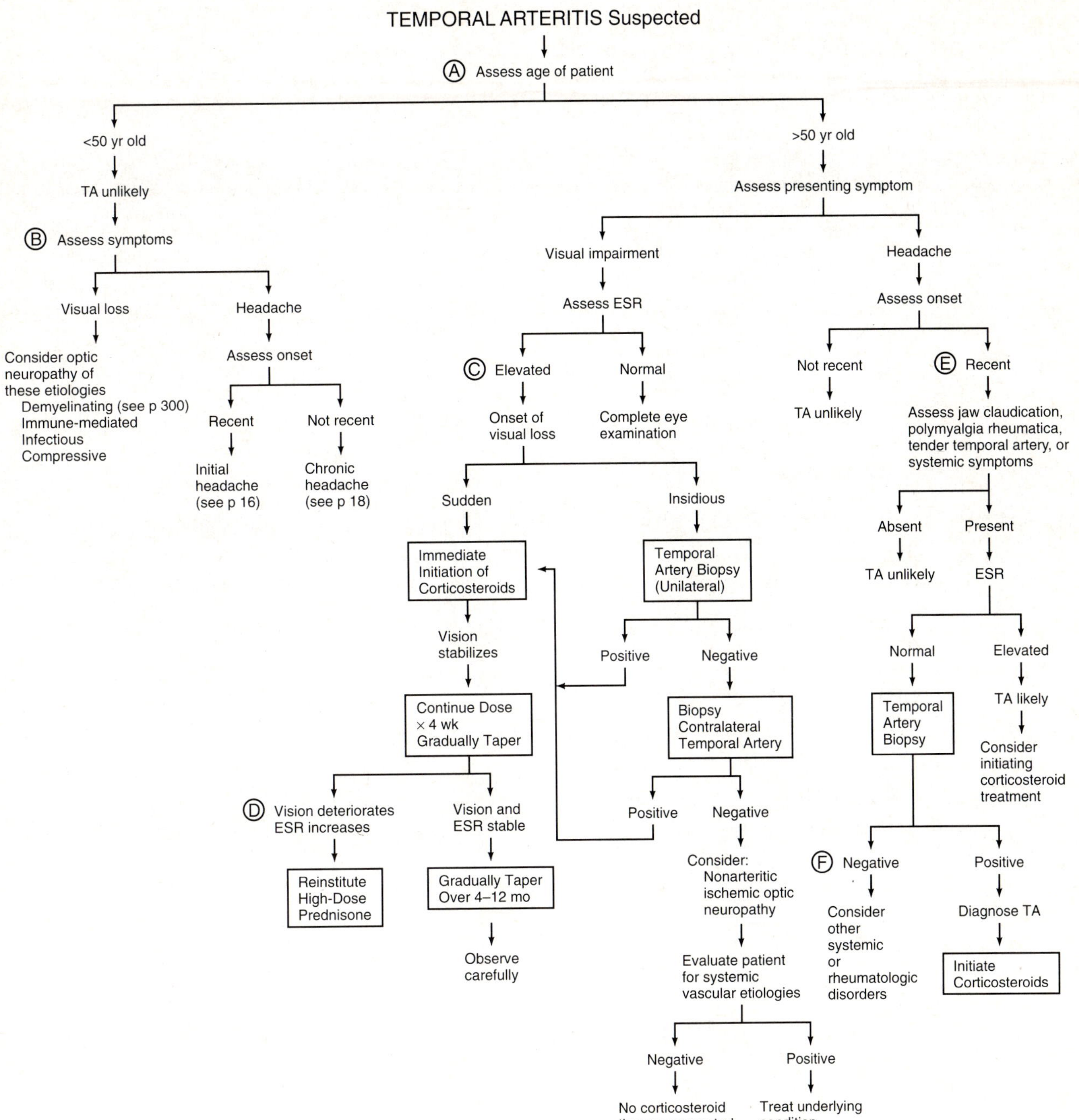

SLEEP DISORDERS

Richard L. Strub, M.D.

Until recently the only commonly known sleep disorder was simple insomnia. Now, with the development of specialized sleep laboratories that record all-night EEG and with television monitoring of sleep behavior, many specific disorders of sleep and wakefulness have been described. Because of the lack of availability of sleep laboratories and the expense of this type of evaluation, the physician usually must arrive at the diagnosis from the history, which must be taken both from the patient and from some other person who can help describe the patient's sleep behavior. The history must include information about the diet; alcohol, drug, or stimulant use; the emotional history; the sleep pattern (time to bed, time up, wakenings, snoring); daytime sleepiness; and the presence of medical illness. Sleep disorders have been divided into four major categories, the insomnias and hypersomnias (excessive daytime sleepiness) being the most important. The others, disorders of sleep-wake schedule (e.g., jet lag or shift work) and sleepwalking, are special cases and do not pose the diagnostic challenge of insomnia or hypersomnia.

HYPERSOMNIA

A. Unemployment, problems at work, and marital difficulties are common causes of daytime sleepiness.

B. Sleep attacks are episodes in which the patient suddenly falls asleep. This can occur while driving, sitting at the dinner table, or waiting in the doctor's office. These attacks are sudden drops into stage 2 sleep. This is the cardinal symptom of the narcolepsy tetrad; the other features are cataplexy (sudden loss of muscle tone with laughter or excitement), sleep paralysis (inability to move when first awakened), and hypnagogic hallucinations (frightening nightmares). Various combinations of symptoms are seen. The diagnosis can be made clinically if the patient has cataplexy; if not, HLA typing (all white narcoleptics have HLA-DR2; black narcoleptics often have HLA-DQw1) and referral to a sleep laboratory for multiple sleep latency test are indicated.

C. In some patients the pharynx is very lax and the throat can close at night. These patients struggle for breath and eventually break through with a loud snore that wakes them up. Such obstructive sleep apnea is dangerous and can lead to hypertension, pulmonary hypertension, daytime sleepiness, nocturnal anoxic seizures, and migraine-type headaches.

References

Association of Sleep Disorder Centers. Diagnostic classification of sleep and arousal disorders. Sleep 1979; 2:1.

Gottlieb GL. Sleep disorders and their management. Am J Med 1990; 88(Suppl 3A):29.

Thorpy MJ. Classification of sleep disorders. J Clin Neurophysiol 1990; 7:67.

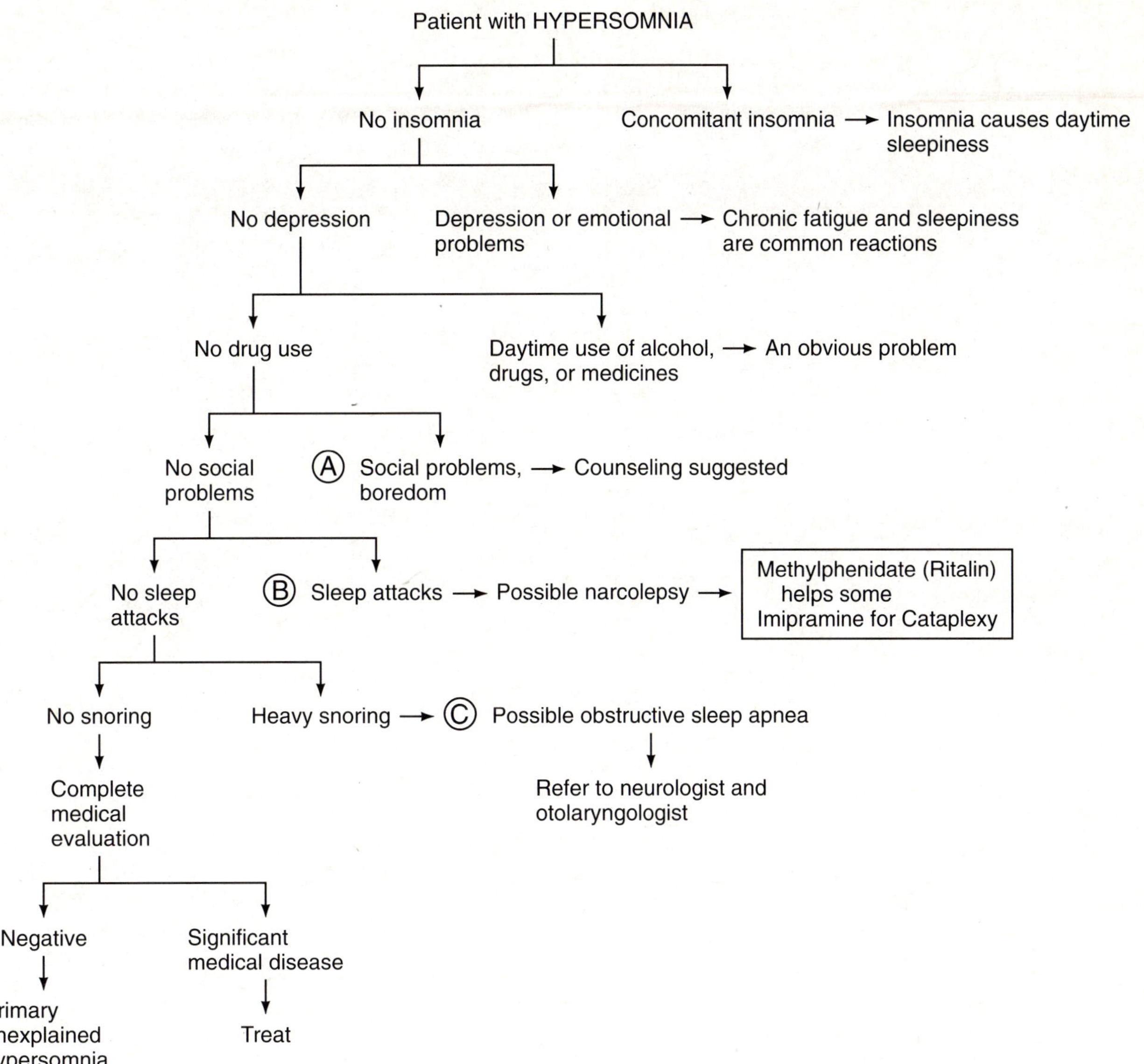

Patient with HYPERSOMNIA
No insomnia
Concomitant insomnia → Insomnia causes daytime sleepiness
No depression
Depression or emotional problems → Chronic fatigue and sleepiness are common reactions
No drug use
Daytime use of alcohol, drugs, or medicines → An obvious problem
No social problems
A Social problems, boredom → Counseling suggested
No sleep attacks
B Sleep attacks → Possible narcolepsy → Methylphenidate (Ritalin) helps some Imipramine for Cataplexy
No snoring
Heavy snoring → C Possible obstructive sleep apnea
Refer to neurologist and otolaryngologist
Complete medical evaluation
Negative
Significant medical disease
Primary unexplained hypersomnia
Treat

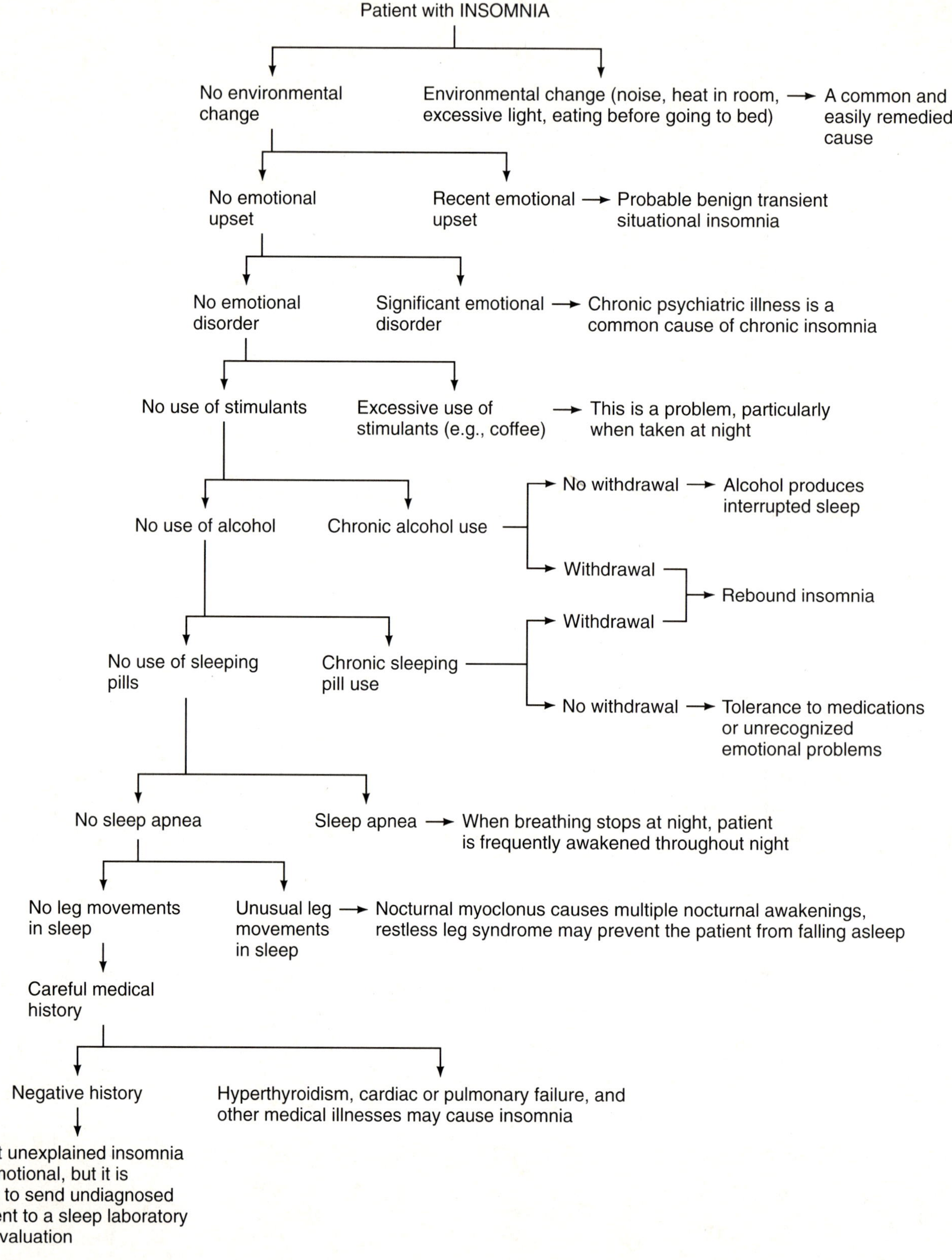

Patient with INSOMNIA
No environmental change
Environmental change (noise, heat in room, excessive light, eating before going to bed)
A common and easily remedied cause
No emotional upset
Recent emotional upset
Probable benign transient situational insomnia
No emotional disorder
Significant emotional disorder
Chronic psychiatric illness is a common cause of chronic insomnia
No use of stimulants
Excessive use of stimulants (e.g., coffee)
This is a problem, particularly when taken at night
No use of alcohol
Chronic alcohol use
No withdrawal
Alcohol produces interrupted sleep
Withdrawal
Rebound insomnia
Withdrawal
No use of sleeping pills
Chronic sleeping pill use
No withdrawal
Tolerance to medications or unrecognized emotional problems
No sleep apnea
Sleep apnea
When breathing stops at night, patient is frequently awakened throughout night
No leg movements in sleep
Unusual leg movements in sleep
Nocturnal myoclonus causes multiple nocturnal awakenings, restless leg syndrome may prevent the patient from falling asleep
Careful medical history
Negative history
Hyperthyroidism, cardiac or pulmonary failure, and other medical illnesses may cause insomnia
Most unexplained insomnia is emotional, but it is wise to send undiagnosed patient to a sleep laboratory for evaluation

INDEX

MPTP, 242
Multi-infarct dementia, 85
Multiple myeloma, neuropathy and, 206
Multiple sclerosis, 8, 12, 50, 62, 225, 300
Muscle biopsy, 226
Muscle cramps, 56, 230, 286
Muscle pseudohypertrophy, 228
Muscle stretch reflexes, 96
Muscular dystrophy, 228, 230, 232
Myalgia, 230
Myasthenia gravis, 12, 42, 44, 104
Myasthenic crisis, 238
Myasthenic syndromes, 238, 239
Mycotic aneurysm, 148
Mydriasis, 102
Myelography; see Back pain.
Myeloma, multiple, 58, 206
Myelopathy, 6, 24, 54, 94
Myoclonic disease, 243, 290
Myoglobinuria, 234
Myokymia, 54
Myopathy, 6, 38, 54, 104, 226
Myositis, 228, 230
Myotonia congenita, 232
Myotonic dystrophy, 232
Myotonic syndromes, 232, 236
Mysoline
    for essential tremor treatment, 248, 249
    for seizure treatment, 158

N

Narcolepsy, 8, 156, 306
Neck stiff, 24, 258, 262
Neck pain, 24
Neck trauma, 24
Nemaline rod disease, 42
Neoplastic meningitis, 204
Neoplastic plexopathy, 210
Neuralgia, trigeminal nerve, 22
Neuralgic amyotrophy, 210
Neuritis
    brachial, 210
    lumbosacral, 212
    optic, 62, 112
Neurologic localization
    lesions above foramen magnum, 4, 5
    lesions below foramen magnum, 6, 7
Neuroma
    acoustic, 64, 68, 69, 190
    trigeminal nerve, 190
Neuromyotonia, 54
Neuropathy, 6, 38, 46, 92, 94, 204
Neurosyphilis, 102, 259
Nightmare, 306, 307
Nocturnal myoclonus, 306
Nonketotic hyperosmolar coma, 118
Nonwilsonian hepatolenticular degeneration, 242
Normal pressure hydrocephalus, 46
Nuchal rigidity, 258, 262
Nystagmus, 110

O

Occipital lobe
    lesion, 4
    phenomenon, 88
Ocular dysmetria, 46
Ocular myasthenia gravis, 106, 238, 239
Oculocephalic test, 36
Oculogyric crisis, 256
Oculomotor paresis, 62, 102, 106, 214

Oculopharyngeal muscular dystrophy, 106, 227, 229
Olfactory nerve, 90
Oligodendroglioma, 186
Olivopontocerebellar degeneration, 242, 243
Ommaya reservoir, 268
Oncocytoma, 192
Ophthalmopathy, dysthyroid, 108
Opisthotonus, 256, 276
Optic atrophy, 8, 112, 274, 302
Optic nerve fenestration, 284
Optic nerve glioma, 108
Optic neuritis, 8, 62, 112, 302
Orbital biopsy, 109
Orbital decompression, 104, 108
Orbital pseudotumor, 108, 109
Orofacial mandibular dystonia, 257, 270
Orthostatic hypotension, 172
Otitic hydrocephalus, 152
Otorrhea, 184
Otosclerosis, 64

P

Pain
    arm, 26
    back, 30
    facial, 22
    hand, 26
    neck, 24
Palatal myoclonus, 66
Palmomental reflex, 100
Pancerebellar syndrome, 46, 200, 262
Papilledema, 104, 112, 152, 198, 284
Papillitis, 302
Paramyotonia congenita, 232, 233
Paraneoplastic syndromes, 92, 94
Paraparesis, 6, 48
Paraphasic aphasia, 74
Paraplegia, 6
Parasellar tumor, 62, 102, 188, 192
Paredrine, for evaluation of Horner's syndrome, 102
Paresthesia, 92
Parietal lesion, 4
Parinaud syndrome, 188
Parkinson's disease, 242
Parkinsonism, 242
Parlodel, 192, 246, 276
Parosmia, 90
Partial complex seizure, 156, 168
Pendular reflexes, 96
Penicillamine, 251
Peripheral polyneuropathy, 213
Peroneal neuropathy, 222
Petit mal seizure, 164
Phalen sign, 26, 218
Phenobarbital, 158
Phenytoin, 158, 174
Phosphorylase deficiency, 234
Photomyoclonic response, 174
Pick's disease, 84
Pinealoma, 188
Pinhole test, 62
Pituitary adenoma, 62, 102, 188, 192
Pituitary apoplexy, 192
Plantar reflex, 98
Plasmapheresis, 240, 241
Pleocytosis, 258, 262
Poliomyelitis, 224, 225
Polyarteritis nodosa, 214
Polycythemia, 58, 132, 153
Polymyalgia rheumatica, 62, 304, 305
Polymyopathy, 226
Polymyositis, 228, 230

Weakness—cont'd
  facial, 70
    symmetric, 38
Werdnig-Hoffman disease, 42
Wernicke's aphasia, 74
Wernicke's encephalopathy, 86
White matter lesions, 4
Wilson's disease, 242, 250, 251

Wrist drop, 214, 215
Writer's cramp, 252

Z

Zidovudine, 293, 296